MANUAL OF ORTHOPAEDICS
Sixth Edition

MANUAL OF ORTHOPAEDICS
Sixth Edition

Editor
Marc F. Swiontkowski, MD
Professor and Chair
Department of Orthopaedic Surgery
University of Minnesota
TRIA Orthopaedics Center
Minneapolis, Minnesota

Associate Editor
Steven D. Stovitz, MD
Assistant Professor
Department of Family Medicine and Community Health
University of Minnesota
Minneapolis, Minnesota

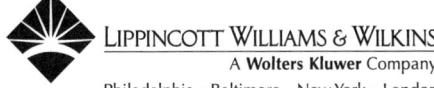

LIPPINCOTT WILLIAMS & WILKINS
A **Wolters Kluwer** Company
Philadelphia • Baltimore • New York • London
Buenos Aires • Hong Kong • Sydney • Tokyo

Acquisitions Editor: Robert Hurley
Managing Editor: Jenny Kim
Project Manager: Nicole Walz
Senior Manufacturing Manager: Ben Rivera
Marketing Director: Sharon Zinner
Design Coordinator: Terry Mallon
Production Services: Laserwords Private Limited
Printer: RR Donnelley–Crawfordsville

6th Edition
© 2006 by Lippincott Williams & Wilkins

© 2001 by Lippincott Williams & Wilkins
530 Walnut Street
Philadelphia, PA 19106

All rights reserved. This book is protected by copyright. No part of this book may be reproduced in any form or by any means, including photocopying, or utilizing by any information storage and retrieval system without written permission from the copyright owner, except for brief quotations embodied in critical articles and reviews.

Printed in the United States

Library of Congress Cataloging-in-Publication Data

Manual of orthopaedics / editor, Marc F. Swiontkowski.--6th ed.
  p. ; cm.
Includes bibliographical references and index.
ISBN 0-7817-5755-X
  1. Orthopedics--Handbooks, manuals, etc. 2. Musculoskeletal system--Wounds and injuries--Handbooks, manuals, etc. 3. Fractures--Handbooks, manuals, etc. I. Swiontkowski, Marc F.
  [DNLM: 1. Musculoskeletal System--injuries--Handbooks. 2. Fractures--rehabilitation--Handbooks. 3. Orthopedics--Handbooks. WE 39 M2938 2005]
RD732.5.I96 2005
616.7--dc22

2005008138

Care has been taken to confirm the accuracy of the information presented and to describe generally accepted practices. However, the authors, editors, and publisher are not responsible for errors or omissions or for any consequences from application of the information in this book and make no warranty, expressed or implied, with respect to the currency, completeness, or accuracy of the contents of the publication. Application of this information in a particular situation remains the professional responsibility of the practitioner.

The authors, editors, and publisher have exerted every effort to ensure that drug selection and dosage set forth in this text are in accordance with current recommendations and practice at the time of publication. However, in view of ongoing research, changes in government regulations, and the constant flow of information relating to drug therapy and drug reactions, the reader is urged to check the package insert for each drug for any change in indications and dosage and for added warnings and precautions. This is particularly important when the recommended agent is a new or infrequently employed drug.

Some drugs and medical devices presented in this publication have Food and Drug Administration (FDA) clearance for limited use in restricted research settings. It is the responsibility of health care providers to ascertain the FDA status of each drug or device planned for use in their clinical practice.

The publishers have made every effort to trace copyright holders for borrowed material. If they have inadvertently overlooked any, they will be pleased to make the necessary arrangements at the first opportunity.

To purchase additional copies of this book, call our customer service department at (800) 638-3030 or fax orders to (301) 824-7390. International customers should call (301) 714-2324. Lippincott Williams & Wilkins customer service representatives are available from 8:30 am to 6:30 pm, EST, Monday through Friday, for telephone access. Visit Lippincott Williams & Wilkins on the Internet: http://www.lww.com.

10 9 8 7 6 5 4 3 2 1

CONTENTS

    Contributing Authors vii

    Preface ix

1   **The Diagnosis and Management of Musculoskeletal Trauma** 1
    Dr. Peter A. Cole

2   **Complications of Musculoskeletal Trauma** 27
    Dr. Andrew H. Schmidt

3   **Prevention and Management of Acute Musculoskeletal Infections** 39
    Dr. Dean Tsukayama

4   **Acute Nontraumatic Joint Conditions** 51
    Dr. Denis R. Clohisy

5   **Pediatric Orthopaedic Conditions** 67
    Dr. Kevin R. Walker

6   **Common Types of Emergency Splints** 93
    Dr. Marc F. Swiontkowski

7   **Cast and Bandaging Techniques** 101
    Dr. Marc F. Swiontkowski

8   **Orthopaedic Unit Care** 119
    Dr. John Stark and Dr. Marc F. Swiontkowski

9   **Traction** 137
    Dr. Marc F. Swiontkowski

10   **Operating Room Equipment and Techniques** 153
    Dr. Marc F. Swiontkowski

11   **Acute Spinal Injury** 183
    Dr. Daryll C. Dykes

12   **Disorders and Diseases of the Spine** 203
    Dr. Ensor E. Transfeldt and Dr. David Polly

13   **Fractures of the Clavicle** 213
    Dr. Peter A. Cole

14   **Sternoclavicular and Acromioclavicular Joint Injuries** 217
    Dr. Peter A. Cole

vi Contents

15 Acute Shoulder Injuries **223**
Dr. Daniel D. Buss

16 Nonacute Shoulder Disorders **229**
Dr. Daniel D. Buss

17 Fractures of the Humerus **239**
Dr. Thomas F. Varecka and Dr. Marc F. Swiontkowski

18 Elbow and Forearm Injuries **251**
Dr. Thomas F. Varecka and Dr. Marc F. Swiontkowski

19 Acute Wrist and Hand Injuries **265**
Dr. Matthew D. Putnam

20 Nonacute Elbow, Wrist, and Hand Conditions **283**
Dr. Matthew D. Putnam

21 Fractures of the Pelvis **299**
Dr. Marc F. Swiontkowski and Dr. David C. Templeman

22 Hip Dislocations, Femoral Head Fractures,
and Acetabular Fractures **307**
Dr. Marc F. Swiontkowski and Dr. David C. Templeman

23 Fractures of the Femur **317**
Dr. Andrew H. Schmidt

24 Knee Injuries: Acute and Overuse **339**
Dr. Elizabeth A. Arendt

25 Fractures of the Tibia **359**
Dr. Mohit Bhandari and Dr. Marc F. Swiontkowski

26 Ankle Injuries **371**
Dr. Fernando A. Pena

27 Fractures and Dislocations of the Foot **383**
Dr. J. Chris Coetzee

28 Overuse and Miscellaneous Conditions of the
Foot and Ankle **393**
Dr. J. Chris Coetzee

29 Aspiration and Injection of Upper and Lower Extremities **403**
Dr. Fernando A. Pena

Appendix A Joint Motion Measurement **411**

Appendix B Muscle Strength Grading **433**

Appendix C Dermatomes and Cutaneous Distribution
of Peripheral Nerves **435**

Appendix D Desirable Weights of Adults **439**

Appendix E Surgical Draping Techniques **443**

Appendix F Electromyography and Nerve Conduction Studies **449**

Index **453**

CONTRIBUTING AUTHORS

Elizabeth A. Arendt, MD
Associate Professor and Vice Chair
Department of Orthopaedic Surgery
University of Minnesota
Minneapolis, Minnesota

Mohit Bhandari, MD, MSc, FRCSC
Assistant Professor, Canada Research Chair
Division of Orthopaedic Surgery
McMaster University
Hamilton, Ontario
Consultant
Division of Orthopaedic Surgery
Hamilton Health Sciences-General Hospital
Hamilton, Ontario

Daniel D. Buss, MD
Adjunct Associate Professor
Department of Orthopaedic Surgery
University of Minnesota
Minneapolis, Minnesota
Shoulder and Elbow Specialist
Sports and Orthopaedic Specialist
Edina, Minnesota

Denis R. Clohisy, MD
Professor
Department of Orthopaedic Surgery
University of Minnesota
Minneapolis, Minnesota

J. Chris Coetzee, MD, FRCSC
Associate Professor
Chief, Foot and Ankle Division
Department of Orthopaedic Surgery
University of Minnesota
Minneapolis, Minnesota

Peter A. Cole, MD
Associate Professor
Department of Orthopaedic Surgery
University of Minnesota
Minneapolis, Minnesota
Chief
Department of Orthopaedic Surgery
Regions Hospital
St Paul, Minnesota

Daryll C. Dykes, MD, PhD
Staff Physician
Twin Cities Spine Center
Minneapolis, Minnesota

Fernando A. Pena, MD
Assistant Professor
Department of Orthopaedic Surgery
University of Minnesota
Minneapolis, Minnesota

David Polly, MD
Professor
Chief, Spine Division
Department of Orthopaedic Surgery
University of Minnesota
Minneapolis, Minnesota

Matthew D. Putnam, MD
Professor
Department of Orthopaedic Surgery
University of Minnesota
Minneapolis, Minnesota

Andrew H. Schmidt, MD
Associate Professor
Department of Orthopaedic Surgery
University of Minnesota
Minneapolis, Minnesota
Faculty
Department of Orthopaedic Surgery
Hennepin County Medical Center
Minneapolis, Minnesota

John Stark, MD
Assistant Professor
Department of Orthopaedic Surgery
University of Minnesota
Minneapolis, Minnesota

Steven D. Stovitz, MD
Assistant Professor
Department of Family Medicine and
    Community Health
University of Minnesota
Minneapolis, Minnesota

Marc F. Swiontkowski, MD
Professor and Chair
Department of Orthopaedic Surgery
University of Minnesota
TRIA Orthopaedics Center
Minneapolis, Minnesota

David C. Templeman, MD
Associate Professor
Department of Orthopaedic Surgery
University of Minnesota
Minneapolis, Minnesota

Ensor E. Transfeldt, MD
Associate Professor
Department of Orthopaedic Surgery
University of Minnesota
Minneapolis, Minnesota
Staff Physician
Twin Cities Spine Center
Minneapolis, Minnesota

Dean Tsukayama, MD
Associate Professor
Division of Infectious Diseases,
    Department of Medicine
University of Minnesota
Minneapolis, Minnesota
Director
Division of Infectious Diseases,
    Department of Medicine
Hennepin County Medical Center
Minneapolis, Minnesota

Thomas F. Varecka, MD
Professor
Department of Orthopaedic Surgery
University of Minnesota
Minneapolis, Minnesota
Director
Hand Trauma
Department of Orthopaedic Surgery
Hennepin County Medical Center
Minneapolis, Minnesota

Kevin R. Walker, MD
Assistant Professor
Department of Orthopaedic Surgery
University of Minnesota
Minneapolis, Minnesota
Staff member
Department of Orthopaedic Surgery
Gillette Specialty Health Care
St. Paul, Minnesota

PREFACE

The sixth edition of the *Manual of Orthopaedics* continues the recent trend of altering the content and the format to be of greater use to a wider audience of students and practicing physicians. This is the second edition which uses this title, which was changed from the *Manual of Acute Orthopaedic Therapeutics* with the fifth edition. The title change reflected a new direction for the manual. The introduction will conclude with a list of new features in the sixth edition. It is worthwhile to review the history of this useful "spiral notebook" to place the continuing changes within the context of history.

The *Manual of Acute Orthopaedic Therapeutics* was the creation of Dr. Larry Iversen who worked out its basic framework and conceptualization with his orthopaedic mentor, Dr. D. Kay Clawson. Dr. Iversen was at the time a senior resident working closely with Dr. Clawson, who was the first professor and Chairman of the Department of Orthopaedic Surgery at the University of Washington. The orthopaedic services at the University Hospital and King County Hospital (later renamed Harborview Medical Center) were active and focused mainly around the management of injured patients. Drs. Clawson and Iversen saw the need for a manual that would improve teaching and patient care in these institutions. These were days when the management of long bone fractures was in transition from traction and casting to operative techniques, and the University of Washington Orthopaedic department was at the forefront with wonderful, dedicated, and creative clinicians like Drs. Robert Smith and Sigvard Hansen. Care was primarily delivered by junior house staff, interns, and students, and they needed information readily at hand. Therefore, the manual provided the "how-to's" for traction, casting, and pre- and postoperative care while explaining the rationale for treatment decisions and providing an excellent reference list for later review and in-depth study. This manual was a labor of love for Drs. Iversen and Clawson; the two would often work on the manuscripts for three straight weeks seated around the dining room table in Dr. Clawson's home. Little Brown publishers liked the concept of the book and added it to its growing list of subspecialty spiral manuals; the book enjoyed broad acceptance.

Each of the first three editions brought a review of the contents and reference list for each chapter as the field continued to evolve. In 1987, I returned to the University of Washington, where I had done my training (and used the second edition), to assume a position at Harborview Medical Center. In 1991, I was a new professor in the department and chief of the orthopaedic service, and Dr. Clawson asked me to assume his place with the manual. It then became Dr. Iversen and I who labored for two weeks in the medical school library revising the chapters, updating the reference lists, adding sections of historical references, changing several illustrations, and adding fresh chapters on infection and rheumatologic conditions. As such we began to broaden the scope of the manual to include conditions that were nonacute and nontrauma-related in order to make the manual more useful for students and interns as well as to provide a more comprehensive tool for primary care physicians. The changes in care delivery moved strongly in favor of attending delivered/supervised care in academic centers where the manual was in widespread use. As such the chapters evolved drastically as the push towards operative management of fractures had dramatically changed the way trauma patients were managed—for the better, we believe.

For the fifth edition, Dr. Iversen, with a mature, busy private practice in Bremerton, Washington, chose to step aside. I moved from the University of Washington to assume the Chair of the Orthopaedic Surgery Department at the University of Minnesota in 1997, and brought the project along. This was the point where we made a major philosophical shift in the manual, changing its title to the *Manual of Orthopaedics*. It became a more comprehensive tool, covering nearly all areas of orthopaedic surgery in new chapters. Members of the Department of Orthopaedic Surgery at the University of Minnesota agreed to support the project by authoring new chapters on pediatric orthopaedics, nontraumatic hand and shoulder surgery, spine, and chronic and nonacute lower extremity orthopaedics. Treatment protocols preferred by the attending staff at Hennepin County Medial Center, where the University of Minnesota has a level 1 trauma rotation, were added. These were placed at the end of appropriate chapters, and the intent was to provide a set of principles for decision making which serve as a starting point for developing individualized treatment plans for patients. The manual at that time moved from a two-author project to a multiple-author, single orthopaedic surgery department project in the evolution towards greater usefulness for students, house staff, and primary care physicians.

In the sixth edition, we continue this trend. New chapters have been added on injection techniques and sections within each individual "nonacute" chapter provide guidelines for primary care physicians to evaluate presenting complaints from patients. In this era of cost containment, we have tried to provide guidelines for primary care physicians as to when expensive diagnostic studies should be requested, and offer direction for how the use of physical and occupational therapy should be utilized. Dr. Steven D. Stovitz was a reviewer or an editor for all chapters to be sure that the entire manual had maximal usefulness for the primary care doctor.

All chapters have been updated and, in some instances, new authors have been involved. The discussion of individual conditions and the reference lists are not meant to be comprehensive, rather they are meant to provide a starting point in approaching an individual patient with his or her problem. Every student, resident, and physician is encouraged to delve more deeply into the study of the condition: both the reference lists and historical references will be useful in gaining more information for personal gratification or for preparing for teaching conference discussions. Generally speaking, there is no single way to manage an orthopaedic injury or condition; we have attempted to provide scholarly discussions which cover the gamut of approaches while informing the reader of what we think is the best current method. We have attempted to be clear about which conditions are appropriately managed by primary care physicians and which need orthopaedic subspecialist care.

No individual in the Department of Orthopaedic Surgery at the University of Minnesota will receive personal remuneration for this project. The funds derived from the sale of this book will be utilized to further student education and research. This principle rings true to the initial motivation of Drs. Clawson and Iversen in creating the manual. The sixth edition continues to be dedicated to these two fine surgeon educators as well as to the many students, residents, and primary care physicians who will benefit from the *Manual of Orthopaedics*.

Marc F. Swiontkowski, MD
Steven D. Stovitz, MD

THE DIAGNOSIS AND MANAGEMENT OF MUSCULOSKELETAL TRAUMA

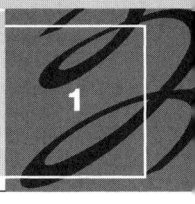

I. **INTRODUCTION AND PHILOSOPHY**
   A. **Epidemiology of orthopaedic trauma.** Musculoskeletal trauma has gained significant and increased attention over the past 10 years for a number of reasons. Such reasons include the realization of its **societal impact** from health care costs and lost workdays in the labor force. These statistics are coupled with an increased realization that the orthopaedic surgeon and health care team can positively influence such statistics, both through excellent intervention as well as education on **injury prevention**. Leadership from key organizations [Orthopaedic Trauma Association (OTA), American Academy of Orthopaedic Surgeons (AAOS), American College of Surgeons (ACS), American Orthopaedic Association (AOA), and many others] has played a major role in lobbying for proactive trauma-related **health care policy** and implementation of public education programs for injury prevention.

   Whereas it is likely that certain of these educational measures such as seatbelt safety, aggressive standards for highway safety, and lower blood alcohol limits for drivers helps to lower accident related injury rates, other forces seem to counter such progress such as the pervasive trend toward faster cars, the burgeoning enthusiasm for extreme sports, and increased numbers of trauma survivors with significant musculoskeletal injuries due to airbags.

   An even greater awareness is emerging regarding the **aging baby boomers** who will account for massive demands on the health care system. The baby boomers will be hitting the 65-year-old age mark in approximately 10 years, and it is estimated that by the year 2040 there will be 35,000,000 more people over the age of 55 than there are now and that the number of hip fractures alone will increase from 250,000 to 500,000 on an annual basis (1). The estimated uptick in **geriatric musculoskeletal trauma** over the next 30 years is due to the vulnerability of the skeletal system from the natural process of relative bone mineral loss manifesting in the condition of **osteoporosis**. Compounding the number of injuries in this group is the increasingly active lifestyle of this aging population. To put it in perspective, it is estimated that one-third of all women reaching the age of 90 will sustain at least one hip fracture (2).
   B. **Definition of musculoskeletal trauma.** Musculoskeletal trauma includes any injury to **bone, joint (including ligaments), or muscle (including tendons)**. Nearly always, such injuries occur in combination, as the energy imparted to breaking a bone or tearing a ligament is also dissipated to impact structures nearby or even distant from the most obvious site. With greater experience, such combinations of injuries become more apparent to the diagnostician, which allows for swifter and more accurate detection of injury characterization.
   C. **Multiple injuries.** The energy it takes to render trauma to the musculoskeletal system can also dissipate to injure other organs. This is particularly common with the high energy mechanisms that are responsible for pelvic, spine, or long bone fractures. Due to the greater density and strength of bone in younger individuals, there is even greater energy required to create fractures in this population. Therefore, it is incumbent upon the trauma team to remain vigilant to the likelihood of injuries to other bones and other organ systems. Often, the dramatic and salient injuries during the initial patient evaluation will attract all the diagnostic and therapeutic attention, while occult and sometimes equally grave injuries remain initially undetected.

For example, it is estimated that only 7% of the patients who die from life-threatening high-energy pelvic fractures actually die from arterial exsanguination related to the pelvic fracture itself (3), while the rest succumb due to injury involving other organ systems. Forty percent of patients with femur fractures have other associated fractures (4), and 90% of patients with scapula fractures have other associated injuries (5). These impressive associated injury statistics demand most heightened awareness when working up the trauma patient to keep the missed injury rate to a minimum.

D. **Missed injury rate.** The missed injury rate in the context of polytrauma has been reported to be 4% to 18% (6). These statistics may be lowered with appropriate protocols and underscore the importance of a most vigilant secondary survey, as well as a re-review of the patient's physical examination each ensuing day after injury. A **secondary survey** is a head-to-toe review by a physician that occurs after the initial **primary survey**, which is defined as the evaluation of the 3 screening trauma films (lateral cervical spine, anteroposterior chest, and pelvic x-ray) and, most importantly, the patient's airway, breathing, and circulation (the ABCs).

It is valuable to understand the main reasons cited for missing injuries: significant multisystem trauma with another more apparent orthopaedic injury, trauma victim too unstable for a full orthopaedic evaluation, altered sensorium, hastily applied initial splints obscuring other injuries, and poor radiographs (6).

E. **Multiple patients.** It is not uncommon, particularly at a Level I trauma center, to require simultaneous evaluation of multiple patients, such as with motor vehicle collisions in which multiple victims are involved. Doctors who have had some training on the fundamentals of trauma surgery and, in particular, **Advanced Trauma Life Support (ATLS),** which includes strategies for triaging patients and resources during a mass casualty situation, must be available in order to effectively **"captain the ship."** ATLS courses have been developed, refined, and sponsored by the American College of Surgeons and have an excellent educational track record. Typically (but not exclusively), in the United States, it is a general surgery trauma surgeon who is running the trauma room. It is beyond the scope of this orthopaedic text to delve into the specifics of ATLS management, however; we will focus on certain of the fundamentals and cover the triage process of multiple orthopaedic injuries that may present during such circumstances. To further master the details of ATLS management, please refer to the ATLS Manual (7th edition) published in 2004 (7).

It is imperative to understand what is an orthopaedic emergency and what is orthopaedically urgent. A review of the **"orthopaedic emergencies"** in a subsequent section of this chapter will help to understand how these injuries need to be prioritized for treatment. Furthermore, it is important to understand what measures can be taken to **stage orthopaedic treatment**. Not all broken bones need definitive treatment right away, and the practitioner must understand how to **titrate the proposed treatment to the physiologic presentation** of the patient. For example, a patient with limited physiologic reserve, due to a great physiologic challenge from hemorrhagic shock and compromised ventilation from a hemothorax, should not spend 10 hours in the operating room getting several fractured bones fixed. In such a case, it may be wiser to place an external fixator across a broken femur rather than to immediately nail the femur and place a plaster splint on a displaced ankle fracture rather than to fix it right away. These measures save a lot of time, blood loss, anesthesia, and fluid challenge during a potentially critical stage in postinjury physiologic evolution.

There are many ways to stage the treatment of injuries, which also gives the orthopaedist more time to solicit expertise, get to know the patient and family, plan the details of an operation, and understand the comorbidities and the likelihood of patient compliance. All these different factors may, in fact, impact the ultimate treatment that the orthopaedic surgeon chooses to render and will most certainly influence positive outcomes.

II. **EVALUATING THE TRAUMA PATIENT FROM THE ORTHOPAEDIC PERSPECTIVE.**
As alluded to already, the patient who presents from an accident scene should receive a much different type of workup than would be called for by a scheduled history and

physical examination, though certainly history and physical examination are part and parcel of the process. The difference in this setting is that the sequence and algorithms in workup, diagnosis, and treatment are very different than that for a patient presenting in a nonemergent setting.

It is important to acknowledge that there is a "captain of the ship," typically an ATLS-trained general surgeon, who will have the clearest overview of the patient and who will be delegating many simultaneous responsibilities. The person taking primary responsibility for the orthopaedic injuries must heed the captain's call and clearly communicate diagnostic or treatment priorities for the orthopaedic conditions and ultimately fit into the context of overall priorities.

Trauma care is organized in three stages: primary survey, secondary survey, and definitive management. The primary survey occurs even before, or at least at the same time as, the history, so it will be discussed here first. Meanwhile other members of the team are simultaneously obtaining the trauma series of x-rays to be readily available for interpretation, drawing blood, or inserting a urinary catheter.

A. Primary survey. The primary survey is concerned with the preservation of life. The first steps in managing the trauma patient follow the **ABCs**. It is important to correct each of these problems in sequence. Another way to think of it is that a competent airway must be established if life is to continue through the rest of the evaluation. These initial steps generally have been performed by the paramedic team, but the surgeon in charge should follow the established ABC sequence.

　1. Airway. The most common cause of preventable death in accidents is airway obstruction, so the trauma leader must immediately check that the patient's airway is adequate and patent. Any obstruction (e.g., vomitus, tongue, blood, dentures) must be removed and the airway secured by a jaw thrust maneuver or tracheal intubation.

　2. Breathing. After airway obstruction has been ruled out or controlled (i.e., intubation), the patient's ventilation should be assessed. The major life-threatening problems are tension pneumothorax, massive hemothorax, and flail chest. Again, this aspect of the physical exam requires the examiner to inspect, touch, and auscultate the patient as this is typically done before roentgenographic diagnosis is available.

　3. Circulation. After breathing has been addressed, cardiovascular status must be immediately evaluated and supported. Prompt determination of vital signs is essential. Control of **external bleeding** is accomplished by direct pressure and bandage. Simple elevation of the lower extremities helps prevent venous bleeding from the limbs and increases cardiac venous return and preload. The classic Trendelenburg (head down) position is not used for more than a few minutes because it can interfere with respiratory exchange. In the critically injured or hemodynamically labile patient, venous blood samples should be taken for **type and cross matching**.

　　Until cross-matched blood is available, rapidly infuse 1 to 2 L of isotonic Ringer lactate or normal saline solution. If **blood loss is minimal**, then blood pressure should return to normal and remain that way with only a maintenance intravenous amount of balanced saline solution.

　　In general, hypotension in a trauma patient should not be assumed to come from a long bone fracture, and another source must be sought. The following gross **estimates of localized blood loss** (units) from adult closed fractures can be useful in establishing baseline blood replacement requirements:

　　　Pelvis　　　　　　　　　1.5–4.5
　　　Hip, femur　　　　　　　1.0–2.5
　　　Humerus, knee, tibia　　　1.0–1.5
　　　Elbow, forearm, ankle　　 0.5–1.0

B. Trauma x-ray series. Recall that the **trauma x-ray series** was being taken in the trauma room while the primary survey was being conducted. Now that the primary survey has been performed and the most critical steps have been taken, even before a thorough history and physical exam, this x-ray trauma series should be reviewed; the examiner is ruling in or out the next most critical clues to saving life and limb. The trauma series consists of three x-rays: **lateral cervical spine**, an **anteroposterior chest**, and an **anteroposterior pelvic** view. Any patient who is involved in high-energy trauma, has head injuries, or is under chemical substance influence should have these views.

The cervical spine roentgenogram must show the inferior endplate of cervical vertebrae 7 (C7), or it should be deemed inadequate and repeated. Both odontoid and C7–C8 pathology are frequently missed injuries even after the secondary survey. **If a spine fracture is detected**, then a complete spinal series including anteroposterior, lateral and odontoid cervical views, and thoracic plus lumbar spine view is mandatory. Computed tomography (CT) may be required to rule out upper cervical fractures. The documented incidence of multiple level spine fractures is 7% to 12%. A full spine series should be obtained in the unconscious trauma victim.

All the x-rays should be taken with excellent technique so as not to obscure the many potential clues to danger which exist on the radiograph. Care must be taken not to be misled by overlying backboards, over- and underpenetrated films, and equipment, clips, and buckles which are frequently left on the x-ray field. Examples abound of subtle femoral neck fractures that were obscured on the x-ray by a belt buckle, a pneumothorax in the upper lobe that was cut out of view due to positioning, or a critical sacral fracture masked by the opacity of a backboard.

C. **History and physical examination.** The **history** should include a careful account of the accident, a description of the mechanism of injury, and a statement of the degree of violence involved. Concomitant medical disease, drug abuse, and alcoholism should be considered as contributing factors. The transporting paramedic team or member of the accompanying family should be interviewed for these details if the patient cannot reliably give an appropriate history. A useful mnemonic to guide the initial history is the word **AMPLE:**

A: Allergies

The physician working up an orthopaedic patient should be particularly aware that open fractures should be treated with certain antibiotics to cover the spectrum of bacteria that are at risk for certain types of wounds (see open fractures below). Furthermore, every patient having an orthopaedic operation should receive perioperative antibiotics, making the question of allergies quite germane. A penicillin allergy is the most common.

M: Medications

Medications can influence surgical decision making. They will also tip off the practitioner to important comorbidities and perhaps imply the need for a general medicine consultation prior to surgery. Patients on anticoagulants should have bleeding and clotting parameters checked as it may be prudent to stop such meds or reverse a coagulopathy prior to surgery.

P: Past illness

Diabetes can influence outcomes of orthopaedic surgery, and heart disease can increase surgical risk. Steroids and nicotine (the use of tobacco products) increases orthopaedic surgical complications as well as outcomes as measured by healing time and healing rates.

L: Last meal

This is important when considering whether or not the patient needs to go to the operating room urgently, as the risk of aspiration of food or vomitus is higher postprandial. Most anesthesiologists opt to hold on administration of anesthesia within 6 to 8 hours of food intake. This concern should not, however, override the emergent nature of certain life- or limb-threatening conditions which will be discussed below.

E: Events of accident

Accident circumstances such as direction of impact, extrication time from vehicle, hours in the field, outside temperature, being trapped under heavy objects, smoke inhalation, and many other possibilities are warning flags to the experienced practitioner, which clue in certain medical or orthopaedic conditions and injury patterns.

Chapter 1: The Diagnosis and Management of Musculoskeletal Trauma

D. Secondary survey. The **Secondary Survey** is a complete **physical examination** from head to toe. By this juncture, the potentially life-threatening pathology of the ABCs has been addressed, and necessary resuscitation is underway. The patient should be completely undressed for the secondary survey for a most thorough exam.

1. **Neurologic mental status.** The **level of consciousness** of the patient should first be noted. A brief **"disability exam"** in an awake patient is a rapid, organized neurologic examination which documents mental orientation, verbal response to questioning, and response to stimuli. Furthermore, each extremity should be examined for motor and sensory function as well; accurate documentation is crucial since neurologic examinations can reveal progressive deficits. The extremity neurologic exam can also be documented with the specific physical exam of each extremity, but it is imperative that all four extremities be included. It is good to develop a pattern of examination and stick with that pattern each time for consistency.

    In the unconscious patient, a **Glasgow coma score** is rapidly conducted based on pupil response to light, motor activity, and withdrawal to painful stimuli (**Table 1-1**). This information is initially obtained by the medics who perform the initial in-the-field evaluation. The Glasgow score therefore is used as the measure of neurologic progress or deterioration. The medics generally also note the position of the patient at the scene of the accident, especially the head, and whether all limbs were actively moving. It is frustrating to the orthopaedic or neurosurgeon to be asked to evaluate a patient who has been sedated and chemically paralyzed in the trauma room, particularly when the initial neurologic exam was not properly documented. In general, the use of **maximal monitoring and minimal medication** is a useful trauma room principle which avoids such frustration by the examiner who relies on accurate neurologic exams.

2. **Head and neck.** Carefully palpate **skull and facial bones** and look for **lacerations** hidden in the hair. **Cranial trauma should raise an immediate suspicion for cervical spine injury** given the sudden and violent force it

TABLE 1-1   Glasgow Coma Scale

Eye opening (E)	
Spontaneous	4
To speech	3
To pain	2
None	1
Verbal response (V)	
Oriented	5
Confused conversation	4
Inappropriate words	3
Incomprehensible sounds	2
None	1
Motor response (M)	
Obeys command	6
Localizes	5
Withdraws to pain	4
Abnormal flexion	3
Extensor response	2
None	1

(E + M + V) = Glasgow coma score between 3–15

takes to injure the face and cranium. Roentgenograms of facial bones are difficult to interpret unless previous clinical examination suggests the presence of trauma. The **association between cervical spine and head injuries** must be emphasized. In a guided fashion with cervical immobility, remove or loosen the C-collar to palpate the posterior cervical spine looking for tenderness or spasm. In a conscious patient, any neck pain or spasm is a cervical spine injury until proven otherwise. In the unconscious patient, the neck must be protected with a hard C-collar until bony injury is ruled out by cervical roentgenography and physical exam. A benign physical exam by itself is unreliable if there are distracting injuries or if the patient is intoxicated. If a cervical spine injury is diagnosed, appropriate orthopaedic or neurosurgical spine consultation should be obtained immediately, and the extremity neurologic exam should be reported and documented.

3. **Thorax and abdomen.** Though the thorax and abdomen are largely the domain of the general surgeon, the examiner must inspect, palpate, and auscultate the abdomen and thorax to determine possible underlying injury. **Hemothorax** and **pneumothorax** often cause preventable death. Therefore, the chest should be examined carefully and the examination repeated frequently. Furthermore, this assessment helps the orthopaedist place musculoskeletal injuries in the broader context of the patient. **Abdominal injury** is also a common cause of preventable death. The imprint of clothes or a contusion of the abdominal wall from the seat belt suggests intraabdominal injury. Airbags have altered patterns of injury in frontal collision (8). Appropriate diagnostic studies should follow the suspicion of injury, and in many centers the spiral "whole body" CT scan of the chest, abdomen, and pelvis has supplanted selective CT scans, ultrasounds, and peritoneal lavage.

4. **Pelvis.** Low back pain, pubic tenderness, or pain with compression of the iliac crest can indicate a pelvic ring injury. Sequential anterior to posterior compression over the iliac wings can help to discriminate gross pelvic motion. Pelvic fractures may cause severe internal bleeding, and as stated earlier, a patient can easily lose four or more units of blood after a displaced pelvic fracture.

    A **rectal examination** must be done in all patients with a spine or pelvic injury, both to **check for bleeding as well as loss of sphincter tone** indicative of neurologic injury. Furthermore, a **high-riding prostate** also indicates major urologic disruption common to high-energy pelvic fractures in men. An inspection of the **penile meatus for hemorrhage** should also be performed, and such a finding is further indication of a genitourinary system disruption. Bloody urine or the **inability to void** raises the suspicion of a urethral injury, so a retrograde urethrogram should be considered before a catheter is inserted (9). In male patients, blood at the penile meatus or a "high-riding" prostate seen on rectal examination is a clear indication for obtaining a retrograde urethrogram before bladder catheterization. If the catheter does not pass easily, then it should not be forced and the urologist should be consulted. If a bladder injury is suspected, then it is essential to insert an indwelling catheter unless the patient is voiding clear urine.

    A **bimanual pelvic examination** is appropriate in female patients to rule out open fractures which can penetrate the vaginal vault. **Perineal inspection** for integument lacerations should be conducted and in the setting of displaced pelvic fractures should be assumed to represent an open pelvic fracture.

5. **Back and spine.** Carefully log roll the patient and **palpate the entire spine** to detect tenderness or defects of the interspinous ligaments. It is very important that a log roll be conducted properly with three assistants controlling simultaneous rotation of the entire body. A fourth assistant should be controlling the cervical spine (while in a hard collar) with gentle traction. An increase in the interspinous distance accompanied by local swelling may signify injury. Occasionally, ecchymosis or kyphosis can be recognized, and their presence or absence should be documented.

6. **Upper and lower extremity examination.** When **gross deformity and crepitation** are present, further examination of the fracture site is not necessary. Otherwise, all four limbs should be palpated thoroughly and each joint placed through a passive range of motion. Look specifically for point tenderness. Any obvious **fractures or deformities are splinted**, and any **open wounds are covered** with sterile dressings. Dressings over open wounds, particularly over fractures, should not be taken down multiple times by multiple examiners. Such repeated exposures will only increase the rate of infection with each exposure to the contaminated environment (10). A more detailed description of fracture wound management is given later in this chapter. Every diagnosed fracture should have properly centered x-rays of the joint above and below. Carefully evaluate the circulation of the limb distal to any fracture and record the presence of all wounds after applying a sterile dressing.

III. **ORTHOPAEDIC EMERGENCIES AND URGENCIES.** Surgical stabilization of fractures is generally not classified as emergent or urgent and typically can be done on a semielective basis. For example, an **isolated, closed fracture which is not threatening local blood supply may wait days to weeks**. There are many considerations, however, which go into the optimal timing of surgery, and **immediate consultation with an orthopaedist clarifies the issue of timing of surgery.**

All the **emergent entities, and most of the urgent injuries, ultimately have a common denominator: blood supply, or lack thereof**. The lack of circulation affects adequacy of tissue oxygenation, and consequently limb or life is threatened. This may occur on a macroscopic level, such as with a hemorrhaging pelvis in which a person's life is threatened, or on a microscopic basis, such as when end-organ perfusion is cut off beginning with occlusion of the venules in a muscle bed due to increased interstitial pressure exceeding intravenous pressure during the condition of compartment syndrome. Threatened blood supply to local tissues can be a more subtle phenomenon that requires further understanding of the vasculature to certain bones. For example, a relatively benign appearing x-ray of a femoral neck fracture to the inexperienced eye may not gain much attention, but the experienced clinician knows that even a nondisplaced femoral neck fracture can threaten the hip joint forever through a process called avascular necrosis. Certain other orthopaedic injuries may not accurately be classified as emergent since life or limb is not immediately at risk, but they still warrant heightened attention. Such injuries may be classified as urgent since they need prompt action by an orthopaedist and surgical timing in the range of 6 to 24 hours. In the next two sections on emergent and urgent orthopaedic injuries, the discussion will address these in descending order from most to least acute.

A. **Orthopaedic emergencies**
  1. **Hemodynamically unstable patient with a pelvic fracture.** This is the one injury in which circulation can be compromised to the extent that a life is immediately at risk and in which an orthopaedic intervention can save such a life. The pelvic ring can be disrupted in high-energy accidents (or low-energy falls in osteoporotic patients) and most always is disrupted in at least two points around the ring. The saying, "it is impossible to break a ring at a single point" nearly always applies to the pelvis. Therefore, the examiner should look for a lesion posteriorly in the sacrum or sacroiliac joint and anteriorly in the pelvic ramii or pubic symphisis.

  When a pelvic fracture is recognized on the anteroposterior x-ray view obtained with the initial trauma series, two more radiographs should be obtained: a pelvic inlet and pelvic outlet view. These are orthogonal views of the pelvis which help to critically evaluate all the pelvic bony landmarks as well as displacement of fractures. If there is significant displacement (more than 5 mm) at any one pelvic fracture line, a pelvic CT scan should be obtained. Many orthopaedists will prefer a CT scan with even lesser displacements to more critically evaluate the injury or preoperatively plan. **If a fracture line enters the acetabulum, then Judet x-ray views should be obtained.** These are 45-degree angled x-ray views from the right and left side of the patient centered on the pelvis, once again giving the examiner orthogonal views to critically assess the bony landmarks of each acetabulum. Note that **it is wasteful to obtain "five views of the pelvis" for every pelvic fracture** as the Judet views are not needed unless the acetabulum is involved. Likewise, it is not necessary to get five views of an acetabular fracture, omitting the inlet and outlet pelvic x-rays when the posterior pelvic ring (sacrum or sacroiliac joint) is not involved.

The pelvis is like a cylinder or sphere of bone that contains many critical soft tissue structures and organs such as the bladder, the iliac vessels, prostate or vaginal vault, and the rectum. All these organs are at risk, but the worrisome life-threatening hemorrhage is what must be diagnosed promptly and addressed. Bleeding typically continues until tamponade can occur and clotting factors take control. **It is highly recommended to tie a sheet around the pelvis of a patient who is hemodynamically unstable until the anteroposterior radiograph of the pelvis rules in or out a displaced pelvic fracture.** The sheet must be tied very snug, and it is recommended to be applied at the level of the greater trochanters for maximal effectiveness in closing down the volume of the broken and separated sphere, thus leading to earlier tamponade of bleeding vessels (11). There is little to lose if the patient does not have such an injury, and the sheet is simply removed. Commercially available pelvic slings, now with pressure calibration, are becoming commonplace in trauma units for such a purpose. There is essentially no role for the trauma room application of an external fixator as this maneuver has been simplified by the more effective use of a pelvic sling.

2. **Extremity arterial injury.** Probably the next most emergent condition which an orthopaedist faces is the extremity that is at risk for limb loss. This can occur due to a torn or lacerated artery or compartment syndrome. Arterial injury can be caused by blunt or penetrating trauma. There are **four "hard signs" of arterial injury which warrant immediate vascular exploration**, and time should not be wasted ordering and performing a diagnostic arteriogram (12). The rationale is that a vascular surgeon knows the proximity of the injury based on the wound or the x-ray that demonstrates the pathology. There is no sense in using precious minutes finding out what is already known when irreversible ischemic damage to nerve and muscle tissue occurs after 4 hours of warm ischemia time. A warm ischemia time interval of less than 6 hours is the generally accepted time interval within which arterial continuity must be restored in order to avoid loss of limb (13).

The Four "Hard Signs" of Arterial Injury:
a. **Pulsatile hemorrhage**
b. **Expanding hematoma**
c. **Audible bruit**
d. **Pulseless limb**

The only time an arteriogram would be warranted in such an acute circumstance is when there is multilevel injury (multiple fractures or shotgun wound) in which the vascular surgeon cannot be sure what level the arterial damage has occurred.

The more difficult diagnostic problem occurs in the majority of patients who present with more subtle clues to vascular injury. Such "soft signs" might include a history of severe hemorrhage at the accident scene, subjectively decreased pulses, a deficit of an anatomically related nerve, or a nonpulsatile hematoma. Other soft signs include the orthopaedic **injury patterns that have been associated with a high incidence of arterial damage:**
a. **Knee dislocations**
b. **Highly displaced tibia plateau fractures**
c. **Medial tibia plateau fractures**
d. **Ipsilateral fractures on either sides of a joint (floating joint)**
e. **Gunshot or knife wounds in proximity to neurovascular structures**
f. **The mangled extremity**

The best screening exam for an arterial injury should be quick, non-invasive, portable, and cost effective, as well as reliable. Determination of the arterial pressure index (API) requires the use of a Doppler machine and a blood pressure cuff. It has been investigated as a screening tool for clinically significant arterial compromise (14). The API has also been referred to in the literature as the ABI (Ankle Brachial Index) or AAI (Ankle Arm Index), and the terms are interchangeable. To conduct an API examination, a blood pressure cuff is placed just above the ankle or wrist in the injured limb so that a systolic pressure can be determined with a Doppler probe at the respective posterior tibial artery or radial artery. The dorsalis pedis or ulnar arteries may logically be used as well, as long as the blood pressure cuff is placed distal to the injury. The same measurement is determined on an uninjured upper or lower extremity limb (**Fig. 1-1**). **The API is simply the calculation of the systolic pressure of the injured limb divided by the systolic pressure of the uninjured limb:**

$$API = \frac{\text{Doppler Systolic Arterial Pressure in Injured Limb}}{\text{Doppler Systolic Arterial Pressure in Uninjured Extremity}}$$

Since pulses have been reported to be palpable distal to major arterial lesions, including complete arterial disruption (15–17), and perception of a pulse is subjective and impossible to quantify, physical exam alone or the detection of a palpable pulse is not appropriate for diagnosis.

As it is impossible to spell out every clinical scenario that may be associated with an arterial injury, it should be reiterated that every case bears

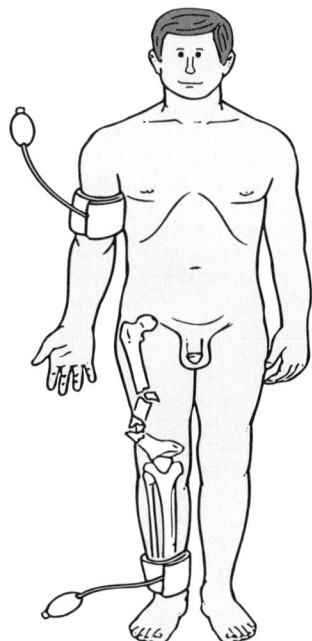

Figure 1-1. The placement of the pressure cuff and the Doppler probe is illustrated. One systolic pressure measurement is taken in an uninjured limb, and the other systolic pressure measurement is taken on the injured limb distal to the injury.

$$API = \frac{\text{Doppler Systolic Arterial Pressure in Injured Limb}}{\text{Doppler Systolic Arterial Pressure in Uninjured Extremity}}$$

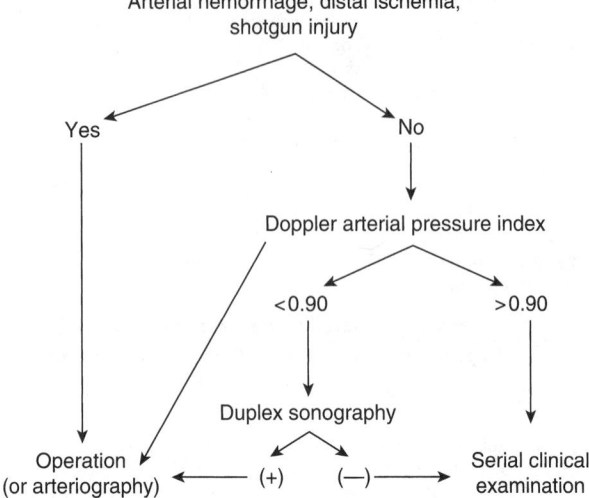

Figure 1-2. The diagnostic algorithm for a patient with a possible extremity arterial injury.

individual judgment, and given the absent morbidity of the API examination, a conservative approach to testing and documentation is the most prudent course. The clinician should approach the patient who has a high-risk vascular injury with a clear diagnostic algorithm (**Fig. 1-2**). Besides the patient with one of the four hard signs of vascular arterial injury who warrants immediate surgical exploration, a patient's API should dictate the next step. If the API is greater than 0.9, then the patient may be followed clinically without any further workup. If the API is less than 0.9, then they should proceed to the next diagnostic step of either an arteriogram or duplex ultrasound, the results of which will dictate the final plan of action.

3. **Compartment syndrome.** Compartment syndrome is a condition in which there is increased pressure within a closed soft tissue space, with the capacity to cause damage or necrosis to such tissues. Therefore, it should be recognized that the condition can occur in any muscular compartment of the body, though it is most commonly encountered in the leg. It is perhaps the most common orthopaedic emergency and often difficult to diagnose. In the awake and alert patient, symptoms include
   a. **Pain out of proportion to the injury** (despite adequate narcotic analgesia).
   b. **Pain with passive stretch** of the muscles within the compartment.
   c. **Paresthesias**

   Furthermore, these symptoms should occur in the setting of swollen tissues. **Diminished or absent pulse is specifically not listed, as it is such a late and subjective sign, that its absence should never be relied upon to exclude the diagnosis of compartment syndrome.** These clinical symptoms obviously cannot be used in the obtunded patient and should not even be relied upon in a patient with altered sensorium due to intoxication, for example. The clinician should have great suspicion for compartment syndrome in the setting of high-energy trauma or comminuted and displaced fractures, and if he or she encounters such a patient with very swollen tissues (often characterized as "tense"), then a pressure measurement should be taken of the suspected compartments. It is important to note that **compartment syndrome is well described in low energy mechanisms and does not have to be associated with a fracture. Chart**

documentation should be rigorous when tracking the possibility of compartment syndrome, and excellent patient examination should occur at intervals no more than 3 hours apart until compartment syndrome can be ruled out.

Most emergency and operating rooms have readily available pressure measuring devices such as the Stryker Quickstick, which can be used to measure suspected compartments. An indwelling catheter rigged with a mercury manometer (18) or an arterial line attached to a pressure transducer can also be used. **If there is ever any doubt as to whether a patient has compartment syndrome, then such measurements must be taken to confirm or rule out the diagnosis. Intracompartmental pressures exceeding the diastolic pressure minus 30 mm Hg warrant emergent fasciotomies (19).** Fasciotomy incisions should extend to nearly the length of the compartment to ensure complete decompression and adequate visualization and assessment of tissues. A text should be reviewed prior to the operation to review recommended incisions which address each and every compartment of the suspected part of the extremity (thigh, leg, foot, hand, antebrachium, brachium, buttock, and more).

4. **Mangled extremity and traumatic amputations.** Another clinical entity that should warrant great concern for limb viability is the so-called mangled extremity. The mangled extremity is not clearly defined, and there is no objective criteria on which clinicians agree on definition. Suffice it to say that it represents the end of an injury spectrum that involves a magnitude of trauma which destroys soft tissue to the extent that limb survival is in question.

The principles of open fracture management as discussed in the next section should be heeded, and the algorithm for a vascular workup should be followed expeditiously as described in the former section (**III.A**). Most importantly, several services should come to bear in assessment, workup, and coordination of care including trauma surgery, orthopaedic surgery, plastic surgery, and, if necessary, vascular surgery. Communication around treatment considerations and timing should be open, clear, and decisive. In the same way, the patient and loved ones should be included in the communication in order to understand the gravity of the injury and that amputation is a real and sometimes optimal solution (20).

An accurate neurovascular exam should be performed and documented. **If an adult patient has a severed tibial nerve, then amputation should be executed**, though absent tibial nerve sensation does not necessarily mean that neurodiscontinuity has occurred. A patient with a mangled extremity should be managed at a Level I Trauma Center where the appropriate expertise and experience is available.

There are several prognostic factors that influence outcome and therefore should be weighed in the consideration for limb salvage versus amputation. A number of scoring systems have been developed to account for these variables, but none has proved reliable in predicting limb viability. A simple and popular grading system is the MESS (Mangled Extremity Severity Score), which helps to guide the clinician. **The MESS yields a score to the variables of injury energy, limb ischemia, shock or hypotension, and age** (**Table 1-2**) (21). A score of more than seven was found to be predictive of the need for amputation. This scale is merely a guide.

Early management includes skeletal stabilization versus amputation, wide and aggressive debridement of all devitalized tissue, abundant irrigation, reestablishing vascular continuity, and reoperations every couple of days for wound management until definitive coverage can be executed by a microvascular team if necessary. An antibiotic bead pouch or perhaps a vacuum-assisted closure system for open wounds are helpful in the interim between cases.

For the **complete traumatic amputation of a finger or entire extremity, the team approach should also be used to assess the possibility of a replantation.** The proximal stump is first dressed with Ringer's

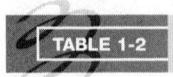

TABLE 1-2 MESS (Mangled Extremity Severity Score) Variables

Component	Points
Skeletal and soft tissue injury	
Low energy (stab, simple fracture, "civilian gunshot wound")	1
Medium energy (open or multiplex fractures, dislocation)	2
High energy (close-range shotgun or "military gunshot wound," crush injury)	3
Very high energy (same as above plus gross contamination, soft tissue avulsion)	4
Limb ischemia (score is doubled for ischemia >6 hours)	
Pulse reduced or absent but perfusion normal	1
Pulseless; parasthesias, diminished capillary refill	2
Cool, paralyzed, insensate, numb	3
Shock	
Systolic blood pressure always greater than 90 mm Hg	0
Hypotensive transiently	1
Persistent hypotension	2
Age (years)	
less than 30	0
30–50.1	1
greater than 50	2

Note: A MESS of greater than 7 warrants immediate transfer to a Level 1 Trauma Center.
From Johansen K, et al. *J Trauma*. 1990;30:568–573.

lactate soaked dressing and pressure is applied. A tourniquet is to be avoided. **The amputated part is wrapped in a Ringer's lactate moistened sterile sponge and placed in a plastic bag. It should be cooled by placing it in a container with ice**, which delays autolysis and thus allows time for transport to a center with a replantation team. The **part must not be frozen or placed in direct contact with ice**. If the travel distance by car is less than 2 hours, then this form of transport can be used. If not, arrangements should be made for air evacuation. **Make no promises to the patient** regarding whether replantation can be attempted or what the outcome will be. **Absolute indications for attempts at replantation include thumb amputations and pediatric amputations, and border digits are a relative indication**. Prognosis is improved when an extremity has been amputated in a sharp cutting mechanism as opposed to a crushing or traction mechanism.

5. **Femoral neck fracture in the nonelderly.** A femoral neck fracture in a young patient is considered an emergency because the blood supply to the femoral head is threatened. **The lateral epiphyseal artery branch off the medial circumflex artery is the dominant blood supply to the femoral head** (the artery of the ligamentum teres supplies 10%). There is an associated risk of **avascular necrosis** (AVN) of the femoral head after a femoral neck fracture, which can lead to femoral head collapse, which is a catastrophic complication in a young active patient in whom a hip replacement or a hip fusion is a dreaded salvage option.

The **risk of AVN exists even in nondisplaced fractures**; therefore all such femoral neck fractures (in a hip which needs to be saved) are regarded as emergent. For the displaced variety, an open reduction is indicated to establish anatomic alignment followed by internal fixation, classically with three large cannulated screws. In the nondisplaced variety, percutaneous fixation may be appropriate, but the hip capsule should still be surgically decompressed.

The **possible mechanisms for arterial insufficiency include** (22)
   a. **Intracapsular tamponade from bleeding into a closed space**
   b. **Kinking of vessels from tenting bone fragments**
   c. **Arterial disruption**

When considering these mechanisms, one can understand that urgent decompression and stable realignment can be helpful in restoring blood flow. In fact, studies indicate that prognosis is related to the time it takes to get to the operating room (23).

6. **Hip dislocation.** For the same reason as for the femoral neck fracture, a dislocated hip is an emergent condition as prognosis and the rate of AVN are directly related to the amount of time dislocated (24,25). One or two attempts at a closed reduction in the emergency room is indicated, but, if unsuccessful, a trip to the operating room for complete anesthesia and muscular relaxation usually suffices.

7. **Threatened soft tissues.** Anytime a fracture or dislocated bone is tenting the skin, and the injury cannot be reduced, the patient should go to the operating room emergently so that a closed reduction with pharmacologic paralysis can be attempted. If that fails, an open reduction should be performed. This scenario commonly occurs with ankle and subtalar fractures or dislocations, wrist fractures, and even fractures and dislocations around the knee. **Leaving any joint dislocated does not make sense when considering the tissues at risk** (even if it is not compromising skin), venous obstruction, and pain.

B. **Orthopaedic urgencies**
   1. **Open Fractures**
      a. **Emergency room management.** Early and careful treatment of wounds is necessary to decrease the chance of infection. Simple limb realignment should be performed for provisional splintage. **Wounds, large or small, should immediately be covered with a sterile dressing, and the temptation for multiple examiners to reexpose the wound must be avoided to decrease the likelihood of infection. Any laceration of the integument in the vicinity of a fracture should be assumed to represent an open fracture and, therefore, should be formally explored in the operating room. Cover the wound with a simple saline-moistened dressing. Do not probe or blindly use surgical hemostats in the wound. Do not push or stuff extruded soft tissue or bone back into the wound.** Externalized material is contaminated and will contaminate deeper recesses if replacement into the wound is attempted outside the operating environment.

      Open fractures are generally **classified** using Gustilo system (**Table 1-3**). With increasing severity, the complications of deep infection, nonunion, and amputation increase. **A Type IIIB open fracture requires a muscle flap for wound closure. A Type IIIC fracture is one which requires a vascular repair for limb viability.** The Gustilo classification is useful but because of its subjective criteria, such as high energy, comminution, and contamination, there is poor intraobserver reliability (26).

      b. **Operating room management. All large wounds, open fractures, nerve disruptions, and most tendon lacerations should be debrided and repaired in the operating room. Debridement** means removal of all foreign matter and devitalized tissue in or about a lesion. Irrigation with large quantities of saline does not replace the need for proper surgical debridement technique. Pulsating saline lavage is a useful adjunct to good debridement.

      The wound should be **debrided from the outside in**. The skin edges are sharply trimmed to viable margins. The debridement is then continued into the depth of the wound until the entire damaged area has been identified and

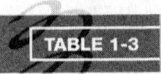

TABLE 1-3	**Gustilo and Anderson Classification of Open Fractures**

Type I	Skin opening of 1 cm or less, quite clean; most likely inside out; minimal muscle contusion; simple transverse or short oblique fractures.
Type II	Laceration more than 1 cm; extensive soft tissue damage; minimal to moderate crushing component; simple transverse or short oblique fractures with minimal comminution.
Type IIIA	Extensive soft tissue laceration associated with muscle, skin, and/or neurovascular injury but with adequate coverage of bone; typically segmental or comminuted fractures.
Type IIIB	Extensive soft tissue injury with periosteal stripping and bone exposure; usually associated with severe contamination.
Type IIIC	High energy features of other type IIIs but with arterial injury requiring repair.

Adapted from Gustilo RB, Mendoza RM, Williams DM. Problems in management of type III open fractures. A new classification of type III open fractures. *J Trauma* 1984;24:742.

resected. Muscle viability is evaluated based on the criteria described by Artz, et al: capacity to bleed, color, contractility, and consistency (27). These are helpful descriptors in determining whether or not to resect muscle.

With an open fracture, **all devitalized bone (bone without enough soft-tissue attachments to maintain adequate blood supply) should be removed**. The exception is pieces with articular cartilage attached that should be saved to attempt to reconstruct a joint surface. Great care must be taken not to devitalize the bone further. Initial internal fixation of open fractures is preferable if rigid stabilization is provided without significantly jeopardizing the blood supply (28). Again, the soft-tissue coverage should not create enough tension to cause any devitalization from a lack of blood supply. **Use monofilament sutures for skin closure**, not braided wire or multifilament synthetic, cotton, or silk sutures. Adequate control of bone bleeding may be difficult, so the surgeon should use either a loose skin closure that allows exodus of some of the hematoma or a skin closure combined with a suction drain.

Open fractures should generally be treated by a **delayed primary closure** (3–5 days). An exception may be made for uncomplicated hand fractures, wounds that enter joints, or small wounds with no extensive hemorrhage. **The burden of proof rests with the surgeon electing to close the wound.** Cover all exposed tendons, nerves, and bone but not at the expense of compromising blood supply to injured skin and subcutaneous tissues. Acute consultation with an orthopaedic or plastic surgeon skilled in myoplasty is indicated if adequate coverage over implants and bone cannot be accomplished. During the interval between debridement and definitive soft tissue coverage, it is wise to cover the wound with an antibiotic bead pouch (29) or a vacuum-assisted wound closure technique (30,31). This aids in maintaining an aseptic environment during the waiting interval (28).

c. **Antibiotic management.** It should be emphasized that **the primary management of an open fracture is surgical and that antibiotics play a strictly adjunctive role.** Furthermore, all patients with an open wound should be up to date with tetanus immunization or be treated with toxoid. Although there are numerous recommended tetanus prophylaxis schedules, the authors generally follow the recommendations of the American College of Surgeons. **Table 1-4** lists the current guidelines. With any open fracture or major wound, start parenteral **bactericidal antibiotics** immediately in the emergency department (28).

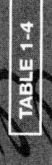

TABLE 1-4 Prophylactic Treatment of Tetanus[a]

		Patient not immunized or immunized in distant past.	
Type of wound	Partially immunized	5[c]–10 yr	>10 yr
Clean minor	Begin or complete immunization per schedule; tetanus toxoid, 0.5 mL	None	Tetanus toxoid, 0.5 mL
Clean major or tetanus prone	In one arm, human tetanus immunoglobulin, 250 units[b] In other arm, tetanus toxoid, 0.5 mL; complete immunization per schedule[b]	Tetanus toxoid, 0.5 mL	In one arm, tetanus toxoid, 0.5 mL[b] In other arm, human tetanus immunoglobulin, 250 units[b]
Tetanus prone, delayed or incomplete debridement	In one arm, human tetanus immunoglobulin, 500 units[b] In other arm, tetanus toxoid, 0.5 mL; complete immunization per schedule thereafter[b], antibiotic therapy	Tetanus toxoid, 0.5 mL; antibiotic therapy	In one arm, tetanus toxoid, 0.5 mL[b] In other arm, human tetanus immunoglobulin, 500 units[b], antibiotic therapy

[a]With different preparations of toxoid, modify the volume of a single booster dose appropriately.
[b]Use different syringes, needles, and injection sites.
[c]No prophylactic immunization required if patient has had a booster within 5 years.
From Walt AJ, ed. *Early care of the injured patient.* Philadelphia, PA: WB Sauders, 1982:70.

Cephalosporins are the drug of choice for prophylaxis of a Gustilo type I and II injury. Patients who are allergic to penicillin (excluding history of anaphylaxis) usually may receive cephalosporins. A small test dose is recommended before giving the entire dose. To obtain an adequate concentration of antibiotics in the fracture hematoma, begin the antibiotic therapy as soon as an open fracture is diagnosed. To avoid many of the side effects of antibiotics, such as superinfections, limit the duration of prophylactic antibiotic to 48 to 72 hours postoperative.

An acceptable alternative is **vancomycin** 1 g intravenously (IV) daily (32). Use this drug only if there is both penicillin and cephalosporin allergy or a history of anaphylaxis since the isolates of resistant strains of bacteria have increased in number recently, and this drug is the mainstay of treatment for methicillin-resistant *Staphylococcus aureus* (MRSA).

For type III open wounds with marked contamination or large exposure, gram negative coverage should be added to the antibiotic spectrum. An aminoglycoside is typically used as an appropriate agent during this short-term period of treatment for gram-negative organisms. If there is a risk for **soil, or sewage contamination, an agent against that acts against clostridium bacterial species is important to add.** Though penicillin may be added to the regimen for this purpose, the antibiotic Zosyn is a good choice offering broad coverage and eliminates the need for administration of three different medications for infection.

d. **Gunshot wounds.** If possible, **identify** the caliber and type of **weapon**. This information helps determine whether the wound was caused by a high- or low-velocity weapon. The majority of civilian injuries are **low velocity and interestingly do not seem to be associated with higher infection rates, even when associated with a fracture** (33–35). Decision making regarding the fracture proceeds as with a closed fracture. If the bullet **enters a joint,** formal **lavage and debridement is indicated.**

The protocol for management of a low velocity gunshot is as follows:
i. **Tetanus prophylaxis**
ii. **1 day of antibiotics** (first-generation cephalosporin)
iii. **Local cleansing**
iv. **Debridement of devitalized skin**
v. **Superficial irrigation**
vi. **Sterile dressing**

High-velocity weapons have a muzzle velocity greater than 610 m/sec or an impact velocity of 2,000 to 2,500 ft/sec. These weapons cause severe cavitation within the wound, which make debridement necessary. Big-game rifles, such as a 0.30 to .030 or a 0.30 to 0.06, can approach this high-velocity impact energy, and wounds from these must be treated accordingly with irrigation and debridement, possibly on a serial basis depending on the cavitation injury. Gunshot wounds of high-impact energy cause marked comminution of the fracture and leave a gaping exit. These are managed like an open fracture and certainly require appropriate vascular screening as previously discussed.

2. **Open joints.** Open joint injuries are also at risk for septic complications. **The surgeon should assume that lacerations over a joint extend into the joint until the contrary is proven in the operating room.** Air in the joint noted on roentgenography is a sign that a laceration extends into the joint. It is a reasonable idea to inject the joint with saline or a methylene blue-enhanced saline to check for communication with the suspected laceration. A healthy volume of fluid under pressure must be used to enhance sensitivity of this test—(for the knee, no >50 mL). This method is not 100% sensitive and should be used with judgment. An operative joint lavage, either open or arthroscopic technique, should be performed if an open joint is suspected. Certainly, if there are foreign bodies in the joint, such as missile fragments from gunshot wounds, these must be evacuated. A course of 48 hours of

gram-positive and gram-negative coverage with parenteral antibiotics (as with a Gustilo type IIIA fracture) is a reasonable and prudent adjunct to surgery.
3. **Talus fractures.** A fracture of the talus is considered a relative operative emergency due to its vulnerable blood supply. Though underpowered, and inconclusive, a recent study seems to suggest that time to operative fixation does not matter, while talar neck comminution and open fractures do correlate with poorer outcomes and a higher rate of AVN (36). Since the talus is at risk for AVN, collapse, and subsequent arthrosis, and since it is a weight-bearing joint, most orthopaedic traumatologists prefer to operate on this fracture urgently for the same reasons described for the femoral neck fracture in a young patient. Certainly the displaced variety of talus fracture, in which soft tissue tenting occurs, is an emergency due to the eventuality of full-thickness skin necrosis, which can lead to catastrophic complications.
4. **Long bone fractures in the face of multisystem trauma.** Patients who present with a femur fracture and other injuries to critical organs such as the lung, brain, or abdomen, or who have extended periods of hypotension, are at risk for complications such as acute respiratory distress syndrome, fat embolism syndrome, extended internsive care unit (ICU) stays, and pneumonia. It is generally well accepted that **early stabilization of femur fractures helps to decrease such complications and will allow for earlier mobility and thus less consequent problems from extended recumbent time periods** on a ventilator in the ICU. Patients with femur fractures and head injury should generally have the femur fracture stabilized (37). It is important that fluid management be well controlled by anesthesia in such a setting. Aggressive stabilization for femur and pelvic fractures has a favorable effect on pulmonary function following blunt trauma (38). In general, fixation of femur fractures with an interlocking nail is indicated in the multiply injured patient (37,39,40). Evidence supports femur fixation within 24 hours of injury in the polytrauma patient (41–43).

Timing and titration of orthopaedic procedures, however, is very important and requires significant judgment. Damage control orthopaedics is a recently espoused philosophy which favors femur stabilization with an external fixator rather than an intramedullary nail in order to prevent the "second hit" or second physiologic insult which occurs from intramedullary reaming and manipulation (44). It is thought that the intramedullary nailing should be delayed further stabilization, if a patient is physiologically challenged from multiple injuries; however, early (less than 24 hours) femur stabilization with an external fixator is still prudent.

IV. PEDIATRIC ORTHOPAEDIC CONSIDERATIONS
A. **General principles of fracture care.** Pediatric orthopaedics is a separate discipline because in part there are many nuances in diagnosis and management that are very different than adult orthopaedic fracture care. Obtaining a history is more difficult and takes significant patience, and often family help to solicit appropriate information. Children have injury patterns that are distinctive, and with an understanding of these recurring patterns, effective management can be learned and applied with greater confidence.

Reducing fractures is frequently more effective in a setting where general anesthesia can be administered as it is otherwise difficult to gain the cooperation of the child. The rule **"one doctor, one manipulation"** should be observed in the emergency room setting. With all types of injuries involving the epiphyseal plate, an accurate diagnosis as to the type of injury is important. Minor residual deformity in Salter-Harris I and II (see below) injuries correct themselves with subsequent growth, so open reduction is not indicated because the operation itself may cause more trauma. What the clinician can accept for angular deformity is more liberal in children because of their remarkable capacity to remodel deformity. For this reason, there are many fewer indications for surgical stabilization with internal fixation than in adults. Helpful treatment principles follow.

1. Up to **30 degrees of angulation** in the plane of joint motion is **acceptable** in metaphyseal fractures in young children. The **younger** the patient, the greater the angulation acceptable. **The closer the fracture is to the dominant growth plate, the more angular deformity, and so the greater the capacity to remodel.** The dominant growth plate is
    a. **Femur–distal**
    b. **Tibia–proximal**
    c. **Humerus–proximal**
    d. **Radius–distal**
2. If a **fracture deformity** is obvious on inspection, it should be **reduced**.
3. Fractured femurs in the 3- to 8-year-old group can be allowed to have **1.0 to 1.5 cm of overlap** due to the potential for overgrowth.
4. Children do not experience stiffness of otherwise normal joints.

B. **Growth plate injuries.** The epiphyseal plate is weakest at the site of cell degeneration and provisional calcification (growth plate zones of calcification and hypertrophy). Children who have undergone a rapid growth spurt, and in those who are excessively heavy for their skeletal maturity, are particularly vulnerable to such growth plate injuries. **Salter** classified traumatic epiphyseal separations into the following functional groups.
    1. **Class 1.** A fracture through the zone of provisional calcification without fracture of bone tissue. Such an injury does not involve a germinal layer unless associated with severe trauma either from the initial injury or from attempted reductions. Growth disturbances are rare but do occur.
    2. **Class 2.** An epiphyseal plate fracture with an associated fracture through the bony metaphysis. Growth disturbance (physeal arrest) is also rare in this category of injury.
    3. **Class 3.** An epiphyseal plate fracture associated with fractures through the epiphysis. These fractures involve the articular surface. Histologically, there is a fracture through the germinal layers. Accurate reduction is essential to prevent subsequent growth disturbance, but even so, alterations in growth are unpredictable. If the articular surface has more than 1 mm of "step off," then open reduction is indicated.
    4. **Class 4.** A fracture through the epiphysis, epiphyseal plate, and metaphysis. Such an injury almost invariably results in significant growth disturbance unless it is anatomically reduced. Open reduction and internal fixation is indicated if there is any displacement.
    5. **Class 5.** This is an impact or "smash" injury that destroys all or part of the epiphyseal plate and results in growth arrest. Close monitoring for remaining growth is essential. Surgical resection of the bone bridge and fat interposition are necessary if growth arrest results.

C. **Diagnostic and therapeutic pediatric pitfalls**
    1. **Treating accessory ossicles as fractures**
    2. **Missing an osteochondral fracture**
    3. **Not following a child long enough to follow effect of growth arrest (valgus or varus)**
    4. **Missing a stress fracture**
    5. **Confusing an epiphyseal fracture for a ligament injury ("kids don't sprain")**
    6. **Missing a tibial spine fracture**
    7. **Overdiagnosing instability of C2–C3 ("pseudosubluxation")**
    8. **Overtreating an upper humeral fracture (tremendous remodeling capacity)**
    9. **Failing to realize the instability of an apparently undisplaced lateral condylar fracture of the humerus**
    10. **Overlooking radial head dislocation (should bisect the capitelum) for both the anteroposterior and lateral radiographs**
    11. **Distal forearm fractures lose initial reduction frequently**
    12. **Overlooking abdominal injury in a child with a thoracolumbar flexion injury**
    13. **Always obtain an opposite limb (joint) x-ray to aid interpretation of a physeal injury, particularly in the injured elbow.**

V. **PRINCIPLES OF RADIOGRAPHIC DIAGNOSIS.** Accurate diagnosis and best orthopaedic treatment is absolutely dependent upon excellent radiological execution and interpretation. **The clinician must, at the very least, demand two good quality, orthogonal, appropriately penetrated, x-ray views centered on the bone or joint of interest without overlying objects obscuring detail.** This basic principle is perhaps the most violated orthopaedic axiom, which leads to mismanagement, frustration, litigious outcomes, and compromised patient care.

A long bone has an **articular surface made up of hyaline cartilage** at each end. **This end of the bone is called the epiphysis in the skeletally immature patient.** In general, a goal of treatment is to ensure that a fracture heals with anatomic alignment of articular fragments. Therefore, **intraarticular fractures deserve a critical radiographic assessment typically with oblique views in addition to an anteroposterior and lateral view.** An alternative to oblique x-rays is the CT scan, but x-rays should never be omitted altogether. Just under the epiphysis is the metaphysis, which is made up of the broad funnel-shaped area of bone with thin cortices and dense trabecular bone. In between each metaphysis is the area of bone called the diaphysis. In general, the metaphyseal and diaphyseal fragments do not need to be reduced anatomically during treatment and healing. The treatment principle in these areas of bone is to restore length, alignment, and rotation of the bone. **Any diaphyseal fracture warrants orthogonal x-rays of the joint above and below the injury to look for associated fractures or luxations.**

Unfortunately, too many young practitioners bypass the radiograph and go directly to a CT scan to interpret fractures. This practice is wrong. Most of the time, radiographs suffice for common orthopaedic injuries and, in fact, contain all the necessary detail the clinician needs for appropriate treatment. The ubiquitous ordering of CT scans is an extremely expensive and wasteful strategy and simply bypasses appropriate diagnostic algorithms. Furthermore, x-rays yield better information about the quality or density of bone and better information about displacement and spatial context of related bones.

The role of **computed axial tomography** might be necessary in complex fractures, particularly those that enter joints. It is also particularly useful for assessment of spine and pelvic injuries. The CT scan helps to assess greater bony detail and often provides a roadmap during preoperative planning. Critical CT findings to look for in certain injuries include:

A. Spine-subluxation of vertebral elements
B. Pelvis-sacral fractures and sacroiliac involvement
C. Acetabulum-intraarticular fragments of the acetabulum or femoral head (which suggests necessary axial traction)
D. Impaction injury to the acetabulum
E. Distal femur-coronal plane (Hoffa) fractures
F. Tibia plateau and pilon-fracture vector and comminution
G. Talus-talar dome and lateral process injuries (often missed on x-ray)
H. Calcaneus comminution at subtalar joint

VI. **PRINCIPLES OF FRACTURE HEALING (45). Factors generally reported with delayed union and nonunion fracture** (46)
   1. **Too much motion** destroys the vascular budding into the fracture hematoma and interferes with revascularization. Adequate stabilization of the fracture, therefore, is mandatory (46).
   2. **Distraction** decreases the surrounding vascularity as well as increases the length of the bony bridge necessary to heal the fracture.
   3. **Patient factors** include smoking, diabetes, steroid medications, and poor nutrition.

VII. **STRESS FRACTURES.** Normal bone might undergo fatigue or stress fractures when subjected to unaccustomed use. This condition can range from a stress fracture of a fibula in a runner who has recently increased his or her training distance or in an older person who is being mobilized after having been confined to a chair or bed. A **history** of having done something out of one's normal routine, followed by pain, should raise the question of stress fracture in the mind of the physician. Common sites of stress fracture include the metatarsals after unusually long walks or running, the distal fibula in runners, the tibia in football players (frequently misdiagnosed as shin splints), and the femoral neck in both young and older patients.

The **physical examination** reveals tenderness to pressure on the bone at the site of the fracture. Occasionally, swelling and erythema are present. Radiographic examination usually is negative in the first 10 to 14 days, after which a small, radiolucent line can usually be seen in association with increasing adjacent bone sclerosis. A bone scan shows radioactive uptake earlier and may be indicated in the competing athlete, particularly if the suspected fracture is in the tibia or femoral neck, both of which have a high incidence of complete fracture if the athlete continues competition. Magnetic resonance imaging (MRI) can definitively identify a stress fracture. Healing stress fractures have been mistaken for bone tumors (47).

Treatment should be based on the relief of symptoms unless there is danger of complete fracture under normal use. Under such circumstances, the injury should be treated like any undisplaced fracture.

VIII. SOFT TISSUE INJURIES
A. Tendon
1. **Diagnosis** (48)
   a. **First-degree strain** (mild)
      i. The **etiology** is trauma to a portion of the musculotendinous unit from excessive forcible stretch.
      ii. Symptoms include local pain that is aggravated by movement or by tension.
      iii. Signs of injury include mild spasm, swelling, ecchymosis, local tenderness, and minor loss of function and strength.
      iv. Complications include recurrence of the strain, tendonitis, and periostitis at the tendinous insertion site.
      v. Pathologic changes cause a low-grade inflammation and some disruption of muscle-tendon fibers by no appreciable hemorrhage.
   b. **Second-degree strain** (moderate) (48)
      i. The **etiology** is trauma to a portion of the musculotendinous unit from violent contraction or excessive forcible stretch.
      ii. **Symptoms and signs** include local pain that is aggravated by movement or tension of the muscle, moderate spasm, swelling, ecchymosis, local tenderness, and impaired muscle function.
      iii. **Complications** include a recurrence of the strain.
      iv. The **pathologic findings** consist of hemorrhage and the tearing of muscle–tendon junction fibers without complete disruption.
   c. **Third-degree strain** (severe) (48)
      i. **Symptoms and signs** include severe pain and disability, severe spasm, swelling, ecchymosis, hematoma, tenderness, loss of muscle function, and usually a palpable defect. An avulsion fracture at a tendinous insertion may mimic a severe strain.
      ii. A **complication** is prolonged disability.
      iii. **Roentgenograms** can demonstrate an avulsion fracture at the tendinous attachment as well as soft-tissue swelling.
      iv. The **pathology** consists of a ruptured muscle or tendon with the resultant separation of muscle from muscle, muscle from tendon, or tendon from bone.
2. **Treatment.** Direct treatment toward immobilization, with the disrupted tissue ends approximated. In some settings, this requires removal of devitalized tissue and repair by the sites and type of suture that will not cause further devitalization. When possible, sutures are placed in the surrounding fascia and not in the muscle itself.

B. Tendon
1. Tendons are relatively avascular structures and do not handle infection well. At sites where they course along long synovial tunnels, **blood supply** is via the long axis of the tendon or vincula. Trauma or sheath infections can jeopardize nutrition of the tendon.

2. As a **general principle**, a lacerated or ruptured tendon should be repaired primarily with a nonreactive material and a suture technique to ensure continued approximation of the tendon ends. Even with prophylactic antibiotics, primary repair of tendons in wounds more than 12 hours old carries considerable risk. A nonreactive synthetic suture or braided wire is the suture of choice. If the tendon is expected to glide subsequently, then handling the tendon with sponges and forceps is avoided because this causes further trauma and may be associated with dense adhesions.
3. Any involved **tendon sheath** should be opened in a longitudinal fashion so that the tendon is unroofed for the entire excursion of a repaired laceration site to
   a. **Prevent "triggering"** of the enlarged sutured site.
   b. **Allow for revascularization** of the tendon at the suture site.
   c. **Prevent fixation** on the relatively immobile sheath.
4. Only those with special training in hand surgery should repair **digital flexor tendons in the hand.**

C. Ligaments
1. **Types of injury**
   a. **First-degree sprain** (mild)
      i. **Signs** include mild point tenderness, no abnormal motion, little or no swelling, minimal hemorrhage, and minimal functional loss.
      ii. **Complications** include a tendency toward recurrence.
      iii. The **pathology** consists of minor tearing of the ligamentous fibers.
   b. **Second-degree sprain** (moderate)
      i. **Signs** include point tenderness, moderate loss of function, slight-to-moderate abnormal motion, swelling, and localized hemorrhage.
      ii. **Complications** can include a tendency toward recurrence, persistent instability, and traumatic arthritis.
      iii. This **pathology** is a partial tear of a ligament.
   c. **Third-degree sprain** (severe)
      i. **Signs** include a loss of function, marked abnormal motion, possible deformity, tenderness, swelling, and hemorrhage.
      ii. **Complications** can involve persistent instability and traumatic arthritis.
      iii. **Stress roentgenograms** demonstrate abnormal motion when pain is adequately relieved.
      iv. The **pathology** is a complete tear of a ligament.
2. **Diagnosis** of the extent of the ligamentous injury presents one of the major problems in orthopaedics. Rupture may be suspected from the mechanism of injury or from physical examination, which reveals tenderness over the ligament. If the patient is seen shortly after injury, a gap may be felt where the ligament is normally located. The injury might be fairly painless, especially if the ligament is completely disrupted. Once hemorrhage and swelling occur, this diagnostic possibility is eliminated. Another diagnostic aid is a stress roentgenogram, but it must be compared with the opposite and normal side. Such films should be made when the pain is inhibited by regional or general anesthesia. Arthroscopy or arthrography can provide pertinent information and a diagnosis, but a skilled arthroscopist should first be consulted. An MRI scan can be used to make the diagnosis.
3. **Treatment** of a complete ligamentous rupture is in essence the treatment of a dislocated joint after the dislocation has been reduced. In general, preserving motion is most important, and early mobilization is the treatment of choice. Ligaments are relatively avascular, so healing is slow. The larger ligaments must be protected until the scar matures (8–16 weeks).
4. There often is no clear answer when operative repair of ligaments is essential, but **open repair** is indicated in the following instances:
   a. Whenever the joint **cannot be anatomically reduced**
   b. When there is reasonable evidence of **infolding or turning of the ligament** on itself so that with any closed treatment the ends of the torn ligament would not be in close proximity

c. When ligaments are injured **about a joint that has no internal stability** (relies primarily on ligamentousvg structure for its stability)
D. Nerves
1. Nerve injuries are of **three types:** contusion or **neurapraxia**, crush or **axonotmesis**, and complete division or **neurotmesis**. Blunt injuries and those associated with fractures tend to be either neurapraxia or axonotmesis. For this reason, the fracture should be treated in its usual manner and the nerve injury observed. If it is neurapraxia, recovery will be complete within 6 to 12 weeks. If it is an axonotmesis, recovery from the trauma site to the next muscle to be innervated should be followed, keeping in mind that the expected recovery rate is 1 mm/day or 1 in./month. If reinnervation does not occur on time, exploration is indicated. When the distance from the site of trauma to the next innervated muscle that can be assessed causes a 6-month delay, early exploration is indicated. An electromyogram shows reinnervation approximately 1 month before it can be detected clinically, but one is dependent on the skill of the electromyographer for interpretation (see **App. F**). A traction injury is usually a mixed lesion with a large element of neurotmesis of individual axons at various places along the nerve. A nerve injury associated with sharp trauma is usually neurotmesis, and surgical repair is indicated. The **brachial plexus** presents a special diagnostic and treatment problem. Injuries from lacerations, especially in children, should be repaired primarily. Most brachial plexus injuries, however, are caused by traction and are either an avulsion of the root from the cord or the typical tearing of the axons at multiple levels along the nerve. MRI is essential for differentiation. If the lesion is an avulsion injury, no recovery is possible, and the patient should be started early on rehabilitation. If the lesion is the typical traction injury, the patient should be followed up to document recovery. If no recovery appears at the appropriate time intervals, exploration and possible suture or nerve graft should be considered.
2. As a general principle, **secondary repair** (3–6 weeks after injury) is preferable to primary repair for the following reasons:
   a. The repair is done as an **elective procedure** by the first team. The surgeon is rested and prepared for the procedure.
   b. There is **less hesitancy in extending the incision** for proper mobilization of the nerve.
   c. It is easier to delineate the **extent of damage** along the nerve.
   d. The **epineurium** has some degree of scarring and hence holds the suture better.
   e. The **distal axon tubules** are open because wallerian degeneration has occurred, and regeneration has a chance to proceed.
3. There are many **exceptions** to the preference for **secondary repair**, such as suturing
   a. A **digital nerve**
   b. A **nerve in the brachial plexus**
   c. An isolated nerve injury **less than 8 to 12 hours old** inflicted by a **razor** or sharp **knife**
4. **Nerve surgery should not be performed at any time by a surgeon inexperienced in microscopic techniques.**
E. Hematomas
1. **Treatment** of large hematomas (large compared to the area of confinement) whether subcutaneous or in muscle usually should consist of evacuation as an elective procedure in the operating room. A hematoma is not absorbed but undergoes organization, fibrosis, and scarring. Aspiration of a clot is not possible, so a large hematoma is evacuated by open drainage. Before considering this, the surgeon must be sure the hematoma is not expanding or is the cause of shock. If it is, vascular surgery consultation is mandatory to consider primary repair.
IX. FROSTBITE (49)
A. **Classification.** Frostbite is a pathologic entity that occurs on a spectrum of severity depending on temperature and duration of exposure. **Frostnip** results in pallor

and numbness but no tissue damage after rewarming. **Chilblain** typically involves the patient's face, pretibial region, or dorsum of the hands, and results from repeated exposure. **Trenchfoot** occurs during water immersion of an extremity in subfreezing conditions.

Frostbite occurs commonly in temperatures less than 2°C and includes the following degrees of severity:

1° = hyperemia and edema
2° = hyperemia and vesicle formation with partial-thickness necrosis
3° = full-thickness skin necrosis
4° = full-thickness skin and underlying structure necrosis

B. Treatment
1. **Prehospital care.** Protection of the frostbitten part from mechanical trauma. Avoid rewarming until it can be done definitively.
2. **Rewarming.** Hypothermia of the patient should be treated first. Stimulation of the vagus or myocardium with Naso-gastric (NG) tubes, Swan-Ganz catheter, or other methods should be avoided. If the patient is breathing, intubation is not appropriate. The patient should be rewarmed in a water bath with mild antibacterial soap at 40° to 42°C (104°–108°F). A flushed appearance indicates reperfusion and the patient should be removed from the bath.
3. **Definitive care.** The goals of definitive care are to preserve viable tissue and prevent infection. If possible, a burn center should be contacted for initiation of thrombolytic therapy to salvage threatened tissue and limbs. The injured limb should be elevated and protected from even mild trauma. Lambs wool should be placed between the toes. Analgesics and ibuprofen 4 mg/kg should be administered 3 times a day. Tetanus prophylaxis is appropriate. Any source of nicotine should be strictly prohibited.

References
1. Cummings SR, Rubin SM, Black D. The future of hip fractures in the united states: numbers, cost, and potential effects of postmenopausal estrogen. *Clin Orthop* 1990;252:163–166.
2. Cummings SR, Kelsey JL, Nevitt MC, et al. Epidemiology of osteoporosis and osteoporotic fractures. *Epidemiol Rev* 1985;7:178–208.
3. Poole GV, Ward EF. Causes of mortality in patients with pelvic fractures. *Orthopedics* 1994;17:691–696.
4. Court-Brown CM, Robinson CM. Femoral diaphysis fractures: Epidemiology. In: Browner BD, Jupiter JB, Levine AM, et al., eds. *Skeletal trauma*, 3rd ed., Vol. 2. Philadelphia, PA: WB Saunders, 2003:1884–1924.
5. Armstrong CP, Van Der Spuy J. The fractured scapula: importance and management based on a series of 62 patients. *Injury* 1984;14:324–329.
6. Ward WG, Nunley JA. Occult orthopaedic trauma in the multiply injured patient. *J Orthop Trauma* 1991;5:308–312.
7. American College of Surgeons' Committee on Trauma, *Advanced trauma life support for doctors® (ATLS®)*, American College of Surgeons, 7th ed, Chicago, IL: 2004:1–391.
8. Loo GT, Siegel JH, Dischinger PC, et al. Airbag protection versus compartmental intrusion effect determines the pattern of injuries in multiple trauma motor vehicle crashes. *J Trauma* 1996;41:935–951.
9. Bone LB, McNamara K, Shine B, et al. Mortality in multiple trauma patients with fractures. *J Trauma* 1994;37:262–264.
10. Tscherne H. Management of open fractures. In: Tscherne H, Gotzen L, eds. *Fractures with soft tissue injuries*, Berlin, Germany: Springer-Verlag New York, 1984:10–32.
11. Bottlang M, Krieg JC, Mohr M, et al. Emergent management of pelvic ring fractures with use of circumferential compression. *J Bone Joint Surg (Am)* 2002;84(S2):43–47.

12. Turcotte JK, Towne JB, Bernhard VM. Is arteriography necessary in the management of vascular trauma of extremities? *Surgery* 1978;84:557–562.
13. Miller HH, Welch CS. Quantitative studies on the time factor in arterial injuries. *Ann Surg* 1949;130:428–438.
14. Lynch K, Johansen K. Can Doppler pressure measurement replace "exclusion" arteriography in the diagnosis of occult extremity trauma? *Ann Surg* 1991;214:737–741.
15. Rose SC, Moore EE. Trauma angiography: the use of clinical findings to improve patient selection and case preparation. *J Trauma* 1988;28:240–245.
16. Snyder WH 3rd, Thal ER, Bridges RA, et al. The validity of normal arteriography in penetrating trauma. *Arch Surg* 1978;113:424–426.
17. Weaver FA, Yellin AE, Bauer M, et al. Is arterial proximity a valid indication for arteriography in penetrating extremity trauma? A prospective analysis. *Arch Surg* 1990;125:1256–1260.
18. Whitesides TE Jr, Haney TC, Hirada H, et al. A simple method for tissue pressure determination. *Arch Surg* 1975;110:1311–1313.
19. McQueen MM, Court-Brown CM. Compartment monitoring in tibial fractures. *J Bone Joint Surg (Br)* 1996;78:99–104.
20. Hansen ST Jr. Technology over reason. *J Bone Joint Surg (Am)* 1987;69:799–800.
21. Johansen K, Daines M, Howey T, et al. Objective criteria accurately predict amputation following lower extremity trauma. *J Trauma* 1990;30:568–573.
22. Swiontkowski MF. Intracapsular hip fractures. In: Browner BD, Jupiter JB, Levine AM, et al. eds. *Skeletal trauma*, 3rd ed. Vol 2. Philadelphia, PA: WB Saunders, 2003:1700–1775.
23. Swiontkowski MF, Winquist RA, Hansen ST. Fractures of the femoral neck in patients between the ages of twelve and forty-nine years. *J Bone Joint Surg (Am)* 1984;66:837–846.
24. Epstein HC, Harvey JP. Traumatic anterior dislocations of the hip. Management and results. An analysis of fifty-five cases. *J Bone Joint Surg (Am)* 1972;54:1561–1562.
25. Herndon JH, Aufranc OE. Avascular necrosis of the femoral head in the adult. A review of its incidence in a variety of conditions. *Clin Orthop* 1977;86:43–62.
26. Brumback R, Jones A. Interobserver agreement in the classification of open fractures of the tibia. *J Bone Joint Surg (Am)* 1994;76:1162–1166.
27. Artz CP, Sako Y, Scully RE. An evaluation of the surgeon's criteria for determining the viability of muscle during debridement. *AMA Arch Surg* 1956;73:1031–1035.
28. Henry SL, Osterman PA, Seligson D. The antibiotic bead pouch technique: the management of severe compound fractures. *Clin Orthop* 1993;295:54–62.
29. Henry S, Ostermann P, Seligson D. The prophylactic use of antibiotic beads in open fractures. *J Trauma* 1990;30:1231–1238.
30. Argenta LC, Morykwas MJ. Vacuum assisted closure: a new method for wound control and treatment: clinical experience. *Ann Plast Surg* 1997;38:563–577.
31. Joseph E, Hamori CA, Bergman S, et al. A prospective randomized trial of vacuum assisted closure versus standard therapy of chronic nonhealing wounds. *Wounds* 2000;12:60–67.
32. Calhoun J. Use of antibiotic prophylaxis in primary TJA. Frontlines. *AAOS Bulletin* August, 2004;52(4):15.
33. Gellman H, Wiss DA, Moldawer TD. Gunshot wounds to the musculoskeletal system. In: Browner BD, Jupiter JB, Levine AM, et al. eds. *Skeletal trauma*, 3rd ed., Vol. 1. Philadelphia, PA: WB Saunders, 2003:1884–1924.
34. Gustilo RB, Anderson JT. Prevention of infection in the treatment of one thousand and twenty five fractures in long bones. *J Bone Joint Surg (Am)* 1976;58:453–458.
35. Patzakis MJ, Harvey JP, Ivler D. The role of antibiotics in the management of open fractures. *J Bone Joint Surg (Am)* 1974;56:532–541.

36. Vallier HA, Nork SE, Barel DP, et al. Operative management of talar neck fractures: outcomes and the effect of timing. *18th Ann Mtg of the Orthop Trauma Assoc, Toronto, Ontario, Canada,* Oct 11–13, 2002;Paper#32, 121–122.
37. McKee MD, Schemitsch EH, Vincent LO, et al. The effect of a femoral fracture on concomitant closed head injury in patients with multiple injuries. *J Trauma* 1997;42:1041–1045.
38. Routt MI, Simonian PT, DeFalco AJ, et al. Internal fixation in pelvic fractures and primary repairs of associated genitourinary disruptions: a team approach. *J Trauma* 1996;40:784–790.
39. Bosse MJ, MacKenzie EJ, Reimer BL, et al. Adult respiratory distress syndrome, pneumonia, and mortality following thoracic injury and a femoral fracture treated either with intramedullary nailing with reaming or with a plate: a comparative study. *J Bone Joint Surg (Am)* 1997;79:799–809.
40. DuWelius PJ, Huckfeldt R, Mullins RJ, et al. The effects of femoral intramedullary reaming on pulmonary function in a sheep lung model. *J Bone Joint Surg (Am)* 1997;79:194–202.
41. Bone LB, Johnson KD, Weigelt J, et al. Early vs. delayed stabilization of femoral fractures. *J Bone Joint Surg (Am)* 1989;71:336–340.
42. Johnson KD, Cadambi BA, Seibert GB. Incidence of adult respiratory distress syndrome in patients with musculoskeletal injuies: effect of early operative stabilization of fractures. *J Trauma* 1985;25:375–383.
43. Riska EB, Bonsdorff HV, Hakkinen S, et al. Primary operative fixation of long bone fractures in patients with multiple injuries. *J Trauma* 1977;17:111–121.
44. Pape HC, Grimme K, Van Griensven M, et al. EPOFF study group. Impact of intramedullary instrumentation versus damage control for femoral fractures on immunoinflammatory parameters: prospective randomized analysis by the EPOFF study group. *J Trauma* 2003;55:7–13.
45. Einhorn TA. Enhancement of fracture healing. *J Bone Joint Surg (Am)* 1995;77:940–956.
46. Weitzel PP, Esterhai JL Jr. Delayed union, nonunion and synovial pseudarthrosis. In: Brighton CT, Friedlaender GE, Lane JM, eds. *Bone formation and repair.* Rosemont, IL: American Academy of Orthopaedic Surgeons, 1994:505–527.
47. Eisele SA, Sammarco GJ. Fatigue fractures of the foot and ankle in the athlete. In: Heckman JD, ed. *Instructional course lectures, 42.* Rosemont, IL: American Academy of Orthopaedic Surgeons, 1993:175–183.
48. Taylor DC, Dalton JD Jr, Seaber AV, et al. Experimental muscle strain injury: early functional and structural deficits and the increased risk for reinjury. *Am J Sports Med* 1993;21:190–194.
49. Mohr WJ. Frostbite injury. *Regions hospital trauma protocol cards*, 2nd ed. Minneapolis, MN: HealthPartners, Inc, 2003.

Selected Historical Readings

Godina M. Early microsurgical reconstruction of complex trauma of the extremities. *Plast Reconstr Surg* 1986;78:285–292.
Gustilo RB, Mendoza RM, Williams DM. Problems in management of type III open fractures. A new classification of type III open fractures. *J Trauma* 1984;24:742–746.
Nash G, Blennerhassett JB, Pontoppidan H. Pulmonary lesions associated with oxygen therapy and artificial ventilation. *N Engl J Med* 1967;276:368–374.
Salter RB, Harris WR. Injuries involving the epiphyseal plate. *J Bone Joint Surg (Am)* 1963;45:587–622.
Shackford SR, Hollingworth-Fridlund P, Cooper GF, et al. The effect of regionalization upon the quality of trauma care as assessed by concurrent audit before and after institution of a trauma system: a preliminary report. *J Trauma* 1986;26:812–820.
Subcommittee on Classification of Sports Injuries. *Standard nomenclature of athletic injuries.* Chicago, IL: American Medical Association, 1976:99.

Tibbs PA, Young AB, Bivins BA, et al. Diagnosis of acute abdominal injuries in patients with spinal shock: value of diagnostic peritoneal lavage. *J Trauma* 1980;20:55–57.

Traverso LW, Lee WP, Langford MJ. Fluid resuscitation after an otherwise fatal hemorrhage: I. Crystalloid solutions. *J Trauma* 1986;26:168–175.

Urbaniak JR, Roth JH, Nunley JA, et al. The results of replantation after amputation of a single finger. *J Bone Joint Surg (Am)* 1985;67:611–619.

COMPLICATIONS OF MUSCULOSKELETAL TRAUMA   2

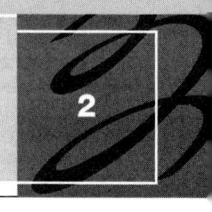

*C*omplications of musculoskeletal trauma are distressingly common. Some complications are a consequence of the injury itself and may be unavoidable, while others are iatrogenic and potentially preventable. Regardless of the etiology of the complication, prompt recognition and appropriate treatment lessen the impact of the complication and improve the outcome.

I. SYSTEMIC INFLAMMATORY RESPONSE SYNDROME (SIRS)
  A. SIRS has many manifestations ranging from occult hypoxemia to multiorgan dysfunction (MOD) (1). Fat embolism syndrome (FES) and the adult respiratory distress syndrome (ARDS) are other clinical manifestations of similar phenomenon that are related to SIRS. FES may be one of the etiologic factors contributing to SIRS, while ARDS is now recognized as the "final common pathway" of the pulmonary consequences of SIRS. The fat embolism syndrome is generally a self-limited pulmonary disease that usually occurs within 3 days of a fracture. The **diagnosis** is suspected if the following symptoms and signs are present in a patient with a fracture (2–4):
    1. **Disturbances of consciousness** (i.e., confusion, delirium, coma)
    2. **Tachycardia and dyspnea**
    3. **History of hypovolemic shock**
    4. **Petechial hemorrhages**

  Any combination of the above symptoms may be present in patients with isolated or multiple fractures. Patients with major long bone fractures should be monitored for occult hypoxemia with continuous, noninvasive pulse oximetry (5). When hypoxia is documented, supplemental oxygen is provided. Patients with hypoxia should be evaluated for coagulopathy and monitored for pulmonary, renal, and hepatic dysfunction that may develop in full-blown SIRS.

  B. Pertinent laboratory findings
    1. Of all the laboratory values, a platelet count of less than 150,000 and an arterial oxygen tension (PaO_2) of less than 60 mm Hg are the **most useful diagnostic tests**. Hypoxemia itself is very common in trauma patients and may or may not suggest pulmonary compromise (5). Recent data suggests that patients with elevated interleukin 6 (IL-6) levels are at increased risk of SIRS, and this is a useful marker to follow in patients with multiple injuries. Patients with multiple injuries and elevated IL-6 levels seem to be at increased risk for complications following surgery, and when possible, nonemergent orthopedic procedures should be deferred until the abnormal systemic inflammatory response has resolved (1).
    2. **Electrocardiographic changes** may be present and include tachycardia, a prominent S wave on lead I, a prominent Q wave on lead II, a shift in the transition zone to the left, arrhythmias, inverted T waves, depressed RST segments, and a right bundle branch block. Serial electrocardiograms are useful.
    3. **Increased serum lipase** is indicative of FES, but is of little practical value.
    4. **Chest roentgenographic changes**, when present, are patchy pulmonary infiltrates. The clinical manifestations of fat embolism usually precede these changes. The pulmonary findings become more severe in those patients that meet criteria for ARDS.

C. Recommended treatment
1. **Respiratory support** is the cornerstone of prevention and treatment of FES, ARDS, and MOD. Respiratory support is provided to keep the PaO_2 between 50 and 100 mm Hg. Patients with ARDS and MOD usually need prolonged ventilatory support with continuous positive airway pressure (CPAP). In patients with isolated fractures, early (within 24 hours) fixation of femur fractures helps limit the incidence of this complication (4,6).
2. **Shock** is treated as outlined in **Chap. 1, I.A.3.**
3. Coagulopathy is monitored and treated with fresh frozen plasma and/or cryoprecipitate. Platelet counts should ideally be maintained above 50,000.

II. NERVE COMPRESSION SYNDROMES
A. Carpal tunnel syndrome (CTS, median nerve entrapment at the wrist)
1. The **diagnosis** is suspected with a history of pain, tingling, and numbness in the first three digits; the symptoms are usually worse at night. CTS is only rarely associated with acute trauma and is generally a chronic condition typically associated with repetitive microtrauma. When occurring as a complication of trauma, the condition may develop and progress rapidly. Acute CTS is most commonly associated with distal radius fractures but can also occur with perilunate dislocation and other more subtle injuries. CTS must be recognized and treated emergently, first with fracture reduction and then with carpal tunnel release if symptoms do not immediately resolve (see **Chap. 20**).

B. Ulnar nerve compression at the elbow ("tardy" ulnar nerve palsy, acute ulnar palsy) is commonly associated with fractures and dislocations about the elbow in children as well as adults. Acute ulnar neuropathy following injury is most often the result of iatrogenic damage such as injury occurring during pinning of a supracondylar fracture in a child, or retraction during internal fixation of a distal humerus fracture in an adult.
1. An early **diagnostic sign** is the inability to separate the fingers (interosseous weakness). There is usually decreased sensation in the fourth and fifth fingers. Light pressure on the cubital tunnel may reproduce the pain. Nerve conduction studies show a slowing of the ulnar nerve conduction velocity as it crosses the elbow (see **App. F**); this test is not useful diagnostically until 3 weeks after injury.
2. If symptoms are minimal, ulnar nerve compression is managed with observation and passive range of motion of the fingers. **Surgical therapy** consists of exploration and transposition of the ulnar nerve beneath the flexor muscle mass anterior to the medial epicondyle when the pattern of injury or fracture permits. This treatment usually stops any progressive neuropathy but does not guarantee complete regression of the neurologic symptoms or signs.

C. Peroneal nerve palsy may be due to **compression of the common peroneal nerve** in the area of the fibular head or as the nerve enters the anterior compartment. Apparent peroneal palsy may also be a manifestation of more proximal **injury to the peroneal division of the sciatic nerve**. Thus peroneal palsy may be a complication of hip or pelvic fracture/dislocation.
1. **Diagnosis** often is based on the motor loss, which includes weakness of dorsiflexion of the ankle and toes as well as eversion of the foot. History of a hip, tibia, ankle, or foot injury is likely. Pain is usually on the lateral aspect of the leg and dorsal aspect of the foot. Pressure over the nerve trunk may cause local pain as well as radiation into the sensory distribution of the nerve. Pressure over the nerve as it courses around the proximal fibula results from patient positioning in the operating room or intensive care unit or from poorly applied splints.
2. **Treatment.** Associated hip, knee, or ankle dislocations are emergently reduced. If there is an operable cause, then neurolysis is indicated. During the recovery stage, a lateral shoe wedge or plastic ankle-foot orthosis maintains eversion of the foot. Tendon transfer may be appropriate for some patients with a permanent foot drop.

D. Sciatic nerve neuropraxia can accompany hip dislocation or fracture dislocation (acetabular fracture). Note that some sciatic palsies may present as an isolated peroneal palsy, as discussed above.

    1. The main differentiating factor in the **diagnosis** of a sciatic neuropathy is an L5 or S1 root injury resulting from pelvic or spine fracture. A sciatic neuropathy must be suspected when multiple neurologic (L5–S3) segments are involved. A helpful differentiating test is straight-leg raising just short of discomfort; pain caused by a sciatic neuropathy is increased by internal rotation and relieved by external rotation of the hips. This reaction is not seen with lumbar radiculopathies.

    2. Treatment is aimed at the cause of the sciatic neuropathy, and the neuropathy itself is treated with observation. If the sciatic nerve is known to be damaged and is not improving, neurolysis may be indicated. In general, the tibial portion of the nerve recovers well, but the peroneal portion does not (7). This may relate to the fact that it is the peroneal portion that lies against the pelvis as it exits through the greater sciatic foramen.

III. COMPARTMENTAL SYNDROMES. A compartmental syndrome is defined as "a condition in which increased pressure within the space compromises the circulation to the contents of that space" (8). Although most commonly applied to the osteomyofascial compartments of the extremities, compartment syndrome can occur in the abdomen and in major muscle groups about the spine and pelvis. Other terms that have been used to describe compartment syndrome are Volkmann ischemia, local ischemia, traumatic tension in muscles, impending ischemic contracture, exercise ischemia, exercise myopathy, anterior tibial syndrome, medial tibial syndrome, rhabdomyolysis, and calf hypertension.

A. Locations

    1. In the **upper extremity**, typical locations include the volar and dorsal compartments of the forearm (**Fig. 2-1**). There are also several intrinsic compartments of the hand.

    2. In the **lower extremity,** typical locations include the anterior, lateral, superficial posterior (gastrocnemius, soleus), and deep posterior compartments of the leg (**Figs. 2-2, 2-3**). Compartmental syndromes are also seen in the thigh, arm, buttocks (gluteal), and foot compartments (9).

B. Etiologies

    1. Decreased compartment volume, such as occurs following closure of fascial defects, application of tight circumferential dressings, and localized external pressure, can precipitate a compartmental syndrome (10).

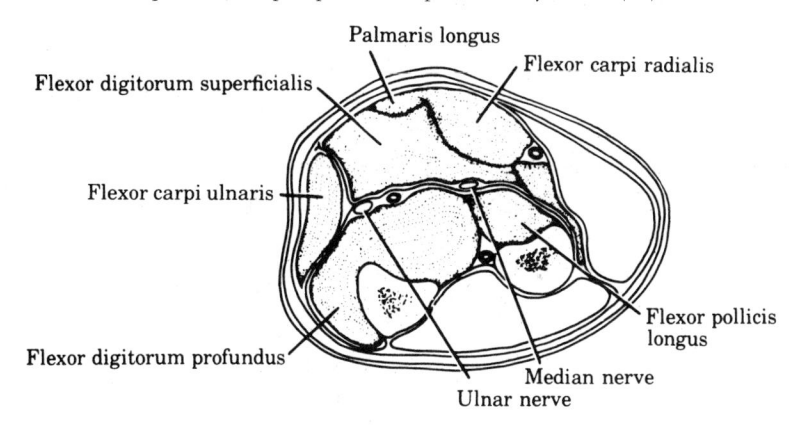

Figure 2-1. Volar compartmental syndrome of the forearm. Symptoms and signs of weakness of finger and wrist flexion, pain on finger and wrist extension, hypesthesia of the volar aspect of the fingers, and tenseness of the volar forearm fascia.

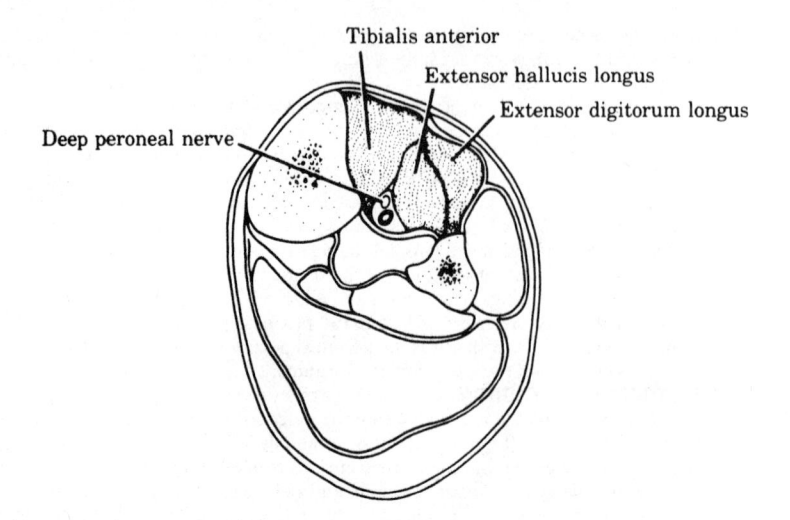

Figure 2-2. Anterior compartmental syndrome of the leg. Symptoms and signs are weakness of toe extension and foot dorsiflexion, pain on passive toe flexion and foot plantar flexion, hypesthesia in the dorsal first web space, and tenseness of the anterior compartmental fascia.

2. **Increased compartment content** arises from:
   a. **Bleeding** caused by a major vascular injury, edema from massive tissue crushing, or a bleeding disorder
   b. **Increased capillary permeability** due to shock, postischemic swelling, exercise, direct trauma, burns, intraarterial drugs, or orthopaedic surgery
   c. **Increased capillary pressure** from exercise or venous obstruction
   d. **Muscle hypertrophy**
   e. **Direct infusion (infiltrated intravenous line, injection gun)**
   f. **Application of excessive traction (Fig. 2-4)**

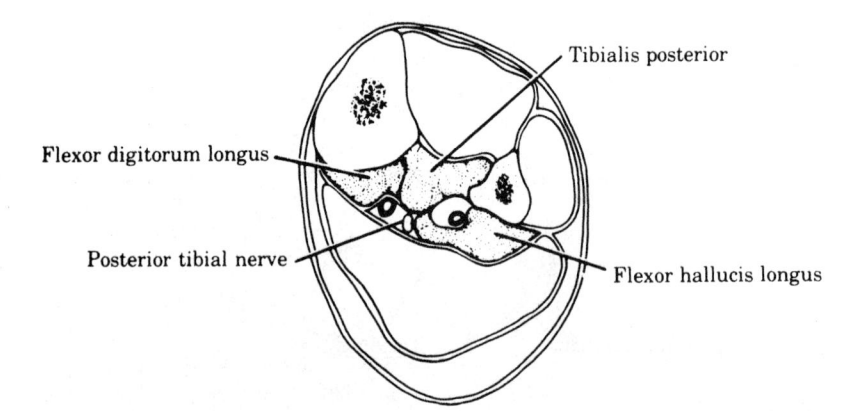

Figure 2-3. Deep posterior compartmental syndrome of the leg. Symptoms and signs are weakness of toe flexion and foot inversion, pain on passive toe extension and foot eversion, hypesthesia of the plantar aspect of the foot and toes, and tenseness of the deep posterior compartmental fascia (between the tibia and Achilles tendon).

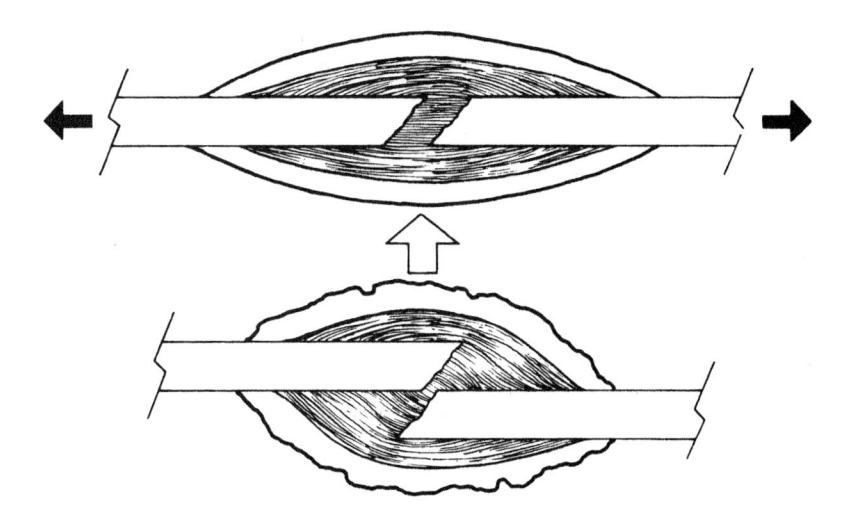

Figure 2-4. Distraction of fracture fragments (excessive traction) can increase compartmental tissue pressure and be a cause of a compartmental syndrome.

- C. **Increased tissue pressure** is the key feature of compartmental syndromes. Once the pressure is elevated, it can compromise the local circulation by at least three mechanisms: decreased perfusion pressure, arteriolar closure, and reflex vasospasm. Muscle cell death and nerve dysfunction begin at approximately 6 hours after the pressure begins to approach 20 mm Hg lower than the patients diastolic pressure.
- D. **The clinical approach.** Note that compartment syndrome may be divided into "chronic" and "acute." Chronic compartment syndromes are related to exertion and tend to occur when a given activity level causes transiently increased tissue pressures that resolve with rest. The topic of this chapter relates to acute compartment syndromes, which are limb-threatening and must be treated as potential emergencies.
    1. **Identify** the patients at risk as early as possible and **examine them frequently.** Continuous real-time monitoring of intramuscular pressure should be done if the patient's mental status and/or the ability to examine the patient is compromised in any way. If the risk is high and the patient is under anesthesia, consider **prophylactic decompression**. Patients who have been hypotensive for any reason are at particular risk.
    2. Carefully **document** the time and findings of each examination.
    3. The appearance of excess **pain, sensory deficits**, or **muscle weakness** demands a thorough examination to rule out a compartmental syndrome (**Table 2-1**). Because the compartmental syndrome is usually progressive, **frequent examination** is indicated in questionable cases. Of the 5 "Ps" traditionally taught to be associated with compartmental syndrome (pain, pulselessness, pallor, paresthesias, paralysis), only pain and paresthesias are useful for the early diagnosis of compartment syndrome. Classically, pain with gentle passive motion is the first sign, and pulselessness is the last. Patients who are at risk for developing compartment syndrome of an injured extremity should not have regional anesthesia. Patient-controlled anesthesia techniques are also capable of masking the pain associated with compartment syndrome and should be used with caution in "at-risk" patients.
        a. Check each potentially involved nerve using **two-point discrimination** and **light touch** because both are more sensitive than the commonly used pin.
        b. Grade the **strengths** of all potentially involved muscles (see **App. B**).
        c. The **passive muscle stretch** test causes severe pain if the muscle is ischemic.

TABLE 2-1 Diagnostic Factors in Compartmental Syndromes of the Lower Extremity

Compartment	Distribution of sensory changes	Muscles weakened	Painful passive movement	Location of tenseness
Anterior	Deep peroneal (first web space)	Toe extensors and tibialis anterior	Toe flexion	Anteriorly between tibia and fibula
Lateral	Superficial and deep peroneal (dorsum of foot)	Peronei	Inversion of foot	Laterally over fibula
Deep posterior	Posterior tibial (sole of foot)	Toe flexors and tibialis posterior	Toe extension in distal half	Posteromedially of leg between Achilles tendon and tibia
Superficial posterior	None	Gastrocnemius and soleus	Foot dorsiflexion	Over the bulk of the calf

From Matsen III, FA. Compartmental syndrome. *Clin Orthop* 1976;113:8, with permission.

   d. Palpation of each compartment is important because tenseness is a specific sign of a compartmental syndrome. This sign is obscured unless the dressing and plaster are adequately opened. Warm and red skin overlying the affected compartment suggests a cellulitis or thrombophlebitis.
   e. The **peripheral pulse** frequently is normal in the presence of a compartmental syndrome. If it is abnormal, the diagnosis of a major arterial occlusion or compartmental syndrome must be entertained.
   f. Laboratory findings are nonspecific.
4. The **tissue pressure** can be accurately measured by the infusion or wick techniques (**Figs. 2-5, 2-6**), which give similar pressure readings (11). A simpler but less reliable measurement can be obtained by the injection technique (**Fig. 2-7**). Tissue pressure readings within 30 mm Hg of the patient's diastolic blood pressure (perfusion pressure <30 mm Hg) are strongly suggestive of a compartmental syndrome (12). The various techniques for pressure measurement are described by Whitesides (10). The anterior compartment is nearly

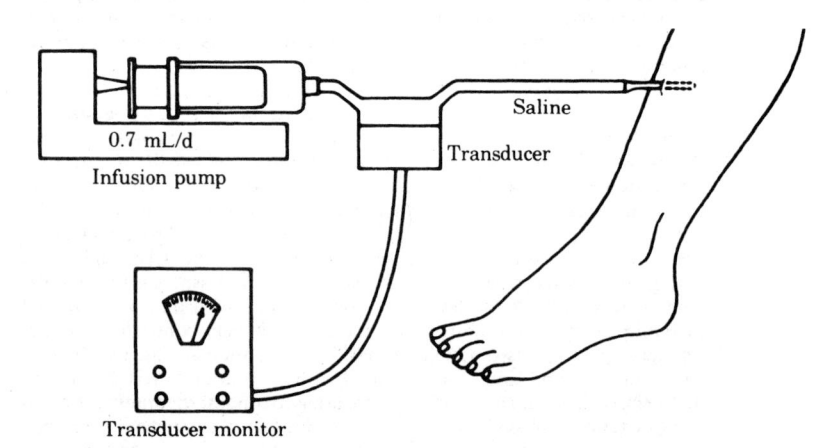

Figure 2-5. Tissue pressure measured by the infusion technique.

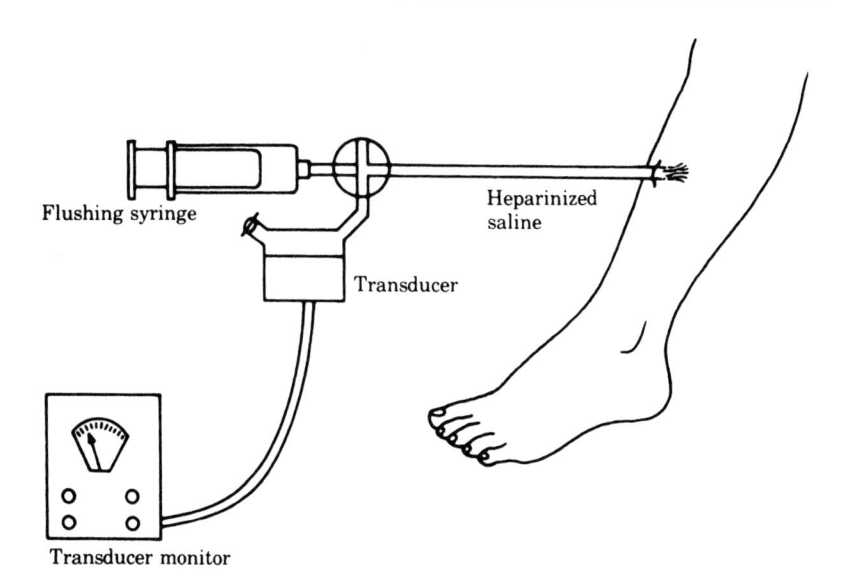

Figure 2-6. Tissue pressure measured by the wick technique.

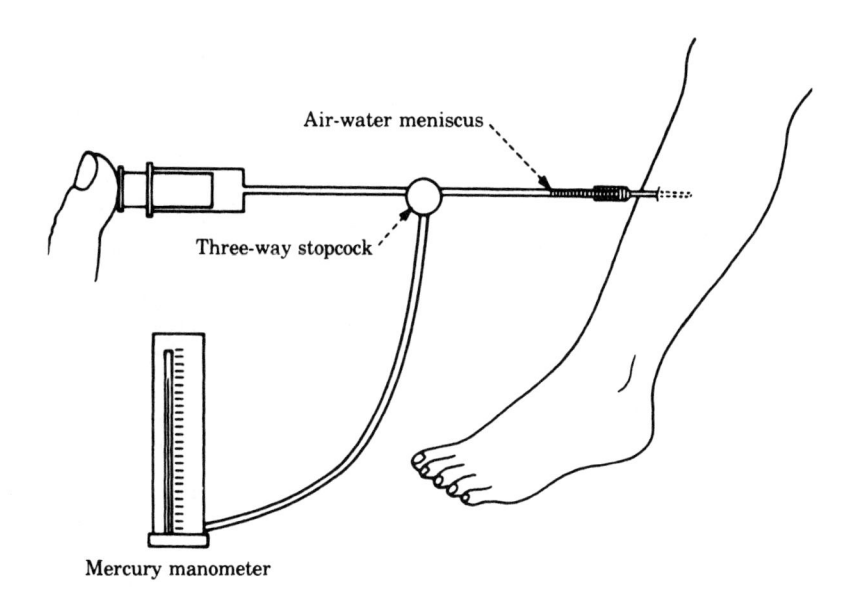

Figure 2-7. Tissue pressure measured by the injection technique.

always involved in patients with compartment syndrome and has been called the "sentinel" compartment. Continuous monitoring of the anterior compartment is simply performed by connecting a saline-filled intravenous (IV) tube to an angiocath inserted into the muscle, which is connected to a standard pressure transducer. A three-way valve allows the line to be flushed periodically. Although these measuring techniques are useful, the clinician should rely largely on the patient's history and ongoing (or repeat) examinations to establish the proper diagnosis and treatment program. In the presence of head injury, intoxication, or an unreliable or unconscious patient, monitoring techniques become indispensable. The evaluation should include measurement of the tissue pressure at multiple levels in the compartment (13).

5. If the examination suggests a compartmental syndrome, **decompression of the involved compartments by fasciotomy** should be performed emergently, ideally within 8 hours of the onset of symptoms. It is very important to perform a longitudinal skin incision that spans the majority of the length of the involved compartment; inadequate skin release does not provide adequate decompression (14) and is a common reason for continued tissue ischemia and poor outcome.

6. If decompression does not produce the expected improvement, one should consider the possibilities of inadequate decompression, another compartmental syndrome, incorrect diagnosis, or secondary arterial occlusion. Careful **reexploration** and possibly **arteriography** are indicated.

7. Because **myoglobinuria** and **renal failure** can complicate compartmental syndromes, adequate hydration and urinary output, with alkalinization of the urine using IV sodium bicarbonate, should be ensured. Dark urine may usually be attributed to myoglobinuria if the benzidine test is positive and in the absence of hematuria.

If the compartment syndrome is recognized more than 24 hours after the onset of symptoms, fasciotomy should not be performed. The risk of deep infection is high and often results in limb loss. When the time of onset is known to be 24 hours or longer, observation with urine alkalinization should be the recommendation (15).

IV. **CHRONIC REGIONAL PAIN SYNDROME [CRPS, ALSO KNOWN AS SYMPATHETICALLY MAINTAINED PAIN SYNDROME; SUDECK ATROPHY; REFLEX SYMPATHETIC DYSTROPHY (RSD)].** Suspect early CRPS in any patient with persistent complaints of pain, especially when associated with hyperesthesia of the skin and/or abnormal pseudomotor response. For example, an excessively sweaty extremity that has severe pain with light touch (such as with bedding sheets or clothing) should be suspected as having CRPS. **For successful treatment, the diagnosis must be made before the classic signs** of thin shiny skin, excessive hair growth, attrition of nails, and diffuse osteoporosis occur. Whenever the diagnosis is suspected, institute treatment immediately. Treatment consists of regional sympathetic nerve blocks plus vigorous active physical therapy to mobilize any edema as well as to increase the muscle activity and the range of joint motion. The condition can occur in the upper extremity as well as in the lower extremity from the knee distally.

V. **VENOUS THROMBOEMBOLISM**
   A. Deep vein thrombosis (DVT) is extremely common in the trauma patients (16). The risk is greatest in patients with spine, pelvic, and hip trauma but is sufficiently high to warrant prophylactic treatment in all injured patients. The risk of DVT is further increased in patients with hereditary (often occult) thrombophilia, women who receive hormone replacement therapy, pregnant patients, and those who are obese, have cancer, or a previous history of DVT.

   The **diagnosis** of DVT should be entertained in any patient with lymphedema and or pain in an injured extremity. Pulmonary embolism (PE) is rarely the first manifestation of DVT. When the diagnosis of DVT is considered, screening the extremities with duplex Doppler venous ultrasound is usually done first. Contrast venography is not usually done except in the research setting because of its invasiveness and potential complications. Magnetic resonance venography is an

emerging technique that is especially promising for diagnosing DVT in the pelvis, whereas ultrasound has been shown to be less reliable.
   B. When DVT is identified, patients are usually **anticoagulated**. Although intravenous therapeutic heparin infusion followed by oral warfarin is the traditional regimen, new data supports the use of intermittent, therapeutic doses (1 mg/kg/day) of low-molecular weight heparin. Treatment is usually provided for 3 to 6 months. When anticoagulation is not possible, often because of associated injuries, a **vena cava filter** should be inserted.

   Prophylactic treatment to prevent DVT is initiated in every trauma patient upon admission. Mechanical devices such as sequential compression stockings or intermittent plantar compression pumps should be applied to both legs of injured persons when possible. Intermittent fixed-dose heparin (5,000 units heparin every 8 hours) or low-molecular weight heparin should be started when possible.

   Screening of patients with venous ultrasound should be done in patients who have had a delay in the initiation of prophylaxis for any reason. Screening can also be considered at discharge to assist with decisions about continuing prophylaxis following discharge.

VI. **MYOSITIS OSSIFICANS**
   A. Heterotopic bone formation often occurs after injury or surgery and can occur in any collagenous supportive tissue of skeletal muscles, tendons, ligaments, and fascia. There are **four clinical types**; three may be seen in injured patients:
      1. **Myositis ossificans progressiva** is rare and can be genetic. It usually occurs between the ages of 5 and 10 years (younger than age 20) and proceeds relentlessly to progressive ossification of skeletal muscles. It is often present in the shoulders and neck as firm subcutaneous masses, which can be hot and tender and can undergo ossification. Often associated are microdactyly of the great toes and thumbs, ankylosis of the interphalangeal and metatarsophalangeal joints, and bilateral hallux valgus. Minor trauma often causes exacerbations. Treatment may include diphosphonate combined with surgery for severe joint malpositioning and functional impairment.
      2. **Myositis ossificans paralytica** occurs in proximal paralyzed muscles. The ossification occurs 1 to 10 months after a spinal cord injury. This process causes decreased passive range of motion. The three classic sites are in the vastus medialis, the quadratus femoris, and the hip abductors. Surgical treatment is indicated only if the position and function of the extremity are unacceptable and when the ossification has matured. After excision, the dead space created must be drained by closed suction and the wound carefully observed for a hematoma.
      3. **Myositis ossificans circumscripta** can be idiopathic but is more commonly caused by focal trauma and is common as a sports injury in the contact setting. It is more common in teenage or young adult males. It presents as an uncomfortable, indistinct mass that shows local induration and a local increase of temperature. The lesion occurs 80% of the time in the arm (biceps brachialis) but also occurs in the thigh (abductors and quadratus femoris). Roentgenograms show fluffy calcification 2 to 4 weeks after injury. In 14 weeks, the calcification has matured, and in 5 months, ossification has occurred. The differential diagnosis includes osteosarcoma and periosteal osteogenic sarcoma. Treatment is by excision, only if the lesion is unusually large or painful and after ossification is mature.
      4. **Myositis ossificans traumatica**, the most common type of heterotopic ossification presents the same way as the circumscripta type except for a clear history of trauma, with ossification of a single muscle group in the traumatized area (17). Treatment is controversial but generally is aimed at the prevention of ossification by immediate application of cold and compression to the area of muscle injury. Later, heat is applied. An operation is indicated only when the ossification causes permanent impairment and only after the process has stabilized, often as soon as 6 to 8 months after injury.
   B. The **precise pathophysiology of myositis ossificans is not known. Preventive treatment** should be designed to stop the sequence of osteogenesis.

1. **Pharmacologic treatment** is generally prophylactic and has historically included bisphosphonates to inhibit hydroxyapatite crystallization, mithramycin to interfere with mobilization of calcium, and cortisone to decrease bone formation at the site of injury. None of these drugs, however, has proved to be an extremely beneficial therapeutic agent. Indomethacin and Naprosyn have been shown to help minimize posttraumatic heterotopic ossification associated with acetabular fractures and arthroplasty (18–20). Similarly, low-dose irradiation with 800 to 1,000 rad has been shown to be very effective at preventing heterotopic ossification (21).
2. When **surgical treatment** is indicated, traditional teaching has been to wait until the ossification is mature—that is, when the bone scan is negative and the alkaline phosphatase level is decreasing. Many authors have recently advocated earlier resection before these tests have returned to normal (22).

References

1. Giannoudis PV, Pape HC, Cohen AP, et al. Review: systemic effects of femoral nailing: from Kuntscher to the immune reactivity era. *Clin Orthop* 2002;404:378–386.
2. Ganong RB. Fat emboli syndrome in isolated fractures of the tibia and femur. *Clin Orthop* 1993;291:208–214.
3. Lindeque BGP, Schoeman HS, Dommisse OF, et al. Fat embolism and the fat embolism syndrome—a double blind therapeutic study. *J Bone Joint Surg (Br)* 1987;69:128–131.
4. Muller C, Rahn BA, Pfister U, et al. The incidence, pathogenesis, diagnosis and treatment of fat embolism. *Orthop Rev* 1994;23:107–117.
5. Wong MWN, Tsui HF, Yung SH, et al. Continuous pulse oximeter monitoring for inapparent hypoxemia after long bone fractures. *J Trauma* 2004;56:356–362.
6. Turen CH, Dube MA, Le Croy MC. Approach to the polytraumatized patient with musculoskeletal injuries. *J Am Acad Orthop Surg* 1999;7:154–165.
7. Fassler PR, Swiontkowski MF, Kilroy AW, et al. Injury of the sciatic nerve associated with acetabular fracture. *J Bone Joint Surg (Am)* 1993;75:1157–1166.
8. Matsen FA III. *Compartmental syndromes.* New York: Grune & Stratton, 1980:162.
9. Manoli A, Fakhouri AJ, Weber TG. Concurrent compartment syndromes of the foot and leg. *Foot & Ankle* 1993;14:339–342.
10. Whitesides TE, Heckman MM. Acute compartment syndrome: update on diagnosis and treatment. *J Am Acad Orthop Surg* 1996;4:209–218.
11. Mubarak SJ, Owen CA, Hargens AR, et al. Acute compartment syndromes: diagnosis and treatment with the aid of the Wick catheter. *J Bone Joint Surg (Am)* 1978;60:1091–1095.
12. McQueen MM, Court-Brown CM. Compartment monitoring in tibial fractures. The pressure threshold for decompression. *J Bone Joint Surg (Br)* 1996;78:99–104.
13. Heckman MM, Whitesides TE, Greve SR, et al. Compartment pressure in association with closed tibia fractures—the relationship between tissue pressure, compartment and the distance from the site of fracture. *J Bone Joint Surg (Am)* 1994;76:1285–1292.
14. Cohen MS, Garfin SR, Hargens AR, et al. Acute compartment syndrome. Effect of dermotomy on fascial decompression in the leg. *J Bone Joint Surg (Br)* 1991;73(2):287–290.
15. Finklestein JA, Hunter GA, Hu RW. Lower limb compartment syndrome: course after delayed fasciotomy. *J Trauma* 1996;40:342–344.
16. Abelseth G, Buckley RE, Pineo GE, et al. Incidence of deep-vein thrombosis in patients with fractures of the lower extremity distal to the hip. *J Orthop Trauma* 1996;10:230–235.
17. Hyder N, Shaw DL, Bouen SR. Myositis ossification: calcification of the entire tibialis anterior after ischaemic injury (compartment syndrome). *J Bone Joint Surg (Br)* 1995;78:318–319.

18. Matta JM, Siebenrock KA. Does indomethacin reduce heterotopic bone formation after operations for acetabular fractures? A prospective randomized study. *J Bone Joint Surg (Br)* 1997;79:959–963.
19. Moed BR, Karzes DE. Prophylactic indomethacin for the prevention of heterotopic ossification after acetabular fracture in high risk patients. *J Orthop Trauma* 1993;7:33–38.
20. Schmidt SA, Kjaersgaard-Andersen P, Pedersen NW, et al. The use of indomethacin to prevent the formation of heterotopic bone after total hip replacement: a randomized, double-blind clinical trial. *J Bone Joint Surg (Am)* 1988;70:834–838.
21. Bosse MJ, Poka A, Reinert CM, et al. Heterotopic ossification as a complication of acetabular fracture: prophylaxis with low-dose irradiation. *J Bone Joint Surg (Am)* 1988;70:1231–1237.
22. Viola RW, Hanel DP. Early "simple" release of posttraumatic elbow contracture associated with heterotopic ossification. *J Hand Surg (Am)* 1999;24:370–380.

Selected Historical Readings

Bivins BA, Boyd CR, Winter WG Jr, et.al. Fat embolism revisited. *South Med J* 1976;69:899–901.

Gelberman RH, Garfin SR, Hergenroeder PT, et.al. Compartment syndromes of the forearm: diagnosis and treatment. *Clin Orthop* 1981;161:252–261.

Gossling HR, Pellegrini VD. Fat embolism syndrome. *Clin Orthop* 1982;165:68–82.

Gurd AR, Wilson RI. The fat embolism syndrome. *J Bone Joint Surg (Br)* 1974;56:408–416.

Liljedahl SO, Westermark L. Etiology and treatment of fat embolism. *Acta Anaesthesiol Scand* 1967;11:177–194.

Matsen FA III, Winquist RA, Krugmire RB Jr. Diagnosis and management of compartmental syndromes. *J Bone Joint Surg (Am)* 1980;62:286–291.

Murray DG, Racz GB. Fat-embolism syndrome (respiratory insufficiency syndrome). A rationale for treatment. *J Bone Joint Surg (Am)* 1974;56:1338–1349.

Paterson DC. Myositis ossificans circumscripta. *J Bone Joint Surg (Br)* 1970;52:296–301.

Peltier LF. Fat embolism. An appraisal of the problem. *Clin Orthop* 1984;187:3–17.

Riska EB, von Bonsdorff H, Hakkinen S, et.al. Prevention of fat embolism by early internal fixation of fractures in patients with multiple injuries. *Injury* 1976;8:110–116.

Rorabeck CH, Bourne RB, Fowler PJ. The surgical treatment of exertional compartment syndrome in athletes. *J Bone Joint Surg (Am)* 1983;65:1245–1251.

Ten Duis HJ, Nijsten MW, Klasen JH, et.al. Fat embolism in patients with an isolated fracture of the femoral shaft. *J Trauma* 1988;28:383–390.

PREVENTION AND MANAGEMENT OF ACUTE MUSCULOSKELETAL INFECTIONS

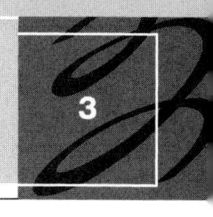

3

*P*revention of infection is the key to successful orthopaedic surgery. Meticulous attention to aseptic technique in the operating room, proper skin preparation and surgical scrub, the use of modern gown and mask techniques, planning the operation to shorten the time the tissues are exposed to air, laminar flow air, and prophylactic antibiotics (1–4) are all important in the prevention of infection. None, however, is as critical as meticulous debridement of wounds and the careful handling of tissues to prevent cell death (4). When infection does occur following an operation or from hematogenous origin, early diagnosis and prompt effective treatment can prevent disastrous complications.

I. PREVENTION
   A. Elective surgery. Refer to **Chap. 1, III,** and **Chap. 10, I,** for techniques described for the prevention of operative and posttraumatic infections.
   B. Early diagnosis
   1. Whenever a patient's postoperative or postinjury status does not follow the normal or expected course, the surgeon should be alert to the possibility of infection. A **respiratory problem** such as mild atelectasis may be a cause for persistent postoperative temperature elevation (this is especially common in patients who smoke), but such a potential diagnosis should not lull the surgeon into complacency. Wound infection may be the cause, or the two could be concurrent. Large hematomas can themselves be the cause of low-grade fever, but hematomas also represent the best culture media for bacteria and hence should be avoided or evacuated if present. Always obtain a culture of any evacuated hematoma.
   2. When there is concern regarding a wound infection, **inspect the wound and document the findings** at least daily, using sterile technique. Inspect the wound for swelling, erythema, and serous or bloody drainage. Culture any drainage. Tense skin, erythema, and abnormal tenderness or swelling frequently are signs of low-grade inflammation and infection.
   3. If the patient does not respond promptly to treatment or if the wound remains indurated, then **aspiration** should be carried out using aseptic technique with a large needle inserted into the wound area but away from the suture line.
   4. A low-grade fever in patients who have had antibiotics is not uncommon. In such instances, the temperature rarely exceeds 37.8°C (100°F) and may show a mild afternoon elevation. The patient frequently feels lethargic and has mild anorexia. If the **low-grade inflammatory process** involves a joint, the patient complains of pain to passive motion of the joint, which should alert the surgeon to the possibility of a septic joint.
   5. Be alert to the possibility of infection. **Establish the diagnosis through cultures** whenever possible, and treat the infection aggressively. If in doubt, the best course is generally to return the patient to the operating room and open the wound, irrigate and debride it to remove hematoma and necrotic wound tissue, and reclose the wound using the most "tissue friendly" suture technique (see **Chap. 10**). Consultation with another experienced surgeon can be helpful.
   C. Treatment. Once the diagnosis of a musculoskeletal infection has been established, treatment proceeds as for acute osteomyelitis or septic arthritis. The principles of

treatment include removal of all dead tissue and any hematoma along with appropriate antibiotic therapy. The wound is nearly always left open for secondary closure except when the infection involves a joint. If the wound is closed, a suction drain is mandatory.

II. BONE AND JOINT INFECTIONS

A. Bones and joints represent special problems for the host defense mechanisms. Normal bone has an excellent blood supply, although there is slowing of the circulation in the metaphyseal region in children. **Once pus forms under pressure, the vascular supply to bone is lost** because of its rigid structure, resulting in areas of infected, devitalized bone. Septic emboli in bone or vascular thrombosis can cause additional devascularization. Ligaments and tendons are relatively avascular structures and do not handle infection well. Joints, with their avascular cartilage and menisci, pose a particular problem. Local phagocytic function can be deficient, and it is often difficult to ensure adequate delivery of humeral factors (antibodies, opsonins, complement). In addition to the direct destructive effect of cell breakdown on cartilage, the pus under pressure interferes with cartilage nutrition and blood supply to the periarticular structures. At particular risk is the epiphyseal blood supply, and avascular neurosis may be the result. Antibiotics can inhibit or cure an infection only when they can reach the infecting organism in bacteriostatic or bactericidal concentrations. Infections producing pressure in a bone or joint as well as in relatively avascular tissues can impede or prevent antibiotics from reaching the primary site of infection.

B. An **acute infection of bone (hematogenous osteomyelitis)**, in its earliest phase, is a medical disease and can often be cured by prompt, appropriate antibiotic therapy. However, the time between initial infection and bone infarct is often short. If effective treatment is delayed and devascularization of the involved tissues results, then surgical treatment is a necessary adjunct to the antibiotic therapy. Even under the best of circumstances, late treatment (perhaps as early as 48 hours after the infection starts) may result in the loss of or abnormal function of the joint. Thus, appropriate antibiotic therapy must be initiated as early as possible. Appropriate therapy requires knowledge of the etiologic agent and its sensitivities. Every effort should be made to obtain a bacterial culture and determine sensitivity. Once the culture specimen is obtained, it is important to institute antibiotic therapy based on a probable diagnosis using the most effective broad-spectrum antibiotics.

C. **Diagnosis**

1. The earliest symptom or sign that may help differentiate a bone or joint infection is usually **pain or localized tenderness in the periarticular region**. In the infant, refusal to move or use an extremity may be noted first. The cardinal signs of infection—redness, heat, and swelling—may appear later than the pain and tenderness, or not at all. When examining a child with a fever of unknown origin, note any pain or alteration of the normal range of motions of a joint and carefully palpate all metaphyseal areas to determine local tenderness. Roentgenograms are of little value in making the early diagnosis, although careful comparison with the opposite side may show abnormal soft-tissue shadows. Roentgenographic evidence of bone or joint destruction is seen during the chronic phase of the disease. Osteomyelitis should always be included in the differential diagnosis for a patient with the radiographic appearance of a bone tumor (5). Radioisotopic bone scanning, especially indium imaging, is helpful in early localization of bone infection (6). Many authorities have advocated the use of magnetic resonance imaging in the diagnosis of osteomyelitis (7–10), but clinical context is of paramount importance in the evaluation of any abnormal findings. Erythrocyte sedimentation rate (ESR) and C-reactive protein (CRP) serum levels are useful in laboratory evaluations (11–14).

2. **Identification of the infecting organism** is essential. In the early stages of the disease, particularly if there is a spiking temperature, blood cultures can often yield the organism. If acute metaphyseal tenderness is present, then the organism can frequently be obtained by inserting a needle into the site of maximum tenderness. A serrated biopsy needle is useful if subperiosteal pus is not

encountered. If a joint is involved, then the effusion should be aspirated before joint lavage. Processing the aspirates should include the following:
   a. **Immediate Gram stain.**
   b. Inoculation of culture broth for aerobic and anaerobic **cultures**.
   c. **White blood cell count.** If thick, purulent material is encountered, then dilution in broth occasionally enhances the growth of organisms by decreasing the concentration of leukocytes and humeral antibacterial factors. This is done routinely in the microbiology laboratory with fluid aspirates.
   d. Determination of the character of the hyaluronic precipitate, the presence of fibrin clots, and any disparity between the glucose in the aspirate and blood **glucose** may prove helpful, but the Gram stain, culture, and cell count are most valuable (see **Chap. 3**).
D. **Differential diagnosis. Care must be taken to differentiate soft-tissue infection, or cellulitis, from an infection occurring in a bone or joint.** This is a particularly important precaution when the infection overlies a joint because any aspiration of a reactive sterile effusion by passing a needle through the soft-tissue infection may create a pyarthrosis. Tenderness and swelling from unrecognized trauma over a bone, particularly with some periosteal reaction, can present a confusing picture, but the absence of fever and systemic signs is helpful. Nonbacterial inflammatory arthritis, including viral and toxic synovitis and rheumatoid arthritis, must be included in a differential diagnosis, but until proved otherwise, think first of septic arthritis. Spontaneous hemorrhages in patients with hemophilia and fractures in paraplegic patients, particularly patients with meningomyelocele, are special situations that can confuse the picture.
E. **Bacterial considerations** (1,4,12)
   1. In **acute hematogenous osteomyelitis**, *Staphylococcus aureus* is the most common etiologic agent in all age groups. In recent years, an increasing number of isolated strains have been found to be methicillin resistant. In infants younger than 1 month, a diversity of other bacteria must also be considered. Group B streptococci and gram-negative organisms such as *Escherichia coli, Proteus* species, *Pseudomonas aeruginosa, Klebsiella pneumoniae,* and *Salmonella* species are all suspect. In infants with a complicated medical history, particularly those who have had prolonged indwelling venous catheters, extensive surgery, or intensive prior antibiotic therapy, coagulase-negative staphylococci and rarely anaerobic organisms such as *Bacteroides fragilis* and fungal agents such as *Candida albicans* (hard to diagnose) must also be considered.
   2. In **septic arthritis and osteomyelitis** among infants younger than 1 month, *S. aureus* is the predominant etiologic agent. After the neonatal period and up to 4 years of age, *Haemophilus influenzae* is also a major cause of septic arthritis. In later childhood, the etiologic agents are the same as for adults, with *S. aureus* predominating. *Neisseria gonorrhoeae* must be seriously considered, particularly among adolescents with single (especially the knee joint) or multiple joint findings. If there has been a preceding infection or if there is a concurrent infection in another organ system, one may suspect that the etiologic agent is the same as that from the initiating focus. But, because this is not always the case, direct culture from the bone or joint infection is advised.
F. **Special considerations**
   1. Infections of the intervertebral discs, or **acute discitis**, may be encountered in children **without antecedent infection or surgery** (15). When organisms have been recovered, they have usually been staphylococcal. Infants may merely refuse to stand or walk, whereas older youngsters complain of pain in the back or lower extremity. The infection usually is low grade, particularly among children younger than 5 years of age. Roentgenograms reveal that the involved disc narrows rapidly over the first 2 to 3 weeks. A bone scan shows increased activity in the adjacent vertebrae. Although the process often appears self-limited, the symptoms and course of the disease can be improved by plaster immobilization and antistaphylococcal antibiotics. The difficulty in

obtaining a bacterial diagnosis, even with needle biopsy, combined with the benign course of this condition, has led many clinicians to ignore efforts at establishing a bacterial diagnosis. The condition must, however, be differentiated from vertebral osteomyelitis with secondary disc destruction; in the latter condition, it is essential to obtain the bacterial diagnosis as an integral part of treatment of what can be a severe disease. The same precaution applies to disc infections following laminectomy. In these cases, an infection should be suspected when a postsurgical patient complains of increasing back pain starting 1 to 2 weeks postoperatively.
 2. Patients with **hemolytic disorders**, particularly those with sickle cell disease, are prone to the development of a subacute form of osteomyelitis. *Salmonella* infections are frequent, but other types of bacterial osteomyelitis are not uncommon (4). Because the diagnosis is usually made late, treatment is difficult and may require extensive surgical debridement and prolonged antibiotic therapy.
 3. Another special problem is presented by the patient who sustains a **puncture wound** in the sole of the foot. Despite initial cleansing and occasional debridement, cellulitis, arthritis, or osteomyelitis involving the foot develops in many patients (11). This occurrence is most commonly caused by *P. aeruginosa*. Early surgical debridement of the infected, including the plantar fascia, combined with preoperative and postoperative anti-*P. aeruginosa* antibiotics, has been the most effective method of management. For a serious infection, treatment is 5 days of antibiotic therapy with an aminoglycoside (e.g., tobramycin) or an antipseudomonal beta-lactam (e.g., ceftazidime) administered parenterally. Recently, ciprofloxacin has been used in gram-negative bone and joint infections (1); it must not be used in prepubertal children, however. Appropriate sensitivities guide antibiotic selection. Duration of therapy is empirical and may be guided by the clinical appearance and the CRP or ESR (11,15). Aminoglycoside doses need to be adjusted according to peak and trough serum levels and monitoring must include weekly Serum Creatinine (Cr) measurements and regular audiologist evaluation. Patients with human immunodeficiency virus or acquired immunodeficiency syndrome can have septic joints, which frequently may be missed because of the relatively weak immune response to the infectious agent. Joint aspiration should be performed in this setting (16).
 4. **Lyme arthritis.** Lyme arthritis, the most common vectorborne infection in the United States, is caused by the spirochete *Borrelia burgdorferi*, which is transmitted to humans primarily via the *Ixodes scapularis* tick from its natural hosts, deer and white-footed mice (17). Arthritis, the most common form of late Lyme disease (other forms being encephalopathy and polyneuropathy), can occur weeks to months after the original infection. Approximately 60% of untreated primary disease will develop arthritis (18). Clinical presentation includes fever and joint effusion, which may be confused with acute septic arthritis, especially in children (19). Treatment with oral antibiotics such as doxycycline for 4 weeks or the parenteral agent ceftriaxone for 2 weeks usually results in lasting cure. However a small percentage of patients experience ongoing symptoms despite antibiotic therapy. Possible reasons include persistent infection, residual joint damage, or a chronic autoimmune synovitis (20).

G. **Requirements and characteristics of appropriate antibiotic treatment** (1,4,21)
 1. For initial treatment of bone or joint infection, choose a **bactericidal antibiotic** effective against the suspected organism and a route of administration that ensures delivery of therapeutic levels to the infected site. The intravenous (IV) route is generally preferred for initial treatment [although some agents such as gentamicin and tobramycin are effective given intramuscularly (IM)]. Recent studies (1) have indicated that oral antibiotics appear in therapeutic concentrations in bones and joints and, if given properly, can substitute for parenteral therapy in children. Most authorities, however, prefer the IV route.
 2. The **duration of parenteral treatment** is 3 to 4 weeks for septic arthritis and 4 to 6 weeks for osteomyelitis (the longer duration for infections caused by *S. aureus*). **In adults** with selected organisms, the treatment may be completed using

oral quinolones after the initial pain, swelling, and fever have resolved with IV antibiotics. Quinolone antibiotics (ciprofloxacin, gatifloxacin, levofloxacin, moxifloxacin) have allowed oral therapy against a broad spectrum of bacteria including *Pseudomonas* (1). **In treating children** with osteomyelitis, treatment may be initiated with an IV agent such as nafcillin (Nafcil or Unipen), and the 4- to 6-week treatment course may be completed with oral dicloxacillin (Dynapen) or trimethoprim (Bactrim or Septra). **For all ages** the dosage of antibiotics (oral or parenteral) is at the upper therapeutic level. When appropriate, adequate bactericidal drug levels for both oral as well as parenteral agents should be documented. Providing parenteral antibiotics through home health care teams greatly reduces the cost of treatment. The differentiation between a mild, well-localized infection and a localized bone tumor can sometimes require a surgical biopsy (5). The CRP or ESR is also a helpful guideline to determine the duration of treatment (11). A summary of antimicrobial agents commonly used in acute bone and joint infections is presented in **Table 3-1**. These agents are known to enter bone and joint sites readily when given in adequate doses.

3. In an acute infection in which the organism is not immediately identified, the **choice of therapy** is determined by the organisms most commonly expected in the various age groups, along with the other factors previously listed. General guidelines are presented in **Table 3-2**.

4. **A local instillation or continuous irrigation with an antibiotic solution is almost never indicated.** Systemic antibiotics, properly administered, achieve adequate levels in viable tissues (1,4). In many posttraumatic conditions, delivery of local antibiotics in methyl methacrylate beads is worthwhile (21). This treatment is indicated especially when a delayed bone graft or soft-tissue muscle flap is planned. Some favorable reports have been published about an implantable pump with a reservoir for antibiotic (generally amikacin).

5. Continue antibiotics until the infection has been eliminated. A normal or declining ESR or CRP is one of the most helpful **laboratory tests** to indicate control of infection.

H. **Adjunctive treatment.** Most orthopaedists believe that the healing process is aided by **immobilizing** the infected area. There is disagreement over casting or splinting. Undoubtedly, however, patients are more comfortable when the infected area is immobilized. If damage to the bone is significant, cast immobilization may be important to prevent a pathologic fracture. If damage to articular cartilage is suspected, motion of the involved joint is recommended after a brief 1- to 2-day period of immobilization.

I. **Surgical intervention.** Appropriate antibiotic treatment instituted within the first 48 hours of acute osteomyelitis or septic arthritis is usually satisfactory. However, early diagnosis is rarely the case. **If treatment is initiated over 48 hours after onset, it is important to determine whether medical treatment alone is adequate.** Err on the side of more aggressive operative drainage. If the patient has been on an appropriate antibiotic for more than 24 hours without significant resolution of pain and temperature, then surgical intervention is indicated.

1. In a **bone infection**, metaphyseal or subperiosteal abscesses must be drained. If metaphyseal point tenderness is present, and there is doubt whether this represents significant metaphyseal or subperiosteal pus, then it is safer to err on the side of a small surgical exploration or aspiration with a biopsy needle. If pus is encountered, then open surgical drainage is indicated.

2. **Joints**
   a. In joint infections, satisfactory evacuation of pus can be achieved by **needle aspiration**. When the joint is easily visible and palpable, such as with the knee joint, repeated needle aspiration is usually adequate to keep the joint decompressed. Aspiration should be done with a 16- to 18-gauge needle. Irrigation of the joint to ensure removal of as much cellular debris as possible is helpful (12). The hip joint presents special problems (12). The blood supply to the femoral head is intraarticular; hence, any increase in pressure can deprive the entire femoral head of its circulation. Because hip

TABLE 3-1   Antimicrobial Agents Commonly Used Initially in Acute Bone and Joint Infections

Antibiotic	Usual susceptible organisms	Daily dosage (IV route)	Comment
Cefazolin (cephalosporins)	Penicillinase-producing *Staphylococcus aureus*; will also treat streptococci, pneumococci, non-penicillinase-producing staphylococci, and *Klebsiella pneumoniae*	0–7 d: 40 mg/kg divided doses q12h Infant: 60 mg/kg divided doses q8h Child: 80 mg/kg divided doses q6h Adult: 3–6 g divided doses of 8h	A drug of choice; IV route preferred, but may be given IM. Adjust adult dosage according to blood urea nitrogen or, preferably, the creatinine clearance
Nafcillin[a]	Same as cefazolin	0–7 d: 50 mg/kg divided doses q12h[a] 7 d–6 wk: 75 mg/kg divided doses q8h 6 wk–3 y: 80 mg/kg divided doses q6h Child: 150 mg/kg divided doses q6h Adult: 2–12 g divided doses of 4–6 h	A drug of choice
Methicillin	Same as cefazolin and nafcillin	No longer commonly used; too many problems	Monitor patients for proteinuria: drug has occasionally been implicated in adverse renal side effects
Clindamycin	*S. aureus*, pneumococci, streptococci (not enterococci), and many *Bacteroides fragilis* strains	Pediatric: 10–20 mg/kg PO or IV or IM in 3–4 doses Adult: 600–900 mg of 6–8 h	Considered an excellent agent for *B. fragilis* infections
Penicillin G (aqueous)	Streptococci (not enterococci), pneumococci, gonococci, and penicillin-susceptible staphylococci	0–7 d: 50,000 unit/kg divided dose q12h greater than 7 d: 75,000–100,000 unit/kg IV or IM divided doses q8h 12 y–adult: 12–24 million units of 4–6 h	Useful for open fractures contaminated with barnyard waste and for treatment of clostridia infection
Ampicillin	Same as penicillin G; also *Haemophilus influenzae*, some strains of *Escherichia coli*, *Proteus*, and *Salmonella*	0–7 d: 50 mg/kg divided doses q12h 7 d–6 wk: 75 mg/kg divided doses q8h Infant: 100 mg/kg divided doses q6h	*H. influenzae* now shows a 10%–20% ampicillin resistance in some areas. Empirin therapy must therefore be with ceftriaxone or cefuroxime

TABLE 3-1 (Continued)

Drug	Indication	Dose	Notes
Ceftriaxone	Select gram-negative organisms or mixed infections	Child: 150 mg/kg divided doses q6h; 12 yr–adult: 8–12 g; 0–12 yr: 50 mg/kg once daily; 12 yr–adult: 2 g q24h	Generally reserved for resistant or mixed infections
Cefuroxime	Select gram-negative organisms or mixed infections	greater than 3 mo–12 yr: 75 mg/kg divided doses q8h; 12 yr–adult: 1.5 g q8h	Generally reserved for resistant or mixed infections
Ceftazidime	Select gram-negative organisms including *Pseudomonas* or mixed infections	less than 12 yr not indicated; 12 yr–adult: 1 g q8–12h	Same as cefuroxime
Gentamicin	Gram-negative infections	less than 12 yr: 6–7.5 mg/kg in three equal doses	Agent of choice for suspected gram-negative infections
Tobramycin		12 yr–adult: 3–5 mg/kg in three equal doses (dose adjusted based on peak and trough levels) can be given as a single daily dose	May be given either IV or IM. Renal function must be carefully checked, and therapy beyond 10 days must be administered cautiously because of potential nephrotoxicity and ototoxicity. May be synergistic with carbenicillin against some strains of *Pseudomonas aeruginosa*; also usually synergistic with penicillin against enterococci. Reduce dosage to 3 mg/kg/d as soon as clinically indicated. Follow with peak and trough serum levels if available

[a]Some authorities recommend that nafcillin not be used in 0- to 7-day-old infants because of poor pharmacokinetics.

From Hansen ST Jr, Ray CG. Antibiotics in orthopaedics. In: Kagan BM, ed. *Antimicrobial therapy*, 3rd ed. Philadelphia, PA: WB Saunders, 1980, with permission.

TABLE 3-2 Tentative Selection of Therapy When Organisms Are Not Immediately Identified

Situation	Organisms suspected	Suggested antibiotic choice
Newborn (1 mo) Osteomyelitis	Staphylococcus aureus Streptococci Gram-negative bacteria including Escherichia coli, Klebsiella pneumoniae, Proteus group, Pseudomonas aeruginosa	Nafcillin plus gentamicin or tobramycin
Septic arthritis	S. aureus	
1 mo–4 yr Osteomyelitis	S. aureus	Second-generation cephalosporin to cover H. influenzae
Septic arthritis	Haemophilus influenzae S. aureus Streptococci	Second-generation cephalosporin to cover H. influenzae
4 yr–12 yr Osteomyelitis Septic arthritis	S. aureus	First- or second-generation cephalosporin
12 yr–adult Osteomyelitis	S. aureus	A cephalosporin (first- or second-generation agent) or nafcillin
Septic arthritis	S. aureus	A cephalosporin or nafcillin (ceftriaxone if gonococcus is strongly suspected)
Special considerations Chronic hemolytic disorders Osteoarthritis Septic arthritis	S. aureus Pneumococci Salmonella group[a]	A cephalosporin (second-generation if salmonella is suspected) or nafcillin until sensitivity results are available
Infections following puncture wounds of the foot	Pseudomonas aeruginosa	Ceftazidime actually achieves better drug levels than aminoglycosides (gentamicin or tobramycin)
Infections following trauma or surgery	S. aureus Streptococci Gram-negative organisms	A first- or second-generation cephalosporin (or nafcillin) plus gentamicin or tobramycin

[a]Infections caused by Salmonella should be documented first by culture and sensitivity testing before empirical treatment with agents such as ampicillin (or chloramphenicol) is initiated.

From Hansen ST Jr, Ray CG. Antibiotics in orthopaedics. In: Kagan BM, ed. *Antimicrobial therapy*, 3rd ed. Philadelphia, PA: WB Saunders, 1980, with permission.

joint effusions are not readily palpable, it is difficult to be certain that repeated aspirations decompress the joint. For this reason, most authorities believe that immediate surgical drainage of a septic hip is indicated, and some believe that the shoulder should be treated similarly. The possible exception is in gonococcal arthritis (22). The hip joint can be drained anteriorly between muscle planes or posteriorly with a muscle-splitting incision. The capsule and synovium are opened and drains are inserted.
- b. At times, the fibrin entering the joint as a transudate forms clots and isolates segments of the joint from decompression. Hypertrophy of synovium and adhesions may also affect the ability of the surgeon to decompress the joint adequately. Under these circumstances, **it is advisable to debride the joint arthroscopically or with an open procedure.** Joints amenable to arthroscopic lavage are the knee, shoulder, and ankle.
- J. **Chronic osteomyelitis** presents a different problem from acute infection. Acute infection in the earliest phase is primarily a medical disease, with surgical techniques used as an adjunct. In chronic infection, the primary problem is **surgical removal** of all dead and poorly vascularized tissue. If this removal is properly done under appropriate antibiotic therapy, it is possible to eradicate most sites of chronic osteomyelitis. The operation must be carefully planned because it often involves significant removal of bone and surrounding tissues. In the case of chronic joint infections, it may mean complete resection of the joint with the creation of a pseudarthrosis or an arthrodesis. Rotational muscle flaps or free-tissue transfer may be required to cover areas of viable but poorly covered bone. Intravenous and oral antibiotics serve as valuable adjuncts. Patient quality of life can be profoundly impacted by chronic osteomyelitis (23); treatment leading to resolution of the infection does improve this impact.
- K. **Gas gangrene**
  1. Gas gangrene can be a fatal process. **Prevention** can be achieved by thorough debridement and removal of all devitalized tissue, delayed wound closure when in doubt, and antibiotic treatment as recommended previously.
  2. *Clostridium perfringens* infections carry a 65% overall mortality rate, which increases to 75% in infants and elderly patients. The **diagnosis** should be suspected when the patient is pale, weak, perspiring, and more tachycardiac than the degree of fever warrants. The patient frequently complains of severe pain. Mental confusion and gas in the tissues are late signs, as are the characteristic mousy odor, jaundice, oliguria, and shock.
  3. Other gas-producing species in addition to *C. perfringens* (ten isolated toxins), include *E. coli, Enterobacter aerogenes,* anaerobic streptococci, *B. fragilis,* and *K. pneumoniae.* Antitoxin does not appear to help much because it is neutralized as rapidly as it reaches muscle. **Treatment** consists of debridement and high doses of antibiotics. Penicillin is usually the best for the *C. perfringens* group; it should be given in amounts of 20 to 50 million units/day. Clindamycin or metronidazole are good alternative antibiotics in patients who are allergic to penicillin. Some clostridia are resistant to clindamycin, making it necessary to check sensitivities carefully. Hyperbaric oxygen is only an adjunct to surgery. Its use allows the surgeon to save more tissue than might otherwise be possible, and it does lower the mortality rate slightly.

     Although exceedingly uncommon, group A streptococcal myonecrosis can have a similar course and results in death in a high percentage of cases. It must be treated with aggressive surgical debridement or amputation in addition to appropriate antibiotic therapy. Toxic shock syndrome has also been noted in orthopaedic patients and is caused by unique staphylococcal strains with unusual phage types. Toxic shock syndrome is also a surgical condition, but it carries a more favorable prognosis. Necrotizing fasciitis can be caused by several bacterial types (most commonly group A streptococcus) and often requires debridement combined with appropriate antibiotic therapy. Infectious disease consultation is indicated for each of these infectious conditions.

III. SUMMARY

A. Infections in the musculoskeletal system present special problems for treatment with antibiotics alone. Cartilage is avascular, tendon and ligaments are relatively hypovascular, and bone is vulnerable to situations that render it avascular. Because antibiotics can be effective only if they are delivered to the site of infection, every effort must be made to preserve a normal blood supply and normal joint fluid dynamics. The **essentials of treatment** are as follows:
  1. **Prompt diagnosis**, with identification of the bacteria through culture and with sensitivity for determining the appropriate antibiotic
  2. **Rapid initial treatment** with the most effective bactericidal antibiotic
  3. **Constant evaluation** to assess the need for surgical drainage of pus or removal of devitalized tissue
  4. **Antibiotic therapy** by a route that ensures adequate blood levels and administration until the signs of infection, as manifested usually by a decreasing ESR, resolve completely
  5. **Judicious use of immobilization and traction** to improve patient comfort and provide the best possible environment for primary healing

B. The greatest benefit of antibiotics in musculoskeletal infection is in **preventing** the mortality and morbidity that result from chronic osteomyelitis and joint destruction from pyarthrosis. Even chronic infection can be controlled and a satisfactory functional result obtained in most patients by the use of surgery and appropriate antibiotics.

References

1. Greenberg RN, Kennedy DJ, Reilly PM, et al. Treatment of bone, joint, and soft-tissue infections with oral ciprofloxacin. *Antimicrob Agents Chemother* 1987;31:151–155.
2. Hendershot EF. Fluoroquinolones. *Infect Dis Clin North Am* 1995;9:715–730.
3. Henry SL, Galloway KP. Local antibacterial therapy for the management of orthopaedic infections: pharmacokinetic considerations. *Clin Pharmacokinet* 1995;29:36–45.
4. Mader JT, Landon GC, Calhoun J. Antimicrobial treatment of osteomyelitis. *Clin Orthop* 1993;295:87–95.
5. Cottias P, Tomeno B, Anract P, et al. Subacute osteomyelitis presenting as a bone tumor: a review of 21 cases. *Int Orthop* 1997;21:243–248.
6. Schauwecker DS. The scintigraphic diagnosis of osteomyelitis. *AJR Am J Roentgenol* 1992;158:9–18.
7. Boutin RD, Brossman J, Sartoris DJ, et al. Update on imaging of orthopedic infections. *Orthop Clin North Am* 1998;29:41–66.
8. Tang JS, Gold RH, Bassett LW, et al. Musculoskeletal infection of the extremities: evaluation with MR imaging. *Radiology* 1988;166:205–209.
9. Tehranzadeh J, Wang F, Mesgarazadeh M. Magnetic resonance imaging of osteomyelitis. *Crit Rev Diagn Imaging* 1992;33:495–534.
10. Unger E, Moldofsky P, Gatenby R, et al. Diagnosis of osteomyelitis by MR imaging. *AJR Am J Roentgenol* 1988;150:605–610.
11. Crosby LA, Powell DA. The potential value of the sedimentation rate in monitoring treatment outcome in puncture wound-related *Pseudomonas* osteomyelitis. *Clin Orthop* 1984;188:168–172.
12. Dagan R. Management of acute hematogenous osteomyelitis and septic arthritis in the pediatric patient. *Pediatr Infect Dis J* 1993;12:88–92.
13. Frederiksen B, Chritiansen P, Knudsen FU. Acute osteomyelitis and septic arthritis in the neonate, risk factors and outcome. *Eur J Pediatr* 1993;152:577–580.
14. Unkila-Kallio L, Kallio MJ, Eskola J, et al. Serum C-reactive protein, erythrocyte sedimentation rate and white blood cell count in acute hematogenous osteomyelitis of children. *Pediatrics* 1994;93:59–62.
15. Cushing AH. Diskitis in children. *Clin Infect Dis* 1995;17:1–6.
16. Malin JK, Patel NJ. Arthropathy and HIV infection: a muddle of mimicry. *Postgrad Med* 1993;93:143–150.

17. Spiro ED, Gerber MA. Lyme disease. *Clin Infect Dis* 2000;31:533–542.
18. Steere AC. Lyme disease. *N Engl J Med* 2001;345:115–125.
19. Willis AA, Widmann RF, Flynn JM, et al. Lyme arthritis presenting as acute septic arthritis in children. *J Pediatr Orthop* 2003;23:11418.
20. Weinstein A, Britchkov M. Lyme arthritis and post-Lyme disease syndrome. *Curr Opin Rheumatol* 2002;14:383–387.
21. Ostermann PA, Seligson D, Henry SL. Local antibiotic therapy for severe open fractures: a review of 1085 consecutive cases. *J Bone Joint Surg (Br)* 1995;77:93–97.
22. Scopelitis E, Martinez-Osuna P. Gonococcal arthritis. *Rheum Dis Clin North Am* 1993;19:363–377.
23. Lerner RK, Esterhai JL Jr, Polomano RC, et al. Quality of life assessment of patients with posttraumatic fracture nonunion, chronic refractory osteomyelitis and lower extremity amputation. *Clin Orthop* 1993;295:28–36.

Selected Historical Readings

Burnett JW, Gustilo RB, Williams DN, et al. Prophylactic antibiotics in hip fractures. *J Bone Joint Surg (Am)* 1980;62:457–462.

Clawson DK, Davis FJ, Hansen ST Jr. Treatment of chronic osteomyelitis with emphasis on closed suction-irrigation technique. *Clin Orthop* 1973;96:88–97.

Ha'eri GB, Wiley AM. The efficacy of standard surgical face masks: an investigation using "tracer particles." *Clin Orthop* 1980;148:160–162.

Hamilton HW, Booth AD, Lone FJ, et al. Penetration of gown material by organisms from the surgical team. *Clin Orthop* 1979;141:237–246.

Lunseth PA, Heiple KG. Prognosis in septic arthritis of the hip in children. *Clin Orthop* 1979;129:81–85.

Monson TP, Nelson CL. Microbiology for orthopaedic surgeons: selected aspects. *Clin Orthop* 1984;190:14–22.

Patzakis MJ, Harvey P Jr, Ivler D. The role of antibiotics in the management of open fractures. *J Bone Joint Surg (Am)* 1974;56:532–541.

Perry CR, Ritterbusch JK, Rice SH, et al. Antibiotics delivered by an implantable drug pump: a new application for treating osteomyelitis. *Am J Med* 1986;80(6B):222–227.

Peterson AF, Rosenberg A, Alatary SD. Comparative evaluations of surgical scrub preparations. *Surg Gynecol Obstet* 1978;146:63–65.

Schurman DJ, Hirshman HP, Nagel DA. Antibiotic penetration of synovial fluid in infected and normal knee joints. *Clin Orthop* 1978;136:304–310.

ACUTE NONTRAUMATIC JOINT CONDITIONS 4

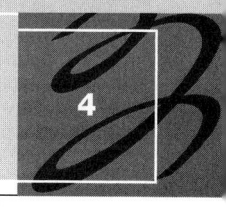

I. **HISTORY.** Document the onset of the symptoms: Did the joint pain begin days, weeks, or months ago? Morning stiffness is important to differentiate inflammatory forms of arthritis (rheumatoid arthritis and ankylosing spondylitis) from noninflammatory forms (degenerative joint disease). The character and duration of the pain are more important. Is the pain only associated with activity or is it present even at rest? Is only one joint involved or are multiple joints affected? Are they symmetrically involved? In the hands, the proximal finger joints are often involved with rheumatoid arthritis and the distal finger joints are more often involved in osteoarthritis (1) (**Table 4-1**). A thorough history of past medical problems and social issues and a current review of systems is essential. One must consider possible exposure to infectious diseases and current systemic symptoms of illness when differentiating the possibilities.

II. **EXAMINATION.** Check for fever because the temperature may be elevated with septic arthritis. Muscle wasting occurs more often with rheumatoid arthritis. Tenderness about the joint and increased warmth are more indicative of inflammatory conditions. The examination should determine the presence of an effusion (fluid in the joint). Severe guarding against joint motion associated with pain usually is indicative of a septic condition (**Table 4-1**).

III. **ROENTGENOGRAPHIC AND LABORATORY DATA**
   A. **Roentgenographic findings.** Look for evidence of periarticular soft-tissue swelling, joint effusion, osteopenia, joint space narrowing, periarticular erosions, joint subluxation, and articular cartilage or bone destruction (1). All of these

TABLE 4-1 History and Examination

History	Rheumatoid arthritis	Septic arthritis	Degenerative joint disease
Onset	Weeks	Day(s)	Months
Morning stiffness	++		−
Pain duration	Hours	Constant	Minutes
Pain with activity	++	+++	±
Number of joints involved	Multiple, symmetric	One (occasionally more)	Variable
Finger joint	Proximal		Distal
Examination			
Febrile	±	++	0
Muscle wasting	++	0	+
Synovial tenderness	+	++	±
Increased warmth	±	++	0
Effusion	+	++	±
Joint range of motion	↓	↓↓↓	↓

+++, extremely important symptom or sign; ++, very important symptom or sign; +, important symptom or sign; ±, symptom or sign might or might not be present; 0, symptom or sign is not present; ↓, decreased; ↓↓↓, markedly decreased.

TABLE 4-2 Roentgenographic Findings

Rheumatoid arthritis	Septic arthritis	Degenerative joint disease
Early		
Periarticular soft-tissue swelling	Joint effusion	Joint space narrowing
Periarticular osteoporosis		Marginal osteophytes
Late		
Joint space narrowing	Articular cartilage and bone destruction	Subchondral sclerosis
Periarticular erosions		Subcortical cysts
Articular cartilage and bone destruction		Marginal osteophytes
Joint subluxation secondary to ligamentous involvement		

findings are evidence of inflammatory (rheumatoid or septic) arthritis. In contrast, marginal osteophytes, subchondral cysts, joint space narrowing, and sclerosis are associated with osteoarthritis (**Table 4-2**). In the lower extremity, weight-bearing radiographs increase the diagnostic value of the study.

B. Laboratory data (Table 4-3)
  1. **Synovial fluid analysis involves assessing the following:**
     a. **Appearance (color)**
     b. **Clot (presence or absence)**
     c. **Viscosity**
     d. **Glucose** (compare with simultaneous serum glucose)
     e. **Cell count per cubic millimeter**
     f. **Differential cell count**
     g. The type of **crystals** that might be present in the joint fluid aspirate as evaluated under a polarizing light microscope
     h. **Gram stain and synovial fluid culture:** aerobic, fungal, acid fast baccilus (AFB)

TABLE 4-3 Synovial Fluid Analysis

Finding	Normal	Rheumatoid arthritis	Septic arthritis	Degenerative joint disease
Appearance	Clear	Cloudy	Turbid	Clear
Clinical viscosity test	High (fluid remains intact when slowly pulled between thumb and index finger)	Watery (fluid breaks into droplets easily)	Very watery	High
Glucose	Within 60% or more of serum glucose	Low	Very low	Normal
Cell count/mm^3	200	2,000–50,000	Usually greater than 50,000	2,000
Differential cell count	Monos	50/50	Polys	Monos

TABLE 4-4 Differential Diagnosis of Inflammatory Polyarthritis

A. **Rheumatoid arthritis (RA)**
   1. Seropositive—female, symmetric joint and tendon involvement, synovial thickening, joint inflammation in phase, nodules, weakness, systemic reaction, erosions on radiogram, rheumatoid factor present, $C'H_{50}$ level depressed in joint fluid that has 5,000–30,000 WBCs/mm^3, approximately 50%–80% polymorphs.
   2. Seronegative—either sex, symmetric joint and tendon involvement, joint inflammation in phase, little or no systemic reaction, usually no erosions radiographically, rheumatoid factor absent, $C'H_{50}$ not depressed in joint fluid that has 3,000–20,000 WBCs/mm^3, approximately 20%–60% polymorphs.
B. **Collagen-vascular**
   1. Systemic lupus erythematosus—female, symmetric joint distribution identical to RA, hair loss, mucosal lesions, rash, systemic reaction, visceral organ or brain involvement, leukopenia, (false-) positive serologic test for syphilis, no erosions radiographically, noninflammatory joint fluid with good viscosity and mucin clot and 1,000–2,000 WBCs/mm^3, mostly small lymphocytes. Serum $C'H_{50}$ often depressed, antinuclear antibody (ANA) titer elevated, anti–native-human DNA antibody titer increased.
   2. Scleroderma—tight skin, Raynaud phenomenon, resorption of digits, dysphagia, constipation, lung, heart, or kidney involvement, symmetric tendon contractures, little or no synovial thickening, radiographic calcinosis circumscripta, positive ANA with speckled or nucleolar pattern.
   3. Polymyositis (dermatomyositis)—proximal muscle weakness, pelvic and pectoral girdles, tender muscles, skin changes, typical nail and knuckle pad erythema, symmetric joint involvement, electromyographic evidence of combined myopathic and denervation pattern, muscle biopsy abnormal, elevated creatine phosphokinase.
   4. Mixed connective tissue disease—swollen hands, Raynaud phenomenon, tight skin, symmetric joint and tendon involvement, may be joint erosions radiographically, positive ANA speckled pattern, antiribonucleoprotein antibody increased, good response to corticosteroid therapy given in antiinflammatory doses.
   5. Polyarteritis nodosa—symmetric involvement, diverse clinical picture of systemic disease, histologic diagnosis.
C. **Rheumatic fever**
   Young (2–40 yr), sore throat, group A streptococci, migratory arthritis, rash, heart or pericardial involvement, elevated antistreptolysin O titers. Migratory joint inflammation responds dramatically to aspirin treatment.
D. **Juvenile rheumatoid arthritis**
   Symmetric joint involvement, rash, fever, no rheumatoid factor, radiographic periostitis, erosions late, can begin or recur in adult.
E. **Psoriatic arthritis**
   Asymmetric boggy joint and tendon swelling, skin or nail lesions may not be prominent or may follow arthritis, distal interphalangeal joints might be prominently involved, radiologic periostitis or erosions, no rheumatoid factor. $C'H_{50}$ usually not depressed in inflammatory joint fluid with polymorph predominance.
F. **Reiter's syndrome**
   Male, urethritis, iritis, conjunctivitis, asymmetric joints, lower extremity, nonpainful mucous membrane ulcerative lesion, balanitis circinata, keratosis blennorrhagica, weight loss. $C'H_{50}$ increased in serum and in joint fluid with 5,000–30,000 leukocytes/mm^3. Macrophages in joint fluid with 3–5 phagocytosed polymorphs (Reiter's cell).
G. **Gonorrheal arthritis**
   Migratory arthritis or tenosynovitis fully settling in one or more joints or tendons, either sex, primary focus urethra, female genitourinary tract, rectum, or oropharynx, skin lesions, vesicles, gram-negative diplococci on smear but not on culture of vesicular fluid, positive culture at primary site, blood, or joint fluid.

(continued)

TABLE 4-4 (Continued)

H. **Polymyalgia rheumatica**
   Elderly patient (>50 yr), symmetric pelvic or pectoral girdle complaints without loss of strength, morning stiffness of long duration, fatigue prominent, weight loss, joints can be involved, especially shoulders, sternoclavicular joints, knees, sedimentation rate markedly elevated, fibrinogen always elevated, alpha 2 and gamma globulin elevation, anemia, response to low-dose (10–20 mg) prednisone, serum creatine phosphokinase normal, elevated alkaline phosphatase (liver).

I. **Crystal-induced**
   1. Gout—symmetric arthritis, flexion contractures, prior history of acute attacks, tophi, joint inflammation out of phase, systemic corticosteroid treatment for RA, hyperuricemia, monosodium urate monohydrate crystals in joint fluid.
   2. Pseudogout—symmetric arthritis, flexion contractures, metacarpophalangeal, wrist, elbow, shoulder, hips, knees, and ankles, prior acute attacks (sometimes), joint inflammation out of phase, calcium pyrophosphate dihydrate crystals in joint fluid.

J. **Other**
   Amyloid arthropathy, peripheral arthritis of inflammatory bowel disease, tuberculosis, subacute bacterial endocarditis, viral arthritis.

Modified from McCarty DJ. Differential diagnosis of arthritis: analysis of signs and symptoms. In: McCarty, DJ, ed. *Arthritis and allied conditions*, 10th ed. Philadelphia, PA: Lea & Febiger, 1985:51–52.

TABLE 4-5 Rheumatoid Arthritis Diagnostic Criteria

1. Morning stiffness
2. Pain on motion or tenderness in at least one joint[a]
3. Swelling (soft tissue thickening or fluid, not bony overgrowth alone) in at least one joint[a]
4. Swelling of at least one other joint[a,b]
5. Symmetric joint swelling with simultaneous involvement of the same joint on both sides of the body[a,b]; terminal phalangeal joint involvement will not satisfy the criterion
6. Subcutaneous nodules over bony prominences, on extensor surfaces, or in juxtaarticular regions[a]
7. Roentgenographic changes typical of rheumatoid arthritis (which must include at least bony decalcification localized to or greatest around the involved joints and not just degenerative changes[b])
8. Positive tests for rheumatoid factor in serum[b]
9. Poor mucin precipitate from synovial fluid (with shreds and cloudy solution)
10. Characteristic histologic changes in synovial membrane[b]
11. Characteristic histologic changes in nodules[b]

Categories	Number of criteria required	Minimum duration of continuous symptoms	Exclusions[c]
Classic	7 of 11	6 wk (No. 1–5)	Any of listed
Definite	5 of 11	6 wk (No. 1–5)	Any of listed
Probable	3 of 11	6 wk (one of No. 1–5)	Any of listed

[a]Observed by a physician.
[b]Refer to original reference for further specifications.
[c]Refer to original reference for listing of exclusions.
From Medsger TA Jr, Masi AT. Epidemiology of the rheumatic diseases. In: McCarty DJ, ed. *Arthritis and allied conditions*, 10th ed. Philadelphia, PA: Lea & Febiger, 1985:11.

2. Helpful **blood tests** include a complete blood count, erythrocyte sedimentation rate (ESR), C-reactive protein (CRP), uric acid, rheumatoid factor, and antinuclear antibody.

IV. DIFFERENTIAL DIAGNOSIS OF ACUTE NONTRAUMATIC JOINT CONDITIONS (Table 4-4) (1–3)

A. Rheumatoid arthritis (Table 4-5)

1. **History** often reveals symmetric joint and tendon involvement, typically in a younger female patient (4).
2. **Examination** shows synovial thickening, joint tenderness, subcutaneous nodules, weakness associated with muscle wasting, and, often, systemic disease.
3. **Roentgenograms and laboratory data show that erosions are usually present, but rheumatoid factor is present in only 75% of patients.** Roentgenograms are often normal in acute forms of rheumatoid arthritis except for signs of swelling or periarticular osteopenia. Joint fluid contains 2,000 to 50,000 white blood cells (WBCs)/mm^3, approximately 40% to 80% of which are polymorphonuclear leukocytes.

B. Septic arthritis

1. **Bacterial**
   a. The **history** may indicate drug or alcohol abuse, systemic illness (e.g., diabetes, chronic renal failure, or poor nutrition).
   b. **Examination** can reveal severe inflammation and often a primary septic focus. Severe splinting (autoprotection by muscle spasm) of the joint is present, and pain is associated with passive motion.
   c. **Laboratory tests** show a purulent joint fluid with polymorphonuclear leukocytes predominating (WBCs: 50,000–300,000/mm^3). The infectious agent may be identified on smear or culture. Synovial glucose is less than 60% of a concurrent serum glucose. The ESR and CRP are elevated. Serial blood cultures obtained before antibiotic therapy often grow the infecting organism.
2. **Tubercular and fungal**
   a. **History** may reveal a focus, chronic immunodeficiency [human immunodeficiency virus (HIV) or acquired immunodeficiency syndrome (AIDS)], drug or alcohol abuse, or poor nutrition.
   b. **Examination** shows marked chronic joint swelling.
   c. **Laboratory tests** reveal predominating polymorphonuclear leukocytes with acid-fast organisms present on smear and culture.
3. **Viral**
   a. **History** often indicates antecedent or concomitant systemic viral illness.
   b. **Laboratory analysis** of joint fluid can mimic inflammatory or noninflammatory conditions. Either mononuclear or polymorphonuclear leukocytes can predominate.

C. Osteoarthritis (nonerosive degenerative joint disease)

1. **History** reveals a middle-aged or elderly patient unless the condition follows trauma.
2. **Examination** reveals that angulatory deformities and osteophytes are frequently present in the later stages of disease (1,5,6).
3. **Roentgenograms** show narrowing of the cartilage space associated with marginal osteophytes. There is often subchondral bone sclerosis and occasionally subchondral cysts, which accompany these findings in the weight-bearing joints.

D. Crystal-induced arthritis (Table 4-6) (5)

1. **Gouty arthritis**
   a. The patient may report a history of similar attacks.
   b. **Examination** can show redness and warmth over the affected joint, typically the first metatarsal-phalangeal joint. Later, symmetric arthritis with contractures and tophi (subcutaneous crystal deposits) may develop.
   c. **Laboratory findings** include hyperuricemia and synovial fluid containing monosodium urate monohydrate crystals. The crystals, which are seen by

TABLE 4-6 Differential Diagnosis of Inflammatory Monarthritis

A. Crystal-induced
1. **Gout**—male, lower extremity, previous attack, nocturnal onset, precipitated by medical illness or surgery, response to colchicine, hyperuricemia, sodium urate crystals in joint fluid with polymorphs predominating, and WBCs 10,000–60,000/mm^3.
2. **Pseudogout**—elderly, knee or other large joint, previous attack, precipitated by medical illness or surgery, flexion contractures, chondrocalcinosis on radiography, calcium pyrophosphate dihydrate crystals in joint fluid with polymorphs predominating, and WBCs 5,000–60,000/mm^3.
3. **Calcific tendonitis or equivalent**—extraarticular, tendon or capsule of larger joints, previous attack same or other area, calcification on radiography, chalky or milky material aspirated from area, polymorphs with phagocytosed ovoid bodies microscopically.

B. Palindromic rheumatism
Middle-aged or elderly male, very sudden onset, little systemic reaction, previous attacks, positive rheumatoid factors, little or no residual chronic joint inflammation, olecranon bursal enlargement.

C. Infectious arthritis
1. **Septic**—severe inflammation, primary septic focus, drug or alcohol abuse, joint fluid with polymorphs predominating, WBCs 50,000–300,000/mm^3 (pus), infectious agents identified on smear and culture, or bacterial antigens identified in joint fluid. Lyme disease must be considered in the differential where possible exposure to tick vector is possible.
2. **Tubercular**—primary focus, drug or alcohol abuse, marked joint swelling for long period, joint fluid with polymorphs predominating, acid-fast organisms on smear and culture.
3. **Fungal**—similar to tuberculosis.
4. **Viral**—antecedent or concomitant systemic viral illness, joint fluid can be of inflammatory or noninflammatory type, either mononuclear or polymorphonuclear leukocytes may predominate.

D. Other
1. **Tendonitis**—as in A.3 but without radiologic calcification, antecedent trauma, including repetitive motion.
2. **Bursitis**—as above, but inflamed area more diffuse, antecedent trauma.
3. **Juvenile rheumatoid arthritis**—one or both knees swollen in preteenager or teenager without systemic reaction, no erosions, mildly inflammatory joint fluid with some polymorphs, and no depression in synovial fluid C'H$_{50}$ levels.

From McCarty DJ. Differential diagnosis of arthritis: analysis of symptoms. In: McCarty DJ, ed. *Arthritis and allied conditions*, 10th ed. Philadelphia, PA: Lea & Febiger, 1985:50.

---

compensated polarized light microscopy (sometimes by ordinary light microscopy), are negatively birefringent, needle-shaped rods.

2. **Pseudogout**
   a. **History** sometimes reveals previous acute attacks.
   b. **Examination** discloses a symmetric arthritis with frequent contractures of the metacarpophalangeal, wrist, elbow, shoulder, hip, knee, and ankle joints. Roentgenograms may reveal the presence of calcium deposits in cartilage or, less often, in ligaments, meniscus, and joint capsules (chondrocalcinosis). The knee is the most common site. Chondrocalcinosis has been classically associated with pseudogout, but this condition is also seen with a high frequency in hyperparathyroidism, hemochromatosis, hemosiderosis, hypophosphatasia, hypomagnesemia, hypothyroidism, gout, neuropathic joints, and aging (1,5,6).
   c. **Laboratory** analysis of the synovial fluid reveals calcium pyrophosphate dihydrate crystals that are regularly shaped and weakly positively birefringent, but have a different extinction angle compared to that of urate crystals (6).

Chapter 4: Acute Nontraumatic Joint Conditions 57

E. Inflammatory polyarthritis other than rheumatoid arthritis (**Table 4-4**)
  1. **Reiter syndrome**
     a. **History** often reveals a sexually active man (chlamydia is the most common organism identified) with urethritis and conjunctivitis accompanying the arthritis. Patients have an equivocal response to antiinflammatory drugs.
     b. **Examination** often reveals urethritis, iritis, conjunctivitis, and nonpainful mucous membrane ulcerative lesions, with asymmetric arthritis of the joints in the lower extremities or back. Roentgenograms may show an asymmetric sacroiliitis as well as isolated involvement of the spine ("skip" areas). Heel pain can be a common associated feature of the presentation.
     c. **Laboratory data.** The joint fluid has 5,000 to 30,000 leukocytes/mm^3 with macrophages that contain three to five phagocytosed polymorphonuclear leukocytes (so-called Reiter cell). Measurement of HLA-B27 antigen is not very useful.
  2. **Psoriatic arthritis**
     a. **Examination** shows asymmetric boggy joint and tendon sheath swelling. Skin or nail (pitting) lesions are generally present. The distal interphalangeal (DIP) joints of the hand are frequently involved (1,5).
     b. **Roentgenographic** periostitis, cortical erosions, or both can be seen along with spinal asymmetric sacroiliitis and isolated vertebral ankylosis (skip areas). The "pencil-in-cup" deformity is typically seen in the DIP joints of the hand. No rheumatoid factor is found. There is polymorphonuclear leukocytic predominance in the joint field.
  3. **Systemic lupus erythematosus** (SLE)
     a. **History** most commonly reveals symmetric joint distribution identical to rheumatoid arthritis in a female patient. Hair loss and Raynaud symptoms (vasospasm of digital arteries) are common.
     b. **Examination** may disclose rash (facial erythema), mucosal lesions, serositis, renal or brain involvement, and a systemic reaction.
     c. **Laboratory evaluation** shows leukopenia, prolonged partial thromboplastin time (lupus inhibitor) with anticardiolipin antibodies, a noninflammatory joint fluid with good viscosity* and mucin[+], and 1,000 to 2,000 WBCs/mm^3, which are mostly lymphocytes. A depressed serum C'H$_{50}$, elevated antinuclear antibody and an increased anti–native-human DNA antibody titer are found.
  4. **Rheumatic fever**
     a. **History** reveals a sore throat, fever, rash, and migratory joint pain that responds dramatically to aspirin treatment in younger individuals (that are beyond the ages of Reye syndrome).
     b. **Examination** shows a rash as well as heart (murmur) or pericardial (friction rub) involvement.
     c. **Laboratory tests** result in group A streptococci isolated on throat cultures and an elevated antistreptolysin O titer.
  5. **Juvenile rheumatoid arthritis** (JRA)
     a. **History** shows symmetric joint involvement. The illness can begin or recur in the adult. Short stature and limb length irregularity generally accompany the most severe forms because the physes are affected by the inflammatory process. Patients with systemic onset (10% of children with JRA) have intermittent fever with rash. Those patients (40% of total) who have involvement

---

*The clinical viscosity test is considered good or high if the fluid remains intact when slowly stretched between the examiner's thumb and index finger.
[+]A good mucin clot is one that occurs after a few drops of glacial acetic acid are added to a supernatant of centrifuged joint fluid and a dense, white precipitate forms.

of five or more joints are characterized as polyarticular onset and are differentiated from pauciarticular-onset patients (7). There is a very high proportion of cervical spine involvement in the patients with JRA. The prevalence of JRA has been estimated to be between 57 and 113 per 100,000 children younger than 16 years of age in the United States (7).
   b. **Examination** may reveal a rash and fever. Cardiac, renal, and ocular abnormalities may be present. Eye involvement occurs in 30% to 50% of early onset JRA patients (7).
   c. **Laboratory tests** show roentgenographic periostitis with erosions later in the course of disease. Rheumatoid factor or FANA may be present. Other causes of arthritis in the child or adolescent must be excluded.
   6. **HIV infection.** Migratory arthralgia and myalgia with accompanying muscle weakness are features of this disease. Radiographic changes are nonspecific.
F. **Inflammatory spondyloarthropathy (Table 4-7)**
   1. **Ankylosing spondylitis**
      a. **History** usually reveals clinical sacroiliitis in a male patient. A positive family history often is present. A good response to antiinflammatory agents is common.
      b. **Examination** reveals limitation of spinal motion, uveitis, and diminished chest expansion. A positive Patrick's test indicative of sacroiliac involvement is typically present (1,5,6).
      c. There is **laboratory evidence** of roentgenographic sacroiliitis and smooth, symmetric spinal ligamentous calcification, often with complete ankylosis (the "bamboo spine") and no skip areas. The HLA-B27 antigen should be present.
   2. **Reiter syndrome** (see **IV.E.1**)
   3. **Psoriatic arthritis** (see **IV.E.2**)
   4. **Spondyloarthropathy secondary to inflammatory bowel disease**
      a. The **history** may not reveal bowel disease as a prominent feature; it can be subclinical.
      b. Bowel disease is found on **examination**.
      c. **Laboratory tests** show roentgenographic evidence of sacroiliitis that is often symmetric and ankylosing.

TABLE 4-7   Differential Diagnosis of Inflammatory Spondyloarthropathy[a]

A. **Ankylosing spondylitis**—male, symmetric sacroiliitis clinically and radiologically, limitation of spinal motion, uveitis, smooth symmetric spinal ligamentous calcification, ankylosis often complete, no skip areas, family history, HLA-B27 antigen often present, good response to antiinflammatory drugs.
B. **Reiter syndrome**—male with urethritis, skin-eye-heel, asymmetric peripheral joint involvement, sacroiliitis often asymmetric and skip areas of involvement in spine, coarse asymmetric syndesmophytes in spine, ankylosis incomplete and asymmetric, HLA-B27 often positive, equivocal response to antiinflammatory drugs.
C. **Psoriatic spondylitis**—skin or peripheral joints involved, asymmetric sacroiliitis, skip areas, may be ankylosing, HLA-B27 often present.
D. **Inflammatory bowel disease**—sacroiliitis, often symmetric, ankylosing, bowel disease may be silent, spinal inflammation, unlike peripheral arthritis, does not vary with and is not responsive to treatment directed at bowel inflammation, HLA-B27 often present.
E. **Other**—infection (bacterial tuberculous, fungal), osteochondritis, multiple epiphysitis in young adult.

[a]Juvenile rheumatoid arthritis spondyloarthropathy occurs almost entirely in HLA-B27–positive boys and is regarded as juvenile ankylosing spondylitis.
From McCarty DJ. Differential diagnosis of arthritis: analysis of symptoms. In: McCarty DJ, ed. *Arthritis and allied conditions*, 10th ed. Philadelphia, PA: Lea & Febiger, 1985:52.

V. TREATMENT (Table 4-8)
A. Rheumatoid arthritis (8–11)

1. **Aspirin** is inexpensive but inconvenient to take because most authorities recommend a range of 10 to 16 five-grain tablets per day to reach an antiinflammatory level. Some patients simply cannot tolerate the medication because of gastrointestinal side effects. Enteric-coated or time-release preparations, 650 mg PO t.i.d or q.i.d, may be taken with meals but not with antacids. These preparations may limit the dyspepsia but do not alter the risk of gastrointestinal bleeding. Tinnitus must be monitored in all patients receiving aspirin-containing compounds; it is an early sign of salicylate toxicity. This therapy is sufficient only for mild, nonerosive forms of rheumatoid arthritis.
2. **Other nonsteroidal, non-aspirin antiinflammatory medications** are much more convenient, but more expensive. Patients who take these medications long term should have biannual laboratory work to look for adverse hepatic, renal, hematopoietic, and other reactions. Physicians should educate their patients as to the potential adverse effects of any medication. One easy education tool is the patient medication instruction sheet. The treating physician may need to experiment with various antiinflammatory medications before finding which preparation is the best suited for the individual patient. Many different preparations are now marketed (4). Physicians prescribing these medications should know their cost. For example, a 1-month supply (120 tablets) of generic ibuprofen, 600 mg, (prescription or over-the-counter) costs between $15 and $20, whereas a 1-month supply (360 tablets) of an over-the-counter brand name form of the same drug (e.g., Advil, Medipren, Anaprox),

TABLE 4-8 Treatment

Rheumatoid arthritis	Septic arthritis	Degenerative joint disease

1. Drugs
  a. Acetylsalicylic acid (first)
  b. Other antiinflammatory prescription medications
  c. Gold or D-penicillamine
  d. Methotrexate
  e. Sulfasalozine
  f. Chloroquine
  g. Steroids
2. Synovectomy. If done, usually should follow 6 months of medical management. (Do not do a prophylactic synovectomy if there is roentgenographic evidence of joint destruction manifested by a severe loss of cartilaginous space.)
3. Joint debridement and synovectomy (for pain relief only)
4. Partial or complete joint replacement
5. Arthrodesis
	1. Antibiotics. Cefazolin (Kefzoi) or nafcillin (Nafcil or Unipen) with gentamicin (Garamycin) or tobramycin (Nebcin) until the culture and sensitivity results are obtained; then specific antibiotic therapy
	2. Surgery. Operative debridement and irrigation of the joint, followed by appropriate drainage
		1. Antiinflammatory agents
		2. Support by bracing and other means
		3. Physical therapy
		  a. Heat
		  b. Exercises
		4. Surgery
		  a. Debridement
		  b. Osteotomy
		  c. Partial or complete joint replacement
		  d. Occasionally, arthrodesis

200 mg, costs the patient between $35 and $36. The dosage of any antiinflammatory drug should be the lowest possible that is effective in relieving symptoms. There are several classes of these drugs, the latest being the COX II inhibitors, which have a decreased incidence of gastrointestinal ulceration and are equally effective (10,12). This therapy is sufficient only for mild arthritis.
3. **Gold** is often effective for treatment of rheumatoid and psoriatic arthritis; however, it is no longer considered to be first-line therapy. Three forms of gold are available. Two are injectable in the form of water-soluble, gold sodium thiomalate (Myochrysine) and an oil-based aurothioglucose (Solganal). The usual treatment required is two test doses of 10 to 25 mg each, followed by weekly doses of 50 mg IM for 20 weeks. A maintenance dosage of 50 mg every 4 weeks may be given for life, but dosage is empirical and smaller doses may be effective. The third form, Auranofin, is administered orally, 3 mg PO b.i.d. The most common toxic reaction to gold is dermatitis or albuminuria. Almost any condition can occur, and gold should be withheld if any unusual symptoms develop. Do not persist with gold if results are doubtful (9).
4. **D-Penicillamine** (Cuprimine), a derivative of penicillin, may be substituted for gold in the treatment of rheumatoid arthritis; it is also no longer considered to be first-line therapy. The drug is marketed in 125- and 250-mg capsules. The starting dosage is 250 mg/day, and it can be increased by 250 mg every 3 months to a maximum of 1 g/day. This slow approach appears to lessen toxicity but retains efficacy. Because the drug is toxic, the patient must be carefully monitored, particularly for bone marrow depression, thrombocytopenia, and albuminuria (9).
5. **Methotrexate.** First-line therapy.
6. **Sulfasalazine.** First-line therapy.
7. **Chloroquine** is available as 250-mg chloroquine phosphate tablets. **Hydroxychloroquine** (Plaquenil), which is available in 200-mg tablets, is more commonly used because it is less toxic, but it is not as effective as chloroquine phosphate (9).
    a. **Dosage**
        i. **Chloroquine phosphate** is given in doses of 250 mg/day PO.
        ii. **Hydroxychloroquine** is given in doses of 200 mg PO b.i.d.
        iii. It may take up to **6 months to achieve a result. Attempt a dose reduction** every 6 months.
    b. **Precautions**
        i. **Do not exceed the recommended dose.** This **dosage schedule** does not apply to children.
        ii. **Inform the patient of toxicity.**
        iii. Have an **ophthalmologist follow up with the patient.**
        iv. **Do not refill a prescription over the telephone; examine the patient first.**
        v. **Stop** therapy whenever there are any complaints of visual disturbance or a question of eye toxicity.
    c. **Side effects**
        i. The **major** side effect is blindness resulting from chloroquine combining with retinal pigment.
        ii. **Other** effects are gastrointestinal upset, skin rash, weight loss, peripheral neuritis, and convulsions.
8. **Azathioprine,** a purine analog with immunosuppressive activity, has been shown to be effective in rheumatoid arthritis; it should be prescribed by rheumatologists (8).
9. Leflunomide (Aravan)
10. **Etanercept** (Enbrel), a tumor necrosis factor alpha (TNF-α) inhibitor, is the first "biologic" agent for use in rheumatoid arthritis. It has been proven to be effective in controlled trials and is generally well tolerated. Rarely, there have been cases of serious infections, and the cost (over $10,000 per year) must be

considered. It has also been shown to be useful in combination therapy with methotrexate. It should be prescribed by rheumatologists (13–15).
11. **Corticosteroids** yield a dramatic effect in the treatment of rheumatic disease. Although steroids can offer dramatic relief, indiscriminate use may actually produce more harm than good. In the treatment of rheumatoid arthritis, steroids do not alter the course of the disease, and in subsequent years, the relief will probably deteriorate because patients may have more than one disease.
    a. **Usage**
        i. **Establish a specific diagnosis before treatment** with steroids.
        ii. **Adjust the dosage** to the situation. For rheumatoid arthritis, start with 10 to 20 mg to control symptoms, then taper over 2 to 4 weeks to the lowest tolerated dose (usually no more than 510 mg/day) and try not to exceed 10 mg/24 hours. For SLE crisis, one might start with 60 mg in a 24-hour period.
        iii. Although more than 20 generic glucocorticosteroids are available, most rheumatologists have settled on **prednisone as the standard.**
        iv. **Monitor serum electrolytes and glucose** because steroids cause increased excretion of sodium and potassium.
        v. **Administer** the steroid **once each morning** to minimize the effect on the pituitary–adrenal axis. If there is good control of the inflammatory process, use alternate-day therapy.
        vi. Obtain a **baseline eye examination** before starting long-term therapy. Steroids can cause cataracts and increased intraocular pressure.
        vii. Beware of **suppressed reaction to infection** as a complicating factor, especially if the patient's general condition is deteriorating while he or she is taking steroids.
        viii. With long-term therapy, be sure to recognize and manage complications of the systemic rheumatic disease as opposed to the **iatrogenic complications** of long-term steroid use, which are managed differently.
        ix. Patients should always **carry information** that they are on steroids.
        x. **Supplemental increased doses** are necessary when stress occurs, even minor stress such as a tooth extraction.
    b. **Undesirable effects**
        i. **Steroid diabetes** that is insulin-resistant, but without ketosis or acidosis
        ii. **Muscle wasting** secondary to a negative nitrogen balance
        iii. **Buffalo hump** and **round face**
        iv. Sodium retention that results in **edema** (especially important for patients with heart disease)
        v. **Hirsutism** and occasional **alterations in menstrual function** in women secondary to adrenal atrophy
        vi. **Peptic ulcer disease** with possible perforation and abscess
        vii. **Suppressed wound healing**
        viii. **Osteoporosis** and avascular necrosis of the femoral or humeral head. Pathologic fractures are often associated.
        ix. **Lymphocytosis** and occasionally a leukemoid reaction
        x. **Subcutaneous hemorrhages and acne**
        xi. **Central nervous system changes** such as psychosis, seizures, and insomnia at higher dose
        xii. **Immunosuppression** with increased risk of infections, candida, herpes zoster, and so on
12. **Surgical treatment**
    a. **Synovectomy**, if done, should follow at least 6 months of nonoperative management. This prophylactic procedure should not be performed if roentgenographic evidence of joint destruction manifested by a severe loss of cartilaginous space exists.
    b. There is still a place for **joint debridement** and synovectomy (open or arthroscopic) in patients with significant joint pain, but not enough joint destruction

to justify surgical joint knee replacement. Recently, arthroscopic synovectomy in the knee and shoulder has been shown to be effective.
  c. **Joint replacement** may be necessary. The most common joints replaced in the patient with inflammatory arthritis are knee and hip, followed by shoulder, metacarpophalangeal, elbow, wrist, and ankle.
  d. Very rarely, **arthrodesis** is indicated, especially with ankle involvement.
  e. **Forefoot surgery** is frequently required and most commonly consists of first metatarsophalangeal joint arthrodesis combined with lesser metatarsophalangeal joint resection with claw toe release.

B. **Septic arthritis**
  1. **Antibiotics** (see **Chap. 3, Table 3-2**). Proper cultures must be obtained before initiating antibiotic therapy. These are obtained either as an aspirate or intraoperatively.
  2. **Drainage** of the joint is usually necessary.
     a. **Needle aspiration and irrigation** are sometimes sufficient if the joint can be easily inspected for an effusion. The joint may need decompression more than once daily. The hip joint always requires open drainage. A knee joint infection can be handled by needle decompression if the exudate is not loculated and if aspiration clearly decompresses the joint. If marked improvement is not noted within 48 hours, then the open (or arthroscopic) irrigation and debridement should be performed.
     b. **Operative irrigation and drainage** of the joint are often necessary with or without debridement. Postoperatively, wounds are usually closed over drains and judicious immobilization is used. Increasingly, arthroscopic lavage is being used for knee and shoulder joint involvement.

C. **Osteoarthritis**
  1. Medical treatment consists of acetaminophen or **nonsteroidal antiinflammatory preparations.** Due to safety concerns, acetaminophen is considered the first-line agent (2,16). There is some evidence that the "nutricuticals" glucosamine and chondroitin sulfate have some efficacy in treating the symptoms of osteoarthritis (17). See **V.A.1** and **V.A.2** for a more complete discussion.
  2. Various **braces** are available to offer joint support (see also **Chap. 6**). Simple neoprene sleeves for the knee or elbow are useful. For unicompartmental knee arthritis, braces that "unload" the diseased compartment are proven to be effective (3).
  3. **Physical therapy** can be helpful, especially in providing exercises to maintain muscle tone. Deep heat treatments provide symptomatic relief. The most effective therapy is patient-directed home therapy, which emphasizes maintaining strength and motion with low-impact exercise routines. Prolonged outpatient therapy is expensive and of limited value.
  4. **Weight loss** is extremely useful for overweight patients with osteoarthritis. This may seem obvious in the weight-bearing joints of the lower extremity due to excessive force on the joints. Still, it is often neglected. Additionally, there is increasing evidence that obesity is associated with an increase in osteoarthritis of the upper extremity, suggesting a systemic effect such as through inflammatory mediators.
  5. Intraarticular steroid injections are helpful. The options available are listed in **D.2.b.** (pseudogout treatment). Recently, injection of hyaluronic acid compounds (Synvisc or Hyalgan) has been proven to be efficacious. This requires serial injections given 1 week apart over either 3 or 5 weeks. The therapy has the same effectiveness as oral antiinflammatory therapy.
  6. Various **surgical procedures** offer relief of joint pain and improved function. These include the following:
     a. **Debridement,** generally arthroscopic
     b. **Osteotomy** for varus malalignment of the knee to move the weight-bearing axis into the lateral, more normal compartment
     c. Partial or complete **joint resurfacing or replacement**
     d. Occasionally, **joint arthrodesis.** This is generally reserved for use in the previously septic joint.

e. Autologous chondrocyte transplantation is a technique that may be used selectively for the management of focal traumatic articular cartilage defects. It is not indicated for diffuse osteoarthritis of the knee (18,19).
D. **Crystal-induced arthritis** (9)
   1. **Gouty arthritis**
      a. **Acute attacks** may be provoked by surgery or trauma or other systemic illness. They generally respond to the following agents:
         i. **Colchicine**, one 0.6-mg tablet initially followed by one tablet per hour until gastrointestinal upset occurs, joint symptoms resolve, or a maximum of ten tablets has been ingested in a 24-hour period; or 2 mg intravenously (IV) initially (avoid injecting outside the vein by injecting into a functioning IV) followed by 1 mg q6h until the flare symptoms resolve or a maximum of 5 mg has been injected in a 24-hour period. A suppository formulation is available for patients who cannot take oral medications. IV colchicine should be avoided in elderly patients and patients with renal disease.
         ii. **Indomethacin (Indocin)**, 50 mg PO q.i.d for the first day, followed by 25 mg q.i.d.
         iii. **Other antiinflammatory drugs**, which can be tried if indomethacin is ineffective or not well tolerated.
      b. The **authors suggest** treatment with **colchicine**, 0.6 mg PO b.i.d, **between acute attacks** until the patient is symptom free for 1 year. Consultation with a rheumatologist is advised.
      c. A xanthine oxidase inhibitor such as **allopurinol** (Zyloprim), 100 to 300 mg/day PO, works by lowering the uric acid pool of the body. The physician should be aware of the serious and possibly fatal adverse reactions to allopurinol, including agranulocytosis, exfoliative dermatitis, acute vasculitis, and hepatotoxicity. These agents should not be initiated during an acute attack, rather after resolution.
      d. **Uricosuric agents:** probenecid and sulfinpyrazone. These agents increase the amount of uric acid excreted in the urine, so their use can be associated with uric acid renal calculi. As with allopurinol, the therapy should be initiated after resolution of the acute attack.
         i. **Probenecid** (Benemid), 0.5 mg PO q.i.d up to 2 or 3 g/day.
         ii. **Sulfinpyrazone** (Anturane), 100 mg PO b.i.d up to q.i.d.
      e. Recommendations for **managing hyperuricemia**
         i. **Confirm** the elevated serum uric acid by repeating the test.
         ii. **Determine** whether the condition is **secondary** to drugs or blood dyscrasia. One should rule out renal disease with a serum creatinine in a 24-hour serum uric acid excretion test. If uric acid excretion is greater than 1 g per 24 hours, consider treating the hyperuricemia. If renal disease is present, then allopurinol may be the drug of choice.
         iii. **Discuss dietary recommendation** to limit foods rich in purines, such as certain beef and fish.
         iv. **Generally withhold therapy** unless there has been one acute attack of gouty arthritis.
         v. **Rule out** hyperuricemia secondary to a lymphoproliferative or myeloproliferative disease.
         vi. Do not treat hyperuricemia secondary to **thiazide diuretics**.
   2. **Pseudogout**
      a. **Differentiate** pseudogout from acute gouty arthritis by joint fluid examination for specific crystals.
      b. Consider **aspirating** the joint fluid or **injecting** insoluble steroids intraarticularly, using 0.1 mL for small joints and up to 1 to 2 mL for most large joints. The types of steroids useful for this application are as follows:
         i. **Hydrocortisone** acetate, 25 to 50 mg/mL
         ii. **Prednisone** tertiary butyl acetate, 20 mg/mL
         iii. **Triamcinolone** hexacetonide (Aristospan), 5 and 20 mg/mL

        iv. Betamethasone acetate and sodium phosphate (Celestone), 6 mg/mL
        v. Methylprednisolone acetate (Depo-Medrol), 20 and 40 mg/mL
    c. Colchicine may provide dramatic relief.
    d. Many patients respond to **antiinflammatory agents** such as indomethacin.
E. Inflammatory polyarthritis (assuming no coexisting chlamydia infection)
    1. Reiter syndrome treatment is symptomatic. The prognosis is guarded because chronic arthritis develops in many people. Sulfasalazine, MTX may be considered for chronic moderate-to-severe disease.
    2. Psoriatic arthritis. Immunosuppressive drugs, such as methotrexate, are useful when administered in doses of 7.5 to 25.0 mg PO or IM once weekly. Methotrexate can induce hair loss, cause oral ulcers, promote teratogenesis, and cause hepatitis and cirrhosis of the liver.
    3. Systemic lupus erythematosus
        a. Do not treat until the diagnosis is established.
        b. Do not overtreat. Mild cases can be handled with reassurance, aspirin, indomethacin, or one of the many nonsteroidal antiinflammatory drugs that are available.
        c. An **occult infection** sometimes is difficult to diagnose and differentiate from an exacerbation of SLE. In these situations, be sure to rule out infections of the genitourinary tract, heart, and lungs.
        d. Advise the patient to **rest** as necessary.
        e. Avoid excessive exposure to the **sun**.
        f. Chloroquine, hydroxychloroquine, and mepacrine (Atabrine) usually control the skin manifestations and arthralgia. Mepacrine should be administered 100 mg per day PO. This medication can cause yellow staining of the skin, but this effect is not considered a reason to discontinue its use.
        g. Prednisone, less than 10 mg/day PO, may be added to the regimen if the patient does not respond to the preceding measures.
        h. Immunosuppressive agents are indicated as steroid-sparing agents for treatment for SLE.
        i. The treatment of this disease is empirical and must be individualized and monitored by the rheumatologist. There are no absolutes.
F. Inflammatory spondyloarthropathy
    1. Ankylosing spondylitis
        a. The most important part of the initial therapy is an **educational effort** by the physician or physical therapist that should cover proper sleeping position, gait, posture, breathing exercises, and "measuring up" every morning (i.e., straightening the spine every day to reach a mark placed on the wall to help prevent kyphosis or at least identify its development).
        b. Nonsteroidal antiinflammatory drugs are the drugs of choice for milder cases. As with treatment for osteoarthritis, trial and error to identify the optimum drug is the rule. After relief is obtained, decrease the dose to the lowest possible effective dose (6).
        c. Ophthalmologic evaluation is indicated because anterior uveitis occurs in 10% to 60% of patients.
        d. Sulfasalazine or methotrexate may be useful in aggressive cases.
        e. Radiation therapy has been abandoned because of late malignancy reports.
    2. Treatment of Reiter syndrome is discussed in **V.E.1.**
    3. Treatment of **psoriatic arthritis** is discussed in **V.E.2.**
    4. Rheumatic fever
        a. Rest is recommended according to the degree of cardiac involvement (8).
        b. Aspirin is used for mild arthritis.
        c. Prednisone is used for patients with carditis and heart failure. Start with 40 to 60 mg per day, and adjust the dosage according to patient response.
        d. Diuretics and digitalis are often needed.
        e. Penicillin is indicated for the initial treatment as well as continued prophylaxis. See **Chap. 3** for the appropriate parenteral dose.
        f. Throat culture family contacts.

5. **Juvenile rheumatoid arthritis** (1,6)
   a. **Salicylates** or nonsteroidal antiinflammatory drugs are the mainstay of therapy; one third of patients can be managed with these drugs alone (7).
      i. For **children** weighing less than 25 kg, use 100 mg/kg body weight per day in four to six divided doses.
      ii. For **adults**, a total daily dose of 2.4 to 3.6 g of aspirin usually is sufficient.
   b. Methotrexate is effective in 70% to 80% of patients with JRA.
   c. **Gold** is used if, after 6 months of adequate salicylate and physical therapy, loss of joint function is progressive owing to active synovitis. See **V.A.3** for a discussion of gold therapy. For children, use 1 mg/kg body weight per week to a maximum of 25 mg/kg body weight per week; injectable therapy is effective in 50% of patients; oral gold therapy is ineffective.
   d. **Antimalarial drugs** such as hydroxychloroquine are used as an alternative to gold. Do not exceed 200 mg/m^2 body surface per day. Ophthalmologic examinations are recommended every 3 months. See **V.A.7** for a more complete discussion of antimalarial drugs.
   e. **D-Penicillamine** is not recommended for routine use in JRA.
   f. **Corticosteroids** are rarely warranted for joint disease alone. If given, they should be administered at the lowest effective dose, preferably on alternate days for very short periods. Steroid injections into troublesome joints for synovitis may be helpful if multiple injections into the same joint are avoided.
   g. **Physical and occupational therapy** are helpful to maintain function, prevent contracture, and optimize motion and muscle strength. Therapeutic maneuvers should be performed twice daily at home. Night splints to prevent deformity are usually essential.
   h. **Orthopaedic surgery**
      i. **Synovectomy plays a limited role** in the early treatment of JRA.
      ii. **Reconstructive surgery** (e.g., soft-tissue releases, osteotomies, and total joint replacement) can be indicated.
   i. **Ophthalmologic evaluation** is necessary for early diagnostic treatment of any iridocyclitis.
   j. **Amyloidosis** is seen in 5% of patients and can be fatal if kidneys fail.
   k. **Do not forget the whole child, the effects of this disease on other organ systems, and the child's mental health.**

References

1. American College of Rheumatology Ad Hoc Committee on Clinical Guidelines. Guidelines for the management of rheumatoid arthritis. *Arthritis Rheum* 1996;39:713–722.
2. Hochberg MC, Altman RD, Brandt KD, et al. Guidelines for the medical management of osteoarthritis: Part II. Osteoarthritis of the knee: american college of rheumatology. *Arthritis Rheum* 1995;38:1541–1546.
3. McCarty DJ. *Arthritis and allied conditions*, 12th ed. Philadelphia, PA: Lea & Febiger, 1993.
4. Fox DA. The role of T cells in the immunopathogenesis of rheumatoid arthritis: new perspectives. *Arthritis Rheum* 1997;40:598–609.
5. Kirkley A, Webster-Bogaert S, Litchfield R, et al. The effect of bracing on varus gonarthrosis. *J Bone Joint Surg (Am)* 1999;81:539–548.
6. Moreland LW, Heck LW, Koopman WJ. Jr. Biologic agents for treating rheumatic arthritis: concepts and progress. *Arthritis Rheum* 1997;40:397–409.
7. Arthritis Foundation. *Primer on rheumatic diseases*, 11th ed. 1999:393–398.
8. American College of Rheumatology Ad Hoc Committee on Clinical Guidelines. Guidelines for monitoring drug therapy in rheumatoid arthritis. *Arthritis Rheum* 1996;39:723–731.
9. Blackburn WD. Management of osteoarthritis and rheumatoid arthritis: prospects and possibilities. *Am J Med* 1996;100:24S–30S.

10. Fries JF, Williams CA, Morfeld D, et al. Reduction in long-term disability in patients with rheumatoid arthritis by disease-modifying antirheumatic drug-based treatment strategies. *Arthritis Rheum* 1996;39:616–622.
11. Moreland LW, Schift MH, Banngartner SW, et al. Etanercept therapy in rheumatoid arthritis. A randomized, controlled trial. *Ann Intern Med* 1999;130:478–486.
12. Celecoxib for arthritis. *Med Lett Drugs Ther* 1999;41:1045.
13. Muller-Fassbender H, Bach GL, Haase W, et al. Glucosamine sulfate compared to ibuprofen in osteoarthritis of the knee. *Osteoarthritis Cartilage* 1994;2:61–69.
14. Shapiro F, Koide S, Glimcher MJ. Cell origin and differentiation in the repair of full-thickness defects of articular cartilage. *J Bone Joint Surg (Am)* 1994;76:579–592.
15. Weinblatt ME, Kremer JM, Bankhurst AD, et al. A trial of etanercept, a recombinant tumor necrosis factor receptor: Fc fusion protein in patients with rheumatoid arthritis receiving methotrexate. *N Engl J Med* 1999;340:253–259.
16. Hochberg MC, Altman RD, Brandt KD, et al. Guidelines for the medical management of osteoarthritis: part I. Osteoarthritis of the hip: american college of rheumatology. *Arthritis Rheum* 1995;38:1535–1540.
17. Drugs for rheumatoid arthritis. *Med Lett Drugs Ther* 2003;5:23–32.
18. Brittberg M, Lindahl A, Nilsson A, et al. Treatment of deep cartilage defects in the knee with autologous chonrocyte transplantation. *N Engl J Med* 1994;331: 889–995.
19. Weaver A, Caldwell J, Olsen N et al. The Leflunomide RA Investigators Group and Strand V. Treatment of active rheumatoid arthritis with leflunomide compared to placebo or methotrexate. *Arthritis Rheum* 1998;41(Suppl. 9);S131(abst).
20. Kelley WN, et al. *Textbook of rheumatology,* 4th ed. Philadelphia, PA: WB Saunders, 1993.

PEDIATRIC ORTHOPAEDIC CONDITIONS   5

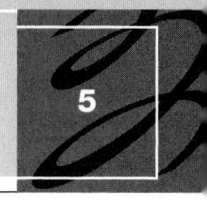

I. **THE LIMPING CHILD.** The limping child is frequently referred to a primary physician's office or an urgent/emergency care center. There is a long list of possible causes to be considered. Important components of the evaluation include a thorough history and a careful physical examination (7).
   A. **History.** Acuteness of onset, pain, history of trauma or injury, constitutional symptoms such as fever, malaise, chills; early morning stiffness and motor milestone development (walked by 15–18 months).
   B. **Past medical history.** Birth history and any previous surgery, injuries, or illnesses.
   C. **Family History.** Family history of childhood lower extremity conditions such as developmental dysplasia of the hip (DDH).
   D. **Physical examination.** The child should be undressed to an appropriate state. Older children and teenagers should be provided with a gown or shorts. Toddlers and small children can be examined in their diaper or underwear. The physical exam should be tailored to each patient depending on the symptoms at presentation. The physical exam of a child with a recent or sudden onset of a painful limp or refusal to walk will be very different from an examination of a child with a chronic, painless limp.
   1. Observation. An **antalgic** gait is characterized by a decreased stance period on the affected limb as well as a trunk shift over the affected limb during stance.
   2. Evaluation for limb length difference: palpate the anterior superior iliac spine (ASIS) with the patient standing. Then, with the patient supine, compare lengths of the lower extremities with the legs extended. Also, compare lengths of the femurs by flexing the hips and comparing the relative heights of the knees.
   3. Physical exam should also include the back, sacroiliac (SI) joints, and abdomen as well as the entire extremity involved.
   4. Palpate the entire length of the limb.
   5. Range of motion of the hip, knee, and ankle joints. Particular attention should be paid to any erythema, warmth, joint effusion, or focal tenderness.
   6. A thorough neurologic examination should also be completed.
   E. The **differential diagnosis** encompasses a broad range and depends on many factors including age, symptoms, severity, acuteness of onset, and clinical findings on physical exam (1,2).
   1. 0 to 5 years old
      a. Septic arthritis
      b. Osteomyelitis
      c. Transient hip synovitis
      d. DDH
      e. Legg-Calvé-Perthes disease/osteochondroses-related conditions
      f. Toddler's fracture
      g. "Nonaccidental injury" (child abuse)
      h. Neurologic disorders (cerebral palsy, Duchenne's Muscular Dystrophy)
      i. Tumor [neuroblastoma, acute lymphocytic leukemia (ALL), benign tumors]
      j. Discitis

        k. Juvenile rheumatoid arthritis
        l. Congenital limb deficiency (femur, fibula, tibia)
     2. **5 to 10 years old**
        a. Septic arthritis
        b. Osteomyelitis
        c. Transient synovitis
        d. Osteochondroses conditions such as Perthes, Kohler, and Osgood-Schlatter disease
        e. Limb length difference
        f. Tumor (ALL, Ewing sarcoma, benign bone tumors)
        g. Neurologic disorders (hereditary motor sensory neuropathy)
        h. Discitis
        i. Juvenile rheumatoid arthritis
        j. Discoid meniscus
     3. **10 to 15 years old**
        a. Osteomyelitis
        b. Slipped capital femoral epiphysis (SCFE)
        c. Osteochondroses conditions such as Perthes and Sever disease
        d. Hip dysplasia
        e. Patellofemoral pain syndrome
        f. Tumor (osteosarcoma, Ewing's sarcoma, benign bone tumors)
        g. Osteochondritis desiccans
        h. Idiopathic chondrolysis
  F. **Radiographic evaluation.** Anteroposterior (AP) and lateral plain radiograph (x-ray) of the entire length of bone involved, including joint above and below the area of concern. **Referred pain** describes pain attributed to one site or location by the patient but the source of the pain is at a different site (e.g., knee pain in a patient with an SCFE involving the hip joint). Referred pain is frequently seen with some childhood conditions.
  G. **Laboratory studies.** Complete blood count (CBC) with differential, erythrocyte sedimentation rate (ESR), and C-reactive protein (CRP). If rheumatologic conditions or spondyloarthropathies are being evaluated, include rheumatoid factor (RF), antinuclear antibody (ANA), anti-streptolysin (ASO) titer, Lyme titer, and HLA B-27.
  H. **Additional imaging studies.**
     1. **Three-phase bone scan.** Useful when source of pain is not easily localizable; sensitive but not specific.
     2. **Magnetic resonance imaging (MRI).** Very sensitive and specific. Able to identify areas of bone marrow edema, soft tissue edema, or fluid collections such as abscesses.
     3. **Ultrasound.** Useful to look for hip joint effusions, subperiosteal or soft-tissue abscesses. May also help guide aspiration of hip joint or soft tissue abscess. **CAUTION:** If septic arthritis is suspected, a **joint aspiration** should be performed without wasting time waiting for the availability of other additional imaging studies.
II. **THE CHILD WHO REFUSES TO WALK/BEAR WEIGHT**
  A. **History**
     1. Fever, lethargy, malaise, or other constitutional symptoms
     2. Pain: location, severity, duration
     3. Trauma/injury
     4. Onset (sudden, gradual, etc.)
  B. **Physical evaluation**
     1. Observe posture of patient/posture of limb
     2. Inspect swelling, redness, deformity
     3. Palpate entire length of extremity, abdomen, spine for sites of pain, mass, warmth
     4. Range of motion (ROM) active/passive, hip, knee, ankle joints

C. Radiograph. Obtain AP and lateral radiographs of the area identified as the location of the patient's pain on physical examination.
D. Laboratory examination. EXTREMELY IMPORTANT:
   1. CBC with differential (may be normal)
   2. C-reactive protein (CRP) (most sensitive)
   3. ESR
   4. Blood culture (particularly in setting of fever/sepsis)
E. Differential Diagnosis. When evaluating a patient with a fever, significant pain with attempted range-of-motion, and/or refusal to bear any weight or to walk, the primary physician should immediately notify the orthopaedic surgeon with whom they wish to consult. As soon as the laboratory studies and x-rays are available, the appropriate disposition of the child can be determined.
   1. **Septic arthritis.** Frequently affects the hip joint in toddlers and young children; may also affect other joints of the lower extremity (knee, ankle) or the upper extremity (shoulder, elbow, wrist). (See **VIII.B** for additional information.)
      a. Symptoms: fever, joint pain, restricted range of motion
      b. Laboratory tests: CBC may be normal, CRP and ESR are elevated
      c. Radiographs: frequently normal, may suggest hip joint effusion
      d. Treatment plan: *immediate referral* to orthopaedist for evaluation and aspiration and/or surgical drainage as well as admission/intravenous (IV) antibiotics
   2. **Transient/toxic synovitis** (see **VIII.C** for additional information)
      a. Symptoms: severity of hip pain may vary, patient usually afebrile
      b. Laboratory tests: normal or minimal elevation of CBC, ESR, and CRP
      c. Radiographs: normal
      d. Hip ultrasound: hip effusion
      e. Treatment: nonsteroidal anti-inflammatory drugs (NSAIDs)/bed rest and re-evaluate in 24 to 48 hours
   3. **Osteomyelitis.** A bacterial infection of the bone (see **VIII.A** for more information).
      a. Symptoms: fever, pain localized over long bone adjacent to joint, pain with joint ROM is less severe than that seen with septic arthritis
      b. Laboratory tests: CBC may be normal, ESR and CRP elevated
      c. Radiographs: early on, normal; later (after 10–14 days), may show a lytic lesion in area of infection. This is frequently adjacent to the physis (growth plate).
      d. Treatment:
         i. Admission to hospital for intravenous antibiotic therapy
         ii. Additional imaging (nuclear medicine vs. MRI)
         iii. Possible aspiration of painful area for culture
   4. **Fracture or other injury.** If patient is too young to provide history, consider possible fracture or other significant injury.
      a. History: patient fell or found lying on floor if injury unwitnessed
      b. Physical exam: area of swelling, deformity, tenderness
      c. Radiograph: look for fracture or physeal separation. Children's x-rays can be difficult to interpret because of the presence of growth plates (physes). If necessary, consider comparison x-rays of opposite limb.
      d. Treatment: splint injured limb and consult orthopaedic surgeon
   5. **SCFE (unstable/acute)** (see **VII.C**)
      a. Symptoms: adolescent child with sudden onset of severe hip pain, inability to walk or bear weight on affected limb. (For stable SCFE, the adolescent patient may complain of hip or thigh pain but may be able to bear weight.)
      b. Physical exam: patient lies with hip flexed and externally rotated. Severe pain with any attempted ROM.
      c. X-ray: obtain AP pelvis x-ray and *cross-table* lateral x-ray of affected hip. Femoral epiphysis is displaced relative to femoral neck.
      d. Treatment: immediate referral to orthopaedic surgery for surgical stabilization.

70   Chapter 5: Pediatric Orthopaedic Conditions

III. LOWER EXTREMITY ALIGNMENT CONDITIONS

A. Intoeing
1. **Definition.** An internal foot progression angle during gait. The foot turns in relative to the line of forward progression during walking. Intoeing is a frequent cause for parental concern. An important part of the evaluation should be listening to the concerns expressed by the parents and answering their questions.

B. Physical examination. The patient should be undressed adequately to visualize the lower extremities.
1. Observation: observe child walk in hallway. Note position of feet relative to line of forward progression (**Fig. 5-1**).
2. Examination: evaluate *rotational profile*. Position patient prone on examination table.
   a. Hip internal (medial) and external (lateral) rotation (see **Fig. 5-1D**). With patient prone and knees flexed to 90 degrees, rotate hip internally and externally until you can feel the position of rotation at which the greater trochanter of the hip is most prominent. Estimate the angle between the tibia and a vertical position in order to estimate *femoral neck anteversion*.
   b. Estimate *thigh-foot axis* and *bimalleolar axis* in order to assess *tibial torsion*.
      Thigh-foot axis: (see **Fig. 5-1C**) angle formed by line down the middle of the foot relative to line down length of thigh.
      Bimalleolar axis: angle formed by a line passing through center of lateral malleolus and medial malleolus relative to line perpendicular to long axis of thigh.
   c. Examine the plantar surface of the foot with the patient still in the prone position. *Metatarsus adductus* is defined as a curvature of the lateral border of the foot (see **Fig. 5-1E**).

C. Causes
1. **Increased femoral anteversion:** rotational twist in femur turns leg in while walking.
2. **Internal tibial torsion:** twist in tibia turns lower leg inward.
3. **Metatarsus adductus:** curvature of foot turns toes/forefoot inward.

D. Discussion. For the majority of children, treatment of these conditions consists of education of the parents, reassurance, and observation. Intoeing is frequently seen in young patients and is a normal part of skeletal development for many children. The most frequent causes are increased femoral anteversion, internal tibial torsion, or metatarsus adductus. Normal **femoral anteversion** in the newborn is 40 to 45 degrees. For most children, this gradually remodels with growth over time and will have improved by age 6 to 8 years old. At skeletal maturity, normal femoral anteversion is approximately 10 to 15 degrees. **Increased femoral anteversion** is femoral anteversion that persists longer than usual and is frequently associated with increased ligamentous laxity. Children with developmental delays or abnormal motor developmental conditions such as cerebral palsy will also frequently exhibit increased femoral anteversion. There are no forms of bracing, shoe-wear, or therapy that will help femoral anteversion resolve. For the vast majority of patients, it does not cause functional nor painful conditions later in life and should simply be observed (3).

E. Internal tibial torsion is frequently seen as a cause of intoeing in infants and toddlers and also gradually corrects with time. It will correct more quickly than femoral anteversion and usually has improved by age 2 to 3 years.

F. Metatarsus adductus refers to a curvature of the lateral border of the foot. This is a frequent finding in newborn children and is often flexible. Simple massage and stretching can be performed by the parents for the first 6 months of life. If no improvement is seen, one may then consider a course of treatment with reverse-last shoes or bracing. If the foot does not appear flexible, a course of serial casting may be considered.

Chapter 5: Pediatric Orthopaedic Conditions **71**

A Foot progression angle

B Examine in prone position

C Thigh foot angle

D Medial rotation   Lateral rotation

E Forefoot adductus

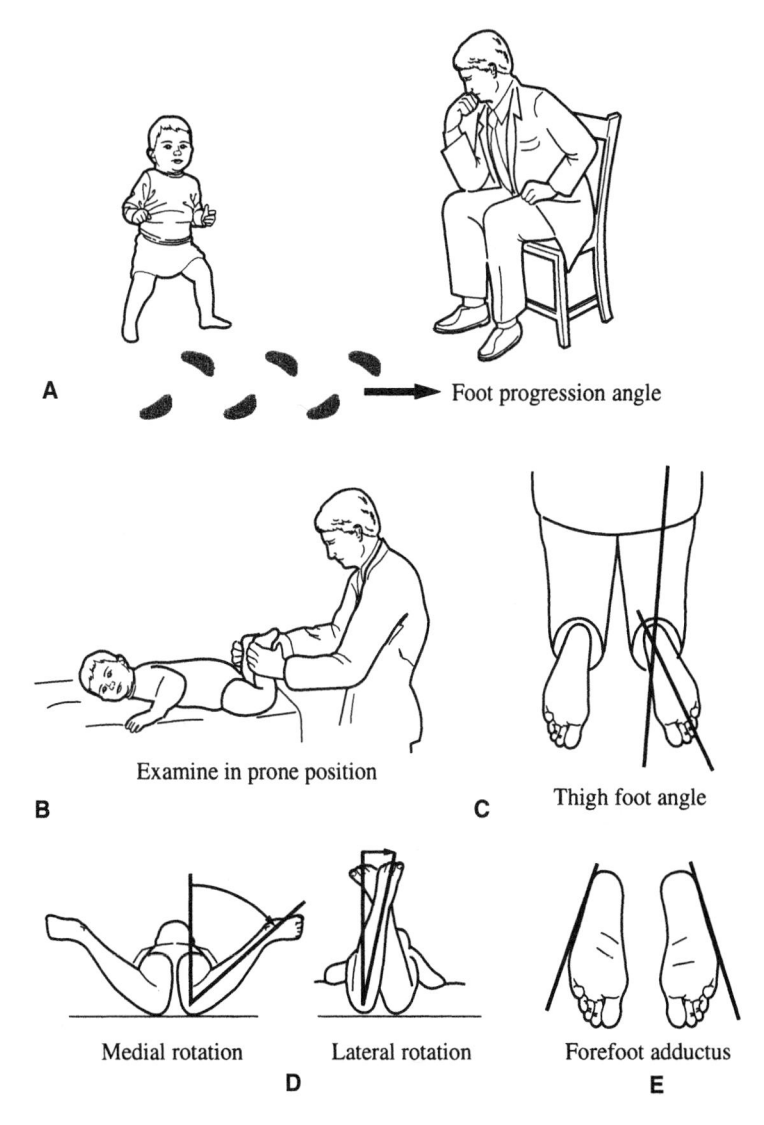

Figure 5-1. Rotational profile. **A:** Observation of foot-progression angle. **B:** Examination of child in prone position to evaluate torsional deformity of the lower extremities. **C:** Thigh-foot angle. **D:** Hip internal (medial) rotation and external (lateral) rotation. **E:** Forefoot (metatarsus) adductus.

IV. LOWER EXTREMITY ALIGNMENT—"BOWED LEGS" OR "KNOCK KNEES"
A. Terminology
   1. **Genu varum** ("bowed legs," genu-knee, varum/varus): the distal segment of the lower leg is aligned toward or close to the midline.
   2. **Genu valgum** ("knock knees," genu-knee, valgum/valgus): the distal segment is aligned away from the midline.

B. **Physical examination.** The child should be undressed appropriately so that both lower extremities can be evaluated. The child should be assessed standing and again supine on the examination table. The amount of angulation at the knee can be assessed in two ways.
  1. **Femoral-tibial angle:** angle between thigh and lower leg
  2. One can also measure and record the distance between bony landmarks.
     a. **Intercondylar distance** (genu varum): the distance between the medial femoral condyles of the knees.
     b. **Intermalleolar distance** (genu valgum): the distance between the medial malleoli of the ankles.
C. **Radiographic evaluation.** For either genu varum or genu valgum, standing AP hip to ankle radiographs of both lower extremities should be obtained. The **mechanical axis** as well as the **anatomic axis** of the lower extremity is measured. In young children with genu varum, the **metaphyseal-diaphyseal angle** is measured.
D. **Causes**
  1. "Physiologic": part of the normal development. Most children who are referred for evaluation have a physiologic form of bowing. Children undergo an evolution of their lower extremity alignment during the first 6 years of life.
     a. Birth to age 2: genu varum
     b. Age 2 to age 4: genu valgum
     c. Age 4 to age 6: continued gradual correction into relatively "mature" alignment of mild genu valgum anatomically (4).
     For children who do not fit this pattern, are of adolescent age, or appear to have asymmetric alignment of their lower extremities, other possible causes should be explored.
  2. **Tibia vara (Blount disease)** is an abnormal varus alignment of the knee due to altered growth of the medial portion of the proximal tibial physis. There is an **infantile form** for children older than age 2 years and **an adolescent form**, frequently associated with obesity.
  3. Other causes could include:
     a. **Coxa vara** (a congenital varus deformity of the proximal femur)
     b. One of the various forms of **skeletal dysplasia.** To help evaluate this, obtain additional radiographs. An x-ray of the hands, shoulders, spine, hips, and knees can help evaluate other potential sights of growth abnormalities.
     c. One of the forms of **rickets** (such as familial hypophosphatemic rickets). To evaluate this further, consider obtaining laboratory studies including vitamin D; parathyroid hormone (PTH); alkaline phosphotase; calcium, magnesium, and phosphorus levels; and consider obtaining an endocrinology consultation.
E. **Treatment**
  1. For physiologic conditions, treatment usually consists of observation. Inform the patient's parents of the expected course and communicate the findings and recommendations to the patient's primary physician. Continued observation can be performed during routine well-child checks. If the child's alignment varies from what is expected, the child can return for reevaluation.
  2. Children with conditions which do not fit the typical "physiologic" pattern should be referred for further evaluation. Further treatment consists of establishing the underlying cause as well as developing an appropriate treatment plan. After the diagnosis has been determined, treatment may consist of:
     a. Observation
     b. Hemiepiphyseal stapling
     c. Hemiepiphysiodesis
     d. Tibial and/or femoral osteotomy
     These should be performed by physicians who are well experienced in planning and performing the appropriate procedures and are able to provide follow-up care.

V. COMMON CHILDHOOD FOOT CONDITIONS

A. Clubfoot (talipes equinovarus)

1. **Description.** A congenital deformity of the foot comprised of ankle equinus, hindfoot varus, and adduction and supination of the midfoot and forefoot. The foot "turns in" and "curves under" compared with the normal.
2. **Incidence.** 1 in 1,000 live births, unilateral in 60% of patients, and the ratio of boys to girls is 2:1. There may be a positive family history.
3. **Etiology.** Multiple theories exist with the most likely cause being **multifactorial**. Theories include arrested fetal development, abnormal intrauterine forces, abnormal muscle fiber type, abnormal neuromuscular function, and germ plasm defects.
4. **Prenatal considerations** include breech position, large birth weight, and oligohydramnios.
5. **Associated conditions** include arthrogryposis, myelodysplasia, congenital limb anomalies, and various syndromes.
6. **Physical examination.** A careful evaluation should include not only examination of the child's feet, but also the child's upper extremities, back, spine, and hips in order to look for other associated conditions. Examination of the foot should include evaluation of the ankle dorsiflexion, the hindfoot position, curvature of the lateral border of the foot, and the forefoot position as well as an assessment of the degree of flexibility of the foot. Deep posterior and medial creases are usually present.
7. **Radiographic evaluation.** Radiographs in the newborn period are not useful because the tarsal bones are not well ossified. Radiographs may be useful after age 3 months for planning or evaluating surgical treatment. They are ordered less often in nonoperative treatment as the physical examination is more useful for clinical decision making. When x-rays are ordered, the most useful images are an AP view and a lateral view in a position of maximum dorsiflexion. **Kite angle** is the angle subtended by the long axes of the calcaneus and the talus on the AP view. This angle is normally between 20 and 40 degrees. In the clubfoot, this angle is less than 20 degrees with relative parallel alignment of the talus and calcaneus. The relationship of the talus and calcaneus should also be assessed on the lateral view. Again, in the clubfoot, this shows relative parallel alignment compared with the normal foot.
8. **Treatment.** The goals of treatment are to achieve a plantigrade, flexible, painless foot. In the early half of the 20th century, Kite published high levels of satisfactory results with his casting technique. The later half of the 20th century saw the emergence and rise in popularity of the surgical treatment of clubfoot as described by such authors as Turco, Carroll, Crawford, Simmons, and McCay (5). The dawn of the 21st century has seen renewed interest in the role of nonoperative treatment using the method developed by Ponseti. His experience has produced impressive results at long-term follow up and is gaining more widespread acceptance and support (6).

B. Flat feet (pes planus)

1. **Definition.** Feet in which the medial longitudinal arch is absent resulting in hindfoot valgus and forefoot supination.
2. **Presentation**
   a. Parental concerns regarding the appearance and shape of the foot
   b. Pain
   c. Difficulties with shoe wear
3. **Patient history.** It is important to note when the foot position was first noticed, whether the foot condition causes problems with function or pain, and any family history of ligamentous laxity or flatfeet.
4. **Physical examination**
   a. Observe the foot while the patient stands and walks. Note presence or absence of medial longitudinal arch.
   b. Inspect the foot for calluses and pressure areas over bony prominences.

74 Chapter 5: Pediatric Orthopaedic Conditions

- c. When the patient is standing, have him or her stand on tiptoe to assess mobility of the hindfoot. If the hindfoot moves from valgus when plantigrade to varus with standing on tiptoe and the foot forms an arch when on tiptoe, then the foot is "**flexible.**" If it does not correct, it is considered "**rigid.**"
- d. Assess the length of the Achilles tendon by examining the range of ankle dorsiflexion.

5. **Radiographic examination.** For young children with a painless, flexible flat foot, no radiographs are indicated. If the flat foot is painful or rigid, then standing AP, lateral, and oblique radiographs of the foot should be obtained.

6. **Flexible flat feet.** The flexible flat foot is a relatively common condition, although the true incidence is unknown. Most young children start with a flexible flat foot before developing a medial longitudinal arch during the first decade of life. Most children are symptom-free, and no treatment is warranted. For the older child or adolescent with a flexible flat foot who experiences aching or discomfort associated with particular activities, one may wish to use an orthotic to support the arch. If the foot is flexible but there is a contracture of the Achilles tendon, one should prescribe a course of physical therapy for a heelcord stretching program. If the patient with an Achilles tendon contracture remains symptomatic despite physical therapy, one may consider injection of Botox into the calf muscle, possibly in conjunction with a stretching cast. For patients that fail conservative therapy, some authors support surgical correction of the hind foot valgus deformity in conjunction with lengthening the tight gastrocnemius (7). This is rarely necessary in the growing child with a flexible flat foot deformity.

7. **Rigid flat feet.** The most common cause for a rigid flat foot is a **tarsal coalition.** This is an incomplete separation of the tarsal bones during fetal development. The two most common types are the **calcaneonavicular** and the **talocalcaneal** coalition. The calcaneonavicular coalition may be best seen on the oblique foot radiograph. The talocalcaneal coalition may be seen on an axial (Harris) radiograph of the foot. If further radiographic imaging is required, a computed tomography (CT) scan of both feet is the study of choice.

8. If tarsal coalition has been excluded as the cause for the rigid flat foot, other possible causes include a **congenital vertical talus**, **juvenile rheumatoid arthritis** (JRA) involving the subtalar joint, **osteochondral fractures** of the subtalar joint, or **neuromuscular** conditions.

9. **Treatment** of the rigid flat foot. The goal of treatment is to achieve a pain-free, asymptomatic foot. Approximately 75% of patients with tarsal coalitions are asymptomatic. Frequently, the onset of pain coincides with the transition of the coalition from a fibrous or cartilaginous junction to a bony bar. For the calcaneonavicular bar, this occurs around ages 8 to 12 years old; for the talocalcaneal bar, this usually occurs between 12 and 16 years of age. Nonoperative treatment consists of applying a short-leg walking cast for 6 weeks followed by use of a molded orthotic. This results in a resolution of the patient's symptoms in a large number of patients. For patients who do not respond to casting treatment or for whom the symptoms recur, surgery is indicated. Operative treatment usually consists of excision of the coalition along with interposition of fat, muscle, or tendon to prevent recurrence. For patients with a talocalcaneal coalition that comprises more than 50% of the subtalar joint surface, some authors have questioned the role of resection of the coalition. For patients with severe degenerative arthrosis of the subtalar joint or persistent pain following previous resection, a triple arthrodesis should be considered (8,9).

C. **Bunions (hallux valgus)**
1. **Definition.** An abnormal bony prominence of the medial eminence of the first metatarsal associated with a hallux valgus deformity of the great toe. It is frequently associated with a medial deviation of the first metatarsal (**metatarsus primus varus**).

2. **Patient history.** These patients are most often adolescent or teenage girls with complaints of pain over the medial eminence, difficulty with shoe wear, or concerns regarding appearance. There may be a positive family history.
3. **Physical examination.** Clinically assess presence of hindfoot valgus and presence of a coexisting flat foot in addition to presence and severity of hallux valgus deformity. Evaluate degree of angulation as well as rotation of great toe.
4. **Radiographic evaluation.** Standing AP and lateral radiographs of the foot are recommended. On the AP radiograph, one can assess the following parameters:
   a. First-second intermetatarsal angle (normal is <9 degrees)
   b. First metatarsal-phalangeal angle (normal is <15 degrees)
   c. Length of the first metatarsal
   d. Congruency of first metatarsophalangeal (MTP) joint
5. **Treatment.** It is important to distinguish the **functional** problems that the patient is experiencing as well as the patient's and the parents' concerns. In the adolescent patient in whom the primary concern is the appearance of the foot, every effort should me made to educate and counsel the family. For patients with a symptomatic hallux valgus deformity, strong consideration should be accorded to postponing any surgical treatment until skeletal maturity is reached because there is a high recurrence rate of bunions in adolescent patients. If surgery is considered, careful examination of the foot is necessary to correct all of the underlying deformities, thus decreasing the risk of recurrence and increasing the likelihood of patient satisfaction. For patients with an underlying flexible flat foot condition, initial treatment should consist of a custom-molded, flexible medial-arch supporting foot orthotic. This will frequently correct the foot deformity and improve the hallux valgus deformity as well.
6. **Surgical options.** There are numerous surgical options.
   a. **Soft-tissue procedures**
      i. Medial capsule advancement of first MTP joint
      ii. Excision of the medial eminence of the metatarsal head
      iii. Adductor hallucis release
   b. **Bony procedures**
      i. Distal first metatarsal osteotomy (Chevron, Mitchell)
      ii. Proximal first metatarsal osteotomy
      iii. First metatarsal double (proximal and distal) osteotomy as described by Peterson (10)
      Geissele reported that the reduction of the intermetatarsal angle is the factor that correlates most highly with both decreased risk of recurrence of angular deformity and with patient satisfaction (11).

VI. **CHILDHOOD KNEE DISORDERS.** Evaluation of patient with knee pain
   A. **History**
      1. Trauma/injury
      2. Swelling of joint
      3. Locking/buckling of knees
      4. Location of pain
      5. Association of pain with specific activities (running, descending stairs, sitting)
   B. **Physical evaluation**
      1. Knee ROM
      2. Hip ROM (remember referred pain from hip)
      3. Effusion of knee joint
      4. Joint line tenderness
      5. Tenderness over patella/tibial tubercle
      6. Assess ligamentous stability
   C. **Radiograph examination.** Obtain AP/lateral radiographs of knee to evaluate for any bony abnormalities. For evaluation of patella alignment or patella-related pain, obtain AP/lateral and "merchant" view or "sunrise" view of knee. For concern regarding possible locking or catching of the knee such as with osteochondritis dessicans (OCD) (see below), obtain AP/lateral and "notch" view radiographs of knee.

D. Differential Diagnosis
1. **Patellofemoral pain syndrome**
   a. **Definition.** Previously termed "chondromalacia patellae" or "anterior knee pain syndrome," it describes a condition in which the pain is attributed to the patellofemoral joint. It typically is characterized by pain localized to the front of the knee.
   b. **Patient history.** Adolescent girls are affected more often than boys. Symptoms may occur gradually or after previous knee injury; usually not associated with specific trauma. There are no symptoms of locking or buckling. Pain is frequently associated with activities such as walking, running, descending stairs, and sitting for prolonged periods.
   c. **Physical examination.** One should include a thorough examination of the knee, paying particular attention to evaluate tracking of the patella, patella mobility medially and laterally, and Q-angle (alignment of extensor mechanism measured by angle of line from ASIS to patella and line from patella to tibial tubercle). Also assess the lower extremity rotational profile (see **III.C.2**)
   d. **Radiographs.** AP, lateral, and patella views should be obtained to evaluate for evidence of patellar tilt as well as to rule out other potential sources of knee symptoms such as OCD and bony lesions.
   e. **Treatment.** Most patients with patellofemoral knee pain respond to a course of conservative treatment consisting of hamstring stretching in addition to closed-chain quadriceps [specifically vastus medialis obliquus (VMO) strengthening]. This may be augmented by use of a patellar-taping program or a patella-stabilizing neoprene knee sleeve in some patients.
2. **Acute patella dislocation**
   a. **Patient history.** Patients may have experienced a traumatic or a nontraumatic patella subluxation or dislocation. The patella dislocates laterally. The patient may be tender over the medial retinaculum and a joint effusion may be present.
   b. **Radiographic evaluation.** AP/lateral/patella views of the knee should be closely evaluated for any evidence of osteochondral fragments. The patella may knock off an osteochondral fragment from the lateral femoral condyle within the process of dislocating or relocating.
   c. **Treatment.** If osteochondral fragments are present, the knee should be evaluated arthroscopically. Very large fragments may need to be replaced and internally fixed; smaller fragments may simply be removed. If no osteochondral fracture is identified, treatment may consist of a short period of immobilization with a soft-sided knee immobilizer followed by a program of quadriceps strengthening exercises.
3. **Chronic patella instability**
   a. **Patient history.** Some patients may have recurrent patella subluxation/dislocation episodes. The initial course of treatment should consist of physical therapy for quadriceps strengthening exercises. If these are not successful in achieving improvement of the instability, surgical stabilization may be indicated (12).
4. **Osgood-Schlatter disease**
   a. **Presentation.** One in the family of conditions known as "osteochondroses," this is an inflammation at the junction of the patellar tendon to the tibial tubercle. It most often occurs in girls aged 10 to 12 and boys aged 12 to 14. The patient usually complains of painful swelling over the area of the tibial tubercle as well as pain associated with activities such as running or jumping sports. **Sinding-Larsen-Johansson syndrome** is a related condition arising at the proximal or distal ends of the patella.
   b. **Treatment.** Consists of hamstring and quadriceps stretching, NSAIDs, periodic ice to the area, and modification of activities.

5. Discoid meniscus
   a. Presentation. Patients with a discoid meniscus may have knee pain as early as age 4 years. Most patients are first seen between ages 6 and 12 years or older. The incidence varies and is estimated to be from 3% to 5% in Anglo-Saxons and as much as 20% in Japanese. The majority of cases involve the lateral meniscus. Patients usually have complaints of snapping or popping of the knee.
   b. Physical examination. Examination of the knee may reveal snapping with flexion of the knee. Unstable menisci may snap or pop in extension.
   c. Classification. There are three principal types. Type I is stable, complete. Type II is stable, incomplete. Type III is unstable because of the absence of the meniscotibial ligament.
   d. Treatment. For stable discoid lateral meniscus, arthroscopic sculpting of the meniscus to a normal configuration is indicated. If it is unstable, stabilization with a capsular suture is recommended (13).

6. Ostochondritis Dessicans (OCD)
   a. Definition. This is a condition of unknown etiology that results in vascular changes of the subchondral bone in the femoral condyle which may lead to fragmentation or separation of the fragment along with the overlying cartilage. It most often occurs in adolescents and is more often in boys than in girls.
   b. History
      i. Nonspecific knee pain
      ii. Knee swelling after activities
      iii. No history of acute trauma or injury
      iv. With or without catching or locking of knee
   c. Physical examination. Mild swelling may be present, tenderness over femoral condyle.
   d. Radiographic examination. AP/lateral/notch views of knee; notch view may show lesion most effectively. Lateral view may also show lesion on posterior aspect of femoral condyle.
   e. MRI: assess "stability" of fragment based on continuity of articular cartilage and subchondral bone.
   f. Treatment depends on age of patient and stability of fragment.
      i. Skeletally immature patient with stable lesion:
         (a) brief period of immobilization
         (b) restriction of activities
      ii. Patient near or at skeletal maturity or unstable lesion: consider arthroscopic evaluation, possible drilling and internal stabilization.

7. Miscellaneous
   a. Referred pain
      i. **Definition.** Pain originating in one location but localized by the patient as arising from a nearby, different location.
      ii. Many children complain of lower extremity pain, and the clinician's challenge is to determine the source of the symptoms. Children and adolescents (as well as adults) may have referred pain in which disorders occurring at one site present with pain at a distal location. A classic example is the overweight adolescent boy with knee pain. An exhaustive evaluation of the knee reveals no obvious cause of his symptoms. However, a careful and thorough examination of the entire lower extremity reveals a SCFE of the hip. To avoid the common pitfalls, one must consider all of the diagnostic possibilities and complete a thorough evaluation.
   b. Tumors
      i. **Definition.** Patients with leukemia or bone tumors often present with bone or joint pain. If history and physical exam are not consistent with other causes of pain, consider possible malignancies including

Ewing sarcoma, osteogenic sarcoma, leukemia, lymphoma, neuroblastoma, etc. Obtain laboratory tests and radiographs/imaging studies appropriately.

VII. COMMON CHILDHOOD HIP DISORDERS
A. Developmental Dysplasia of the HIP (DDH)
1. **Definition.** A spectrum of disorders ranging from complete dislocation of the femoral head to a reduced hip joint with acetabular dysplasia.
2. **Incidence.** Approximately 1 in 1,000 live births.
3. **Risk factors:** include first born, female, breech position in utero, oligohydramnios, and a positive family history. It has also been associated with other congenital conditions including congenital muscular torticollis, metatarsus adductus, and clubfeet.
4. **Physical examination.** In the newborn child or young infant, physical examination should start with a careful evaluation of the other parts of the child other than the hips, including the spine, neck, and upper and lower extremities. Then, focus examination on the hips, trying to detect any evidence of instability. The clinical tests performed include the Barlow/Ortolani and Galeazzi tests. The **Barlow** and **Ortolani** tests are performed with the clinician stabilizing the pelvis with one hand and grasping the child's femur with the other, placing the thumb over the medial femoral condyle and the long finger over the greater trochanter. The hip is flexed to 90 degrees and held in neutral abduction. The Ortolani maneuver consists of abducting the hip and trying to detect the "clunking" sensation of the dislocated femoral head relocating into the acetabulum. Likewise, the Barlow test consists of two maneuvers. The first consists of adducting the hip with gentle longitudinal pressure to provoke the hip to dislocate or subluxate. The second maneuver is the same as that described for the Ortolani maneuver to achieve reduction of the dislocated hip. The **Galeazzi** test consists of comparing the height of the knees with the hips flexed to discern any apparent femoral shortening. One should also check for symmetric degrees of hip abduction as well as for asymmetry of the perineal skin folds. Finally, DDH can be bilateral, which can be easily missed clinically because there is no apparent asymmetry. These children may first come to attention after walking age, with increased lumbar lordosis, limb length difference, or a "waddling gait."
5. **Radiographic evaluation.** In the young infant, ultrasound is the modality of choice to detect any evidence of hip abnormality. The ultrasound allows a static assessment of acetabular development (alpha and beta angles) and percentage of femoral head coverage as well as dynamic assessment of femoral head stability with stress maneuvers. In children older than 6 months, plain AP radiographs are sufficient.
6. **Treatment**
   a. **Age 0 to 6 months.** In the newborn child up to 6 months of age, treatment consists of abduction bracing, usually performed with a **Pavlik harness**. This is usually applied at the time the instability is noted. It may also be used for children with a clinically stable hip but who have significant acetabular dysplasia noted on ultrasound. Moreover, the adequacy of the reduction or positioning in the Pavlik harness can be evaluated with ultrasound. There have been several reports in the literature of "Pavlik harness disease" in which the femoral head was not adequately reduced in the acetabulum while in the harness, leading to progressive deformation of the posterior wall of the acetabulum and exacerbation of the dysplasia. If an adequate, concentric reduction of the femoral head cannot be achieved by 4 weeks after the harness has been applied, treatment with the Pavlik harness should be abandoned (14,15).
   b. **Age 6 to 18 months or the child who fails Pavlik harness treatment.** Treatment for this group is aimed at achieving a satisfactory, congruent, stable reduction. This is achieved by performing either a **closed** or an **open** reduction. Historically, traction has been employed preoperatively in

order to decrease the risk of avascular necrosis of the femoral head after closed reduction. An arthrogram is frequently performed at the time of the closed reduction. If the hip is noted to have a narrow "stable zone," a limited adductor release may be performed to improve stability. If a concentric reduction is not achievable or if excessive force is required to maintain the reduction, then an open reduction may be performed. Popular methods for performing the open reduction include an anterolateral approach and the medial approach (14).
- c. **Age older than 18 months.** Some authors still advocate a trial of preoperative skin traction followed by attempted closed reduction. Alternatively, one can consider open reduction performed in conjunction with femoral shortening to reduce soft-tissue tension and thereby decrease risk of avascular necrosis. If significant acetabular dysplasia is present, a pelvic osteotomy may also be performed (16).
- d. **Secondary procedures.** For older children with persistent acetabular dysplasia or persistent hip subluxation, secondary procedures may take the form of femoral or pelvic osteotomies. Adolescents or young adults may present with hip pain from previously undiagnosed dysplasia. They may be candidates for a redirectional pelvic osteotomy.

B. Legg-Calvé-Perthes disease
1. **Definition.** Idiopathic avascular necrosis to the femoral head in children.
2. **Presentation.** Most often affects children aged 4 to 8 years; however, it may affect children as young as 2 or as old as 12 years. The ratio of incidence in boys to girls is 4:1. The disease may be bilateral in 10% of patients. Patients frequently have younger skeletal age than cohorts. Frequently, the disease presents as a painless limp (**Fig. 5-2**).
3. **Etiology: idiopathic.** It has been associated with abnormalities of thrombolysis as well as deficiencies of protein C, protein S, or thrombolysin.
4. **Differential diagnosis.** If bilateral hip involvement is present on radiograph, then other possible etiologies should be excluded, including renal disease, hypothyroidism, multiple epiphyseal dysplasia or spondyloepiphyseal dysplasia, systemic corticosteroid use, storage disorders, and hemoglobinopathies.
5. **Stages.** Waldenström originally described evolutionary stages that the disease course follows. These have been modified from the original description to include the following:
    - a. **Initial stage.** Femoral head appears sclerotic early in the course of the disease.
    - b. **Fragmentation stage.** Presence of subchondral fracture (Salter sign) is hallmark of onset. The femoral head develops "fragmented" appearance on radiograph as necrotic bone undergoes resorption.
    - c. **Reossification stage.** There is evidence of healing; coalescence of femoral head fragmentation begins to occur.
    - d. **Healed stage.** Reossification is complete. Femoral head returns to predisease density. Any remaining deformity is permanent.
6. **Classification systems.** To describe and to compare the results of treatment, various classification systems have been described.
    - a. **Catterall.** Four-part system (I–IV) based on the amount of femoral head involvement
    - b. **Salter-Thompson.** Two part system (A, B) simplified to less than 50% or greater than 50% involvement of femoral head.
    - c. **Herring:** Recently revised to a four-part system (A, B, BC, C) based on height of lateral "pillar" (lateral one third of femoral epiphysis).
7. **Treatment.** For patients with Legg-Calvé-Perthes disease, it is important to determine which patients will benefit from treatment as well as how to treat them. Risk factors for a poor prognosis include:
    - a. Older age at presentation (>8 years old)
    - b. Greater degree of involvement of the femoral head using any of the above classification systems.

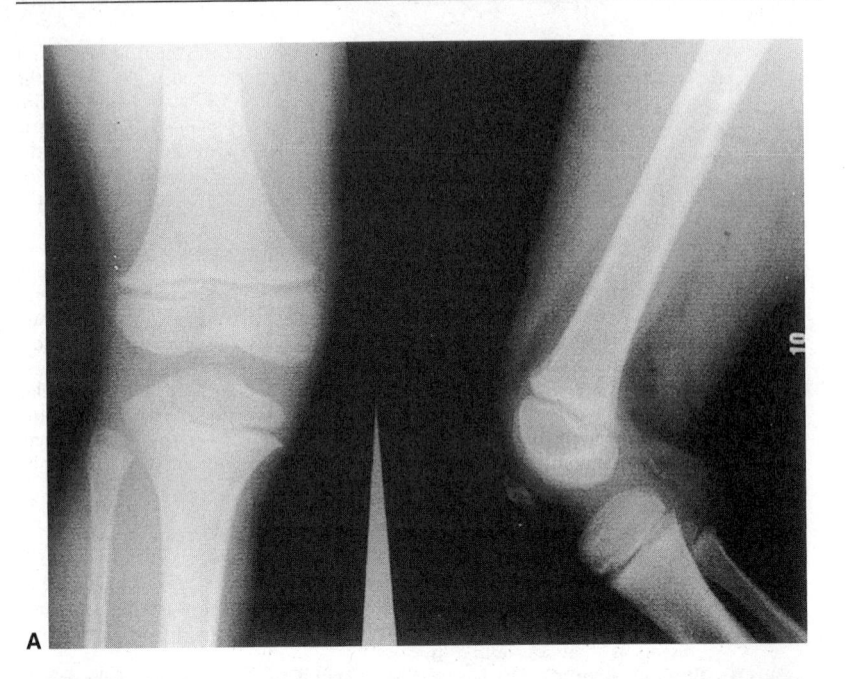

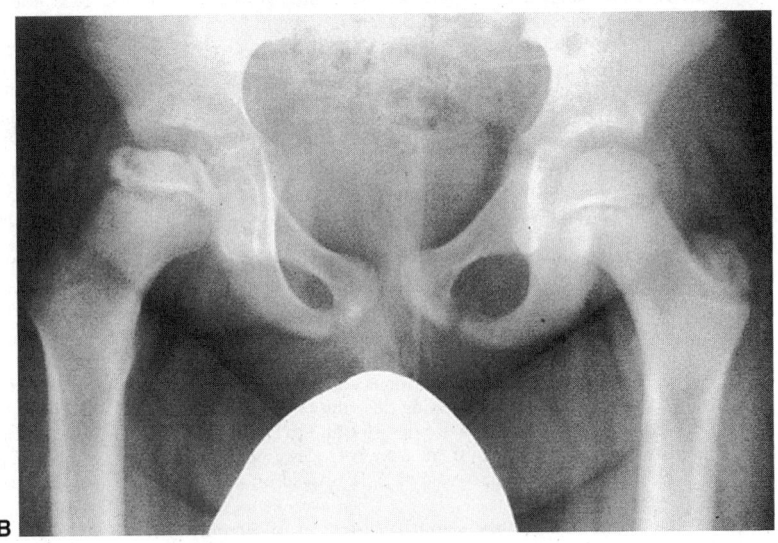

80　Chapter 5: Pediatric Orthopaedic Conditions

Figure 5-2. A 6-year-old boy with a 1- to 2-month history of limping and right knee pain. **A:** Radiographs of the knee are normal. **B:** An AP pelvis radiograph reveals changes in the right hip consistent with Legg-Calvé-Perthes disease.

The hallmarks of treatment consist of:
  a. Maintaining hip range of motion
  b. "Containment" of the femoral head in the acetabulum.

  For younger patients or patients with less involvement of the femoral head, treatment may consist primarily of NSAIDs, physical therapy, and restriction of activities to maintain hip range of motion. For older children, especially those who have more involvement of the hip (and therefore a worse prognosis), treatment may consist of surgical containment of femoral head by femoral and/or pelvic osteotomies (17). Abduction bracing was used historically but now is used very rarely.

C. **Slipped Capital Femoral Epiphysis (SCFE)**
  1. **Definition.** A disorder of the upper femur in which there is a separation (acutely or chronically) of the femoral epiphysis from the femoral neck through the region of the physis (growth plate). The femoral head becomes positioned posterior and inferior relative to the femoral neck.
  2. **Incidence.** Approximately 3 in 100,000; boys more frequently than girls. Bilateral involvement occurs in between 20% and 60% of cases. SCFE is seen most frequently in boys aged 12 to 16 years and in girls aged 10 to 14 years. SCFE is associated with obesity, with more than half of affected individuals weighing greater than the 95th percentile. (Note: Not all patients with SCFE are obese.) Patients with an underlying hormonal or endocrine disorder have an associated increased risk for development of SCFE. For patients with an unusual presentation such as atypical age (before age 10), bilateral involvement at presentation, or with other signs of possible endocrine abnormalities, a careful evaluation for endocrine disorders including hypothyroidism, hypopituitarism or hypogonadism should be conducted.
  3. **Classification**
     a. **Temporal.** One method of classification is based on duration of symptoms. Acute is less than 3 weeks, chronic is greater than 3 weeks, and acute-on-chronic is a sudden exacerbation of subclinical symptoms of long-standing duration.
     b. **Stability.** This classification system has gained greater popularity because it appears to be clinically more useful. A patient with a **stable SCFE** is able to walk without assistance, with mild pain, or a slight limp. Patients with an **unstable SCFE** are unable to walk or to bear weight. Unstable SCFEs are associated with a higher rate of complications (18).
     c. **Displacement.** Classified according to the amount of displacement of the femoral head. This may be represented as a percentage of the femoral neck width or as an angular value measured by the lateral head-shaft angle.
  4. **Treatment.** The most widely recommended form of treatment is surgical stabilization with **percutaneous pinning** *in situ*. For a stable SCFE, this can usually be accomplished with a single, cannulated screw inserted under fluoroscopic control (19). The aim of the procedure is to insert the screw perpendicular to the femoral head in both the AP and lateral planes with close attention to avoid penetrating the femoral head and entering the hip joint. In cases of an unstable SCFE, a second screw may be inserted to further stabilize the femoral head (**Fig. 5-3**).
  5. **Complications.** The primary complications associated with SCFE are **avascular necrosis** and **chondrolysis**. Avascular necrosis is uncommon with stable SCFE treated with pinning *in situ*. There is a greater incidence of avascular necrosis associated with unstable SCFE. A vigorous attempt at reduction of an unstable SCFE should **NOT** be performed. Chondrolysis is a gradual loss of the joint space following stabilization of the SCFE. It has been associated with treatment with one or more pins as well as with a spica cast in which no internal fixation was used.

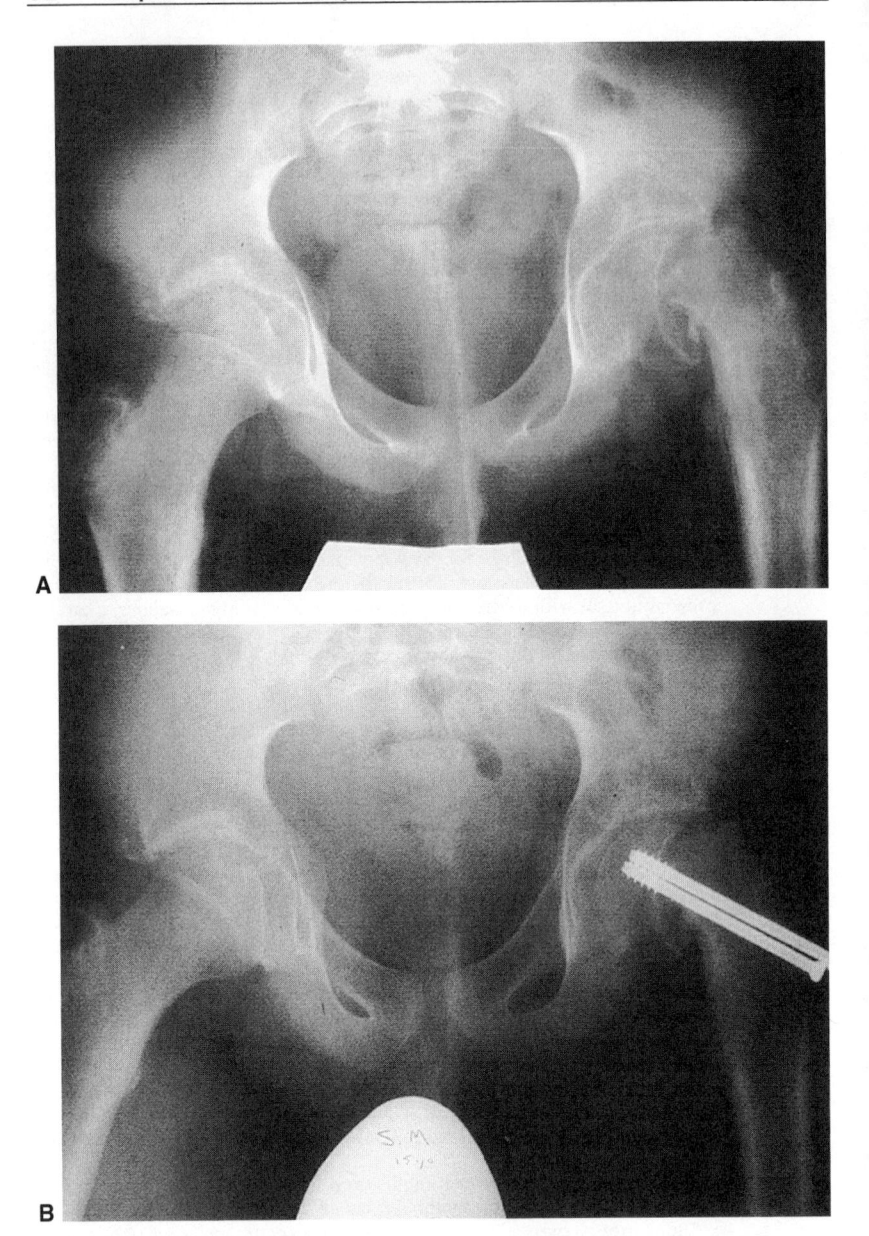

Figure 5-3. Slipped capital femoral epiphysis. **A:** A 13-year-old boy with a severe, unstable left SCFE. **B:** Two cannulated screws were inserted for stabilization.

VIII. INFECTIOUS AND INFLAMMATORY CONDITIONS
A. Osteomyelitis
1. **Definition.** A bacterial infection of the bone.
2. **Etiology.** Bacterial seeding can occur through several methods: direct inoculation (open fractures, penetrating wounds), local extension from adjacent sites, or hematogenous spread from distant sites. Children are skeletally immature and have physes at the ends of their long bones. The metaphyseal region of the bone just below the physis is a frequent location for osteomyelitis to occur.
3. **Presentation.** Patients may present with pain, limping, or refusal to walk or bear weight on the affected lower extremity. Constitutional symptoms of fever, malaise, and flu may or may not be present. One should inquire about immunization status as well as history of recent illnesses [e.g., otitis media, chicken pox, strep pharyngitis, upper respiratory tract illness (URTI)].
4. **Physical examination.** Site of involvement may or may not be easy to identify, particularly in younger patients. Careful palpation of entire extremity and the metaphyseal regions in particular is important. All joints should be placed through a range of motion. Inspect for areas of redness, swelling, or warmth.
5. **Laboratory studies.** CBC with differential, ESR, CRP, and blood cultures are helpful in making the diagnosis. The CRP has been recognized as a more rapidly responsive test than the ESR, increasing more quickly early in the evolution of the condition and declining more rapidly in response to treatment. If the diagnosis remains unclear, consider other diagnostic possibilities such as JRA, Lyme arthritis, and poststreptococcal arthritis.
6. **Radiographic studies.** Plain radiographs of the affected area should be obtained. In osteomyelitis they may frequently be normal for the first 7 to 14 days. However, the radiographs may also be useful to rule out other diagnostic possibilities. In patients with normal radiographs in whom the diagnosis is still unclear, a technetium bone scan is a sensitive test for acute osteomyelitis. It is particularly helpful in cases involving the pelvis, proximal femur, and spine. MRI is also very sensitive and has the added benefit of having greater soft-tissue detail allowing assessment of marrow involvement, soft-tissue extension or abscess formation, and presence of joint effusions. However, an MRI may require significant sedation or anesthesia for younger patients.
7. **Aspiration.** In patients with an identified focus of infection, an attempt at aspiration is recommended by many authors to identify the organism. This may be done with sedation in the emergency department or the fluoroscopic suite or, alternatively, under anesthesia in the operating room.
8. **Organisms.** On the basis of patient age:
    a. **Younger than 1 year old**
        i. *Staphylococcus aureus*
        ii. Group B *Streptococcus*
        iii. *Escherichia coli*
    b. **1 to 4 years old**
        i. *S. aureus*
        ii. *Haemophilus influenzae*
    c. **Older than 4 years old**
        i. *S. aureus*
    d. **Adolescent**
        i. *S. aureus*
        ii. *Neisseria gonorrhoeae*
9. **Treatment.** Appropriate intravenous antibiotic based on culture or most likely organism. Duration of antibiotic coverage is typically 6 weeks. After 2 to 3 weeks of IV treatment, the patient may be switched to oral antibiotics if the following criteria are met: (a) the organism has been identified, (b) there is

a satisfactory oral antibiotic to which the organism is sensitive, (c) the child will take the oral antibiotic, and (d) satisfactory serum levels can be achieved with oral therapy (20).
   10. **Surgical treatment.** If the patient does not respond to antibiotic treatment after the first 24 to 48 hours, consider the possibility of a subperiosteal or intraosseous abscess as well as other diagnostic possibilities. Consider surgical drainage of abscess or intramedullary canal if necessary (21).
B. **Septic arthritis** (22)
   1. **Definition.** An infectious arthritis of a joint, usually bacterial in nature.
   2. **Etiology.** Most frequently, it occurs as a result from adjacent osteomyelitis in which the metaphyseal portion of the bone is intraarticular (e.g., hip, shoulder, elbow, ankle). When pus from metaphysis decompresses itself through cortex, joints can become infected. Infection is also possible through hematogenous spread or direct inoculation.
   3. **Joints most commonly involved:** knee (41%), hip (23%), ankle (14%), elbow (12%), wrist (4%), and shoulder (4%).
   4. **Presentation.** Young children usually refuse to walk or bear weight on the lower extremity. The child will usually be febrile and may show signs of sepsis. If infection is in the upper extremity, children refuse to use the affected extremity. Septic arthritis may also occur in the newborn child; babies in the neonatal intensive care unit (NICU) may present with pseudoparalysis of the affected limb with failure or refusal to move it.
   5. **Physical examination.** If the joint involved is superficial, classic signs of joint redness, swelling, and warmth are present. However, if the joint is not superficial (hip, shoulder), no visible abnormality may be detectable. However, the patient will hold the affected limb in a position of maximum comfort (e.g., keep the hip in flexion and external rotation). Any attempt at passive range of motion is painful and restricted because of guarding.
   6. **Laboratory studies** include CBC with differential, ESR, CRP, and blood culture. The CRP and ESR will become significantly elevated. The CBC may remain normal.
   7. **Radiographic studies.** Plain radiographs of the affected joint should be obtained to look for any evidence of bony destruction or erosions. For patients with suspected hip pain, an ultrasound of the hip may confirm the presence of a hip joint effusion. In some institutions, aspiration is performed under ultrasound guidance.
   8. **Joint aspiration** is mandatory to confirm the diagnosis. Joint fluid should be sent for cell count, Gram stain, and culture and, if quantity permits, glucose and total protein. If the patient is a teenager in whom gonococcal infection is suspected, the laboratory should be notified in order to perform cultures on chocolate agar in addition to the routine media. The Gram stain may be positive for bacteria in only approximately 50% of patients. The cell count most often has greater than 50,000 white blood cells (WBCs) and/or greater than 90% polymorphonuclear neutrophils (PMNs).
   9. **Organisms.** On the basis of patient age:
      a. **Younger than 1 year old**
         i. *S. aureus*
         ii. Group B *Streptococcus*
         iii. *E. coli*
      b. **1 to 4 years old**
         i. *S. aureus*
         ii. *H. influenzae* (less common now with *H. influenzae* B vaccination)
         iii. Group A *Streptococcus*
         iv. *Streptococcus pneumoniae*
      c. **Older than 4 years old**
         i. *S. aureus*
         ii. Group A *Streptococcus*

Chapter 5: Pediatric Orthopaedic Conditions

   d. **Adolescent**
      i. *S. aureus*
      ii. *N. gonorrhoeae*
   e. **Less common** organisms include *Kingella kingae, Salmonella,* and *Neisseria meningitidis.*
10. **Treatment.** In patients suspected of septic arthritis, treatment consists of surgical incision and drainage of the affected joint. Surgical decompression of the adjacent bone may also be indicated if there is evidence of an intraosseous abscess. Intravenous antibiotics should be administered once intraoperative cultures have been obtained. Empiric coverage should be started initially based on the most likely organism involved. Once culture and sensitivities have been identified, antibiotic coverage can be tailored accordingly. The duration of antibiotics is usually 4 to 6 weeks. An initial course of intravenous antibiotics is followed by oral therapy until the patient's symptoms and laboratory studies have returned to normal.

C. **Transient synovitis**
   1. **Definition.** An inflammatory, noninfectious process resulting in joint swelling and pain.
   2. **Presentation.** Transient synovitis most frequently occurs in young children aged 3 to 8 years. Patients often may have had a recent upper respiratory tract illness or other viral illness in the 2 to 3 weeks before onset of symptoms. Patients are usually afebrile with a history of several days of pain or limping. The physician must differentiate between transient synovitis and a truly infectious process such as septic arthritis or osteomyelitis.
   3. **Laboratory studies.** CBC with differential, ESR, and CRP are usually within the normal range.
   4. **Radiographic studies.** Plain radiographs are usually normal or may show evidence of a joint effusion. Ultrasound is helpful for confirming the presence of a joint effusion.
   5. **Aspiration.** Because the clinician is often confronted with having to exclude septic arthritis, joint aspiration can be helpful in order to examine the joint fluid. A Gram stain, cell count, and culture should be obtained. The Gram stain should be negative and the cell count should have between 5,000 and 15,000 WBCs with less than 25% PMNs.
   6. **Treatment.** The primary treatment objective in the treatment of transient synovitis is to ensure that septic arthritis has been excluded. Once septic arthritis is excluded, then the condition can be treated expectantly with reduction in activity, NSAIDs, and careful observation (23).

IX. BACK PAIN AND SPINE-RELATED CONDITIONS
A. **Evaluation of the patient with back pain**
   1. **History**
      a. Location of pain (neck/thoracic/lumbar)
      b. Radiation of pain into lower extremities
      c. Associated symptoms such as numbness, tingling, weakness, change in bowel or bladder function, pain at night, etc.
      d. Onset of pain (acute/gradual)
      e. Frequency and duration of symptoms
      f. Any improvement with NSAIDs/aspirin
      g. Is patient involved in athletic activities that are associated with repetitive hyperextension of back such as figure skating, gymnastics, dance, football (particularly lineman) or hockey?
   2. **Physical exam.** Have patient dressed in examination gown or other appropriate clothing.
      a. Back ROM: flexion/extension/side bending/rotation
      b. Pain with palpation along spine
      c. Radicular pain associated with straight-leg test
      d. Complete neurologic exam including:
         i. Motor strength
         ii. Sensation

iii. Deep tendon reflexes
iv. Signs of upper motor neuron abnormalities: clonus, Babinski, etc.
v. Abdominal reflexes
  e. Adam's forward bending test (see below)
  f. Hip ROM: possible referred pain from hip pathology
3. **Radiologic tests.** If pediatric patient describes significant back pain and/or any abnormal findings are present on physical exam, it is appropriate to obtain plain radiographs.
  a. AP and lateral radiograph of thoracic and lumbar spine if pain is localized to thoracic or thoracolumbar region or any findings to suggest scoliosis.
  b. AP/lateral and oblique images of lumbar spine if patient localizes pain to lumbar region of back or pain radiates into lower extremities.
  c. Evaluate radiographs for signs of:
     i. Scoliosis
     ii. Spondylolysis/spondylolisthesis
     iii. Loss of disc space
     iv. Vertebral end-plate changes (erosions, Schmorl nodes)
     v. Other bony changes (absent pedicle, curvature without rotation, etc.)
4. **Additional imaging tests.** If neurologic abnormalities are identified on physical exam, consider MRI of spinal canal. If no neurologic findings are present but pain presentation is worrisome for underlying bone tumor or structural abnormality, consider three-phase nuclear medicine bone scan.
5. **Differential diagnosis**
  a. Mechanical low-back pain
  b. Spondylolysis/Spondylolisthesis
  c. Discitis
  d. Lumbar Scheuermann disease
  e. Herniated intervertebral disc
  f. Spine-related bone tumors
6. **Mechanical low-back pain**
  a. Definition: back pain usually localized to the lower back without radiation to lower extremities and without neurologic findings on physical exam or radiographic abnormalities. Previously thought to be rare in children, it remains less common in children than in adults but can be a source of back pain if other causes have been excluded. Symptoms most often occur after sitting for long periods of time, tend to be vague or non-specific, and occur sporadically.
  b. Physical exam: notable for lack of abnormal findings.
  c. Radiographic exam: plain radiographs are normal. No specialized radiographic studies are recommended at the time of the initial evaluation.
  d. Treatment:
     i. Referral to physical therapy for home-based exercise program of back strengthening and posture retraining.
     ii. Prescription for NSAIDs.
     iii. Return to clinic in 1 to 2 months for follow-up. If symptoms not improved or have changed, reconsider diagnosis.
7. **Spondylolysis/spondylolisthesis.**
  a. **Spondylolysis:** a structural defect in the bone in the posterior elements of the spine. Most often in the "pars interarticularlis" region of the L5 vertebra. Associated with hyper-extension activities such as dance, gymnastics, figure skating; presents as low-lumbar back pain without radiation into the lower extremities but exacerbated by hyperextension activities.
  b. **Spondylolisthesis:** a translation or slippage of one vertebra on the next lower vertebra. The most common cause in children is an "isthmic spondylolisthesis" in which a lesion or defect in the pars interarticularis permits forward slippage of the superior vertebra.
8. **Discitis.** A condition in which children develop back pain that arises from a presumed bacterial infection of the intervertebral disc. They may present

with gradual onset of pain, loss of lumbar lordosis, and progressive decline in activity level potentially to the point of refusing to walk. The child may remain afebrile. Current theories of etiology suggest it may start as a vertebral osteomyelitis that spreads to the adjacent disc space. If suspected, laboratory tests should be obtained including CBC with differential, ESR, CRP, and blood cultures. The CBC may be normal but some elevation of the ESR and CRP is frequently present. Initial radiographs may be normal or may show vertebral end-plate irregularities. Later radiographs may show a narrowing of the disc space involved. The diagnosis may be confirmed with specialized imaging tests such as nuclear medicine bone scan, CT, or MRI. Treatment consists of antibiotic therapy and, when appropriate, back immobilization with a removable spinal orthosis for symptomatic support.

9. **Lumbar Scheuermann disease.** A condition in which patients present with lumbar back pain without radicular symptoms. There are end-plate changes termed "Schmorl nodes" in the lumbar vertebra on plain radiographs. In contrast to Scheuermann's disease of the thoracic spine (see below), which is associated with significant thoracic kyphosis and vertebral wedging, these changes are not found in the lumbar spine.

10. **Herniated intervertebral disc.** A herniation of the central portion of the disc, the "nucleus pulposus," into the spinal canal. Occurs in adolescent and teenage patients. Symptoms usually have an acute, specific onset and are associated with radicular symptoms of pain radiating down into the lower extremity. Neurologic exam is helpful to look for signs of motor weakness. An **avulsion fracture of the vertebral ring apophysis** may also present with sudden onset of back pain with radicular-type symptoms radiating into the lower extremities. This may be visible on plain films as a small triangular fragment of bone displaced from the lower end plate of the vertebra. If a herniated disc or a vertebral ring apophysis avulsion-type fracture is suspected, an MRI scan can help confirm diagnosis.

11. **Bone tumors involving the spine.** There are a number of bone tumors that may arise from the vertebral body or the posterior elements of the spine. They may present with pain, particularly night pain, deformity, or other associated symptoms. Physical exam may reveal findings of scoliosis, however, radiographs may reveal a curvature of the spine without any rotational component present. This suggests that the curvature is postural, due to the painful process, rather than a structural, scoliosis-type curve. Benign tumors that arise in the spine most frequently include osteoid osteoma, osteoblastoma, and hemangioma. Primary malignant tumors of the bone that arise in the spine are relatively rare.

B. **Idiopathic adolescent scoliosis**
1. **Definition.** A deformity of the spine consisting of a lateral curvature measuring greater than 10 degrees on a spine radiograph that also has a rotational component. The word "idiopathic" suggests no identifiable, underlying cause. There may be a genetic component.
2. **Presentation.** Most often patients are adolescent girls who have been detected either on school screening examination or by an observant primary physician. Boys are affected less often and have a lower incidence of progressive curves. The deformity may occasionally be seen in younger children. Family history is frequently positive. Idiopathic scoliosis should be **painless**. The examiner should inquire about any neurologic symptoms including weakness, numbness, radicular symptoms, or bowel or bladder changes.
3. **Incidence.** For curves greater than 10 degrees, the overall incidence is 2%. However, for curves measuring greater than 20 degrees and requiring treatment, the incidence is 0.2%.
4. **Physical examination.** All patients should be examined in a gown so that the back can be well visualized. Inspect pelvic height for evidence of limb

length difference. Examine shoulder height and trunk position for evidence of asymmetry or truncal imbalance. With the patient standing, have the patient bend forward at the waist. Observe the patient's back for evidence of rib hump deformity. This is the **Adam forward bending test**. Finally, complete a thorough neurologic examination, including abdominal reflexes and tests for long tract or upper motor neuron lesions.

5. **Radiographic evaluation.** PA and lateral spine radiographs on a long cassette to include the thoracic, lumbar, and sacral regions of the spine. The curvature of the spine can be measured using the COBB method.
6. **Characteristics.** For true idiopathic scoliosis, the curve is most often:
   a. Painless
   b. Convex to the right in the thoracic spine
   c. Not associated with any neurologic changes

   If a curve does not fit this pattern, one must exclude other possible causes. If the curve is convex to the left, painful, has associated neurologic changes, or is rapidly progressive, one should consider obtaining an MRI scan in order to rule out possible underlying spinal cord abnormalities such as syringomyelia, tethered cord, diastematomyelia, or spinal cord tumor.
7. **Risk factors for progression** include young age, female gender, prepubertal status, and curve greater than 11 degrees. The spine curve is at greatest risk for progression during periods of accelerated skeletal growth (24).
8. The **goal of treatment** is to prevent further progression of the curve.
9. **Treatment** of idiopathic scoliosis depends on the size of the curve as well as the age of the patient at the time of detection. Typically, for curves greater than 11 degrees and less than 20 degrees, treatment consists of **observation** with repeat spine radiographs obtained in 4 to 6 months. The younger the child at the time of curve detection, the greater the risk for future progression of the curve. If the curve is greater than 20 to 25 degrees in a skeletally immature patient, **brace treatment** is indicated. Brace treatment is most effective in moderate-sized and flexible curves in growing adolescent patients. The goal of brace treatment is to arrest any further progression of the curve. For patients in whom a large curve of greater than 45 to 50 degrees is already present or for whom the curve progresses despite brace treatment, treatment is **surgical spinal fusion with instrumentation**.

C. **Kyphosis**
   1. **Definition.** An increased curvature of the thoracic spine in the sagittal plane, either from the side or on the lateral radiograph, producing a rounded-back appearance.
   2. **Characteristics.** Normal thoracic kyphosis is 20 to 45 degrees. **Scheuermann disease** is a condition in which the thoracic curve on the lateral radiograph is greater than 45 degrees and associated with wedging of three adjacent central vertebral bodies of 5 degrees or more. It may be associated with endplate changes of the vertebral bodies such as Schmorl nodes. It should be distinguished from postural kyphosis, in which the vertebral bodies do not exhibit changes and the curvature resolves with improvement of the patient's posture.
   3. **Presentation.** Patients usually have one of two complaints: pain or concerns regarding appearance.
   4. **Physical examination.** Careful examination of the back with the patient standing, on forward bending, and with hyperextension in the prone position can help determine the flexibility of the kyphosis. Increased thoracic kyphosis is frequently associated with increased lumbar lordosis. The possibility of hip flexion contractures should be assessed. A careful neurologic examination should also be performed.
   5. **Radiographs.** Standing PA and lateral thoracolumbar spine radiographs should be obtained.
   6. **Treatment.** Options include observation, bracing, and surgery. For patients who are asymptomatic with a relatively small curve, one may consider

continued observation. For symptomatic patients who are skeletally immature with curves greater than 45 to 50 degrees, one may consider brace treatment. The indications for surgical treatment include kyphosis greater than 70 degrees, progressive deformity, recalcitrant pain, and concerns regarding patient appearance in the setting of significant deformity (25).

D. Lordosis
  1. **Definition.** An increase in "swayback" appearance of the lower lumbar spine.
  2. **Presentation.** The patient may complain of low back pain, concern regarding appearance, or both.
  3. **Etiology.** Possible causes include posture (especially in younger patients), bilateral congenital dislocation of the hip, hip flexion contracture, hamstring weakness, increased thoracic kyphosis, spondylolysis/spondylolisthesis, and congenital spinal deformity.
  4. **Physical examination** should include careful evaluation of the back, hips, and lower extremities and should also include a thorough neurologic evaluation.
  5. **Radiographs.** PA and lateral thoracolumbar spine radiographs should be obtained.
  6. **Treatment.** Careful exclusion of underlying abnormalities should be undertaken. If other underlying causes have been excluded and the cause is thought to be postural, then treatment may consist of further observation.

X. NEUROMUSCULAR DISORDERS
  A. Cerebral palsy (26,27)
    1. **Definition.** A nonprogressive disorder resulting from an injury to the brain, usually within the first year of life, and resulting in impairment in motor function.
    2. **Classification** can be geographic (part of body most affected) or by type of motor dysfunction.
      a. **Geographic**
        i. **Hemiplegia.** Arm and leg on one side only affected
        ii. **Diplegia.** Major spasticity in lower limbs, less in upper
        iii. **Triplegia.** Three-limb involvement
        iv. **Quadriplegia.** All four limbs, "total body involved"
      b. **Motor type**
        i. **Spastic.** Increased stretch reflexes (pyramidal)
        ii. **Athetoid.** Fluctuating motor tone, often with spontaneous, involuntary rhythmic motor movements (extrapyramidal)
        iii. **Dystonia.** Similar to athetoid; intermittent or inconsistent tone
        iv. **Mixed.** A combination of spasticity and dystonia
    3. **Causes**
      a. **Prenatal.** Intrauterine infection, for example, TORCH (toxoplasmosis, rubella, cytomegalovirus, and herpes simplex), genetic or chromosomal abnormalities
      b. **Perinatal.** Premature birth, low birth weight, asphyxia, erythroblastosis fetalis
      c. **Postnatal.** Infection, stroke, cardiac arrest, near drowning
    4. **Hierarchical approach to problems**
      a. **Primary problems** include abnormal muscle tone, poor selective muscle control, and poor balance.
      b. **Secondary problems** include muscle and joint contractures and bony deformities (increased femoral anteversion, tibial torsion, and foot deformities).
      c. **Tertiary problems** include compensatory mechanisms for primary and secondary problems.
    5. **Treatment**
      a. **Physical therapy**
      b. **Orthotics**
      c. **Assistive devices:** wheelchair, walker, crutches
      d. **Tone-reducing agents or medications:** oral (e.g., baclofen, Valium, dantrolene) or focal (e.g., Botox, phenol)

- e. **Neurosurgical options:** selective dorsal rhizotomy, intrathecal baclofen pump
- f. **Orthopaedic surgery:** soft-tissue lengthening procedures, bony realignment procedures
6. **Nonambulatory patients.** The principal difficulties that affect patients with total body involvement are hip dislocation and neuromuscular scoliosis. These are important issues for these patients because they are wheelchair bound and frequently mentally handicapped. Painful sitting or difficulty with sitting balance resulting from scoliosis or pelvic obliquity can interfere significantly with their activities of daily living, personal care, and activity level. Patients should be monitored regularly for early detection of either hip dislocation or scoliosis.
7. **Ambulatory patients.** If children have independent sitting balance by age 2 years old, then there is approximately a 95% chance that they will eventually be able to ambulate. Children with cerebral palsy who can ambulate usually have difficulty because of increased motor tone, poor selective motor control, which results in co-contracture of muscle groups, and poor balance. Frequently, muscle contractures and bony deformities develop over time. Three-dimensional gait analysis is useful to assess walking in these children in order to identify a problem list of orthopaedic issues or deformities that are contributing to the patients difficulty in walking. Orthopaedic surgery usually consists of muscle lengthening or transfer procedures combined with bony realignment procedures for underlying torsional deformities of the lower extremities. Most often, these are combined in one surgical setting to minimize recovery time and to speed the child's return to activities. The **selective dorsal rhizotomy** is a procedure to decrease lower extremity tone by cutting approximately 30% to 40% of the dorsal afferent sensory nerve rootlets. It is indicated for children with spastic diplegia who have pure spasticity, no contractures, and good balance. It is usually performed in children between the ages of 4 and 8 years old. For children with cerebral palsy, optimum treatment consists of a combined approach involving the physiatrist, the neurosurgeon, the orthopaedic surgeon, the physical and occupational therapists, and the orthotist.

B. **Spina bifida** (28)
   1. **Definition.** A malformation of the spine, resulting from incomplete closure of the posterior elements of the spine as well as of the neural tube in which the meninges and neural elements are exposed at birth.
   2. **Etiology** is multifactorial. There is a genetic component in that there is increased risk for first-degree relatives of patients with spina bifida. There is also an environmental role linked to insufficient dietary folic acid for women of childbearing age.
   3. **Classification** is based on the level of neurologic deficit.
   4. **Associated disorders** include hydrocephalus requiring ventriculoperitoneal shunting, tethered spinal cord, Arnold-Chiari malformations, syringomyelia, and urologic problems.
   5. **Orthopaedic conditions** include scoliosis for patients with high thoracic level deficits, excessive spinal kyphosis, hip dislocation, and foot deformities.
   6. **Ambulatory function** is determined primarily by level of deficit. Patients who ambulate are usually patients who maintain active control of knee flexion and extension. Many children ambulate when young, but as they get older, it takes greater energy and oxygen consumption, and many resort to using a wheelchair.

References
1. Flynn JM, Widmann RF. The limping child: evaluation and diagnosis. *J Am Acad Orthop Surg* 2001;9(2):89–98.
2. Phillips WA. The child with a limp. *Orthop Clin North Am* 1987;18:489–501.
3. Staheli LT. Rotational problems in children. *Instr Course Lect* 1994;43:199–209.
4. Heath DH, Staheli LT. Normal limits of knee angle in children, genu varum and genu valgum. *J Pediatr Orthop* 1993;13:259–262.

5. Cummings RJ, Davidson RS, Armstrong PF, et al. Congenital clubfoot. *J Bone Joint Surg (Am)* 2002;84A:290–308.
6. Cooper DM, Dietz FR. Treatment of idiopathic clubfeet. *J Bone Joint Surg (Am)* 1995;77:1477–1489.
7. Mosca VS. Calcaneal lengthening for valgus deformity of the hindfoot. *J Bone Joint Surg (Am)* 1995;77:500–512.
8. Comfort TK, Johnson LO. Resection of symptomatic talocalcaneal coalition. *J Pediatr Orthop* 1998;18:283–288.
9. Swiontkowski MF, Scranton PE, Hansen S. Tarsal coalitions: long-term results of surgical treatment. *J Pediatr Orthop* 1983;3:287–292.
10. Peterson HA, Newman SR. Adolescent bunion deformity treated with double osteotomy and longitudinal pin fixation of the first ray. *J Pediatr Orthop* 1993;13:80–84.
11. Geissele AE, Stanton RP. Surgical treatment of adolescent hallux valgus. *J Pediatr Orthop* 1990;10:38–44.
12. Fulkerson JP, Shea KP. Disorders of patellofemoral alignment. *J Bone Joint Surg (Am)* 1990;72:1424–1429.
13. Stanitski CL. Meniscal lesions. In: Stanitski CL, DeLee AB, Drez CD, eds. *Pediatric and adolescent sports medicine*, Philadelphia, PA: WB Saunders, 1994:382–384.
14. Weinstein SL, Mubarak SJ, Wenger DR. Developmental hip dysplasia and dislocation. Part I. *J Bone Joint Surg (Am)* 2003;85:1824–1832.
15. Viere RG, Birch JG, Herring JA, et al. Use of the Pavlik harness in congenital dislocation of the hip, an analysis of failures of treatment. *J Bone Joint Surg (Am)* 1990;72:238–244.
16. Weinstein SL, Mubarak SJ, Wenger DR. Developmental hip dysplasia and dislocation. Part I. *J Bone Joint Surg (Am)* 2003;85A:2024–2035.
17. Herring JA. Legg-Calve-Perthes disease: a review of current knowledge. In: Barr JS Jr, ed. *Instructional course lectures 38*, Park Ridge, IL: American Academy of Orthopaedic Surgeons, 1989:309–315.
18. Loder RT, Richards BS, Shapiro PS, et al. Acute slipped capital femoral epiphysis: the importance of physeal stability. *J Bone Joint Surg (Am)* 1993;75:1134–1140.
19. Ward WT, Stefko J, Wood KB, et al. Fixation with a single screw for slipped capital femoral epiphysis. *J Bone Joint Surg (Am)* 1992;74:799–809.
20. Dagan R. Management of acute hematogenous osteomyelitis and septic arthritis in the pediatric patient. *Pediatr Infect Dis J* 1993;12:88–92.
21. Morrisy RT, Haynes DW. Acute hematogenous osteomyelitis: a model with trauma as an etiology. *J Pediatr Orthop* 1989;9:447–456.
22. Kocher MS, Mandiga R, Murphy JM, et al. A clinical practice guideline for treatment of septic arthritis in children: efficiency in improving process of care and effect on outcome of septic arthritis of the hip. *J Bone Joint Surg (Am)* 2003;85:994–999.
23. Haueisen D, Weisner D, Weiner S. The characterization of transient synovitis of the hip in children. *J Pediatr Orthop* 1986;6:11–17.
24. Lonstein JE, Carlson JM. The prediction of curve progression in untreated scoliosis during growth. *J Bone Joint Surg (Am)* 1984;66:1061–1071.
25. Murray PM, Weinstein SL, Spratt KF. The natural history and long-term follow-up of Scheuermann's kyphosis. *J Bone Joint Surg (Am)* 1993;75:236–248.
26. Bleck EE. Orthopaedic management in cerebral palsy. *Clinics in developmental medicine Nos 99/100*. Philadelphia, PA: JB Lippincott, 1987.
27. Gage JR. Gait analysis in cerebral palsy. *Clinics in developmental medicine no. 121*, New York: Mac Keith Press, 1991.
28. Broughton NS, Menelaus MB, eds. *Menelaus' orthopaedic management of spina bifida cystica*. Philadelphia, PA: WB Saunders, 1998.

COMMON TYPES OF EMERGENCY SPLINTS 6

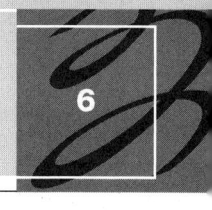

I. **EMERGENCY SPLINTING OF THE SPINE**
   A. Patients with spinal injuries should be splinted with a **backboard** before they are moved, as shown in **Fig. 6-1**. Immobilize patients with suspected cervical spine injuries by placing sandbags, rolled towels, or rolled blankets on each side of the head. Then put a cravat through or around the backboard and over the forehead. **In this way, the patient's head, neck, and backboard can be moved as one unit.** Commercial foam as well as plastic neck collars are available in different sizes and are carried by emergency medical technician (EMT) units. One can also make an adequate neck collar by placing foam or felt of the appropriate width, thickness, and length inside a tubular stockinet and then fastening the stockinet about the patient's neck. This method is particularly useful for immobilizing the neck of injured children where correct sizing is critical so as to immobilize the neck without extension or flexion. The only emergency indication for moving the neck of an individual with a suspected injured cervical spine is to improve an inadequate airway by aligning the neck with the torso and opening the airway with a jaw thrust.
   B. Be aware of possible **neurogenic shock,** which is treated by elevating the lower end of the backboard to improve venous return in the reverse Trendelenburg position.
   C. If complete evaluation identifies a cervical spine fracture, then the patient is usually placed in **traction** or hard collar immobilization. The direction of traction depends on the injury. If there is no dislocation, then a neutral or slightly extended position is preferred (see **Chap. 9**).

II. **UPPER EXTREMITY SPLINTING**
   A. **Remember to remove rings from an involved hand!** Swelling can make them impossible to remove without cutting them off and they obscure x-rays. Petroleum jelly can be useful for ring removal.
   B. Figure-of-8 splint
      1. The **principal use** is for **clavicular fractures** (see **Chap. 13**).
      2. **Application.** The factory-made figure-of-8 clavicular strap is recommended because it is a webbed fabric and does not stretch. If a properly fitting factory-made strap is not available for children younger than 10 years old, make a figure-of-8 strap with a tubular stockinet filled with felt or cotton padding, as shown in **Fig. 6-2**. These should be used only if they make the patient more comfortable. A sling is generally more effective in this regard. Generally, the figure-of-8 splint does not improve fracture reduction.
      3. **Precautions**
         a. **Prevent skin maceration** with a **powdered pad** in the axilla.
         b. In the adult, restrict the use of the sling and encourage glenohumeral motion after 2 weeks to **prevent shoulder stiffness**.
         c. Do not tighten the figure-of-8 strap to the point that the **axillary artery or brachial plexus is compressed**.
   C. Velpeau and sling-and-swathe bandages
      1. These bandages are **used** for **shoulder dislocations, proximal humerus fractures, and humeral fractures**.
      2. One **application** of Velpeau bandage using bias-cut stockinet is seen in **Fig. 6-3**. The common application of the typical sling-and-swathe bandage is shown in

94 Chapter 6: Common Types of Emergency Splints

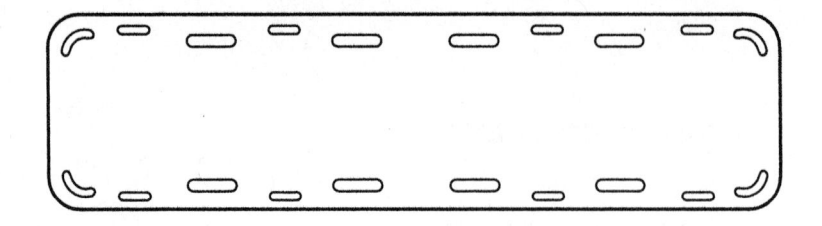

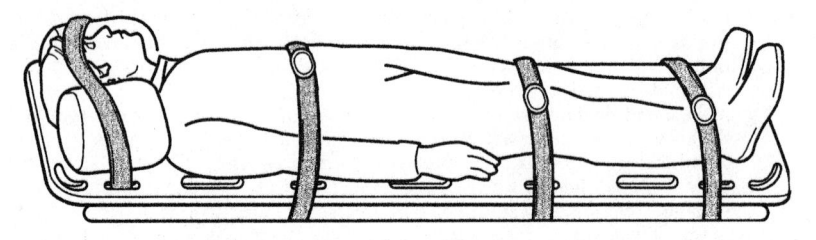

Figure 6-1. A backboard may be used in an emergency to transport a patient with a spinal injury.

Fig. 6-4. Either type of bandage can be covered with a light layer of fiberglass or plaster to prevent unraveling of the material.
3. **Precautions**
   a. **Prevent skin maceration** with a **powdered pad** in the axilla and between the arm and chest.
   b. **Prevent wrist and finger stiffness** with active exercise.

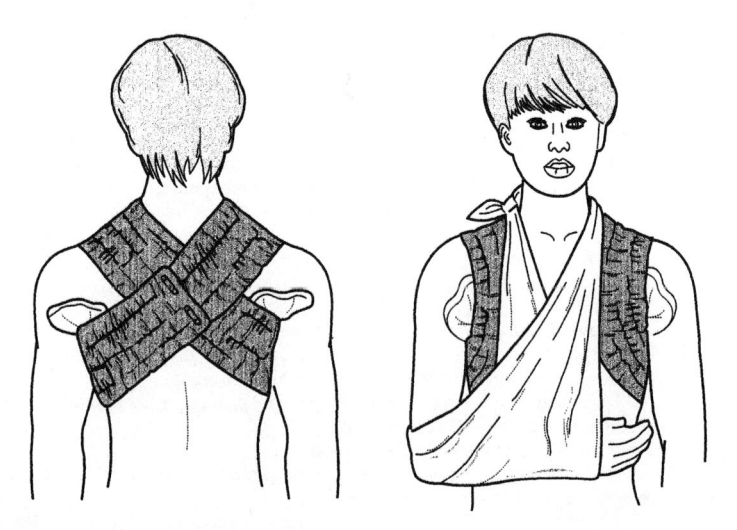

Figure 6-2. Typical figure-of-8 splint made for a child younger than 10 years old with a fractured clavicle. In adults, use a factory-made splint when possible.

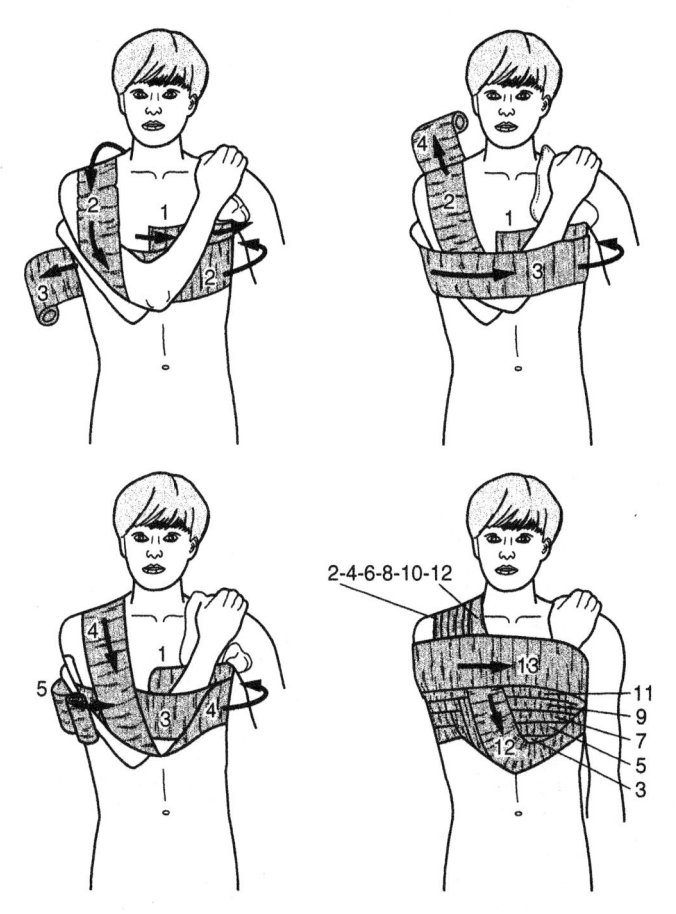

Figure 6-3. Method for applying Velpeau bandage.

4. A number of commercial **shoulder immobilizers** are available. Although they provide less secure immobilization than the Velpeau and sling-and-swathe bandages, these ready-made items have proved satisfactory. Commercial straps for acromioclavicular (AC) separations are also available; they have straps which go over the distal one third of the clavicle and lift up on the elbow in order to reduce the AC separation.
D. Use **air splints** in emergency situations for the distal extremity. The air splint is closed over the extremity by its zipper and inflated by flowing air into the mouth tube. High pressure from mechanical pumps can produce circulatory embarrassment and should not be used. Skin maceration occurs if air splints are used for any extended period. Cardboard or magazines can be used with tape of any sort to achieve temporary immobilization.

III. **LOWER EXTREMITY SPLINTING**
   A. **Thomas splint**
      1. Use for **femoral shaft fractures** and, **occasionally, knee injuries.** The following description is for the emergency situation. The Thomas splint may also be used as fixed skeletal traction, as described in **Chap. 9, VII.F.3**.

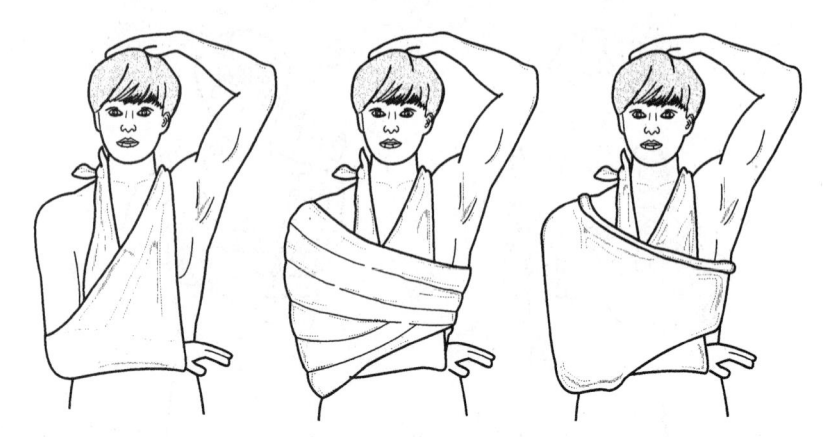

Figure 6-4. Sling-and-swathe bandage, covered by a single layer of plaster to help prevent unraveling of the material.

   2. The ideal Thomas splint **application** uses a full ring splint that measures 2 in. greater than the circumference of the proximal thigh. If a full ring splint is not available, use a half ring splint with a strap placed anteriorly. The ring engages the ischial tuberosity for countertraction, and traction is applied to the end of the splint with an ankle hitch, as shown in **Fig. 6-5**. A Spanish windlass is made by taping several tongue blades together. These twist the material used to secure the ankle hitch to the end of the splint, producing a traction force. The half ring splint still engages the ischial tuberosity, and the strap buckles down across the anterior thigh. Towels or a tubular stockinet placed on the Thomas splint with safety pins support the leg, as shown in **Fig. 6-6**.
   3. **Hare splints and Roller splints** are also commercially available. They differ from the Thomas splint only by the foot attachments and leg supports. They are in widespread use by emergency medical technicians.
   4. Most **precautions** relate to complications of fixed skeletal traction and are discussed in **Chap. 9, VII**. Do not leave the temporary splint on for more than 2 hours, whenever possible, because the ankle hitch places significant pressure on the skin and may produce necrosis.
B. Jones compression splint
   1. Use in **acute knee trauma** (patellar, knee, and some tibial fractures) and **acute ankle injuries**.
   2. Apply by wrapping the injured leg from the toes to the groin in rolled cotton. Next, add a single layer of elastic bandage. Apply 5- × 30-inch plaster splints posteriorly, medially, and laterally to keep the ankle in a neutral position. Medial and lateral splints support the knee in the desired degree of flexion. Do not overlap the splints, or a circumferential plaster will be created about the extremity. The splints are then overwrapped with bias-cut stockinet in a herringbone fashion.
   3. **Precautions**
      a. Do not apply **wraps too tightly**.
      b. Do not make **upper wraps tighter than lower wraps** or venous return will be impeded, causing swelling and circulatory problems.
   4. Although they provide less satisfactory compression, commercial **knee immobilizers** are acceptable in most cases.
C. Short-leg or modified Jones compression splint
   1. Use in **acute ankle and foot trauma** such as ankle sprains, calcaneal fractures, and other foot injuries.

Chapter 6: Common Types of Emergency Splints 97

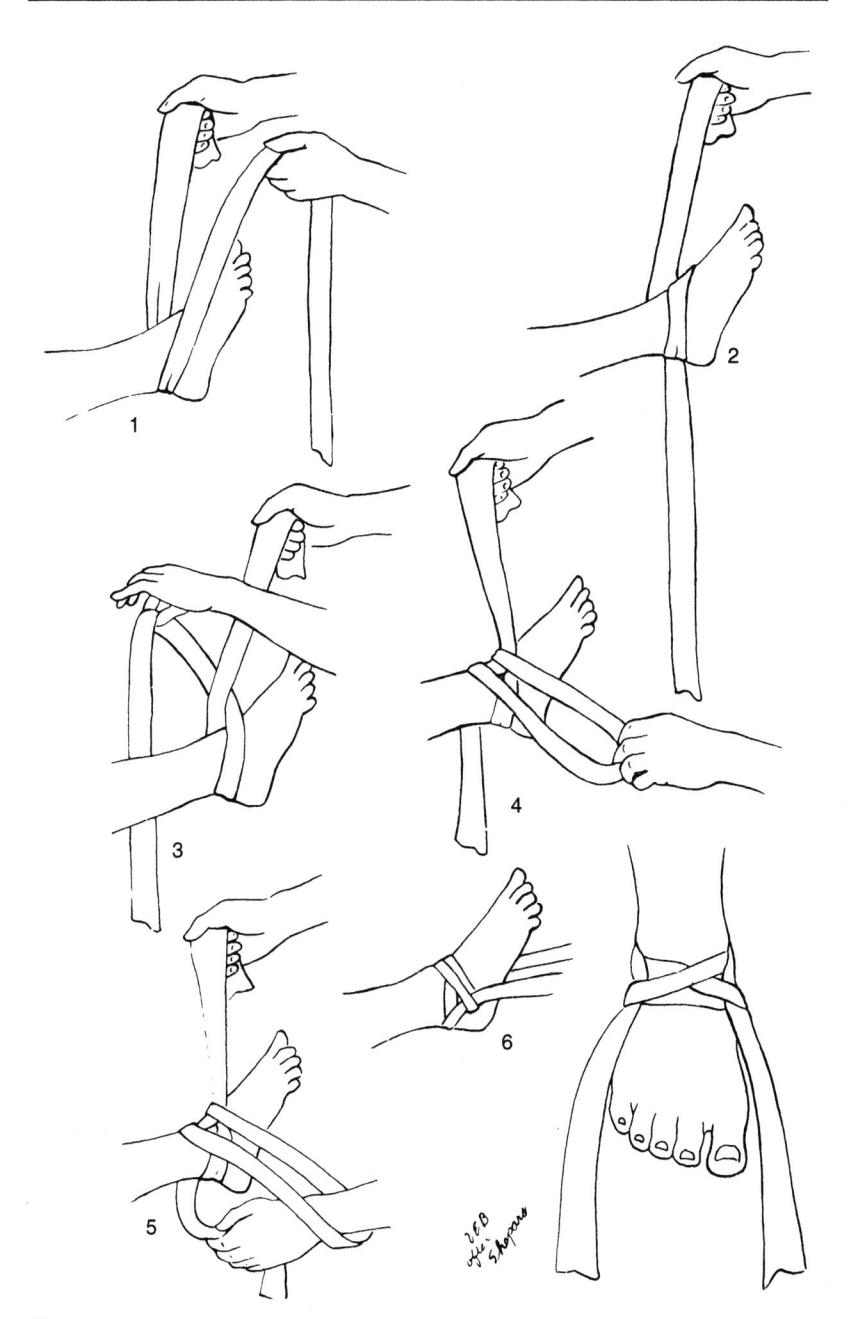

Figure 6-5. A Collins hitch is a means of applying traction from the ankle to the end of the Thomas splint, but it is used only in emergency situations.

98 Chapter 6: Common Types of Emergency Splints

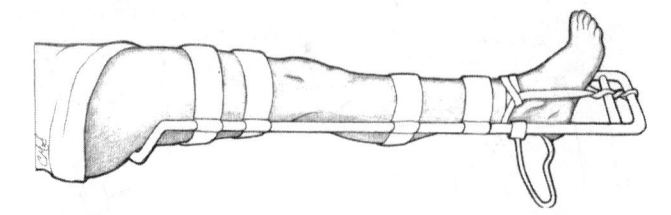

Figure 6-6. A Thomas splint may be used at the scene of the accident for a fracture of the femur.

2. The splint is **applied** in a fashion similar to that described for the Jones splint except that it does not extend above the tibial tubercle.
3. **Precautions** are the same as those for the Jones compression splint.

D. **Commercial leg and ankle braces**
   1. **Short leg walkers** constructed of a rigid foot piece and double uprights and secured with Velcro fasteners are available for conditions not requiring more rigid cast immobilization.
   2. **Lace-up canvas ankle supports** with removable aluminum stays are also often convenient and useful for ankle sprains and instability.
   3. **Air splints** with inflatable medial and lateral supports have recently proven extremely useful as supports for ankle sprains and stable fractures that are well along in the healing process.

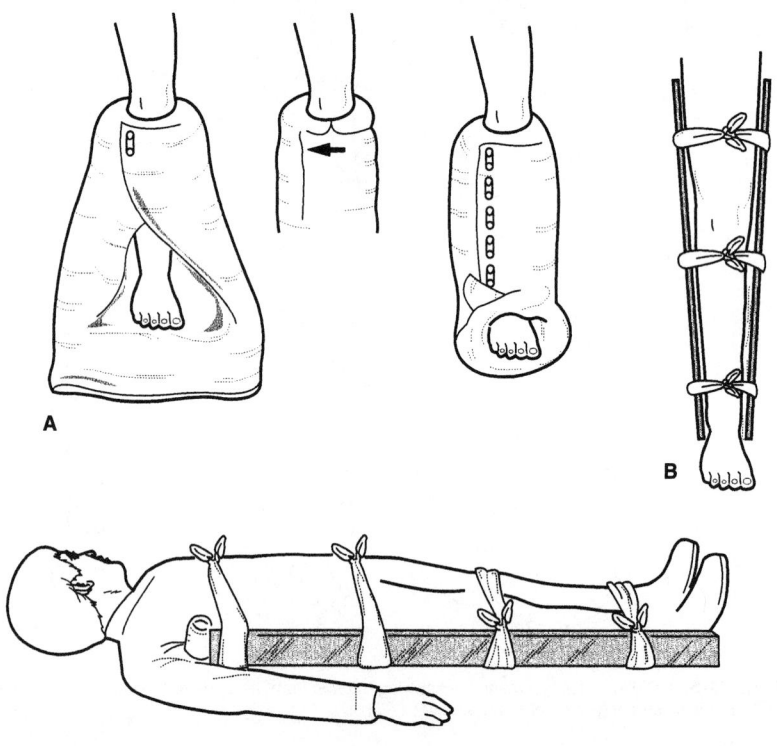

Figure 6-7. A: A pillow splint may be applied to a leg with a distal injury as a temporary measure. **B:** Board splints may be used for lower-extremity fractures in emergency situations.

E. Other emergency splints
 1. **Make-do splints** may be used as a temporary measure. One may apply a pillow splint, rigid cardboard, magazine, or a wooden splint to the upper or lower extremity. A pillow splint for the ankle is shown in **Fig. 6-7A**.
 2. **Precautions**
    a. **Avoid circulatory embarrassment** by applying splint straps or wraps in such a way as to prevent pressure on the skin over a bony prominence or a tourniquet effect to the extremity.
    b. **Splint**
       i. For **closed fractures**, restore gross limb angulation into better alignment before the splint is applied by using gentle traction first in the direction of the angulation and then in the long axis of the limb.
       ii. Restore alignment in the same manner if there is **tenting of the skin** over the injury.
       iii. For **open fractures**, gross limb alignment should be restored, the wound inspected and dressed with sterile technique, and a splint applied.
    c. Cover **exposed bone** with a saline- or betadine-moistened sterile dressing as first aid treatment.

CAST AND BANDAGING TECHNIQUES 7

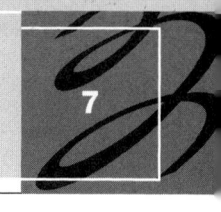

I. MATERIALS AND EQUIPMENT
A. Plaster (1,2)
1. Plaster bandages and splints are made by **impregnating crinoline with plaster of paris** [$(CaSO_4)_2H_2O$]. When this material is dipped into water, the powdery plaster of paris is transformed into a solid crystalline form of gypsum, and heat is given off:

$$(CaSO_4)_2H_2O + 3H_2O \leftrightarrows 2(CaSO_4 \times 2H_2O) + heat$$

Anhydrous calcium sulfate: Hydrated calcium sulfate:
plaster of paris gypsum

2. The amount of heat given off is determined by the amount of plaster applied and the temperature of the water (3,4). The more plaster and the hotter the water, the more heat is generated. The interlocking of the crystals formed is essential to the strength and rigidity of the cast. Motion during the **critical setting period** interferes with this interlocking process and reduces the ultimate strength by as much as 77%. The interlocking of crystals (the critical setting period) begins when the plaster reaches the thick creamy stage, becomes a little rubbery, and starts losing its wet, shiny appearance. Cast drying occurs by the evaporation of the water not required for crystallization. The evaporation from the cast surface is influenced by air temperature, humidity, and circulation about the cast. Thick casts take longer to dry than thin ones. Strength increases as drying occurs.
3. Plaster is available as bandage **rolls** in widths of 8, 6, 3, and 2 inches and **splints** in 5- × 45-inch, 5- × 30-inch, 4- × 15-inch, and 3- × 15-inch sizes. Additives are used to alter the setting time. Three variations are available. Extra-fast setting takes 2 to 4 minutes, fast setting takes 5 to 6 minutes, and slow setting takes 10 to 18 minutes.

B. Fiberglass cast.
In recent years, a number of companies have developed materials to replace plaster of paris as a cast. Most of these are a fiberglass fabric impregnated with polyurethane resin. The prepolymer is methylene bisphenyl diisolynate, which converts to a nontoxic polymeric urea substitute. The exothermic reaction does not place the patient's skin at risk for thermal injury (2,5,6). These materials are preferred for most orthopaedic applications except in acute fractures in which reduction maintenance is critical. Fiberglass casts do not provide higher skin pressure when compared to plaster casts when properly applied (7).
1. **Advantages.** These materials are strong, lightweight, and resist breakdown in water; they are also available in multiple colors and patterns.
2. **Disadvantages.** They are harder to contour than plaster of paris, and the polyurethane may irritate the skin. Fiberglass is harder to apply, although the newer bias stretch material is an improvement. Review in detail the instructions from each manufacturer before using the casting materials. Patients are commonly under the impression that fiberglass casts can be gotten wet. This is incorrect; if submerged, they need to be changed to avoid significant skin maceration.

C. The water.
Warm water causes more heat to be given off and affords faster setting. Cold water allows for less heat and for slower setting. Plaster of paris in the water

bucket from previously dipped plaster accelerates the setting time. The water used for dipping should be deep enough to cover the material rolls standing on end.
- **D. Cast padding**
    1. **Webril** has a smooth surface and less tendency for motion within the thickness of the padding than some of the other padding materials. It requires the most practice to achieve a smooth application, however.
    2. **Specialist** is softer than Webril and contains wood fiber. It has a corrugated appearance, and there is more tendency for sliding to occur within the material. It is easier to apply without wrinkles than Webril, but it becomes very hard if caked with blood.
    3. **Sof-Roll** is a soft padding similar in appearance to Webril but slightly thicker. It has greater tear resistance and is therefore easier to stretch.
    4. **Stockinet**
        a. **Bias-cut** stockinet may be used under a cast as a single layer. It is easy to apply without wrinkles and is better than tubular stockinet if there is a large difference in the maximum and minimum diameters of the extremity. Bias-cut stockinet can be made snug throughout, in contrast to tubular stockinet, which can be snug in the large diameter of the extremity but very loose in the narrow diameter. Plaster sticks to the stockinet, so there is no sliding between the cast and the stockinet padding.
        b. **Tubular** stockinet is made of the same material as the bias-cut type and is available in varying tube sizes from 2 to 12 inches.
    5. **Felt or Reston** should be used to pad bony prominences and for cast margins. When padding over bony prominences, such as the anterior superior iliac spine, make a cruciate incision in the felt for better contouring.
    6. **Moleskin adhesive** can be used to trim cast margins.
- **E. Adherent materials.** Adherent substances (such as Dow Corning medical adhesive B) are applied to prevent slipping and chafing between the skin and the padding. They can contribute, however, to an increased amount of itching inside the cast. Tincture of benzoin compound should not be used in this situation because of fairly frequent skin reactions. Commercial adhesive removers are available.
- **F. Equipment**
    1. Use a clean **bucket**. Plaster residue and other particles in the water can alter the setting time.
    2. **Gloves** keep hands clean and prevent dry skin if one applies many casts. They also make a smoother finish than is achieved by bare hands. They are mandatory for working with fiberglass materials.
    3. **Shoe covers and aprons or gowns** keep shoes and clothes clean to prevent one from appearing sloppy in plaster-covered attire.
    4. Use appropriate **draping** to maintain the dignity of the patient as well as to keep plaster off all areas not casted.
    5. **Cast cutters**
        a. **The cast-cutting electric saw** has an oscillating circular blade that cuts firm rigid surfaces, such as casts or bony prominences. When lightly touched, the skin vibrates with the blade but the blade does not cut. If the blade is firmly pressed against the skin or dragged along it, then it will cut. The saw is noisy and causes considerable anxiety, especially in children. Therefore, it is wise to show younger patients that cast saws are safe by touching the blade to the palm of the hand. The cast saw causes dust to fly; consequently, use of this tool is best avoided in clean operating rooms. In addition, cast saws can cut skin if applied with excessive force, so it is unwise to use them on anesthetized patients.
        b. **Hand cutters** are useful when a saw is not available or to avoid frightening a child with the noise of the saw, to lessen the amount of plaster dust in the operating room, and to remove damp plaster.
    6. **Cast spreaders** are used to open the cut edges of a cast for access to underlying cast padding, which is then cut with scissors. Spreaders come in various sizes for large and small casts.

7. **Cast knives** have sharp blades, and preferably have large handles for better control. Sharp blades are essential; therefore, most practitioners prefer to use no. 22 disposable surgical blades.
8. **Cast benders** adjust cast edges to relieve skin binding and pressure.
9. **Cast dryers** blow warm to hot air around a plaster cast. They are generally not necessary. An exposed cast and a fan work just as well and are safer. Cast dryers can burn skin and tend to hasten the drying time of the outer layers only.

II. **BASIC PRINCIPLES OF CAST APPLICATION**
   A. **Casts are used** for the following **purposes**:
      1. **To immobilize** fractures, dislocations, injured ligaments, and joints; to provide relief from pain caused by infections and inflammatory processes; and to facilitate healing
      2. **To allow earlier ambulation** by stabilizing fractures of the spine or lower extremities
      3. **To improve function** by stabilizing or positioning a joint, such as for wrist drop after a radial nerve injury, which also allows more useful hand function
      4. **To correct deformities,** as in serial casting for clubfoot or joint contractures
      5. **To prevent deformity** resulting from a neuromuscular imbalance or from scoliosis
   B. **Principles.** Although plaster of paris has been used extensively in the treatment of fractures for more than 100 years, there is no unanimity of opinion as to the best technique for application. It can be safely concluded that even the tightest of skintight casts allows some motion at the fracture site, whereas a loosely fitted, well-padded cast with proper three-point fixation can provide satisfactory immobilization. Three points of force are produced by the practitioner, who molds the cast firmly against the proximal and distal portions of the extremity (two of the points) and locates the third point directly opposite the apex of the cast, as shown in **Fig. 7-1**. Periosteal or other soft-tissue attachments usually are required on the convex side of the cast to provide stability. In this way, a curved cast can provide straight alignment of the extremity within it. Charnley has stated, "If a fracture slips in a well-applied plaster, then the fracture was mechanically unsuitable for treatment by plaster, and another mechanical principle should have been chosen." Another method for providing immobilization by plaster is based on hydraulics. Fractures of the tibia do not shorten significantly when placed in a "total contact" cast. The leg is a cylinder containing mostly fluid, and when this water column is encased in rigid plaster, the cylinder does not shorten in height because tissue fluid is not compressible.
   C. The following **application techniques** have been satisfactory in our hands:
      1. The patient is **informed** of the procedure and instructed in whatever cooperation is necessary.

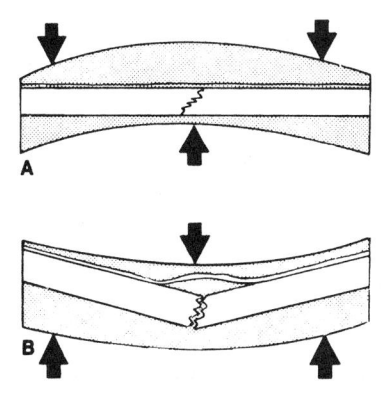

Figure 7-1. A: Three-point plaster fixation will stabilize a fracture when the soft tissue bridging the fracture acts as a hinge under tension. **B:** If the three forces are applied in the wrong direction, the fracture displaces.

2. The surgeon or cast technician must have clearly in mind **what to do and what will be required** (the position of the patient and assistants, how many rolls of plaster will be needed, tools to trim the cast edges, etc.). All material and equipment required to do the job properly should be assembled. (Once cast application starts, it is difficult to stop and obtain something that was forgotten.) The patient's position must be comfortable and must allow the surgeon and assistant to apply the cast expeditiously. Special maneuvers required to perform and hold the reduction are rehearsed.
3. **A circular cast should not be used in fresh trauma or postoperatively** when one anticipates swelling, **unless** the cast is bivalved or split initially and provisions are made for adequate observation.
    a. **Adequate observation** means an examination by a competent observer at least once hourly until any swelling begins to recede. Signs of compartmental syndrome, in order of importance, are the following: increasing pain and discomfort in the extremity, increasing tenseness or tenderness in the involved compartment, pain with passive range of motion of the muscle in the involved compartment, decreasing sensation—especially to two-point discrimination and light touch—in the distribution of the nerves that travel through the involved compartment, increasing peripheral edema, and, finally, decreasing capillary filling. **Good peripheral circulation with distal arterial pulses is no assurance that a compartmental syndrome is not developing** (see **Chap. 2, III**).
    b. An excellent alternative to plaster casts in this situation is a Jones compression splint, as described in **Chap. 6, III.B** and **C.**
4. **If unexpected swelling occurs** in a circular cast, **bivalve or split** the cast immediately all the way to the patient's skin as described in **IV.B** and **C.**
5. Unless specifically contraindicated, **clean** the part to be casted with soap and water, then dry it with alcohol. Apply the cast over a single layer of cast padding with edges of the material minimally overlapping. Protect unusual bony prominences with a 1/4-inch felt or foam rubber padding.
6. **Dip the plaster or fiberglass rolls in water** by placing them on end, which allows air to escape and results in complete soaking of the plaster. The bandages are sufficiently soaked when the bubbling stops. They can be left in the water up to 4 minutes without decreasing the strength of the cast, but the setting time decreases the longer they are immersed. Therefore, for maximum working time, remove bandages soon after the bubbling stops. Lightly crimping the ends of the plaster bandages helps prevent telescoping of the roll.
7. Except for very large casts (e.g., body casts, spicas), **all plaster bandages should be dipped and removed from the water at the same time**. Thus, all the plaster in the cast is at the same point in the setting process. This scheme maximizes the interlocking of the crystals between the layers of plaster, thereby maximizing the strength of the cast. In addition, delamination between the bandages is decreased.
8. Use **cool water** for larger casts when more time is needed to apply all the plaster or fiberglass, and use **warm water** for smaller casts or splints. **Never use hot water** because enough heat can be generated to burn the patient (8). Similarly, do not place limbs with fresh casts onto plastic-covered pillows; these tend to hamper heat dispersion significantly and may result in burning. If the patient complains of burning, it is prudent to remove the cast immediately and reapply using cooler water.
9. Keep the plaster bandage on the cast padding, lifting it off only to tuck and change directions—that is, to push the plaster roll around the patient's body or extremity. Use the largest bandages, usually 4- and 6-in. bandage rolls, that are consistent with smooth, easy applications. Using large bandages allows the fastest application of plaster and provides sufficient time for molding before the critical setting period. **Six or seven layers of plaster** or two to three layers of fiberglass usually are sufficient, except in individuals who are particularly hard on casts. The cast should be of uniform thickness (seven layers or

1/4 in.). Avoid concentrating the plaster about the fracture or the middle of the cast. Avoid placing two circumferential rolls directly on top of each other while wrapping the plaster on the patient's extremity. Reinforce casts where they cross joints by incorporating plaster or fiberglass splints longitudinally. Incorporate reinforcing plaster splints into body and spica casts as described later in this chapter (**III.B** and **C**).

10. During application of the cast, **turn the padding back at the edges of the cast and incorporate it.** Another method of finishing the edges is to turn back the padding after the cast has set and to hold the padding down with a single, narrow, plaster splint; a row of ordinary staples; or moleskin.
11. **Apply all the material rapidly** so there is time to work and mold it before the critical setting period. The cast should have a sculptured look, not only for cosmetic reasons but also for comfort. If the fracture is to be stabilized by the three-point fixation principle, it is more important to maintain the three forces of pressure on the cast during the critical setting period than to have a perfectly smooth surface on the cast. This step is more difficult for fiberglass casts.
12. Once the critical period of interlocking of crystals begins, **molding and all motion should stop** until the material becomes rigid. Otherwise, the cast is weakened considerably.
13. After the cast sets and becomes rigid, **trim the edges** using a plaster knife or cast saw. Use the knife by supporting the cutting hand on the cast and pulling the portion of the plaster to be trimmed up against the knife blade rather than blindly cutting through the plaster and possibly cutting the patient. If the cast is too thick or hard, an oscillating cast saw is preferred.
14. Apply **forearm casts** to allow full 90 degrees flexion of all metacarpophalangeal joints and opposition of the thumb to the index and little fingers.
15. Extend **leg casts** to support the metatarsal heads but not to interfere with flexion and extension of the toes. This rule is invalid when the toes need support (as with fractures of the great toe or metatarsals) or when there is a motor or sensory deficit. In these situations, the cast is extended as a platform to support and protect the toes. Place a 1/2-inch piece of sponge rubber beneath the toes and incorporate it into the plaster for walking casts, or supply the patient with a commercial cast shoe.
16. Immobilize as few joints as possible, but as a general rule, one **immobilizes the joint above and below a fresh fracture.**
17. Instruct the patient regarding
    a. **Signs and symptoms of compression** from swelling within the cast
    b. **Elevation** of the injured part above the level of the heart for 2 to 3 days after the injury
    c. **How soon to walk** on the cast (never sooner than 24 hours)
    d. **Instructions for weight bearing and ambulation**; this should include crutch or walker training
    e. **How to exercise** joints not incorporated in plaster
    f. **Date of the next appointment**
    g. **Person to call** in case of cast problems or evidence of a compression syndrome

III. SPECIAL CASTING/SPLINTING TECHNIQUES
A. Use **plaster splints** when rigid immobilization is not required or when significant swelling of the extremity is anticipated.
  1. **Upper extremity**
     a. Usually splint the **wrist** dorsally by applying a 3-in.-wide plaster splint over cast padding from the metacarpophalangeal joints to the proximal forearm. While the plaster is still wet, wrap the arm with bias-cut stockinet or a single layer of an elastic bandage so that the plaster conforms to the extremity as it hardens. A dorsal splint may be preferable to a volar splint because it allows easier finger and hand function. Combined dorsal and volar splints are frequently used together; this is preferred and gives better support of the limbs.

b. Splint the **elbow** with 5- × 30-in. plaster wraps applied posteriorly with enough distal extension to support the wrist. The splint should not go further distally than the distal palmar crease in order to facilitate metacarpalphalangeal motion. Apply 3-in. plaster strips medially and laterally across the elbow for reinforcement. Wrap the arm and plaster splint with bias-cut stockinet or a single layer of an elastic bandage while the plaster is wet.

2. **Lower extremity.** Usually make posterior plaster splints in the lower extremity by applying a standard cast (knee cylinder, short-leg, or long-leg, cast, as described in **III. D, E, F**) and then bivalving the cast and retaining only the posterior shell. Hold the posterior splint to the leg with bias-cut stockinet or an elastic bandage wrap. Alternatively, use 5- × 30-in. posterior and medial/lateral splints, leaving the anterior aspect of the leg covered only by soft roll.

B. Body casts
1. Apply the **basic body jacket** over large tubular stockinet. Place 1/8- to 1/2-in. felt pads over the shoulders (if suspenders are used), costal margins, iliac crests including anterior iliac spine, and the dorsal spine. Make a cruciate cut in the felt placed over the crests to distribute pressure uniformly over the bony prominence. Apply a single layer of plaster snugly over the padding. Splints may be used, as shown in **Fig. 7-2**. If suspenders are required, make a "V" with 5- × 30-in. splints. Place the point of the "V" between the scapulae and bring the ends over the shoulders. Snugly apply rolled plaster over the splints and mold. Usually extend the jacket posteriorly from the top of the sacrum to the inferior angle of the scapulae and anteriorly from the symphysis pubis to the sternal notch. Body jackets may be applied with the lumbar spine in flexion or extension as well as the neutral position. For hyperextension body jackets, often used in thoracolumbar fractures, use the Goldwaithe iron apparatus for positioning, as in **Fig. 7-3**.

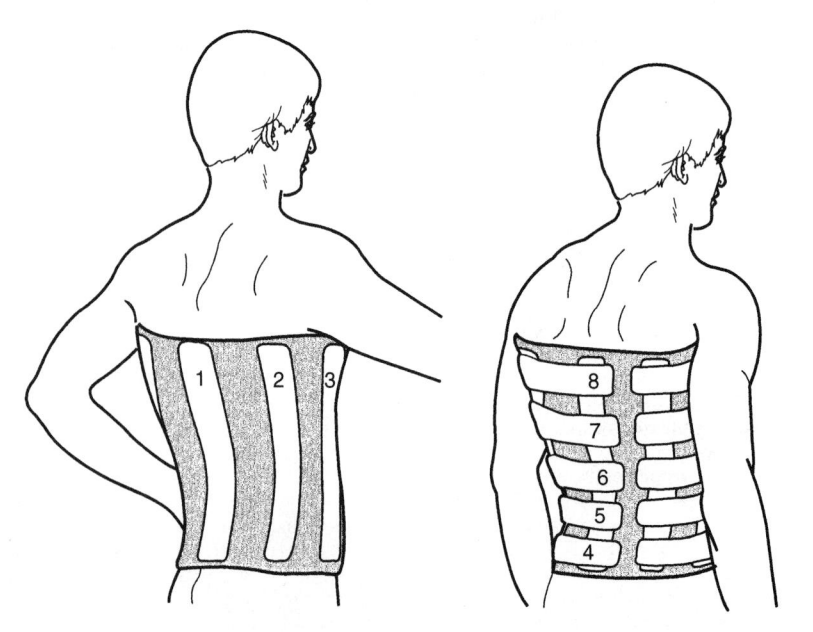

Figure 7-2. Typical application of plaster splints for a body jacket. The splints are placed closer together in the lower aspect of the body jacket. The splints are numbered in order of application.

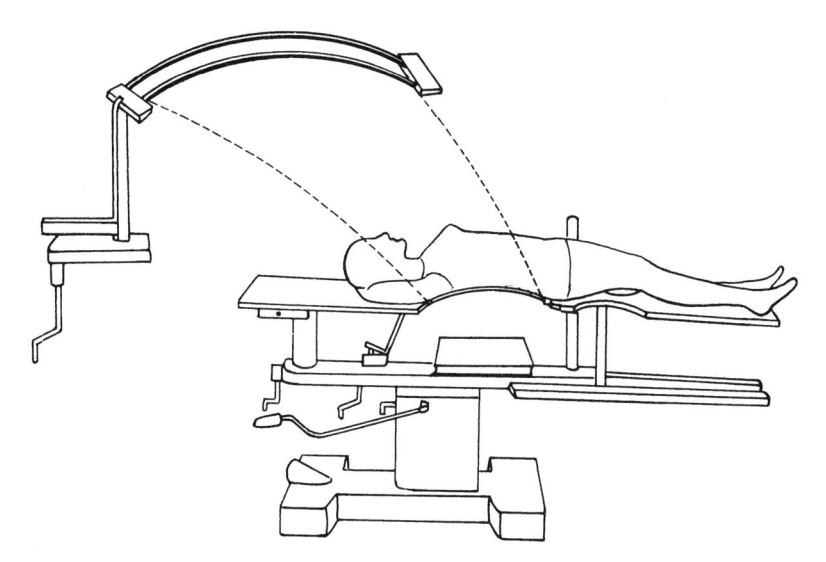

Figure 7-3. Goldwaithe irons, used to make a hyperextension plaster body jacket. The irons are removed after the cast is set.

2. The **Minerva body jacket** is named after the goddess Minerva, who sprang forth from Jupiter's head when it was cleaved by Vulcan in an attempt to relieve Jupiter's headaches. Minerva appeared chanting a triumphant song and wearing a large metal headdress. The Minerva body jacket incorporates the skull and is used to immobilize the cervical spine; its most frequent application is in children. This type of jacket is applied in the same manner as the body jacket but also calls for the following steps. Place a fluted felt pad around the entire neck, with the neck halter traction over the padding. Tie the halter straps at ear level to prevent the halter's slipping off the head. Place another felt pad along the length of the spine and the occiput. Wrap the rest of the head with 3-in. sheet cotton padding. At least two operators are necessary for even application of the plaster, one for the head and one for the body. Roll 3-in. plaster bandages about the head and neck. Apply narrow splints around the chin, neck, occiput, and forehead. Use wide splints all the way from the sacrum to the occiput, with another wide splint extending from the chest to the chin. Incorporate these splints into the cast by snugly wrapping plaster bandages over them. Then mold together the plaster about the head, neck, and body at the same time. Carefully mold beneath the mandible. Cut the plaster in a "V" to release the chin and also cut out about the ears and the face (**Fig. 7-4**, inset). Trim the plaster above the jaw line and leave the eyebrows exposed. A Minerva body jacket is useful in children and when cervical or halo vests (**Fig. 7-4**) orthoses are not appropriate.
3. **Other types of body jackets**
   a. A **Risser localizer cast** is occasionally used for scoliotic spines or for patients with thoracolumbar fractures. Apply a pelvic plaster mold first; then attach pelvic and head halter traction. Make a pressure pad with felt backed by four to six layers of plaster. Produce or hold correction of the scoliosis by applying this pad against the apical ribs and incorporating it into the body jacket that incorporates the jaw, neck, and occiput, but not the head. Make the surface of the pressure area large enough to avoid local necrosis of the skin.

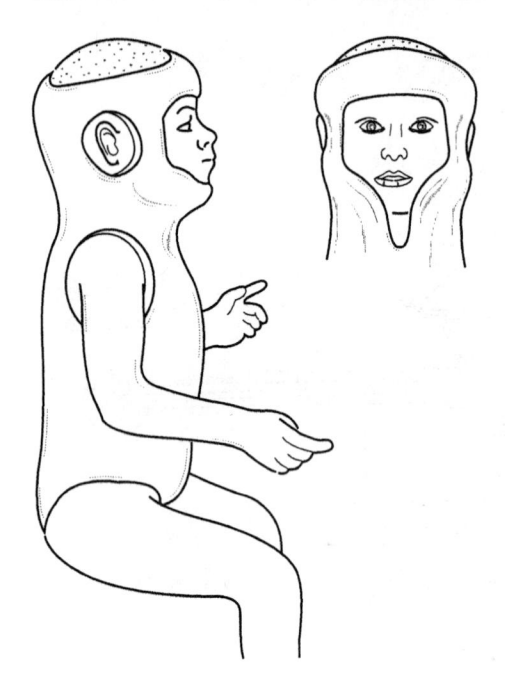

Figure 7-4. Completed Minerva body jacket.

    b. Halo traction can be incorporated into a plaster or fiberglass body jacket with suspenders, and it provides continuous or fixed cervical traction (**Fig. 7-5**). The halo traction is more commonly incorporated into a sheepskin-lined plastic body jacket, which is more lightweight and comfortable (**Fig. 7-6**).

C. Spica is a Latin word that means "ear of wheat," because a spica wrap was used to wrap sheaves of wheat in the fields. The same type of wrap is used to

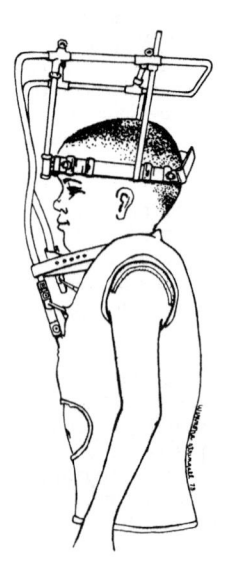

Figure 7-5. Halo traction cast. (From Bleck EE, Duckworth L, Hunter N. *Atlas of plaster cast techniques,* 2nd ed. Chicago: Year Book, 1978, with permission.)

Chapter 7: Cast and Bandaging Techniques   **109**

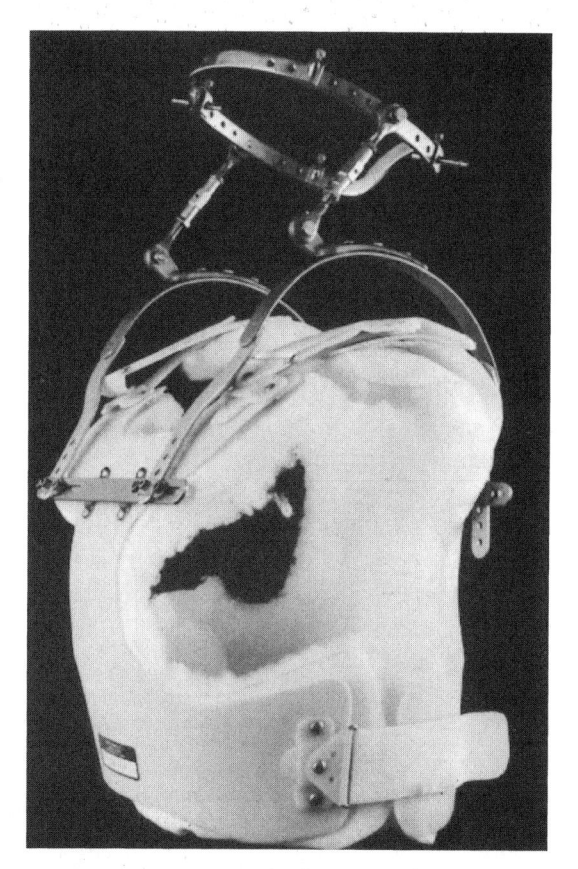

Figure 7-6. A commercially available malleable polyethylene jacket may be substituted for the plaster cast for use with the halo apparatus. Patients report this is significantly more comfortable than the plaster jacket.

immobilize proximal joints with the **spica cast.** Various types of spica casts are described here.

1. Pad a **bilateral short-leg** (panty) **spica** in much the same way as for the body jacket but include the legs. These casts are generally applied on fracture tables (adults) or spica boards (children). Use tubular or bias-cut stockinet. Pad bony prominences with 1/8- to 1/2-in. felt with cruciate incisions. Apply plaster or fiberglass to the upper portion of the cast as is done with the body jacket. Reinforce the hips with splints as shown in **Fig. 7-7**. Apply plaster or fiberglass well next to the perineal post under the sacrum to avoid weakness in the area (the intern's triangle). Snugly tie the splints in with plaster or fiberglass bandage rolls extending to the supracondylar portion of the femurs. Mold the material well over the iliac crests. The patient may be lifted from the table with the sacral rest still in the plaster. Turn the patient on his or her abdomen and cut out the sacral rest. Trim the edges of the cast in the usual manner.
2. Examples of long-leg hip spicas are shown in **Fig. 7-8**. Apply the leg portion of the cast like any other long-leg cast, using the special splints about the hips as described for the short-leg spica. Support the casted extremities with struts. These are usually made of wooden stakes (1/4 × 2 in. or 3/4 × 1/2 in.) or

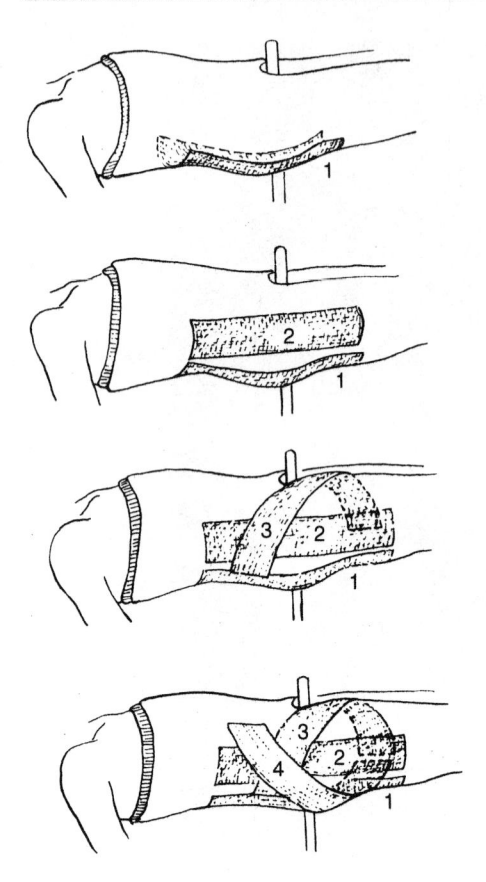

Figure 7-7. Plaster splints to reinforce hip spicas, in addition to those used in the body jackets.

dowels. Cover with plaster or fiberglass and attach them to the casted extremity by wrapping a bandage in a cordlike figure-of-8 fashion about the strut and cast; then roll the bandage around the strut and cast to create a well-molded cast. Sedate or anesthetize infants and small children before spica cast application; they are generally applied in the operating suite.

   3. Apply the **shoulder spica** with the patient standing or supine on a spica table that has a metallic backrest. The arm may be supported with finger traps, or, with a cooperative patient in the sitting or standing position, the cast may be applied while an assistant holds the arm. The principles of padding and cast application for body jackets and long-arm casts are combined to produce a shoulder spica. In addition to the splints normally used for body and long-arm casts, apply a wide splint from the lateral chest, up under the axilla, to the medial side of the arm. Place other splints across the posterior aspect of the arm, over the shoulder, to the opposite side. Tie in the splints with rolled plaster or fiberglass and place a strut between the arm and trunk.

D. Knee cylinder casts. Remove all hair from the medial and lateral aspects of the lower leg. Spray the leg with a nonallergenic adhesive. Place medial and lateral strips of self-adhering foam, moleskin adhesive, or adhesive tape on the skin with 6 to 12 in. of the material extending distal to the ankle. Then place a cuff of 1/4-in. sponge rubber or felt padding measuring 1 in. in width over the strips just above the malleoli. When the strips are turned back and incorporated into the fiberglass or

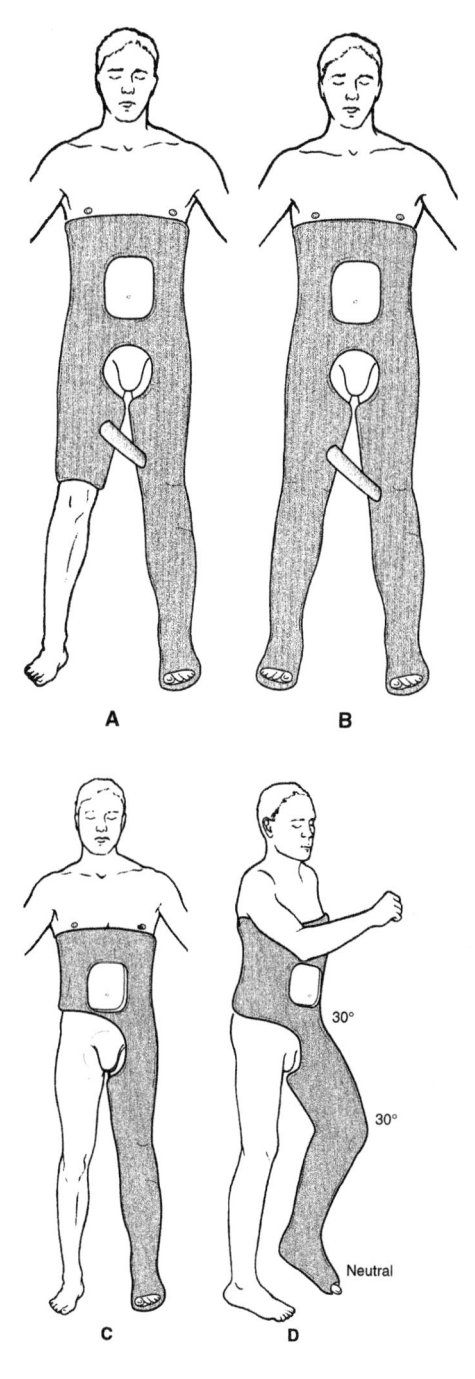

Figure 7-8. Long-leg hip spicas. **A:** One and one-half spica. **B:** Double spica. **C:** Single spica. For all long-leg spica casts, it is important to keep the hip and knee gently flexed for patient comfort and ease of positioning. The ankle must be kept in neutral dorsiflexion **(D)**. In children, it is often advisable to stop the cast at the malleoli distally, leaving the foot free.

plaster, they suspend the cast, and with the thick padding, they prevent pressure on the malleoli. Wrap the leg with a single layer of cast padding and apply the plaster with the knee flexed 5 degrees. Extend the cast proximally as far as possible and distally to just above the flare of the malleoli; the length of the cast provides for lateral and medial stability. Mold the plaster or fiberglass medially and laterally above the femoral condyles to help prevent the cast from sliding distally.

E. Short-leg casts
1. Apply the **short-leg cast** with the patient sitting on the end of a table with the knee flexed 90 degrees. Alternatively, apply it with the patient supine, the hip and knee flexed 90 degrees, and the leg supported by an assistant. The type of padding matters little, except that Webril and stockinet tend to shear less and therefore may allow for a tighter cast over a longer period of time. Use only one layer of padding except over the malleoli, where extra padding frequently is required. For most casts, have the ankle in a neutral position. Two plaster bandages usually are required, and the width selected (3, 4, or 6 in.) varies with the size of the patient. Fold 4-in. splints longitudinally in half, and place one splint on all four sides of the ankle for reinforcement before applying the second plaster bandage. Extend the cast distally from the metatarsophalangeal joints and proximally to one finger breadth below the tibial tubercle. Trim the edges and pad as previously described.
2. If desired, a **walking cast** may be made with either a rubber rocker walker or a stirrup walker. Place either one in the midportion of the longitudinal arch of the foot in line with the anterior border of the tibia. With a rocker walker, the medial longitudinal arch is filled with plaster splints to make a flat base. Then the walker is secured with a third plaster bandage. Commercially available walking shoes (or boots), which fit over the casted foot, are more widely used. A flat plaster base on the plantar aspect of the cast is required for these shoes. If the ankle must be held in equines (such as required for cast treatment of an Achilles tendon rupture), a stirrup walker is advantageous, and the patient's opposite shoe should be adjusted to the appropriate height for walking. All walking casts should dry for at least 24 hours prior to weight bearing.

F. Long-leg casts
1. First apply a **short-leg cast** as described earlier (**III.E**). Then extend the knee to the position desired and continue the cast padding to the groin. Two 6-in. plaster or fiberglass bandages usually are required for the upper portion of this cast except in patients with heavy thighs. After the first bandage is applied, fold 4- or 5-in. splints longitudinally and place them medially and laterally across the knee joint for reinforcement. After the second plaster or fiberglass bandage is applied, mold the cast medially and laterally in the supracondylar area to help prevent the cast from slipping distally when the patient begins to stand.
2. The long-leg **walking cast** is made as described in **III.E.2**, but the knee must be flexed no more than 5 degrees.

G. Casting techniques of Dehne and Sarmiento
1. The cast treatment programs made popular by Dehne and Sarmiento (see Selected Historical Readings) are designed to allow early weight bearing of a fractured tibia. The affected leg is placed in a very snug cast that maintains the tissue and fluids of the leg within a rigid container. Shortening is prevented by the **hydraulic principle** that fluids are not compressible. Thus, the patient can bear weight soon after a fracture without excessive further shortening, and fracture healing is benefitted by the improved vascularity derived from ambulation. The advocates of these casting techniques describe a "total contact cast." The authors believe, however, that all casts to the lower extremities should be total contact casts.
2. The **long-leg total contact cast** as described by Dehne is applied like a long-leg walking cast with only minor modifications.
    a. **Cast the knee in extension.** Some patients, however, find this position uncomfortable and may require a position with 3 to 5 degrees of flexion.

b. This cast may need to be **wedged** to correct angular deformities of the fracture site. For this reason, apply one or two extra layers of the Webril at the fracture site.

3. The **below-the-knee total contact**, or patellar tendon-bearing, **cast** is applied much as a regular short-leg walking cast is, with the following modifications (**Fig. 7-9**):
   a. Keep the affected limb in a long-leg cast or a Jones compression splint until the **swelling subsides** (2–4 weeks).
   b. Apply the **cast padding to the lower leg and extend** to 2 in. proximal to the superior pole of the patella.
   c. First apply a short-leg cast and extend it to just inferior to the tibial tubercle. Sarmiento suggests molding the cast into a **triangular shape**, with the sides of the triangle formed by the anterior tibial surface, the lateral peroneal muscle mass, and the posterior aspect of the leg.
   d. Then have the assistant position the knee in 40 to 45 degrees of flexion. The quadriceps muscles must be completely relaxed. Use a 4-in. bandage of plaster to extend the cast to the superior pole of the patella. Mold carefully

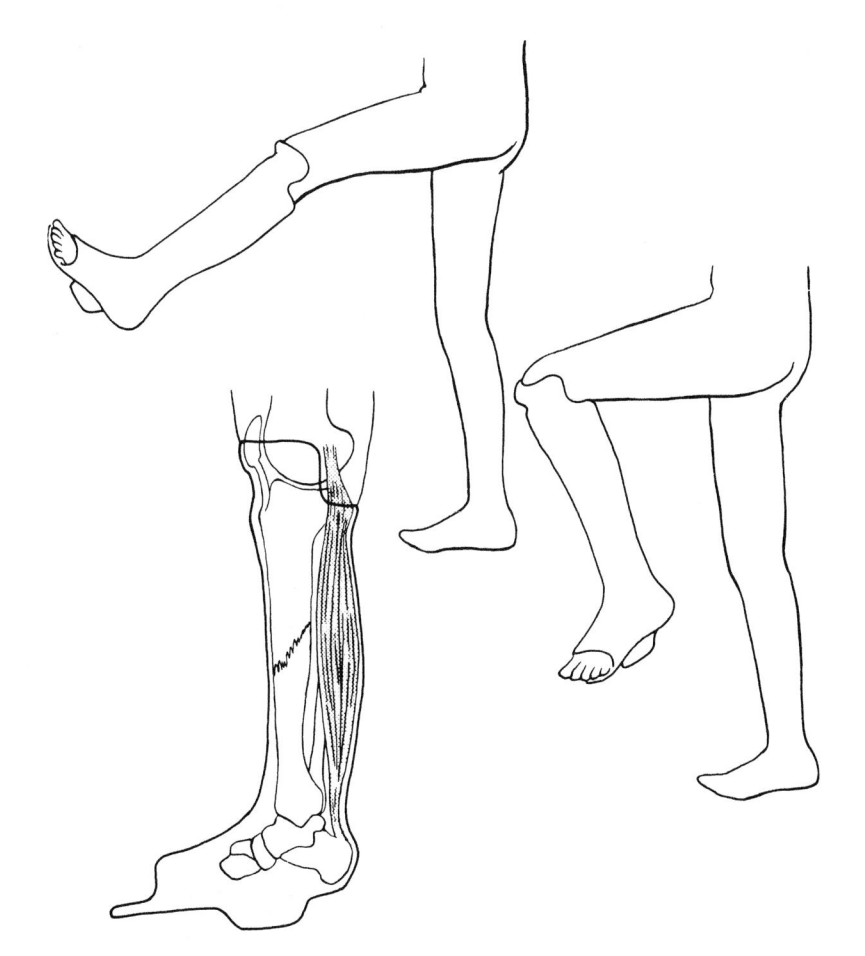

Figure 7-9. Completed below-the-knee total contact cast.

over the medial tibial flare as well as into the patellar tendon and the popliteal fossa. The lateral wings should be as high as possible. Trim the posterior portion of the cast to one fingerbreadth or 1/2 in. below the level of the cast indentation that was made anteriorly into the patellar tendon. The posterior wall of the cast should be low enough to allow 90 degrees of knee flexion without having the cast edge rub on the hamstring tendons. These casts generally require the use of plaster because of the critical molding involved, which is difficult with fiberglass.

    e. If **angulation** occurs at the fracture site with this cast, replace rather than wedge the cast. If the patient ambulates well enough to maintain muscle bulk, the original cast may not need to be replaced.

    f. **Do not switch from a below-the-knee total contact cast to a regular short-leg cast** at some point midway in the healing phase of the fracture, because a regular short-leg cast offers no rotational stability. Recent evidence has shown that this type of cast is no more effective in immobilizing tibia fractures than a standard short-leg cast (9).

4. **The authors believe that a long-leg weight-bearing cast is easier and safer (in regards to skin and fracture complications) for most individuals to apply than the below-the-knee total contact cast.** Comparing the treatment results published in the literature provides no evidence that one technique is superior to the other. The theoretic advantage of providing knee motion with the Sarmiento technique is offset by the expertise required to apply this cast properly.

5. Begin **weight bearing** at 24 to 36 hours after plaster cast application when the patient can tolerate it; patients with fiberglass casts can be encouraged to weight bear 3 to 6 hours after casting.

H. Knee cast-brace

1. A **cast-brace** is a casting device for the treatment of fractures of the distal femur or tibial plateau, which are not considered appropriate for operative management, generally in high-risk patients. Occasionally a cast-brace is applied after 1 to 3 weeks of traction, with the patient remaining in the hospital for a short period after the brace is applied. Thus, the hospital stay can be as long as 2 to 4 weeks. In addition, this technique allows mobility of the knee during the healing phase, so less physical therapy is needed to regain knee motion when the fracture is healed. These devices have generally been replaced by commercially available hinged knee braces.

2. **Technique**

    a. Two people are required for **application**. After the patient is lightly sedated, roll an elastic tubular stockinet over the leg. While an assistant holds the leg, apply plaster over the thigh to within 2 1/2 cm of the ischial tuberosity and the perineum. Extend the plaster distally to the superior pole of the patella but with enough clearance for full knee extension and flexion to 70 degrees. Then apply a short-leg cast. Make the plantar aspect of the cast flat for ambulation in a walking shoe.

    b. Position **two polycentric or cable knee hinge joints** 2 cm posterior to the midline of the limb at the level of the abductor tubercle. Use large hose clamps to secure the hinge joints to the cast temporarily. A jig is helpful to keep these joints parallel. Evaluate knee motion and make adjustments before securing the uprights with plaster.

        i. If the roentgenograms show **satisfactory alignment** of the fracture, start the patient on progressive ambulation with "touch down" weight bearing. If a knee effusion develops, instruct the patient to elevate the limb for 15 minutes of every hour. Once adequate fracture consolidation is demonstrated, the patient can be encouraged to bear weight.

        ii. If the **alignment** of the fracture is **not satisfactory**, remove the cast-brace and temporarily reinstitute traction treatment. Consider continuing standard traction therapy, reattempting a cast-brace again in 2 to 3 weeks, or performing internal fixation.

IV. CUTTING, BIVALVING, AND SPLITTING CASTS
A. General techniques
1. In removing or splitting casts, use the **oscillating saw**. Reassure the patient by giving a cast saw demonstration before actually cutting the cast. Stabilize the hand holding the electric saw on the cast, and push the blade through just the plaster with short repetitive strokes, as shown in **Fig. 7-10**. Avoid bony prominences as the cast saw can cut into the skin over them.
2. **Windows** may be cut from the cast to expose wounds. The windows must be replaced, however, and rewrapped with either a new plaster or an elastic bandage to prevent local edema.

B. Should unexpected swelling occur, **bivalve the cast. Bivalving is superior to simply splitting the cast.** The technique consists of cutting the plaster as well as the cast padding on both sides of the extremity. The anterior and posterior parts of the cast can be held in place with bias-cut stockinet or an elastic bandage. Advantages of this technique are that the anterior half of the cast may be removed to inspect the compartments and that complete anterior, posterior, and circumferential compression is relieved.

C. Splitting a cast requires cutting a 1/2-in. strip of plaster from the full length of the cast; otherwise, the proximal aspect of the plaster may act as a circumferential tourniquet (2). Again, divide the plaster and padding down to the skin because soft dressing might also cause constriction. In the case of the lower extremity, the cast is split anteriorly with a diamond-shaped section of plaster removed from the anterior aspect of the ankle. Spread the cast for relief of the symptoms. Pad the area with felt where the strip of plaster was removed and overwrap with a rubber elastic bandage to avoid local edema. **This technique is not as satisfactory as bivalving a cast but is often appropriate for managing postoperative swelling.**

V. ADHESIVE STRAPPING AND BANDAGING
A. Terminology
1. Use **adhesive strapping** (taping) for the possible prevention and treatment of athletic injuries. Use strips of adhesive tape instead of one continuous winding.
2. **Bandaging** (wrapping) uses nonadhesive materials (gauze, cotton cloth, and elastic wrapping) in the treatment of athletic injuries. Employ one continuous unwinding of material.

B. Adhesive strapping
1. **Purposes of strapping**
   a. **To protect and secure protective devices**
   b. **To hold dressings in place**
   c. **To limit motion**
   d. **To support and stabilize**

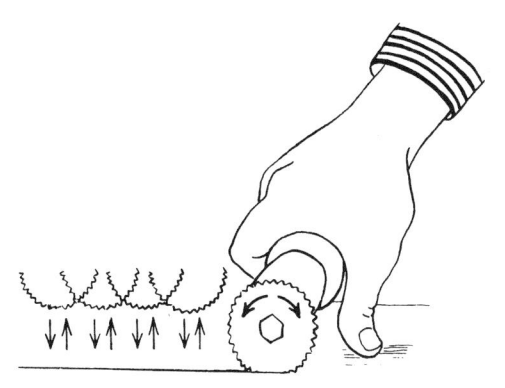

Figure 7-10. Saw-cutting technique that avoids skin laceration.

2. Construction factors
a. Tape grade
(backing material). Heavy backing materials have 85 longitudinal fibers per square inch and 65 vertical fibers per square inch. Lighter grades have 65 longitudinal fibers per square inch and 45 vertical fibers per square inch. **Store** the tape in a cool, dry place. Keep the tape standing on end and not on its side.
b. Adhesives.
Use a rubber-based spray-on adhesive primarily with athletes because strength of backing, superior adhesion, and economy are needed. Use acrylic adhesives in surgical dressing applications because a high degree of backing and superior adhesion are not the primary requirements.

3. Application and removal
a. Preparation
i. **Clean the skin** with soap and water and dry.
ii. **Remove all hair** to prevent irritation.
iii. **Treat** all cuts and wounds.
iv. **Apply** a nonallergic **skin adherent.**
v. **Position** properly.

b. Size of tape
i. Use 1/4- to 1-in. tape on **fingers, hands,** and **toes**.
ii. Use 11/4- or 11/2-in. tape on **ankles, lower legs, forearms,** and **elbows**.
iii. Use 2- or 3-in. tape on **large areas, knees,** and **thighs**.

c. Rules of application
i. **Avoid continuous strapping** because this causes constriction. Use one turn at a time and tear after overlapping the starting end of the tape by 1 in.
ii. **Smooth and mold the tape** as it is laid on the skin.
iii. **Overlap** the tape at least one half its width over the tape below.
iv. Allow the tape to **fit the natural contour** of the skin—that is, let it fall naturally and avoid bending around acute angles.
v. Keep the tape roll in one hand and **tear** it with the fingers.
vi. Keep constant and even **unwinding tension**.
vii. For **best support**, strap directly over the skin.

d. Techniques for removal
i. **Remove** the tape along the longitudinal axis rather than across it. If near a wound, **pull toward the wound,** not away from it.
ii. **Peel** the tape back by holding the skin taut and pushing the skin away from the tape rather than by pulling the tape from the skin.

4. Skin reactions.
Most tape reactions are **mechanical,** not allergic. Allergic reactions are characterized by erythema, edema, papules, and vesicles. Test for an allergic reaction by patch testing. If the test is positive, the above signs manifest themselves within 24 to 48 hours.
a. Mechanical irritation
is produced when tape is removed from the skin. It frequently occurs as a result of shearing the skin when the tape is applied in tension or used for maintaining traction. Such application induces vasodilation and an intense reddening of the skin, which disappears shortly after tape removal. The reaction is due to simple skin stripping—that is, direct trauma to the outer skin layers resulting in loss of cells.
b. Chemical irritation
occurs when components in adhesive mass or the backing of the tape permeate the underlying tissues. This irritation is largely eliminated through tape construction.
c. Another irritative effect
is localized inhibition of sweating, which is corrected by the use of nonocclusive (porous) tape.

C. Bandaging
1. Purposes of bandaging
a. To hold dressing in place
over external wounds
b. To apply compression pressure
over injuries and thus control hemorrhage

c. **To secure splints** in place
d. **To immobilize** or limit motion of injured parts
2. **Materials**
   a. **Gauze,** which holds dressings in place over wounds or acts as a protective layer for strapping
   b. **Cotton cloth** for support wrapping or dressing
   c. **Elastic wrapping** for compression wrapping or dressing

D. **Medicated bandage**
   1. The medicated bandage (Unna boot) **contains** zinc oxide, calamine, glycerine, and gelatin and **usually is indicated** for lower extremity areas of skin loss that require protection and support. This type of support dressing prevents edema and allows ambulation in patients with known venous conditions at the time of cast removal.
   2. **Application**
      a. **Cleanse** the area and position the ankle at a right angle.
      b. **Make a circular turn** with the medicated bandage **around the foot** and direct the bandage **obliquely over the heel.** Then cut the bandage. This procedure ensures a flat surface.
      c. **Repeat** until the heel is adequately covered. Make the first layer snug and apply the roll in a pressure-gradient manner; that is, apply the greatest pressure distally with progressively diminishing pressure over the upper leg.
      d. **Do not reverse any turns** because the ridges formed may cause discomfort as the bandage hardens. Overlap each turn one half of a preceding turn. Avoid winding the bandage on too tightly.
      e. **Cover the leg** approximately three times and extend the bandage 1 to 2 in. below the knee; otherwise, the bandage may slip toward the ankle. Allow the bandage to harden. Prevent soiling of clothing with gauze or stockinet over the medicated bandage. Leave the bandage on for 3 to 7 days, and repeat treatment if necessary.

VI. **JOINT MOBILIZATION**
A. **Following cast removal**
   1. **While the cast is still on,** range-of-motion exercises of the adjacent joints not immobilized and isometric exercises for the immobilized muscles (e.g., weight bearing in a cast) serve both to improve nutrition and to decrease atrophy of articular cartilage, bone, and muscle. Edema and the rehabilitation required after cast removal are also minimized.
   2. **Warn the patient that after removal of any cast from a lower extremity, some swelling is normal.**
   3. **Once the cast is removed,** an elastic stocking or bandage is desirable for support.
      a. Prescribe a **specific exercise program** to increase range of motion. Moist heat, such as a bath or whirlpool, may help mobilize the joint.
      b. If swelling appears to be a problem, **contrast baths** may be indicated (the 3-3-3 treatment): rest 3 minutes in cool water, exercise 3 minutes in warm water, repeat 3 times; follow with 30 minutes of elevation. Repeat the entire process three times daily.
      c. **Active exercise** is the key to success. Passive range-of-motion exercise too frequently becomes a repeated manipulation. Manipulation under anesthesia is occasionally necessary, but this should be followed with an aggressive inpatient therapy program.

B. It is not always true that the sooner **joints adjacent to a fracture** are mobilized, the better the range of motion obtained. The following factors must be considered:
   1. **Fractures not involving articular surfaces**
      a. Joint movement is slow to return and poor in range if attempted movement produces **pain,** associated muscle spasm, and involuntary splinting.
      b. **Early joint movement can delay fracture healing if fixation is not rigid.**
      c. **A normal joint tolerates longer periods of immobilization.** The "safe" period of immobilization coincides well with the normal time necessary for

adjacent fracture healing. Only in the older patient with degenerative changes in the joint is there a likelihood of intraarticular adhesions and periarticular stiffening, even with short periods of immobilization.

   d. **Some joints may tolerate immobilization better than others**, but this presumption is not well documented.
   e. Postinjury or postcasting **edema is "glue."** The area is soon infiltrated with young fibroblasts. Excessive formation of collagen causes early and frequent permanent stiffness, especially when collateral ligaments are immobilized in a shortened position (e.g., metacarpophalangeal joints).
   f. **Isometric exercises** within the cast are recommended. Allow the muscles to move within the limits of the cast.
2. **Fractures involving articular surfaces**
   a. **Reduce intraarticular fractures anatomically if possible.** If operative intervention is indicated, then a goal of internal fixation is to allow range-of-motion exercises or continuous passive motion within the first 2 or 3 days postoperatively.
   b. **If anatomic restitution cannot be achieved**, then early motion may allow mobile fragments to be molded into a better position. This motion should improve the potential of fibrocartilage resurfacing. Early movement is difficult to define, but some movement should be started within the first week.
3. **Between these two groups** is a considerable degree of overlap. If it is anticipated that a complicated and often incomplete open reduction and internal fixation is not secure enough to allow early movement of the joint, then it may be better to treat the fracture nonoperatively. The **objective** is the **best possible final range of movement.**

References

1. Bingold AC. On splitting plasters. *J Bone Joint Surg (Br)* 1979;61:294.
2. Pope MH, Callahan G, Lavarette R. Setting temperatures of synthetic casts. *J Bone Joint Surg (Am)* 1985;67:262–264.
3. Callahan DJ, Carney DJ, Daddario N, et al. The effect of hydration water temperature on orthopaedic plaster casting strength. *Orthopedics* 1986;9:683–985.
4. Lavalette R, Pope MH, Dickstein H. Setting temperature of plaster casts. *J Bone Joint Surg (Am)* 1982;64:907.
5. Callahan DJ, Carney DJ, Daddario N, et al. A comparative study of synthetic cast material strength. *Orthopaedics* 1986;9:679–681.
6. Wytch R, Mitchell C, Ritchie IK, et al. New splinting materials. *Prosthet Orthot Int* 1987;11:42–45.
7. Davids JR, Frick SL, Skewes E, et al. Skin surface pressure beneath an above-the-knee cast: plaster casts compared with fiberglass casts. *J Bone Joint Surg (Am)* 1997;79:565–569.
8. Wehbe MA. Plaster uses and misuses. *Clin Orthop* 1982;167:242.
9. Aita D, Bhave A, Herzenberg J, et al. The load applied to the foot in a patellar ligament-bearing cast. *J Bone Joint Surg (Am)* 1998;80:1597–1602.

Selected Historical Readings

Charnley J. *The closed treatment of common fractures*, 3rd ed. Baltimore, MD: Williams & Wilkins, 1972:179–183.

Connolly JF, King P. Closed reduction and early cast-brace ambulation in the treatment of femoral fractures. *J Bone Joint Surg (Am)* 1973;55:1559.

Dehne E, et al. Nonoperative treatment of the fractured tibia by immediate weight bearing. *J Trauma* 1961;1:514.

Sarmiento A. A functional below-the-knee cast for tibial fractures. *J Bone Joint Surg (Am)* 1967;49:855.

ORTHOPAEDIC UNIT CARE 8

I. The orthopaedic unit must present a warm, friendly, and quiet atmosphere as an essential part of the treatment program. Most patients who enter the hospital are frightened and need reassurance from everyone on the unit. To have an effective team, it is necessary for each individual to understand the goals of the treatment program for each patient. Therefore, careful communication is required, as is recognition that the best run orthopaedic services are those that involve all of the personnel in the decision-making process. To maintain the best possible environment for most patients and to ease the problems of communication, it is helpful to schedule and standardize activities and procedures. This principle is even more important with the current emphasis on shortened length of hospital stay.

II. **ROUNDS.** Rounds are important in that they constitute an evaluation for the benefit of the patient and an educational experience for all of the participants. Be certain that the best interests of the patient are not sacrificed for education. The knowledge that any word, *or non-verbal cue,* uttered in the presence of the patient can stimulate a reaction in him or her is fundamental to the art of healing. The focus of the language must center on the treatment of the patient and the disease process. Fascination, preoccupation, or engagement of the disease (or language to that effect) must be avoided. The patient must be regarded and respected, and all allusions to the disease or the treatment must be framed as a focus on the patient. The patient must be made to feel that he or she is receiving sympathetic attention as a living human being rather than being scrutinized like a specimen. This does not necessarily mean that scientific discussion is inappropriate at the bedside. However, in general, highly technical debate or lengthy discussion should be conducted away from the bedside and out of the patient's hearing range.

   A. The **approach to the patient** must also be direct and personal. Properly conducted, it can be an excellent teaching experience for those in attendance and help the patient understand his or her problems more completely. If the leader of the rounds addresses the patient with friendly words of inquiry or explanation, and with permission enters into the discussion, the patient tolerates or welcomes clinical discussions. Indeed, when managed along these lines, most patients, instead of resenting visitations from large groups, may relish the attention they are attracting and enjoy participating in the process.

   B. **Present case histories at bedside only with the patient's permission.** Devote attention to examining the patient, giving advice, or obtaining further history. The medical student, resident, and nurse who are to report on or present the case should take a position opposite that of the attending physician at the bedside. Refer to patients by name. References to age, sex, or race are out of place unless essential to the discussion and cannot be perceived by those in attendance.

   C. **Sensitive humor** can be beneficial if the patient shares it. This is an art, carefully administered. Laughter can be cruel when the patient thinks it is directed toward him or her.

   D. **The head nurse should be an integral part** of rounds. The nurse prepares for rounds as well as participates in them. When the patient is examined, the nurse should take a station at the head of the bed to promote the comfort of the patient during the examination. The doctors and students have much to learn from the nurse in charge. Personal privacy is very important, and is becoming more so; before starting rounds, the nurse or the assistant should ask visitors (except close adult members of the family) to leave the patient's bedside. The radio or television set is lowered in volume or turned off. Each member of the team performs his or her role with dispatch so that the whole activity runs smoothly and gives an impression of efficiency and dignity to patients and visitors.

E. **Consultations** are an important part of patient care and usually are ordered by the attending physician with a statement as to the current care, opinions, and so on. Make every effort to assist the consultant. Frame the question, anticipate the need, and provide the data When the consultant enters the patient's room, the resident or nurse assigned to the case should introduce the patient and explain the purpose of the visit. The resident should know the relevant findings, plan, and appropriate controversies. Discuss the plan with resident or staff before rounds.

III. **WORKUP ROUTINES**
  A. Either before or as soon as possible after admission, the house officer should conduct a **complete history and physical examination** of the patient. This workup should be reviewed, corrected, amended, and signed by the chief resident and attending physician within 24 hours. The authors prefer problem-oriented medical records. An example of the initial record follows:
    1. **Database**
    2. **Chief complaint**
    3. **History of present illness, including relevant aspects of the injury mechanism, which can explain and anticipate elements of the soft tissue and bony injuries**
    4. **Patient profile**
       a. **Past medical history**
       b. **Medications**
       c. **Allergies**
       d. **Family history**
       e. **Social history (include smoking, alcohol and drug use history)** (1,2)
       f. **Relevant vocations and avocations**
       g. **Hand dominance, as appropriate**
    5. **Review of systems**
    6. **Physical examination**
    7. **Laboratory reports**
    8. **Imaging findings, remaining imaging (pending), or imaging plan**
    9. **Inpatient problem list,** which should be maintained in the outpatient care record
    10. **An initial plan** keyed by number to the inpatient problem list
        a. **Diagnostic** plan
        b. **Therapeutic** plan
           i. **Lesion-specific (splinting, protections, weight-bearing status)**
           ii. **General orthopaedic (infection considerations, anticoagulation, rehabilitation and discharge contingencies)**
        c. **Patient education**
  B. Anticipate any **side effects or complications** from either the primary problems or the treatment plans and make appropriate provisions for prophylactic medications or other measures. **Plan ahead**, to keep the patient as comfortable as possible. **Use** every moment of hospitalization optimally.
  C. **Write progress notes** as often as there is any change in the patient's condition or when a consultation is obtained. The patient should be seen daily and an entry made in the medical record after each visit. The authors prefer the problem-oriented style of progress notes. The note should be accompanied by a date and time of the entry. After initial impressions have been advanced, if there are later complex considerations, trade-offs and major evolutions in the plan will be better understood if dictated as an "Interim Summary," which may look very much like a history with physical, or be reduced to a summary of thoughts, trade-offs, discussions, and explanations on progress.

1. **Narrative notes** are numbered and titled according to the inpatient problem list and are organized as follows:
   a. **Subjective** data
   b. **Objective** data
   c. **Assessment**
   d. **Plan**
      i. **Diagnostic**
      ii. **Therapeutic**
      iii. **Patient education**
2. **Flow sheets** are used when data and time relationships are complex
3. **Discharge summary**
   a. **Identifying data**
   b. **Dates of admission and discharge**
   c. **Master problem list** with the appropriate dates
      i. Use two columns, one headed **active problems** and one **inactive problems**.
      ii. Give each problem a number. Once a problem is assigned a number, whether on an inpatient list or on a master list, do not use the number again.
   d. List of **operations and procedures**, including the dates
   e. **Description** of the inpatient problems
   f. **Physical examination**
   g. **Laboratory data**
   h. **Hospital course** for each problem, including laboratory data, treatment, and plans when appropriate
   i. **Discharge medications and disposition**

IV. **ROUTINE ORDERS AND MANAGEMENT OF INPATIENTS**
   A. The **initial orders** should state
      1. The **condition** of the patient
      2. The type of **activity** desired
   B. **Diet**, an important part of the overall treatment program (3–5).
   C. Wise use of consultants. Contemporary teaching hospitals are staffed with professionals of many kinds, including pharmacists, dieticians, discharge planners, and social workers. Use them; anticipate their needs and communicate freely. Help them help you care for the patients.
   D. **If preoperative preparation is necessary:**
      1. The injury, the patient's general health, and the specific needs of the surgical and anesthesia team must be met. Know and understand the local preferences on preoperative protocols when writing for skin preps, specific labs, and tests [electrocardiogram (ECG), coagulation examinations, etc.]. Anticipate the need for the surgical consent and help to obtain it, if appropriate.
      2. **The surgical prep sometimes includes a** 10-minute chlorhexidine (Hibiclens) or povidone-iodine (Betadine) scrub before surgery (6). If the patient is ambulatory, then the scrub is most easily accomplished by a shower with chlorhexidine or hexachlorophene soap at home the night before surgery. The authors advise that shaving of any hair from the operative field be done in the operating room with mechanical shavers. Small nicks or lacerations often occur with standard razors and can become colonized and increase the risk of a postoperative infection (6). Fracture blisters should be kept intact and dressed sterilely preoperatively (7–9).
      3. **Laboratory data.** Patients undergoing a surgical procedure usually have a hemoglobin test within 30 days of surgery. The erythrocyte sedimentation rate (ESR) and C-reactive protein (CRP) should be determined for all patients with a history of infection. If the age of the patient (generally older than 50 years of age) or the history indicates, then a chest roentgenogram and ECG are appropriate. Whenever blood transfusion is deemed likely, autologous blood donation should be considered (10). This can be set up through the local blood bank. Up to three units of blood can be drawn and stored over a

3-week period. Generally, a fourth week before the scheduled procedure is allowed for recovery. Because this is not possible for acute trauma cases, the use of intraoperative suction-collection-filtering-retransfusion (Cell-Saver) should be considered. Help your team anticipate these needs.

Many lab values and imaging reports are within hospital computer systems. Learn these systems (if you do not know them already). Be prepared to retrieve critical reports and results, anticipating for your team what will be necessary for the smooth running of the ward, preop preparation, and diagnostic problems. Help your team to refocus and address the changing needs of the patients.

E. **Antibiotics are used for open fractures and should be used prophylactically for many types of orthopaedic procedures** (11). For the most part, cephazolin is used, approximately 1 to 2 g before the skin incision, and continuing 1 g every 8 hours for 24 hours postoperatively. For those adults who are allergic to penicillin or cephalosporins, clindamycin [600–900 mg intravenously (IV) every 8 hours] or vancomycin (750–1000 mg every 12 hours) is appropriate. Vancomycin can be associated with hypotension, tachycardia, or flushing, so give it slowly. Also, renal toxicity is a major concern, and drug levels must be monitored if given for more than a few days. Know well the characteristics of the antibiotics used, and obtain a careful history to ascertain possible allergies to antibiotics before administration. The use of surgical drains does not appear to decrease the risk of deep infection. Careful attention to skin preparation at the initiation of the procedure can limit the risk to the patient.

F. **Analgesics, sedatives, and hypnotics.** Virtually all orthopaedic patients admitted for acute problems have pain and anxiety. It is important to make the patient comfortable through adequate medication as quickly as possible. Take into consideration the size of the patient, the amount of medication received previously, and the type of orthopaedic problem or operation causing the pain.

1. Ideally, the analgesic and sedation regimen should keep the patients on a **diurnal schedule** so that they stay awake during the daytime and sleep at night. Sleeplessness is itself debilitating. Patients can tolerate considerably more pain or discomfort during the daytime (when there are distractions) than at night. For this reason, it is frequently helpful to use lighter analgesics during the daytime hours. Allow the nurses latitude in administration of such medications. Give ranges and seek input for the problems and questions which inevitably occur. Consider augmenting narcotics with nonopiate analgesics or nonsteroidal anti-inflammatory drugs (NSAIDs) to decrease narcotic use, remembering that the NSAIDs can interfere with the metabolic pathways of bone healing. Remember that many interfere with platelet activity as well, which is important in the posttraumatic and postoperative situations.

2. **Analgesics.** It is best if the physician can anticipate a patient's pain and its severity because standing orders may then be written on a time-related basis to provide adequate patient comfort. However, these guidelines must be written conservatively, with enough provision for oversight and management to avoid overdosage. Most helpful in this regard has been the development of patient-controlled, parenteral, opiate administration systems. Consider monitoring the patient with respiratory monitors or pulse oximetry. When patients are allowed to titrate small doses of analgesia, they avoid toxicity yet keep their blood levels above the minimum effective analgesic concentration. Morphine, meperidine, (Demerol), and hyromorphone (Dilaudid) are the most widely used drugs with these systems (12). Since the effect and risk of these drugs is higher (though theoretically more precise) with "patient-controlled analgesia," know the doses and ranges. Be conservative and ask about changing recommendations. Many narcotics have similar adverse side effects and produce addiction after approximately 4 weeks. The beneficial effects (analgesia and hypnosis) as well as the adverse side effects vary among patients (13).

3. **Chronic pain.** Narcotics are invaluable in the control of pain but should be **used by experts only** for chronic pain problems (14). Consider pain clinic

consultation for complex problems, conflicting needs, atypical use problems, or demanding patients. Sharing the responsibility for such decisions in highly charged environments is often wise. Anticipate the undesirable side effects (such as reducing the cough reflex and level of respiration, depressing bladder tone, lowering bowel motility, producing nausea and, occasionally, vomiting) and initiate measures to counteract them. Counsel the patient to relieve apprehension regarding these side effects. The patient will then require lower doses. The reduced dose, in turn, decreases the undesirable effects of the analgesics. Patients with chronic pain need the help of an anesthesia or pain consultant.
4. **Sedatives and hypnotics**
    a. For patients with severe anxiety, it is frequently helpful to combine the analgesics with a **sedative or tranquilizing drug**. If a patient is to undergo physical therapy, then avoid muscle relaxants during the day. Hydroxyzine (Vistaril), 50 mg by mouth (PO) or intramuscularly (IM), is useful in conjunction with analgesics, such as the major narcotics or one of the codeine derivatives (e.g., Tylenol No. 3), to control the anxiety and decrease the need for large doses of analgesics.
    b. Generally provide a hospitalized patient with a **hypnotic** for sleep. The need for sleep and the need for pain relief are separate but interrelated. Confer with the nurses about specific needs to avoid overmedication. These drugs need to be used with caution in the elderly.
G. **Prevention of thromboembolism**
    1. The risk of thrombophlebitis and thromboembolism attends every patient at rest and is compounded by physical (venous flow) and hematologic changes of inactivity (15–17). Elderly patients and those undergoing bed rest for longer than a day should be put on a prophylactic program (18). This program **may** include slight elevation of the foot of the bed, application of elastic bandages or stockings, application of sequential compression devices, and initiating an active muscle exercise program (foot pumps) to stimulate circulation through the lower extremities (19,20). **High-risk patients** include those with a history of previous thromboembolic disease, previous surgery to the lower extremities, or chronic venous disease; patients on oral contraceptives; patients with a history of cancer or significant fractures (of the pelvis or femur); patients who smoke; or patients undergoing a lower extremity replacement arthroplasty (18). These high-risk patients should have prophylactic therapy. Spinal or epidural anesthesia may decrease the incidence of deep vein thrombosis (DVT) (21,22). Duplex ultrasound is an accurate method for DVT screening (23).
    2. **There are many options for the prevention and treatment of the patient at risk for thromboembolic phenomena. Warfarin, aspirin, dextran, heparin, low-molecular-weight heparin and sequential compression devices have been used in prophylactic treatment.** Coumadin acts against the vitamin K-dependent clotting factors. Heparin and dextran-related (fragmented heparin) drugs are based on the polysaccharides which anticoagulate via heparin-based mechanisms (24). A third alternative, a pentasaccharide (Arixtra), works by similar mechanisms. Generally, the more effective anticoagulation, the greater the risk of bleeding-related complications, and treating physicians are constantly evaluating this fundamental trade-off. Even after many years (even decades), there is no consensus on optimal treatment. Furthermore, otherwise effective treatments are complicated by administration and technical problems. Coumadin, though easily administered, is difficult (and expensive) to monitor, whereas the low molecular weight dextrans (enoxiparin) require less monitoring but require needle-based injections. Any of these problems may be complicating (or disqualifying) in a given treatment situation. For the most part, a plan based on the contingencies of the local realities and preferences will exist when the student's service rotation starts. The actual treatment selected is largely up to the surgeon because current studies

do not provide conclusive evidence to support or discredit any particular therapeutic regimen. Evidence has supported the prophylactic use of warfarin, low-molecular-weight heparin, or aspirin. The relative risks of embolic disease versus the complications of anticoagulants (hemorrhage, subsequent infection) must be weighed for each patient undergoing treatment.

    a. If **warfarin** is chosen for DVT prophylaxis for elective surgery, it may be started before or after the procedure. The dose will depend on the situation, the patient's underlying comorbidities such as renal or hepatic disease, or preoperative need (such as atrial fibrillation, valvular disease, or coagulation disorder). The starting dose may be 2.5 to 10.0 mg (depending on the patient). Thereafter, alter the dose to maintain the prothrombin time, as determined by International Normalized Ratio at roughly 1.5 to 2 times the normal control. Although this time is difficult to regulate, when properly managed it gives a very satisfactory method in the prevention of fatal pulmonary embolism.

    b. If **aspirin** is chosen, it is started at the surgeon's discretion based on technical consideration of perioperative considerations and risk. The student must ask about proper timing. Generally, if aspirin is used for chronic anticoagulation, a pediatric-sized aspirin (81 mg) daily is enough. Keep in mind the mechanism of aspirin-related platelet effects is different and may complicate the use of other methods of anticoagulation, either vitamin-K based or heparin based.

    c. If **low-molecular-weight dextran** is selected, check with the pharmacist or hospitalist for proper dosing.

    d. If **heparin** is selected, then the usual dosage is 5,000 IU SQ q8h. It has also been given in combination with dihydroergotamine, 0.5 mg IM. The treatment is often started at operation. For patients who have pelvic or femoral fractures, use subcutaneous heparin preoperatively and warfarin to maintain the prothrombin time at 1.5 times control level postoperatively (25).

    e. If **low-molecular-weight heparin** is chosen, the usual starting dose is 30 mg SQ q12h (24,26,27). The advantage of this therapy is that no monitoring of hematologic parameters is usually necessary. If this is to be continued after discharge, then ask the nursing staff to teach the patient family home administration techniques.

  3. **Check with the orthopaedic team, the hospitalists, or pharmacists regarding recommendations on monitoring methods, follow-up, and guidelines for cessation** (28).

H. **Posttraumatic and postoperative urinary retention is not uncommon.** Indications for bladder catheterization include prolonged anesthesia. Prolonged would be easily defined as a case longer than 3 hours, but many surgeons will want a catheter for cases much shorter than this. The decision for a catheter is a joint decision between the surgeon and the anesthesia team. This decision is more easily made if there is good communication between the surgeon and anesthesia about case length, comorbidities, expected blood loss, fluid parameters, trauma status, postoperative nursing needs, and so on. If the bladder has been overdistended, it takes several days to regain normal tone. For this reason, if the patient requires catheterization, it should be done with a small catheter that has a 5-mL balloon. Leave the catheter in the bladder and attached to closed gravity drainage. Some state that the catheter should be left in place until the patient is ambulatory or is off narcotics during the daytime; others argue that the catheter should be removed as soon as the patient is alert enough to urinate in order to limit possible urinary tract infections (29). As common as catheter usage is, literature-based guidance on catheter usage is lacking.

I. **Bowel.** Bowel problems are best addressed if anticipated. A mix of bulking agents, stool softeners, lubricants, and laxatives may make the patient's course more comfortable if given before there is a problem. This is particularly true of at-rest patients on narcotics. Docusate sodium (Colace), 100 mg b.i.d, usually is satisfactory, but it may be necessary to supplement this with 30 to 60 mL of milk of magnesia at bedtime. Mineral oil is a useful stool softener/lubricant, but it should be administered with caution because it may interfere with vitamin absorption.

J. **Skin.** Pressure sores are often prevented by good nursing care (30). Pressure problems are common over the sacrum and the heels. Patients who are unable to change position frequently following surgery or trauma must be turned frequently by the staff. Dressings which cover these common areas must be applied anticipating the inability to move or protect. When exposed, skin checks for redness are critical, especially on newly injured patients, unconscious patients, patients with dementia, patients with spinal cord injury or spina bifida, splinted extremities, and extremities in traction. *The problem is especially acute* in paraplegic and quadriplegic patients or in patients with concomitant head injury. If the orthopaedic condition does not allow frequent change in position, consider using special flotation mattresses or rotating beds (31). Check the skin during rounds. Consider the pressure areas at the same time that the other areas at risk in surgery are considered (calf tenderness, wound complications, etc.).

K. **Activities and physical therapy.** The postoperative activity/physical therapy plan should be recorded in the written operative note. Weight-bearing status and allowable use of the hand below a dressing or splint (whether long arm or short arm) are technical decisions related to many specific orthopaedic considerations (injury, prosthesis, surgical confidence), so ask. Also ask for the rationale so that the student will learn. Each morning on rounds the staff decides what activity or therapy the patient should have that day. Activities may take diverse forms from minor diversions to a full-scale physical therapy program. Dumbbells and pulleys can be used to toughen the hands and strengthen triceps and shoulder muscles in preparation for crutch ambulation. Dumbbells are also useful in increasing chest muscle activity and improving cardiopulmonary exchange (32). All muscles, except those immediate to the injured or operative area, should be exercised in a set daily program. This exercise provides excellent distraction as well as a general sense of improved well-being. In addition, it may help prevent a thromboembolic episode. Regularly scheduled turning, the use of an incentive spirometer, coughing, deep breathing, and leg exercises are integral to any early physical therapy program. It is essential to turn all patients and inspect any areas of potential pressure at least once every 4 hours.

L. **Common *preoperative* orders** for a general orthopaedic procedure
   1. **Diagnosis**
   2. **Condition**
   3. **Diet**—nothing by mouth before surgery, usually 12 hours before, or after midnight for a case the following day
   4. **Activity**
   5. **Vital signs**
   6. **Enema** (optional for hip and back surgeries)
   7. **Laboratory data and other testing. Check with specialists and anesthesia**
      a. **Hematocrit/hemoglobin, as appropriate**
      b. **Urinalysis**
      c. **Chest roentgenogram if patient is older than 50 years**
      d. **ECG if patient is older than 50 years and no recent ECG results are available**
      e. **ESR (and/or CRP) if there is history of infection**
      f. **Roentgenogram of operative area, if indicated**
      g. **Blood typed and cross matched if significant loss is anticipated. The use of an intraoperative suction, collection, and transfusion system such as the "cell saver" should be anticipated and used when blood loss is anticipated to be more than 500 to 600 mL. Similarly, the efficient use of a tourniquet can limit blood loss and should be planned** (33)
      h. **Culture, of wounds which will require treatment**

8. **Antibiotics** if indicated
9. **Analgesics** if indicated
10. **Hypnotic**
11. **Instruction in physical therapy** that may be required postoperatively

M. *Postoperative orders* for a general orthopaedic procedure
1. **Operation performed**
2. **Patient condition**
3. **Diet or IV orders**
4. **Activity or position**
5. **Vital signs**—record intake and output if indicated
6. **Patient turned, coughing, incentive spirometry, and deep breathing encouraged** q1–4h
7. **Small urinary catheter** inserted **if no urine** is produced within 8 hours postoperatively
8. **Analgesic** (as appropriate) prescribed on a time-related basis or patient-controlled system
9. **Hypnotic**
10. **Multivitamin** and supplements IV or PO
11. **Postoperative hematocrit/hemoglobin** (if indicated, preferably at least 8 hours postoperatively)
12. **Postoperative roentgenogram** if indicated
13. **Physical therapy orders**
14. **Physician notified** typical guidelines include: if blood pressure is less than 90/60, pulse is greater than 100, or temperature is greater than 38°C
15. **When a diet is tolerated, appropriate diet, including considerations for diabetes** (3)
16. **Iron** (therapeutic doses) **if anemic or if anemia is anticipated and transfusion is not necessary. Review the contraindications of iron therapy and ask for preferences**
17. **Anticoagulation therapy** if indicated (see above, remember to ask for particular preferences)
18. **Postoperative antibiotics, including those for treatment or for general prophylaxis**
19. **Bowel program including softeners (Docusate sodium) and laxatives (milk of magnesia) as needed**
20. **Social service consultation** if needed for disposition

V. **ORTHOPAEDIC TIPS FOR STUDENTS AND INTERNS:** *Discuss with your residents and staff at the beginning of the rotation*
   A. **Regarding the involvement of medical students on the orthopaedic team:**
   1. To what extent should the student be actively involved with patient care decisions, patient communications, and so on? At what level should the student show initiative?
   2. Ensure a balance between exposure to the clinic, hospital rounds, and operating room.
   3. Are there office staff who will have schedules, knowledge of the other services, and related educational opportunities? To whom should the student report or ask questions?
   4. Would a presentation to the group be of interest? Such presentations, and the interest that they convey, are great ways to get a deeper insight into orthopaedic decisions, thought processes, and priorities. It makes the cases that present especially relevant. What is learned in this exercise will last with the student for his or her entire practice career.
   5. Ensure exposure to the various areas of orthopaedics. Discuss how each of the subspecialists makes decisions about what to care for and what to refer.
   B. **Regarding patient care and ward decisions.** Remember that orthopaedic patients, though they have many of the same general needs as medical surgical patients, have other important needs specific to orthopaedics. These include prophylactic antibiotics, prophylactic anticoagulation, imaging needs (which are specific and evolving as

the case progresses), and physical therapy (including weight-bearing status and protective activities). The student helps the care tremendously by considering these factors, questioning them, and reevaluating them in light of comorbidies, pending surgeries, and interactions with other services. Some of these issues include:
1. How are prophylactic antibiotics used? What are the typical first-line, second-line, and back-up drugs?
2. What will be used for prophylactic anticoagulation? Who will monitor any necessary lab values?
3. Ask about guidelines for preoperative workups and indications for ECGs, labs, chest x-ray. Who will obtain necessary informed consent?
4. What are the indications for urinary catheters? What are the indications for using them or discontinuing them?
5. How are narcotics to be used? What is the role of respiratory monitors and pulse oximeters?

C. **Advice to the student on how to be useful and get the most out of your rotation**
1. Be around the ward, clinic, and operating rooms. They are all important.
2. Start early. If possible, round and review before the team.
3. Know the plan. The plan is dynamic and will evolve. Know the contingencies which would change the plan. Help to anticipate these contingencies.
4. Communicate with all. Ask the nurses, the staff, the residents, and the consultants.
5. Provide for the needs of the patient. Know the necessary steps to **get them ready** for the next stage of their care.
   a. **For surgery**, check on the completion of the preparations. Check and confirm NPO status, pending lab values, pending imaging, surgical consents, and consultant evaluations.
   b. **For the postoperative situation**, ensure adequate pain medication and follow-up on postoperative images and lab values (e.g., hemoglobin, electrolytes). Question the need for urinary catheters and discontinue as early as possible.
   c. **For discharge and follow-up**, help get them ready. When appropriate, involve the therapists, nurses, and social workers with the orthopaedic team.
6. Contribute energy. Be lighthearted but earnest about the priorities and stresses of patient care. Be willing to contribute on those small but unavoidable tasks (e.g., fetching x-rays, changing dressings, removing sutures).
7. Be careful about what information you give directly to the patient. Err on the side of caution. **Never** be the first one to give the patient bad news (unless specifically directed otherwise by the staff physician).
8. Read, study, and ask. Reading is best done immediately surrounding the teaching event, whatever it is.

D. **Maturing as a student of orthopaedics**
"Becoming is superior to being."—Socrates
Orthopaedic deformity is alarming. The pain is deep and visceral, and for the uninitiated there is something untouchable about it. The patient's pain is accompanied by a fear of new injury. This fear and the deep special quality of the distress touch the patient and the caregiver alike.

However common and understandable, a student's personal sensations may be of hindrance to the proper evaluation of these patients. In other specialities the medical evaluation is often not painful, but a fracture or sprain cannot be examined or treated without pain. The fear, which we see in our patients' eyes, can push us away and may result in the lack of the necessary touch toward the consolation, proper examination, necessary positioning, or dressing of the limb.

Intervening takes risk. It takes time to know the patterns of injury, the resources (e.g., imaging, referral expertise), and to know the patterns of response. Like any refined art, it is actually a mix of science and art, which requires a mix of subjective and objective proficiencies to physically execute. There is no place for a lack of courage, lack of humanitarian concern, or energy.

The medical student who chooses to rotate through orthopaedics has a challenging mix of skills, relationships, and resources to develop. What the student takes with him or her will be deeply personal based on his or her own investment. Face time with staff is important. Reading is critical. Student involvement results in a buzz of staff interaction and worthy debate about pathophysiology, social expense, and techniques of surgery. As in the rest of medicine, everyone benefits, including (and especially) the students and patients.

If you are interested, there is no substitute for actually being there. Unfortunately, these interactions may occur at odd hours of the night or very busy periods of the day. They occur in the operating room, the ward, and in the conference room. The student must invest that time.

If the student is interested in procedures or the kind of in-depth experience that helps him or her in a career decision, he or she should say so. Just like other disciplines, the learner will need to put in more time, and a greater physical effort will pull available learning opportunities to them. This means standing in surgery, watching in clinic, running for x-rays, or making the necessary phone calls. Closed reductions (and the snap or crepitation that go with them) or the insertion of a screw may be routine for staff, but it could be life-changing for the right student. Every regular in a teaching institution is there because of prior teaching experience and wants to reward interest.

The student should be proud of his or her contribution. Students may look or feel lowly but they contribute energy, enthusiasm, and concern to each situation in which they are involved. Orthopaedic situations require as much of each of those as it can get. Students are valuable for their present value and future value for all the patients that their staff and residents will never see. We, as teachers and physicians, know that. Socrates said "becoming is superior to being," and it is as true now as it was then. The staff respects what the student is becoming.

Having stated the philosophical truth about the value and interest of students, some principles are common to all areas of medicine and education; some are unique to orthopaedics:

1. **Dealing with patients**
   a. Address their expectations. A patient's satisfaction is, in large part, a function of his or her concept of the treatment and reasonable expectations.
   b. Communicate, reassure, and assuage. When communicating with a patient, strike a balance between the self-justifying catharsis and arrogant selfishness with the facts and reality. You are there because of all the needs you can provide, not just the technical execution of what you know. Even if you are not the final authority to do what may be necessary, your contribution can become a light post to the patient from which he or she may venture from reluctantly.
   c. Exert the necessary energy. There is physicality to being with orthopaedists. The internist may surmise the fluid status of the patient by the strain on the ECG, but the orthopaedist will never know the status of the wound without removing the dressing or the nature of the fracture pattern without digging up and looking at the x-rays ourselves. We will never learn without taking a stab at identifying, describing, and classifying the injury or disease.
   d. Recognize the helplessness of orthopaedic patients. The damaged limb is painful and requires help at several levels (pain medication, splinting, judicious surgery) to make it less so. Orthopaedic patients will not be able to walk out of a hospital in a fire. For the most part, they are truly helpless during the injury and perioperative periods. The student is there to develop a perspective on sensitivity and knowledgeable contribution. Maximizing the function and accelerating the recovery of such patients is a demanding process.

E. **Principles specific to orthopaedics**
   1. Handle bone with the care it needs. It may look hard and impenetrable, but we know it is living tissue. Protect it from inflammation, infection, avascularity, and abnormal (either excessive, inadequate, or malaligned) stresses and motions.

2. Handle joints with the care they require. Restore alignment, anatomy, and soft tissue. Support structure, and consider cartilage stresses. Restoration of anatomy and physiology (stresses and motion) to the joint, its blood supply, its motor control, and its cognitive control are all vital to the function of the joint. Remember that the implications for bone injury, whether diaphyseal, metaphyseal, or periarticular, have specific implications for each of the joints of the limb.
3. Be precise in your understanding of pain. The high incidence of pain as a presenting complaint makes orthopaedics unique. There are many types of pain including classic orthopaedic pain, acute and chronic depression, muscle spasm, and neuralgia. Patients may have more than one, and treatments for one of these may not be good treatments or substitutes for another. The pattern of pain, the physical exam, and the imaging are the methods by which the lesions are mostly separated out. Attack it at every level: the painful lesion, the transmission, and the central pathways. Minimize its effect by addressing the dysfunction and the depression.
4. Remember the soft tissues. Anticipate what the soft tissues will do. Know the difference between disease and disuse. Understand weakness, adhesion, incoordination, and soft-tissue blocks to function.
5. Have a plan of attack and know what you are attacking. Know what is primary (often fracture deformity) and what is secondary (usually inflammation and pain). Know the difference between primary interventions (fracture repair for pain relief) and palliative ones (control of inflammation, control of pain).
6. Appreciate anatomy. Usually the return of function parallels the restoration of anatomy. It makes some sense, intuitively, that this would be true, but sometimes the anatomic relationships are not easily restored. Closed reductions require a level of abstract consideration because they are out of site, but such considerations are also common of open reductions, joint replacement surgery, and balancing operations.
7. Appreciate balance. Much of fracture orthopaedics occurs within the acute situation, but the responsibilities of the orthopaedic intervention are related to the acceleration of the restoration of normalcy. This cannot be considered complete without a consideration for the social situation as well. Balancing these considerations is at the essence of orthopaedics and is dependent on a number of individual factors including those particular to the patient (personal fear of surgery, age), the medical environment (facilities and surgical interest), and those of society (funding priorities, long-term care).
8. Restore the physiologic milieu. Set in place the timeline and processes for that physiologic milieu. With a fracture, reduction of the fracture may be the method. In rheumatoid arthritis, control of inflammation may be the method. Surgery may look like a technical exercise in the restoration of anatomy, but it is at least that and, more fundamentally, a manipulation of physiology. We see and easily relate to the visible deformity, but no technical situation will respond to an ignorant assault on that alone. Anatomy relies on biochemistry, and the successful surgeon thinks of, respects, and protects the physiology of the entire process.
9. Anticipate future problems. For the most part, those deformities that are known to be associated with late problems are understood by the orthopaedist.
10. Know pathophysiology and physiology of each of the processes, including the different forms of pain, inflammation, soft-tissue repair, scar, and regeneration. This includes the fracture healing and patient-human response of anxiety and depression. The treating doctor will be a better physician and the best practitioner if he or she anticipates and attacks pathophysiology at every opportunity. Every patient wants his or her surgeon to be a true physician in every sense of the word.
11. Look for and treat an underlying pathophysiology. Social impairment or lack of access to resources may be at the root of the patient's inability to thrive, which may be the real reason for the bone disease that leads to the fracture.

12. Understand the unique demands of orthopaedic tissues, physiologic loading (valgus/varus, longitudinal, and rotational alignment), stress-strain relationships, cyclic loading, vascular support, and bony congruity. Know the difference between the biologic needs of orthopaedic tissues (respiration, vascular supply) and the mechanical ones (strain rates, cyclic loading and catastrophic failure, and incremental failure).
13. Recognize the interrelationship of the biologic/biophysical and the mechanical. The mechanical and biologic needs of orthopaedic tissues are linked, affecting both the onset of lesions (like stress fractures and tennis elbow) and also the healing rates (incorporation of bone graft, etc). It is fundamental and unique to orthopaedics to consider these interactions and protect the patient from adverse effects of whatever may affect this interaction, such as smoking or premature weight bearing.
14. Have a plan B. Have a way out. Save tissue. Create options.
15. Study what is visible on the x-ray. Know the normal alignments and landmarks.
16. Protect the patient who is distracted by pain elsewhere, is unconscious, or unable to express or describe the symptoms.
17. Minimize the secondary injury. Stiffness, weakness, and autonomic dysfunction all follow the orthopaedic injury and may be as related to treatment (unnecessary immobilization, poor patient support) as the original injury.
18. Learn and execute excellent dressing techniques. Covering a wound or an injured limb is not the same as caring for it or protecting it. The dressing usually has a series of responsibilities, including alignment, immobilization, and compression (to minimize venous stasis and swelling). Apply the dressing knowledgeably and thoughtfully, cognizant of how much patient comfort and care depends on your dressing. Your goal is to ease the patient's transition to the next stage.
19. Recognize that children are different, their problems are different, and their needs are different. Things happen in kids that do not happen in adults, and the injuries and their responses are age and site dependent.
    a. The anatomy is different. The supracondylar area of the elbow goes through a narrow remodeling phase between ages 4 and 8, hence all the fractures in this age group. There are other classic patterns (tri-plane fractures and Tillaux fractures of the ankle). There is no substitute for simply knowing the patterns which occur, watching for them, and treating their idiosyncrasies.
    b. The physiology is different. The blood supply to certain areas (femoral head, epiphyseal fragments) passes through a period of vulnerability. Their ability to heal is different, but the implications of maltreatment, malalignment, or corollary damage (i.e., avascularity, growth plate injury) may be magnified over time. The dynamism of growth is directly related to motor use and function.

F. Principles of the mature care giver
1. Be a clinician. Suppress and delay the inclination to define the problem with an x-ray. Take a history, know the patient, and **examine** the patient.
2. Remember that you must confirm the significance of imaging changes and the absence of other changes **not** reflected by the images.
3. Act but recognize an economy of motion, resources, and time. As a student, you may just have to ask. Know where your opportunity is in the timeline of the pathophysiology. Timing in orthopaedics is everything.
4. Know what you are treating. Know the difference between the valid goals of palliation, temporizing, buying time, using time, allowing healing, mental relief, and cure.
5. Remember the simple things like ice, heat, rest, elevation, and reassurance.
6. Understand inflammation. Understand what it is and is not in orthopaedics. Know when it is primarily part of the pathology (rheumatoid arthritis, bursitis) and when it is part of the healing (fractures, sprains). Know how its treatment may assist the treatment of the orthopaedic problem (reduce pain, augment narcotics) and how that treatment may interfere with the desired outcome

(with fracture healing). When inflammation is the component of the disease process that you want to manage, manage it, but remember that in other situations it is an initial component in the normal processes and pathophysiology including fractures, infection, neoplasia, soft tissue trauma, and pain.
7. Study the problem from all angles, perspectives and depths, mechanisms, and pathophysiologies. Look for referred pain. Look for missed injuries. Know the classic associations.

G. Work well with others
1. Be an effective part of a team. Know the roles of the professionals around you. As expectations have improved, the precise management of the patient in the hospital is scrutinized and overseen by many specialists. They will help us to anticipate the needs of the patients, communicate, and administer cost-efficient care. The same goes for nurses, physician assistants, pharmacists, and a host of experts who can teach and guide through the host of problems our patients will face. The same admonitions about humor, principles, and wisdom that govern our actions in conference are appropriate for our relationships with these other professionals.
2. Follow the trends of the rest of medicine. Right now, these are precision, biologic management, patient involvement, natural (common sense) nutrition, health, etc. The practice and the expectations are not created in a vacuum. Fit yourself within the context of society and its direction; cling to the principles that have formed your education and those things that you know to be true.
3. Do what is necessary to facilitate orderly transfer of care. This is by direct communication with those assuming the care. It is not by hospital note or by the assumption of the role of others. Most specifically, it is not by voice mail or email. Nothing substitutes for direct knowledge that the care and decision making is really transferred, questions are asked, and responsibility is accepted.
4. Do not expect to be the judge of your contribution. Know that, however trivial or ungratifying something such as a follow-up or phone call may seem to you, you may be the only person in the world with the knowledge, insight, or time to make it. It may be your major contribution toward relieving patient suffering that day, however, it may not seem that dramatic. As Emerson said, "The grandeur of character acts in the dark." Much of what you do will be silent and unrecognized. That is the nature of the healing arts. No one will ever be able to appreciate the depth of your preparation or the depth of your considerations. Your rewards will often need to be internal.

H. Presenting at rounds.
It is one of the great exercises in the study of medicine to learn by presenting a case. The exercise puts the patient out there and gives the student presenters a focus to bring principles and practice together, which they will do innumerably during their careers. It gives the expert an opportunity to illustrate specifics and generalities. It gives everyone an opportunity to interact. There should be a hint of reverence to the ideas, a deference to the history and leadership, an excuse to ask questions, and a chance to become friends and better orthopaedists.

There **is** a natural strain in the room. There is pride, anticipation, and excitement. There is conscious and subconscious activity. The best rounds become a mix of energies, humanitarian concern, and academics, dripping with pearls of experience and humor. Obviously, if the student is interested in orthopaedics, it is important to present one's self professionally. The staff wants to see grace and poise, real knowledge, humility, and compassion in someone that they like to work with. This presumes a certain competence, but it is much more than that. The personality of the student must fit the group, and there is a cadence, humanity, confidence, and character aspects to all of this. There is little room for showing off, name-dropping, esoteric article references, or deliberate sandbagging.
1. Be organized. Know the case. Know the radiographs. Be sure to have reviewed them before the case because you can be sure that as soon as they are presented, a roomful of very smart, conscientious, very experienced people will

begin to critique them for orderliness, quality, relevance, subtle cues, and missed lesions.

2. Know the point of the case. You can be sure that if someone wants you to show the case, there is a point. If it is a controversial point or some unexpected outcome, the person should be willing to step in when things get interesting. That does not keep the student presenter from knowing or appreciating the interest of those who want to see it, but if the questions get too pointed, show your interest and stay deferential.

3. Keep control of the case. It makes a room of orthopaedists very anxious and unpleasant if the critical elements of the case are missing and are not available to help them toward a reasonable decision. Know the local feeling about certain classic controversies (if appropriate) including closed versus open methods, approaches, borderline circumstances, etc. Know what is necessary. Ask your fellow residents and mentors for the issues likely to come up.

4. Listen for the pearls to drop. The best conferences are a mix of academics and practical considerations playing off of one another. There will be insights about diagnosis, technique, decision making, and people. The subjective reward for presenting is an incremental professional growth in thinking, problem solving, and interpersonal skills. The objective benefit is that the student will learn something specific about the problem at hand.

5. Know the controversies. The average medical student (and some early residents) will not really know how to interpret all the data. The inability to anticipate questions makes for a very uncomfortable presentation, especially if someone in the room might be waiting for you to speculate your way onto the attending's hot button. On the contrary, presenting the case in a context of what is known so that the attending (for example) can teach some hard-won lesson is appropriate and may be the exact reason for the presentation. If the information is to be meted out for the purposes of some teaching exercise, know this and do it appropriately.

6. Keep it positive. Do not "sandbag." Purposely leading the conference astray may have a point in very specific circumstances, but it is a job for experts. Never upstage the staff, and make the points reachable with insight and experience. Misleading the staff with mismarked films, coincidental shadows, and technical obstructions can make things fun, but it cannot be done at anyone's expense.

7. Watch for the pace of the conference. Some participants will want it to move along, and it will certainly be a different conference if it attempts to instruct residents and not staff. Know which it is.

8. Speak the language. There is a language of fractures. Valgus, varus, proximal, distal, fracture type and classification, and soft tissue injury class are within the point of the presentation exercise. If you use a name ("Colles," "Barton's," "Bennetts"), expect to be asked the derivation of the name. If a fracture class (Schatzker) or injury class (Gustilo, Tscherne, etc.) is used, it is imperative that the student can describe why it is that class and what the definition of the other classifications are. This is basic: **expect to be asked**. Almost all classification systems have inadequacies or shortcomings; be prepared to discuss these. Be prepared to show additional studies that define, if the plain films cannot, why they represent the case. Remember that the best classification systems also include mechanism, pathophysiology, and treatment considerations.

9. Use humor if appropriate, or if someone else does, laugh along with everyone else.

10. Show courage. If you are in trouble, do not expect to be rescued too early. Orthopaedists love what they do and they love people who love what orthopaedists do. This means that they will enjoy watching a competent student struggle with forming a concept or discovering a truth, but it will never be sadistic. Do not bail or defer to the staff or teachers too early. Though it is the first time for you (perhaps), you are probably one of hundreds of students that

the members of the conference have seen in this circumstance, and they will want you to succeed, overcome, and grow. This will take some sweat on your part, but it is the way medicine and the fraternity/sorority of caregivers has been handled for centuries. Remember, if someone asks you to present, it is a compliment of sorts; live up to it.
11. Recognize "roundsmanship." Know where the power is. Know which of the staff **really** knows. The senior staff may lead or save the last word for good reasons. The interaction of the junior staff may be fun to watch. The last comment, particularly if it is poignant or insightful, may be where the wisdom comes from. Be ready to discern technical input from true wisdom.
12. **Never** lie or fudge. If you are presenting a case that you have never seen, say so early. If there is missing data, say that too. This can be very embarrassing at times. Orthopaedists get fussy if their opportunity to lead to a logical conclusion is robbed from them. If there is no point to the presentation, or they cannot be brought logically to that point, they get fussy about that too.
13. Ask what was learned, what was decided, and whether the goals were achieved. Know if there is a relationship of the case you are presenting to the other cases that are being presented. It will come off better if there is an underlying theme, principle, or deeper insight. Learners at all levels appreciate the observation, the obscure lesson, and the surgical trick. However, they will **really** appreciate the principle, wisdom, or a depth of understanding. These higher level lessons leave a mark. The useful is what they come for; the profound is what they hunger for. Enable this, if you can, by priming the staff. Know it when you see it. Associate with those who can do it; learn their methods and insights. Probe the depths a little.
14. Be ready to apply what is learned. If nothing is learned, at least put a note in the chart that documents that it was presented. How much of the controversies go into the chart is decided by the staff and residents on the case.

I. **Working with orthopaedists.** On the ward and in the clinics, medical and professional principles apply to your behavior. Orthopaedists love what they do, especially the creative and inventive aspects of it. The orthopaedic story behind each injury makes the cases interesting. Know it.

J. **Final Thoughts**
1. *Primum non nocere.* For a student on orthopaedics, this means be there, be sensitive, ask questions, and follow through.
2. Know your limitations. This is closely related to *primum non nocere.* One of the great hazards in medicine is the practitioner who rises to a level of incompetence and does not pull back from it. Periods of growth (including being a medical student) carry risks of failure for both patient and doctor. The practitioner takes his or her patient from the realm of the unknown with him or her to the known. Seek and ye shall find. If asking for help is uncomfortable, use that as an opportunity for growth too.
3. Take good medical care of your patients. There is no substitute for seeing (actually seeing) your patients. Remember that they need touching and interaction.
4. Respect patients as humans. Communicate respectfully and honestly. If you do not know, "I don't know, but I'll check" is a useful thing to say. Apologize when late and give a reasonable explanation when it is appropriate. Make eye contact. Touch the patient lightly in a neutral-safe area; shake hands often; and give consolation, sympathy, empathy, and sensitivity to what they may be feeling emotionally and physically. These subjective elements are inestimable in our society, especially today and especially for the less fortunate.
5. Have reverence for the history and process that put you in this remarkable circumstance. The principles you apply were discovered at great cost over centuries. When the exam room door closes, it will be you, the patient, and those principles.
6. Be supportive of your colleagues. It may be your feeling that the patient has been poorly or inadequately served somehow, but it may only add to their suffering to give them misgivings or guilt about how they may have or should

have done things differently. Conversely, if you like or have confidence in, or appreciate certain consultants, assistants or referral primaries, say so. Patients like to be part of a team that works.
7. Do not let anything about your personal limitations or emotions detract from your accomplishments (or those of the profession or department). Remember that you are there to learn professionalism in addition to orthopaedics.
8. Remember, most fundamentally, you are there to relieve suffering of any kind.

References

1. Ewing JA. Detecting alcoholism; the CAGE questionnaire. *JAMA* 1984;252:1905–1907.
2. O'Connor PG, Schottenfeld RS. Patients with alcohol problems. *N Engl J Med* 1998;338:592–602.
3. Herrman FR, Safran C, Levkoff SE, et al. Serum albumin level on admission as a predictor of death, length of stay and readmission. *Arch Intern Med* 1992;152:125–130.
4. Klein JD, Hey LA, Ya CS, et al. Perioperative nutrition and postoperative complications in patients undergoing spinal surgery. *Spine* 1996;22:2676–2682.
5. Smith TK. Prevention of complications in orthopaedic surgery secondary to nutritional depletion. *Clin Orthop* 1987;222:91–97.
6. Gillam DL, Nelson CL. Comparison of a one-step iodophor skin preparation vs. traditional preparation in total joint surgery. *Clin Orthop* 1990;250:258–260.
7. Giordano CP, Koval KJ, Zuckerman JD, et al. Fracture blisters. *Clin Orthop* 1994;307:214–221.
8. Giordano CP, Scott D, Koval KJ, et al. Fracture blister formation: a laboratory study. *J Trauma* 1995;38:907–909.
9. Varela CD, Vanghan TK, Carr JB, et al. Fracture blisters: clinical and pathological aspects. *J Orthop Trauma* 1993;7:417–427.
10. Benli IT, Akalin S, Duman E, et al. The results of intraoperative autotransfusion in orthopaedic surgery. *Bull Hosp Jt Dis* 1999;58:184–187.
11. Boxma H, Braekhuizen T, Patka P, et al. Randomized controlled trial of single-dose antibiotic prophylaxis in surgical treatment of closed fractures: the dutch trauma trial. *Lancet* 1996;347:1133–1137.
12. Drugs for pain. *Med Lett Drugs Ther* 1993;35:1.
13. Jamison RN, Ross MJ, Hoopman P, et al. Assessment of postoperative pain management: patient satisfaction and perceived helpfulness. *Clin J Pain* 1997;13:229–236.
14. Haddox JD, Joranson D, Angasola RT, et al. The use of opioids for the treatment of chronic pain: a consensus statement from the american academy of pain medicine and the american pain society. *Clin J Pain* 1997;13:6–8.
15. Abelseth G, Buckley RE, Pinco GE, et al. Incidence of deep-vein thrombosis in patients with fractures of the lower extremity distal to the hip. *J Orthop Trauma* 1996;10:230–235.
16. Brasel KJ, Borgstrom DC, Weigelt JA. Cost-effective prevention of pulmonary embolus in high-risk trauma patients. *J Trauma* 1997;42:456–462.
17. Paiement GD, Beisaw NE, Harris WH, et al. Advances in prevention of venous thromboembolic disease after elective hip surgery. *Instr Course Lect* 1990;39:413–421.
18. Khan FM, Moran CG, Pinder IM, et al. The incidence of fatal pulmonary embolism after knee replacement with no prophylactic anthoagulation. *J Bone Joint Surg* 1993;75:940–941.
19. Brandjes DPM, Buller HR, Heijboer H, et al. Randomized trial of effect of compression stockings in patients with symptomatic proximal vein thrombosis. *Lancet* 1997;349:759–762.
20. Fordyce MJF, Ling RSM. A venous foot pump reduces thrombosis after total hip replacement. *J Bone Joint Surg (Br)* 1992;74:45–49.
21. Wiklund RA, Rosenbaum SH. Anesthesiology. *N Engl J Med* 1997;337:1132–1141.

22. Williams-Russo P, Sharrock NE, Mattis S, et al. Cognitive effects after epidural vs. general anesthesia in older adults. *JAMA* 1995;274:44–50.
23. Froehlich JA, Dorfman GS, Cornan JJ, et al. Compression ultrasonography for the detection of deep venous thrombosis in orthopaedic patients who have a fracture of the hip. A prospective study. *J Bone Joint Surg (Am)* 1989;71:249–256.
24. Bergquist D, Benoni G, Bjorgell O, et al. Low-molecular weight heparin (enoxaparin) as prophylaxis against venous thromboembolism after total hip arthroplasty. *N Engl J Med* 1996;335:696–700.
25. Gould MK, Dembitzer AD, Doyle RL, et al. Low molecular weight heparins compared with unfractionated heparin for treatment of acute deep venous thrombosis: a meta-analysis of randomized, controlled trials. *Arch Intern Med* 1999;130: 800–809.
26. Geerts WH, Jay RM, Code KI, et al. A comparison of low-dose heparin with low-molecular weight heparin as prophylaxis against venous thromboembolism after major trauma. *N Engl J Med* 1996;335:701–707.
27. Knudson MM, Morabito O, Paiement GD, et al. Use of low molecular weight heparin in preventing thromboembolism in trauma patients. *J Trauma-Injury Infect Crit Care* 1996;41:446–459.
28. Anard SS, Wells PS, Hunt D, et al. Does this patient have deep vein thrombosis? *JAMA* 1998;279:1094–1099.
29. Carpiniello VL, Cendron AM, Altman HG, et al. Treatment of urinary complications after total joint replacement in elderly females. *Urology* 1988;32:186–188.
30. Maklebust J. Pressure ulcers: etiology and prevention. *Nurs Clin North Am* 1987;22:359–377.
31. Allman RM, Walker JM, Hart MK, et al. Air-fluidized beds or conventional therapy for pressure sores: a randomized trial. *Ann Intern Med* 1987;107:641–648.
32. Reilly DE, McNeely MJ, Doerner D, et al. Self reported exercise tolerance and the risk of serious perioperative complications. *Arch Intern Med* 1999;159:2185–2192.
33. Bono JV, Carl AL, Schneider JM. Exsanguination: gravity vs. esmarch. *Contemp Orthop* 1995;30:117–119.

Selected Historical Readings

Harris WH, Athanasoulis CA, Waltron AC, et al. Prophylaxis of deep-vein thrombosis after total hip replacement, dextran and external pneumatic compression compared with 1.2 or 1.3 grams of aspirin daily. *J Bone Joint Surg (Am)* 1985;67:57–62.

Henny CP, Odoom JA, Ten Cate H, et al. Effects of extradural bupivacaine on the haemostatic system. *Br J Anaesth* 1986;58:301–305.

Jensen JE, Jensen TG, Smith TK, et al. Nutrition in orthopaedic surgery. *J Bone Joint Surg (Am)* 1982;64:1263–1272.

Kay SP, Moreland JR, Schmitter E. Nutritional status and wound healing in lower extremity amputations. *Clin Orthop* 1987;217:253–256.

McKenzie PJ, Wishart HY, Smith G. Long-term outcome after repair of fractured neck of femur: comparison of subarachnoid and general anaesthesia. *Br J Anaesth* 1984;56: 581–585.

Means JH. *The amenities of ward rounds and related matters.* Boston, MA: Massachusetts General Hospital Print Shop, 1942.

Michelson JD, Lotke PA, Steinberg ME. Urinary bladder management after total joint replacement surgery. *N Engl J Med* 1988;319:321–326.

Schaeffer AJ. Catheter-associated bacteriuria. *Urol Clin North Am* 1986;13:735–747.

Thorburn J, Louden JR, Vallance R. Spinal and general anaesthesia in total hip replacement: frequency of deep vein thrombosis. *Br J Anaesth* 1980;52:1117–1121.

Weed LL. *Medical records, medical education, and patient care,* 2nd ed. Chicago, IL: Year Book, 1970.

TRACTION   9

I. **OBJECTIVES.** Although traction is being used with decreasing frequency for fracture care in the Western world, a knowledge of these effective principles is necessary for special indications or situations in which equipment or expertise is not available or patient comorbidities do not permit operative intervention.
   A. Traction maintains the **length** of a limb as well as **alignment and stability** at the fracture site. Treating femoral fractures with fixed skeletal traction is an example.
   B. Traction can **allow joint motion** while maintaining alignment of the fracture. For example, the Pearson attachment on a Thomas splint allows knee movement during traction treatment of a femoral fracture; overbody or lateral skeletal traction allows elbow motion while maintaining alignment of a humeral fracture.
   C. Traction can **overcome muscle spasm** associated with bone or joint disease. An example is Buck traction, which is sometimes recommended for patients with hip injuries.
   D. **Edema is reduced** in an extremity by a traction unit that elevates the affected part above the heart.

II. **ESSENTIAL MATERIALS.** The bed must have a firm mattress or a bed board. Elevate the head or the foot of the bed by using either shock blocks or the bed's intrinsic elevation system. Attach an overhead frame, trapeze, and side rails to the bed so the patient can shift position. Traction equipment includes bars, pulleys, ropes, weight hangers, skeletal traction apparatus, and, in some instances, plaster cast materials. Various figures in this chapter show the type and placement of equipment about the bed.

III. **SKIN TRACTION**
   A. Skin traction may be used as a definitive method of treatment as well as a first aid or temporary measure. The **traction force** applied to the skin is transmitted to bone via the superficial fascia, deep fascia, and intermuscular septa. Skin damage can result from too much traction force. The maximum weight recommended for skin traction is 10 lb or less, depending on the size and age of the patient. If this much weight is used, then discontinue the skin traction after 1 week. If less weight is used and if the skin is inspected biweekly, then skin traction may be safely used for 4 to 6 weeks. Pediatric patients need skin inspection on a more frequent basis.
   B. **Application**
      1. **Carefully prepare the skin** by removing the hair as well as washing and drying the area.
      2. **Avoid placing adhesive straps over bony prominences.** If bony prominences are in the area of strap application, cover them well with cast padding before the adhesive straps are applied. Always use a spreader bar to avoid pressure from the traction rope on bony prominences.
      3. Make the **adhesive straps** from adhesive tape, moleskin adhesive, or a commercial skin traction unit consisting of foam boots with Velcro straps. Place the straps longitudinally on opposite sides of the extremity, with free skin left between the straps to prevent any tourniquet effect. Attach the free ends of these straps to the spreader bar. Hold the straps in place by encircling the extremity with an adhesive or elastic wrap. Then apply the traction rope to the spreader bar.
      4. Support the leg in traction with pillows or folded bath blankets to **prevent edema and irritation of the heel.**

IV. SKELETAL TRACTION

A. Definition. Skeletal traction is applied through direct fixation to bone.

B. Equipment

1. **Kirschner wire** is a thin, smooth wire that is 0.0360 to 0.0625 in. in diameter. The advantages of Kirschner wire are that it is easy to insert and that it minimizes the chance of soft-tissue damage or infection. The disadvantage is that it rotates within an improper bow and can cut through osteoporotic bone. These complications are minimized by using the proper traction bow. Even though Kirschner wire is small in diameter and flexible, it can withstand a large traction force when the proper traction bow is used. This special bow (Kirschner bow) provides the wire with rigidity by applying a longitudinal tension force (**Fig. 9-1**). If properly placed and not improperly stressed, the wire does not break and causes less bone damage than the larger Steinmann pins.

2. **Steinmann pins** vary from 0.078 to 0.19 in. in diameter and come in smooth and threaded forms. Because they are large enough to have inherent stability, the Steinmann pin bow (Böhler bow), which attaches to these pins, does not exert tension along the pin as does the Kirschner traction bow. The two types of pins should be readily recognized and used with the appropriate bow (**Fig. 9-1**).

3. **Factors to be considered**
   a. A **nonthreaded wire or pin** is smaller, more uniform, less easily broken, more easily inserted, and removed with less twisting than the threaded type. A disadvantage is that it can slide laterally through the skin and bone. Even with careful attention, it can move enough to disturb the traction or predispose to a pin tract infection.
   b. The **threaded wire or pin** has stress risers at each thread, breaks more easily, must be larger in diameter to gain the same strength, and takes a longer time to insert. In inserting a threaded pin, one is tempted to go rapidly with the hand drill, which creates an undue amount of heat. On the other hand, because the threads prevent lateral slippage of the pin, this type is preferable to the nonthreaded variety for long-term (longer than 1–2 weeks) traction.

4. The wires and pins are available with two types of points. One is a **trocar**, a blunted point that tends to grind through the bone with relatively little cutting ability. The other is a **diamond-shaped point**, a modified type of drill that passes through bone more easily and with less heating. Wires and pins that are dull, sharpened off-center, or bent should not be used. These wander during insertion and create a hole that is too large.

5. Note that pins and wires are frequently used as **internal fixation** devices for fractures; such use is discussed in **Chap. 10** and the chapter on hand fractures.

C. Pin and wire insertion guidelines

1. Pin or wire insertion is a surgical procedure, so **some form of consent** is needed, at least with a witness in attendance who signs a note in the chart attesting that informed consent was obtained. A signed, witnessed surgical consent is preferred.

2. Establish the **status of neurovascular structures** before inserting the pins. Placement of the pins requires knowledge of the specific anatomy and the location of vital structures. **Rule:** Always start the pin on the side where the vital structures are located. This gives better control and better avoidance of these structures. For instance, start an olecranon pin on the medial side to avoid the ulnar nerve.

3. **Skin preparation.** The skin should be free of signs of infection. Follow aseptic procedures, using a topical germicidal antiseptic, drapes, mask, and gloves.

4. It is difficult to obtain enough **anesthesia** to block the periosteum completely. Anesthetize the skin and subcutaneous tissue with 1% lidocaine on the starting side of the bone. Go down to the periosteum with the needle tip and insert enough lidocaine around this area to produce some anesthesia. If there is pain as the pin is inserted and approaches bone, then inject more anesthetic.

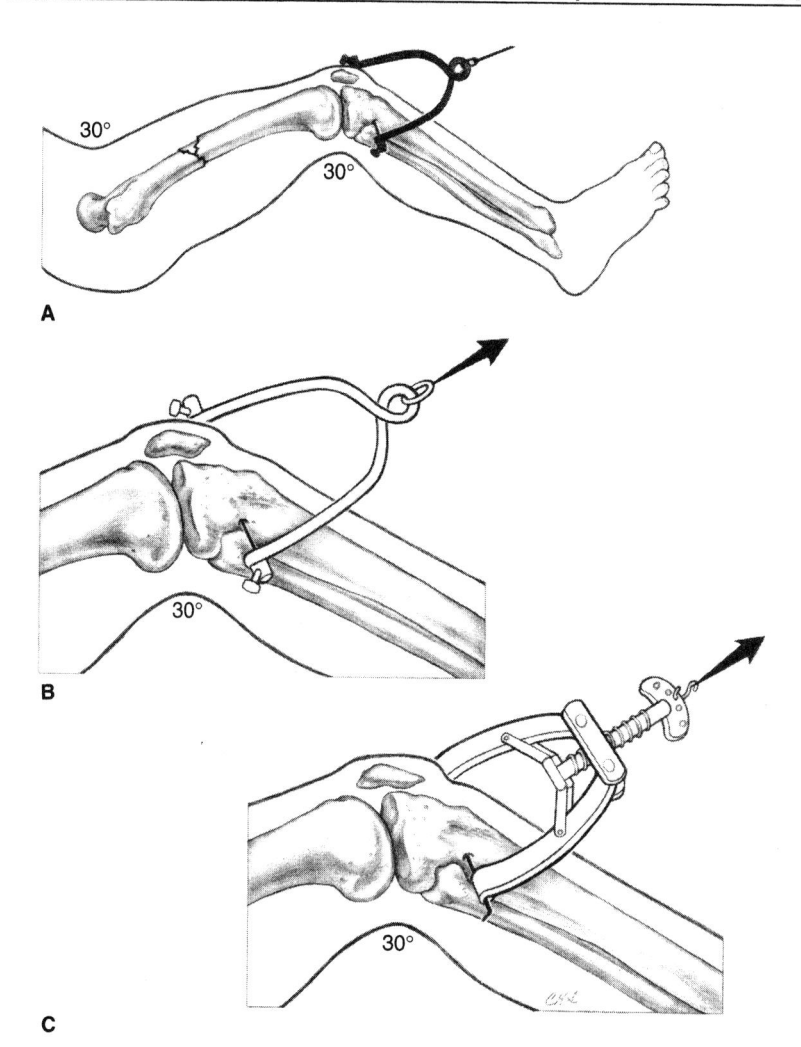

Figure 9-1. Traction bows. When using skeletal traction to treat femoral fractures, the knee is kept in slight flexion **(A)**. Proximal tibial traction is reserved for adults. To avoid physeal injury in children with resultant recurvation deformity, distal femoral traction proximal to the distal femoral physis is used. For larger Steinmann pins, a Böhler bow is used **(B)**. The tensioning capabilities of the Kirschner bow allows the use of smaller Kirschner wires **(C)**.

Drill the pin approximately halfway through the bone, get an idea where it will come out, and then anesthetize the opposite side. In a case in which the wire penetrates two bones, such as the tibia and fibula, it is impossible to anesthetize the area between the two bones. Tell the patient ahead of time that this may be painful for a few seconds but that as soon as the drilling stops, the pain will cease. If done in the emergency department, conscious sedation should be utilized.

5. **Skin incision.** When starting the procedure, pass the wire or pin through a stab wound made with a no. 11 blade. If only a puncture wound is made by

the pin, then **tight** skin adherence to the pin predisposes to an infection. If an infection with abscess does occur, then drain it by extending the stab wound. Dress the pin site with sterile 4 × 4s on each side with Betadine solution applied.
6. Pins and wires should be inserted using a **hand drill** rather than a power tool. The time saved by using power equipment is expended in preparation time. There is also a tendency to use too high a speed with power drills and generate too much heat, thereby promoting development of bone necrosis around the pin insertion, resulting in a ring sequestrum. The smaller the pin and the slower the rotation of the hand drill, the faster the pin is inserted. Adequate support of the limb from adequate help must be available so that, as the pin is being inserted, the limb does not shift and cause the patient further pain.
7. Traction wires or pins are **best placed in the metaphysics**, not in dense cortical bone. Use caution to avoid epiphyseal plate damage, which can result in a growth disturbance. In skeletally immature patients, the pin should be inserted under fluoroscopic control to avoid the physis. In the area of the tibial tubercle, assume in female patients younger than 14 years old and in male patients younger than 16 years old that the epiphyseal plate is open. Because of the risk of physeal injury in the proximal tibia, choose the distal femur for skeletal traction in younger patients if possible. Ideally, pass the pin through only skin, subcutaneous tissue, and bone. Avoid muscles and tendons.
8. **Do not violate a fracture hematoma** by skeletal wires or pins for traction or else the equivalent of an open fracture will result.
9. **Do not penetrate joints** with traction wires or pins as pyarthrosis can occur. Do not enter the suprapatellar pouch with distal femoral wires or pins. Here again, inserting the pin under fluoroscopic control can avoid these complications.
10. **Points to remember** about wire or pin insertion:
    a. Chuck the wire or pin so that just **2 to 4 in. are exposed** to prevent wandering and bending.
    b. **Tighten chuck sufficiently** to prevent score marks that are sources of metal corrosion and fracture.
    c. Be certain the wire **does not bend** as it is inserted.
    d. Use the proper traction bow (**Fig. 9-1**).

D. Specific areas of insertion
1. **Metacarpals.** Place the wire through the metaphyseal diaphysed junction of the index and middle metacarpals. To facilitate insertion, push the first dorsal interosseous muscle in a volar direction and palpate the subcutaneous portion of the bone. Angle the wire to pass through the index and middle metacarpals and to come out the dorsum of the hand, so as to preserve the natural arch.
2. **Distal radius and ulna.** Usually place the wire or pin through both the radius and the ulna. This site is rarely used.
3. **Olecranon.** Take care to avoid an open epiphysis. Do not place the pin too far distally because this causes elbow extension, and it is more comfortable to pull through a flexed elbow than an extended elbow. Use a moderate-sized wire or pin and insert from the medial side to avoid the ulnar nerve. Use a very small traction bow.
4. **Distal femur.** Start on the medial side, anterior enough to avoid the neurovascular structures. This insertion is best accomplished by placing the pin 1 in. inferior to the abductor tubercle. If the pin will be used for traction on a fracture table for delayed intramedullary nailing, make sure it is placed far anterior, off the coronal midline to avoid incarceration by the intramedullary nail. Fluoroscopy should be used to help the surgeon avoid an open physis.
5. **Proximal tibia.** Place the wire or pin 1 in. inferior and 1/2 in. posterior to the tibial tubercle, starting on the lateral side to avoid the peroneal nerve. Take extreme care to avoid an open epiphysis; if the anterior portion of the proximal tibial epiphyseal plate is violated, genu recurvatum can occur.
6. **Distal tibia and fibula.** Start the pin 1 to 1 1/2 fingerbreadths above the most prominent portion of the lateral malleolus to avoid the ankle mortise. Insert it

parallel to the ankle joint and angulate it slightly anteriorly. The surgeon should feel the pin pass through the two fibular cortices and then the two tibial cortices. Pass the pin through both bones to avoid the tendons and neurovascular structures. If the pin is placed too far proximally, the foot rests on the bow, and a pressure sore may occur.
7. **Calcaneus.** Generally select a large diamond-point pin. The preferred insertion site is 1 in. inferior and posterior from the lateral malleolus or 1 3/4 in. inferior and 1 1/2 in. posterior from the medial malleolus. Because of the position of the tibial nerve, the medial starting site is preferred. If the pin is placed too far posteriorly, it causes a calcaneal position of the foot. If the pin is placed too far inferiorly, it may cut out of the bone. If the pin is placed too far superiorly, it can enter the subtalar joint and also spear the flexor tendons or tibial nerve and/or artery. Infections that are difficult to treat often occur when the calcaneus is used for long-term traction.

V. CERVICAL SPINE TRACTION
A. **Neck halter traction** is the simplest of the different types of cervical spine traction but usually is not used in the treatment of acute cervical spine fractures or dislocations, being reserved for chronic conditions such as a cervical radiculopathy. Apply the traction to the mandible and occiput with a soft, commercially made halter.
  1. When **continuous traction** is used with the patient in the supine position, do not exceed 10 lb (5 lb is usually sufficient). With the patient sitting, approximately 8 lb may be added to the attached weight to account for the weight of the head. The total attached weight should not exceed 15 lb with the patient in the sitting position. The traction should not be strictly continuous but used for 1 to 3 hours followed by rest intervals to allow jaw motion and to relieve pressure on the skin.
  2. If **intermittent traction** for short periods of time is used three times daily, then up to 30 lb may be used.
  3. **Problems** associated with head halter traction are related to the weight used and the position of the neck. The optimum position is usually neutral or in slight flexion. Temporomandibular joint discomfort can ordinarily be relieved by changing the direction of traction force or decreasing the attached weight. Symptoms from local skin pressure may be relieved by the above methods or by appropriate padding.
B. **Skull tong traction** is a form of cervical spine traction and is applied by one of the many types of skull calipers (tongs) (**Fig. 9-2**). The most satisfactory caliper is

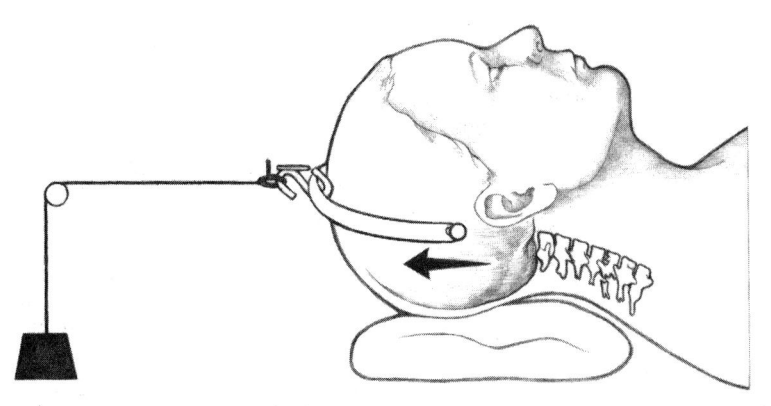

Figure 9-2. Tong traction. This treatment is used for most cervical fractures and dislocations. The points are positioned just above the ear pinnae. Padding can be used to generate more flexion or extension of the cervical spine as is indicated for reduction based on lateral cervical roentgenograms.

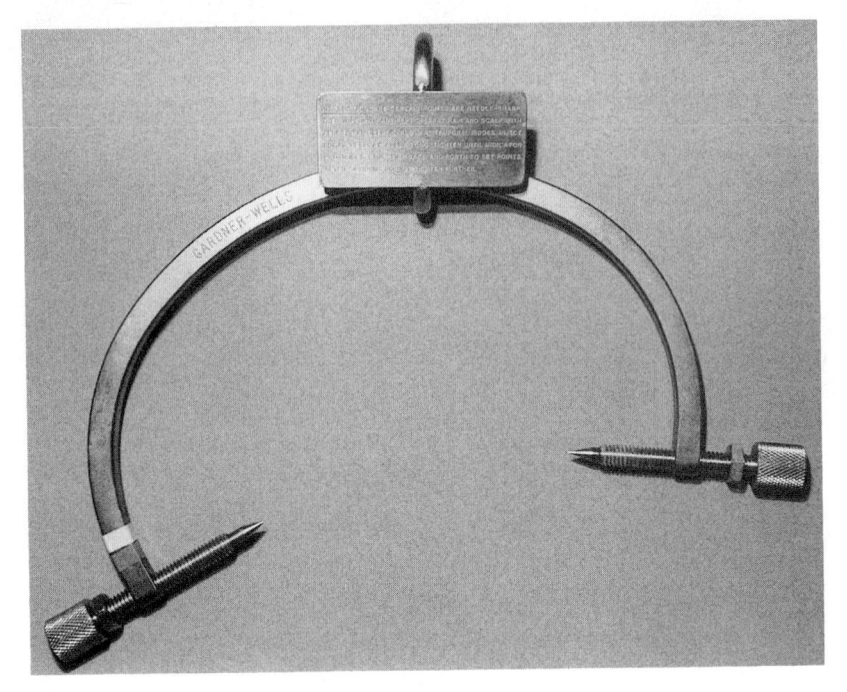

Figure 9-3. Gardner-Wells tongs.

screwed into the skull without the need for previous trephining and does not penetrate more than a preset depth. The Gardner-Wells tongs are recommended (**Fig. 9-3**) (1). With this type of apparatus, heavy traction can be applied to the skull for as long as required. It is especially useful for cervical spine fractures and dislocations. Perform the following procedures after the scalp is cleaned and draped; local shaving is sufficient but is not absolutely mandatory.
  1. The **Gardner-Wells skull traction tongs** are easy to insert. After preparing the skull, position the tongs below the temporal crest and tighten. A spring device within the tong points automatically sets the correct depth and tension. Then the indicator protrudes 1 mm from the knob of the tong, at which time the correct pressure (equivalent to 6–8 in./lb) is exerted. Retighten these pins in a sequential manner to the same value the next day, and then do not tighten them again unless loosening occurs.
  2. Keep the head end of the frame slightly elevated so the patient's body acts as countertraction.
  3. Initiate cervical traction at 10 to 15 lb and incrementally increase only after checking the appropriate roentgenograms. Initiating traction at higher weights can occasionally result in marked distraction of ligamentous injuries. For definitive traction, **Crutchfield's rule of 5 lb/level** starting with 10 lb for the head allows for a maximum range of 30 to 40 lb for a C5–C6 injury.
C. **Fixed halo skull traction.** The halo device, originally introduced by Nickel and Perry (2,3), can be used alone for traction or combined with a vest or cast.
  1. **Materials**
     a. **Halo ring** (five standard sizes available). Carbon fiber rings are preferred because radiographs and magnetic resonance imaging (MRI) scans can be obtained without distortion.
     b. **Five skull pins** (one spare included)

c. **Two torque screwdrivers**
d. **Four positioning pins**
e. **A wooden board** (4 × 15 × 1/4 in.)
2. **Application** procedures are modified from those described by Young and Thomassen (4) and Botte et al (2).
    a. **Shave and trim hair** around the pin sites (optional). The pin sites should be 1 cm above the lateral third of the eyebrow and the same distance above the tops of the ears in the parietal and occipital areas. Place the halo just inferior to the greatest circumference of the head (**Fig. 9-4**).

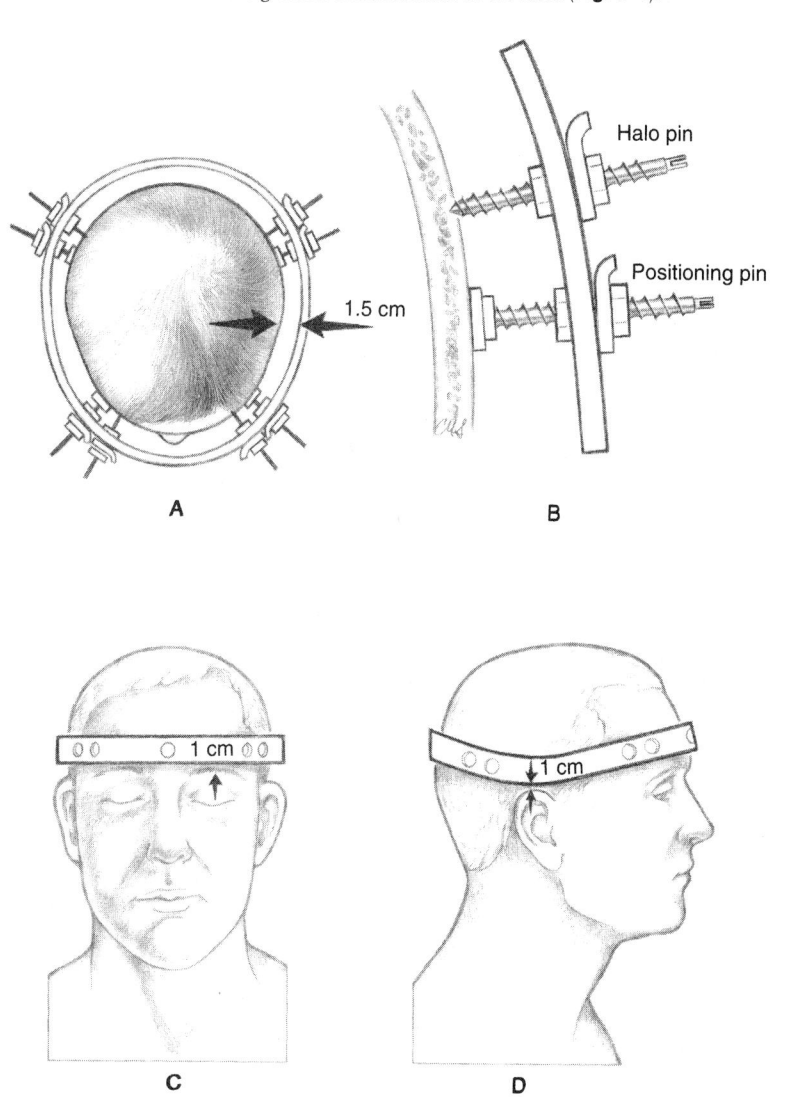

Figure 9-4. Principles of a halo ring application. The correct ring size allows for 1.5 cm of clearance **(A)**. Positioning pins are used to stabilize the ring while the skull pins are inserted **(B)**. The proper position of the ring is 1 cm above eyebrows and ear pinnae **(C, D)**.

b. Position the patient supine on a bed with the head extended beyond the edge. **Have the head supported** by an assistant's hands or by a 4-in. wide board placed under the head and neck.
   c. Place a **sterile towel** under the patient's head. This step is not necessary if an attendant is holding the head.
   d. Select a halo ring that allows for **1.5 cm clearance**. If MRI studies are anticipated, then an MRI-compatible ring and pins must be used (carbon fiber material).
   e. The halo ring, skull pins, and positioning pins should be autoclaved or gas sterilized.
   f. The assistant, wearing gloves, **positions** the halo ring around the head with the raised portion of the ring over the posterior part of the skull. Use positioning pins and plates to place the ring in the proper attitude and to equalize the clearance around the head.
   g. Infiltrate the skin with an **anesthetic** at the four pin sites.
   h. The **skull pins** should be at a 90-degree angle to the skull and turned to finger tightness. The skull pins are designed so that no scalp incisions or drill holes are needed. The shape of the point draws the skin under it and does not cause bleeding. Try to avoid puckering of the skin at the pin site. If puckering does occur, then remove the pins, flatten the skin, and repenetrate.
   i. Both operators use the **torque screwdrivers** simultaneously, turning opposing skull pins. Gain increments of 2 in./lb evenly up to the maximum desired by the physician. A suggested maximum is 4 1/2 in./lb for children and 6 to 8 in/lb for adults.
   j. **Remove the positioning pins.**
   k. Incorporate the **support rods** of the halo apparatus into the plaster body jacket, as shown in **Fig. 7-5**, or use a sheepskin-lined molded plastic body jacket that is commercially available or custom made by an orthotist (**Fig. 7-6**).
   l. **Tangential roentgenographic views** of the skull or a computed tomography (CT) scan can be ordered to check the depth of the skull pins but are not routinely necessary.
  3. **Care of pin sites**
   a. **Clean** around the pins with peroxide solution using a cotton swab twice daily.
   b. **Check the torque** of the pins for the first few days. **Note:** If the patient complains of repeated looseness or if the proper torque cannot be gained, then move the pin to another place on the ring by the aforementioned method. Do not remove a loose pin until the fifth replacement pin is inserted.

VI. UPPER EXTREMITY TRACTION
  A. **Dunlop or modified Dunlop skin traction.** This type of traction is occasionally useful for the management of supracondylar humeral fractures (5). Place the patient supine and suspend the arm in skin traction with the shoulder abducted and slightly flexed. In addition, slightly flex the elbow. Modification of this type of traction provides counteraction on the humerus, which can be achieved with the arm over the edge of the bed and counterweight suspended from a felt cuff over the humerus, or with a felt cuff over the forearm pulling laterally with the elbow flexed (**Fig. 9-5**). Two disadvantages of Dunlop traction are that it cannot be applied over skin injuries and that elevation of the humeral fracture above the level of the heart is not possible with this method.
  B. **Overbody or lateral skeletal traction**
   1. In the management of extraarticular humeral shaft and metaphyseal fractures, it is occasionally desirable to maintain the shoulder in flexion without abduction but with the elbow at a right angle by placing the arm over the body. Maintain this position through olecranon skeletal traction, which allows some flexion and extension of the elbow if the traction pin is properly inserted. Because the

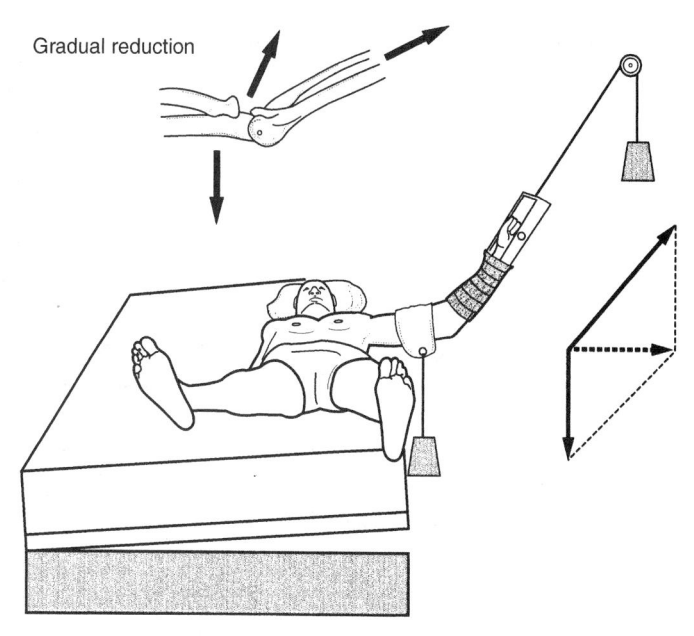

Figure 9-5. Modified Dunlop traction. A weight of 1 to 5 lb is usually required. Associated circulatory embarrassment might be aggravated by increasing elbow flexion.

        hand and wrist usually tire in this position, support the wrist with a plaster splint. Skeletal traction through the olecranon may also be used in the lateral position (**Fig. 9-6**).
    2. A special, rarely used adaptation of upper extremity olecranon traction may be made by **placing the patient in a shoulder spica cast** that incorporates an olecranon pin into the plaster to apply fixed skeletal traction. This adaptation allows the patient to be ambulatory.

VII. LOWER EXTREMITY TRACTION
    A. Apply Buck extension skin traction (**Fig. 9-7**) to the lower extremity to reduce muscle spasms about the knee or hip. However, do not use this form of traction for back conditions. Control rotation to some extent by placing the leg on a pillow with sandbags on the lateral side of the ankle. Although Buck traction is commonly recommended for hip fractures, its use should be limited in duration. For intracapsular fractures, keep the hip flexed to increase hip capsule volume and thereby limit pain. The effectiveness of this type of traction in decreasing pain has not been demonstrated (6,7).
    B. Hamilton-Russell traction (**Fig. 9-8**) may be used for hip or femoral fractures, especially in children weighing 40 to 60 lb. Accomplish the traction with either skin traction or distal tibial skeletal traction plus a sling placed beneath the posterior distal thigh (avoid pressure in the popliteal fossa). A rope is attached to the sling and goes first to an overhead pulley, then to a pulley at the foot of the bed, next to a pulley on the foot plate attached to the spreader bar, then to a fourth pulley at the end of the bed, and finally to the attached weight. Analysis of the vector forces shows that the traction applied to the leg is increased considerably by moving the overhead pulley toward the foot of the bed. If this type of traction is used on a child, one usually attaches 3 lb to the traction apparatus. Produce a countertraction with the patient's body weight by elevating the foot of the bed.

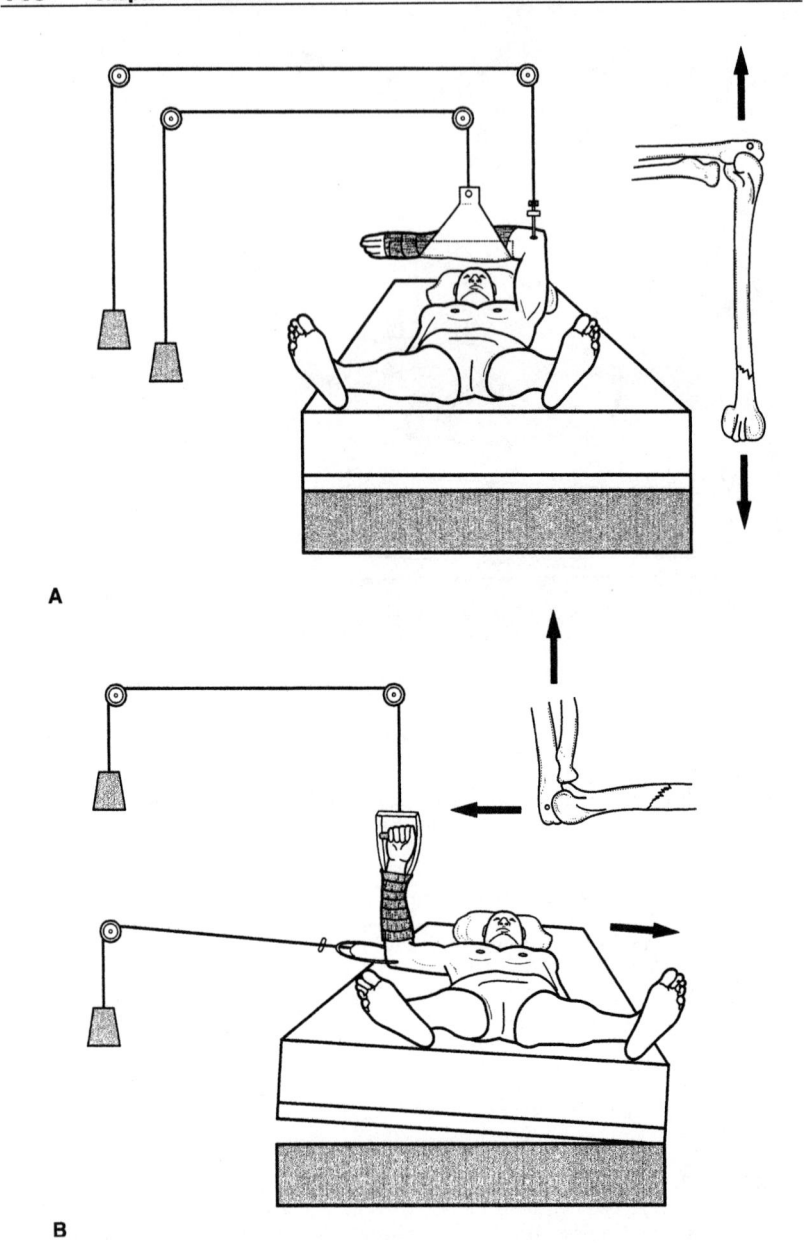

Figure 9-6. Olecranon pin traction. **A:** Overbody traction. Note that the elbow joint can move without disturbing the fracture. The hand and wrist rest in a plaster splint. **B:** Lateral traction.

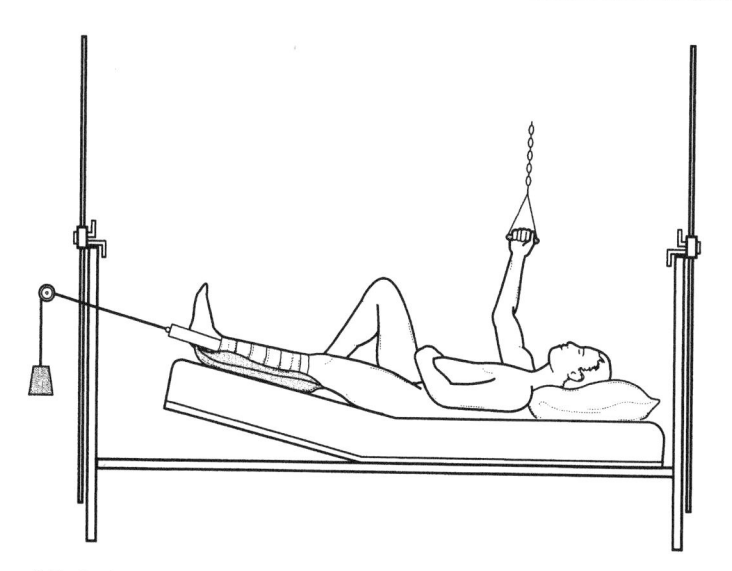

Figure 9-7. Buck extension skin traction. Note elevation of the foot of the bed and support under the calf. Protect the fibular head and malleoli. A weight of 5 to 7 lb of traction is sufficient.

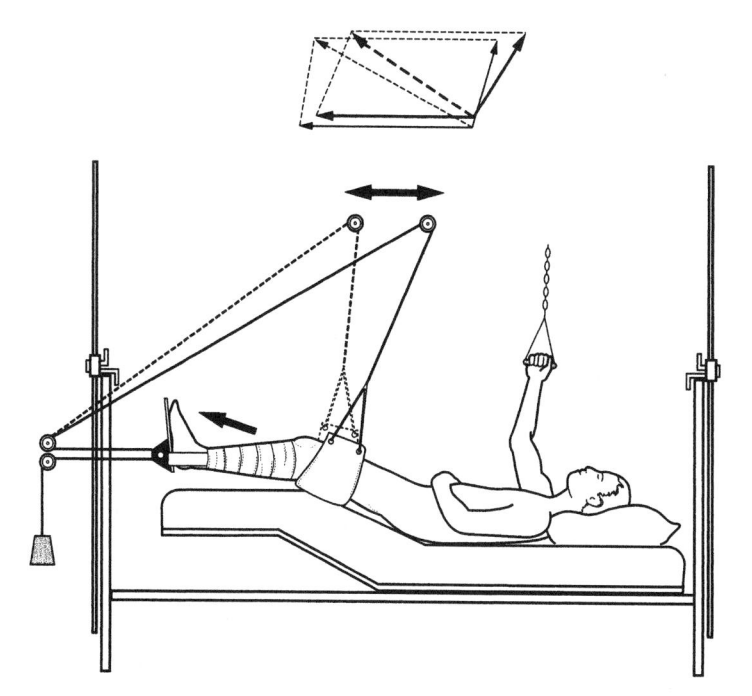

Figure 9-8. Hamilton-Russell traction. Note that the resultant force on the femur is a summation of vector analysis and depends on the position of the overhead pulley. Change the angulation of the distal fragment by moving the single overhead pulley.

C. **Split Russell traction** has the same indications and vector forces as Hamilton-Russell traction. The difference is that split Russell's traction uses two separate ropes and weights, as shown in **Fig. 9-9**.
D. **Charnley traction unit** (boot) is useful for applying skeletal traction to a lower limb and is recommended for routine use (**Fig. 9-10**). This limits rotational forces on the limb controlling alignment, maintains the ankle in neutral position, and limits the stress on the traction bow. The unit is assembled by inserting a wire or pin through the proximal end of the tibia and then incorporating the wire or pin in a short-leg cast. The advantages are as follows:
   1. The foot and ankle are maintained in a neutral **functional position**.
   2. The limb is suspended in a cast, and there is no pressure on the calf muscles or peroneal nerve.
   3. **Movement** of the skeletal pin or wire is **reduced** to a minimum.
E. **Balanced suspension skeletal traction** provides a direct pull on either the tibia or the femur through a wire pin. Rest the lower extremity on a stockinet or a cloth towel stretched over a Thomas splint. The splint, with or without a Pearson attachment, is balanced with counterweights to suspend the leg in a freely floating system. Attach separate suspension ropes to both sides of the proximal full ring

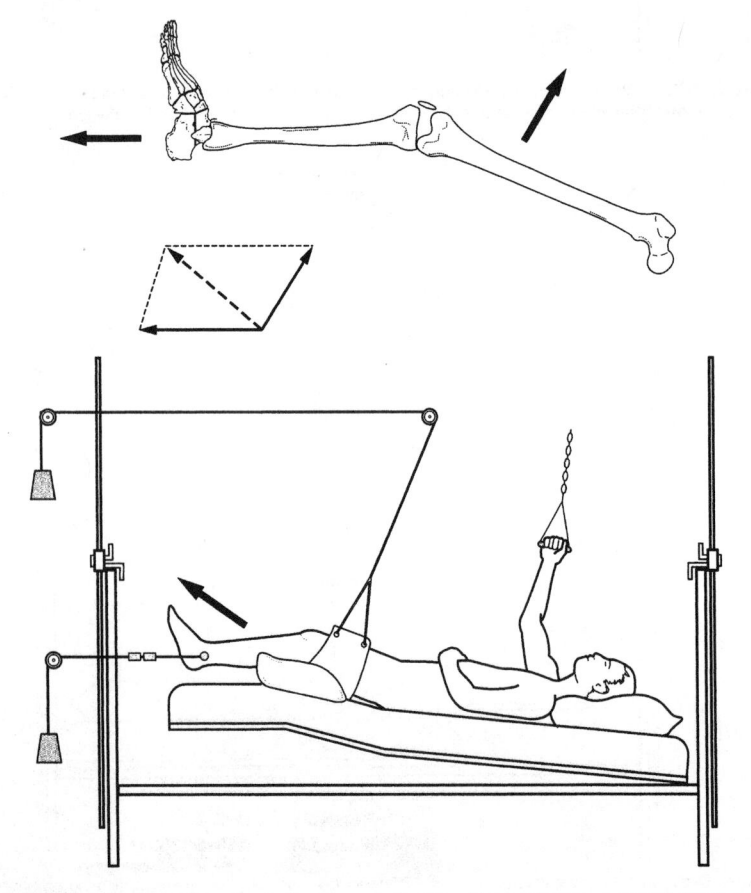

Figure 9-9. Split Russell traction is the same as Hamilton-Russell traction except that two separate ropes and weights are used instead of one.

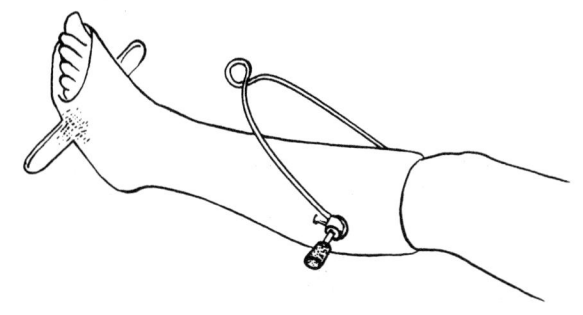

Figure 9-10. Charnley traction unit consisting of a skeletal wire or pin incorporated into a short-leg cast, which has a crossbar fixed to the sole. The unit is commonly employed for femoral fractures treated with skeletal traction.

Thomas splint, run the ropes through overhead pulleys, and fasten weights to ropes at either end of the bed but not over the patient. Control rotation of the ring by individually adjusting the amount of attached weight. Suspend the distal end of the splint from a single rope to an overhead pulley, with the weight attached to the rope at one end of the bed. For safety reasons, place no weights over the patient. Control rotation of the extremity by a light counterweight attached to the side of the splint or by a crossbar attached to the plaster cast. The Charnley traction unit (boot) is ideally suited for both balanced suspension and fixed skeletal traction (which is discussed next) (**Fig. 9-11**). A **Pearson attachment** allows for flexion motion of the knee joint, which is an advantage, especially for those in traction for a long period of time or for those who have a comminuted tibial plateau fracture.

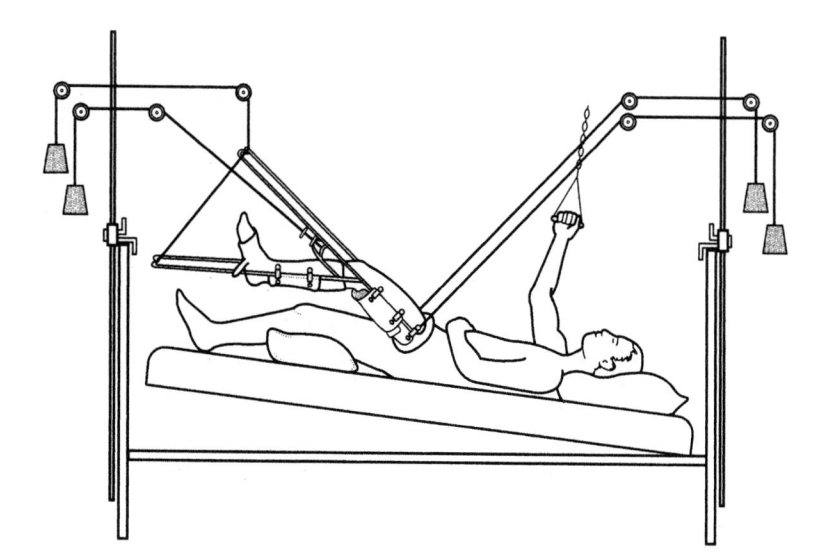

Figure 9-11. With balanced suspension traction, the various weights are adjusted until satisfactory alignment and suspension of the femoral fracture are achieved within the Thomas splint. Note the Charnley traction unit, firm mattress, bed board, and master pad. Wrap an elastic bandage about the thigh and splint to minimize the acute swelling.

F. Use **fixed skeletal traction** in the initial treatment of femoral fractures in patients who will go on to intramedullary nailing or who need to be transported either in the hospital or to another facility.
   1. **In the rare situation in which the fracture must be reduced**, the apprehensive patient or the patient with a transverse fracture usually requires general or regional anesthesia.
   2. Apply the **Charnley** traction unit to the lower leg.
   3. Select a **full or half ring Thomas splint** that is 2 in. greater than the proximal thigh (8). This leeway is critical because a ring that is too tight causes distal edema and one that is too loose is ineffective. The ring must fit against the fibrofatty tissue in the perineum and the medial arch of the buttocks. The half ring is placed against the ischium and the strap tightened loosely against the anterior thigh.
   4. While the leg is supported in traction, place the ring on the limb. Attach a single **master sling** of nonextensible cloth (a double-thickness cloth towel is ideal) measuring 6 to 9 in. long to the splint beneath the fracture. Adjust tension to support the limb. If the sling is too tight, then it causes excessive flexing of the proximal fragment; if it is too loose, then it does not control the fracture. Attach this sling to the splint with several clamps.
   5. Make a supporting or master pad that is 1 to 1 1/2 in. thick and 6 to 9 in. long from an abdominal dressing or a folded towel. Insert a safety pin into the pad to assist localization of the pad on roentgenograms. Place this pad beneath the fracture and adjust it to maintain the normal anterior bow of the femur. A single sling is placed on the Thomas splint distally to support the short-leg cast.
   6. **Check the reduction.** End-on reduction for transverse fractures is ideal in the adult; take care to avoid distraction of the fracture. If the patient will have delayed intramedullary nailing, maintain some distraction, which will aid in intraoperative reduction. In the child, bayonet apposition is preferred. With the oblique fracture, it is important to feel bone-on-bone contact to be certain there is no soft-tissue interposition. If there is interposition, then it can usually be dislodged by manipulation. Then assess length, alignment, and rotational positions and attach traction to the end of the splint. Extend two ropes from the Steinmann pin around the sides of the splint and attach them to the splint end. Tape two tongue blades together to form a Spanish windlass to adjust tension. After the first day or two, when muscle spasm subsides, only slight traction is necessary to maintain the appropriate alignment. It might not be possible to gain full length initially because of unusual tense swelling of the thigh. Attach a second pad or C-clamp to add cross-traction if needed for better alignment, particularly in the more transverse fracture patterns.
   7. **Suspend the splint** to allow patient mobility in bed and to reduce edema. **Figure 9-12** depicts the completed setup.
   8. **Follow-up care**, particularly in the first few weeks, is important. Wash the skin beneath the ring daily with alcohol, dry thoroughly, and powder with talc every 2 hours. The conscious patient may perform this care each hour and massage the skin to improve blood supply. If it is necessary to relieve skin pressure under the ring, then apply traction directly from the end of the splint; slight distraction is preferred when intramedullary nailing is to be delayed for more than 24 hours. Be careful, however, not to cause distraction at the fracture site when using fixed skeletal traction as the definitive treatment. Start quadriceps exercises within the first few days and continue on an around-the-clock basis. All the elements outlined earlier are essential for effective utilization of fixed skeletal traction.

VIII. COMPLICATIONS OF SKELETAL TRACTION
   A. An **infection** of the pin tract is a common complication, but its incidence is reduced when the previously stated guidelines for pin and wire insertion are carefully followed. If an infection with a small sequestrum occurs, it is wise to

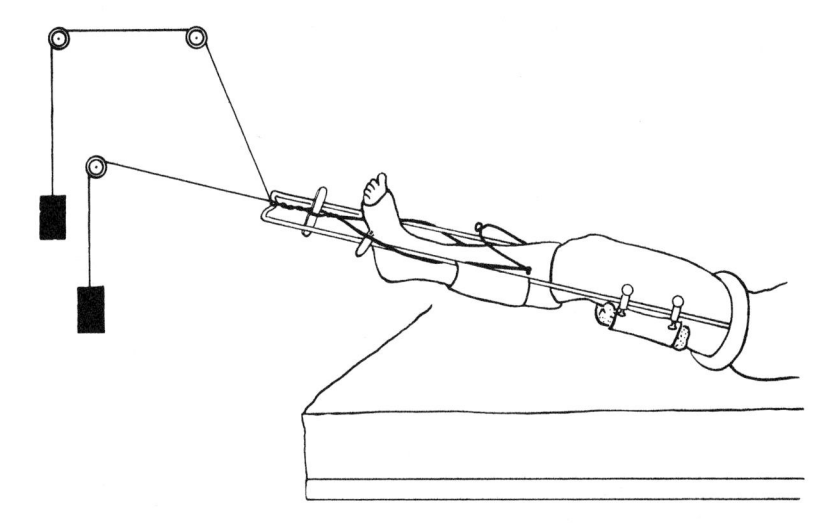

Figure 9-12. Fixed skeletal traction. Note the Charnley traction unit, the method of adjusting traction force via the windlass, the position of the master pad, and the traction on the end of the Thomas splint to relieve skin pressure on the proximal thigh. Place an elastic bandage around the thigh and splint to help control edema.

remove the pin, curette the pin tract, and replace the pin in the operating room under adequate anesthesia. The infection usually subsides satisfactorily with antibiotic therapy.
- **B. Distraction** of bone fragments at the fracture site is avoided by frequently measuring extremity length, by using roentgenograms to check the position of fragments, and by keeping traction to a minimum. Distraction is best assessed by lateral roentgenograms because anteroposterior roentgenograms may not be perpendicular to the fracture and may underestimate the distraction. Distraction can predispose to a delayed union or nonunion of the fracture.
- **C.** Use heavy traction with care and close observation to avoid **nerve palsy**. If paralysis does occur, adjust and possibly abandon the traction.
- **D. Pin breakage** is unusual but can occur if very heavy traction is used for long periods, especially in a restless patient. To protect the pin, incorporate it into plaster in the manner of the Charnley traction unit. Decrease the potential of metal corrosion and fracture by using a wire or pin that is not scored.

References
1. Gardner W. The principle of spring-loaded points for cervical traction. *J Neurosurg* 1973;39:543–544.
2. Botte MJ, Byrne TP, Garfin SR. Application of the halo device for immobilization of the cervical spine utilizing an increased torque pressure. *J Bone Joint Surg* 1987;69A:750.
3. Garfin SR, Botte MJ, Enteno RS, et al. Osteology of the skull as it effects halo pin placement. *Spine* 1985;10:696–698.
4. Young R, Thomassen EH. Step-by-step procedure for applying a halo ring. *Orthop Rev* 1974;3:62.
5. Prietto CA. Supracondylar fractures of the humerus. A comparative study of Dunlop's traction versus percutaneus pinning. *J Bone Joint Surg* 1979;61:425–428.
6. Finsen V, Borset M, Buvik GE, et al. Preoperative traction in patients with hip fractures. *Injury* 1992;23:242–244.

7. Jerre R, Doshé A, Karlsson F, et al. Preoperative skin traction was not useful for hip fractures. *J Bone Joint Surg* 2001;83:303.
8. Henry BJ, Vrahas MS. The Thomas splint: questionable boast of an indispensable tool. *Am J Orthop* 1996;25:602–604.

Selected Historical Readings

Charnley J. *The closed treatment of common fractures,* 3rd ed. Baltimore, MD: Williams & Wilkins, 1972.

Nickel VL, Perry J, Garret A, et al. The halo. *J Bone Joint Surg* 1968;50A:1400.

OPERATING ROOM EQUIPMENT AND TECHNIQUES   10

I. PREPARATION FOR SURGERY
A. Scheduling surgery
1. **Prepare the patient** so that the risks, goals, and benefits of the selected procedure are understood. The patient or legal next of kin should know the nature of the patient's condition, the nature of the proposed treatment, the alternative treatments, the anesthetic risks, the anticipated probability for success, and the possible risks. Explain the postoperative dressings, casts or splints, exercise program, and other special requirements. When the patient has been so informed and has all questions answered, obtain a signed operative permit.
2. **Review the technique** of the proposed operation. At the time surgery is scheduled, be confident that the patient's condition meets the appropriate indications for the proposed surgery. Know the anatomy and the surgical approaches involved in the selected surgical procedure. Carefully plan the procedure with the proper alternatives to reduce the length of time the wound is open. Be sure that all special equipment, implants, assistance, and time are available as expected. Complete any necessary templating of roentgenograms and preoperative planning drawings (1).

B. Before surgery
1. **Patient preparation.** Check to make sure the physical examination, chest roentgenogram, electrocardiogram, hematocrit, and other indicated preoperative studies do not contraindicate surgery. Obtain a preoperative consultation from a specialist in internal medicine for all patients with unstable medical conditions. Order blood, tetanus prophylaxis, and special medications as indicated. If an extremity operation is planned, be sure that the nails are properly trimmed and cleaned. Have the patient, family, and support system begin planning early for postdischarge or postoperation disposition needs, such as transportation home, wheelchairs, hospital beds, wheelchair access to the home, and commodes.
2. **Antibiotics** (2)
   a. **Preoperative antibiotics** should be administered for surgery that is associated with a high risk of postoperative deep wound infection, that is, when any implant is inserted, the operation results in a hematoma or dead space, the anticipated operating time is greater than 2 hours, or the surgeon is operating on bones, joints, nerves, or tendons. Various studies have shown immediate preoperative and postoperative antibiotics to be beneficial with surgery involving musculoskeletal tissues (2–4). See **Chap. 1** for utilization of antibiotics with open wounds. The duration of antibiotic therapy can be limited to 24 hours postoperatively without increasing the risk to infection.
   b. The **timing** of the antibiotic therapy is as important as **dosage**. Ideally, the antibiotic level should be highest when the tourniquet is inflated or the surgical hematoma (potential culture medium) is formed. Thus, the antibiotics **must be given before surgery**. Because the highest blood levels with intravenous (IV) administration are achieved immediately, the ideal time to give IV antibiotics is when the patient is in the preoperative area or operating room during the 10- to 15-minute period just before the tourniquet is

inflated or before the surgical incision is made. Some surgeons who believe that the tissue concentration of antibiotics is more important than the blood levels administer the first dose approximately 2 to 6 hours before surgery. Either way, the antibiotics are readministered at the recommended intervals throughout the operative procedure except when a tourniquet is used. The surgeon must also be aware of the effect of blood loss on the antibiotic levels. If the blood loss equals one half of the patient's volume, then approximately one half of the effective amount of the antibiotics has also been lost. The interval between the recommended doses for that patient, therefore, must be cut in half.

    c. The authors recommend using one of the **first-generation cephalosporins**, which are bactericidal for bacteria usually found in wound infections following musculoskeletal surgery: staphylococcal and streptococcal specimens. The recommended antibiotics are listed in **Table 10-1**.

3. Patients who have been on long-term steroid therapy may need adjustments made in their **steroid dosage** when they undergo surgery or other major stress. The following is the simplest published regimen that the authors have found (5).

    a. On the **day of surgery**, order hydrocortisone sodium succinate (Solu-Cortef), 100 mg IV, to be given with the premedication before surgery.

    b. Use the **same dose** on the **first postoperative day**.

    c. Use 50 mg of **hydrocortisone** on the **second postoperative day**.

    d. Use 25 mg of **hydrocortisone** on the **third postoperative day**, and then continue only with the patient's normal oral daily dose.

4. **Surgery in patients with insulin-dependent diabetes mellitus**

    a. **In the morning before surgery**, the patient should omit breakfast and take about one half of the normal insulin dose subcutaneously (SQ).

    b. **After surgery**, use a **glucose measuring instrument every 4 to 6 hours** to monitor blood glucose levels. The following **sliding scale** is useful: If the glucose level is greater than 350 mg/dL, give 15 units regular insulin SQ. If the level exceeds 250 mg/dL, give 10 units regular insulin SQ.

    c. Return patients to their usual insulin dosage regimen as soon as they return to their normal activity level and to their usual American Diabetic Association diet.

5. **Surgery in patients with hemophilia**

    a. Medical management of a patient with hemophilia who needs surgery requires precise assays of **factor levels** and **prior survival studies** of replacement factors to learn the effect of inhibitors and the biologic half-life in a particular patient. Aim to achieve 100% plasma levels just before anesthetics for surgery are administered. Maintain the level at 60% of normal for the first 4 days and more than 40% for the next 4 days. A level of 100% is also necessary for manipulation of a joint under anesthesia and for removal of pins. A 40% level is needed for suture removal. Levels of 20% are maintained for postoperative physical therapy as long as 4 to 6 weeks after major joint surgery. Forty units of factor per kilogram of body weight administered just before anesthesia (unless survival studies done before surgery show that higher doses are needed) usually achieve close to 100% plasma factor levels.

C. Day of surgery

1. Be sure the **anesthesia** technique proposed is adequate in terms of duration, muscle relaxation, and ability to position the patient properly (6,7). Supervise **positioning, preparing, and draping** so that the planned procedure could be accomplished without difficulty (8). While the assistant prepares the patient, the surgeon can go to the instrument table with the scrub nurse and review major instruments required and implant from start to finish, outlining the planned procedure. The surgeon can also indicate what may be needed if any

TABLE 10-1 Recommended Prophylactic Antibiotics for Orthopaedic Surgical Procedures (Open Trauma, Joint Replacement, Bone, Joint, Tendon, Ligament, and Nerve Surgery)[a]

Bactericidal antibiotics	Dosage for adults	Notable contraindications	Possible complications
Cefazolin[b] (Kefzol or Ancef)	1–2 g q6–8h	History of an anaphylactic reaction to a penicillin drug requires careful usage; with renal insufficiency, the dose must be adjusted to the creatinine clearance	Cephalosporins occasionally cause a false-positive furine reaction with the Clinitest tablets (use test tape instead) and rarely cause blood dyscrasias, overt hemolytic anemia, or renal dysfunction; cephalothin frequently causes a positive Coombs' test
Vancomycin[c]	1 g initially, then 500 mg, q6h	With impaired renal function, dose must be adjusted to patient's creatinine clearance	Rapid IV administration can cause hypotension, which could be especially dangerous during induction of anesthesia, so administer at rate of no more than 10 mg/min

[a]Antibiotics should be given immediately postoperatively and then one dose (IV) or up to 24–48 hr after surgery.
[b]Cefazolin can also be given intramuscularly (IM).
[c]For hospitals in which *Staphylococcus aureus* and *Staphylococcus epidermis* frequently cause wound infection or for patients allergic to cephalosporins.

complications arise. The idea is to ensure that all equipment is immediately available, to review the procedure in the surgeon's mind, and to prepare the nurse so that nurse and surgeon can work together efficiently. See **App. E** for the position and draping of the patient. See **4.c** for a discussion of skin preparations.

2. **Pneumatic tourniquets** (9–11)
   a. When a tourniquet is to be used, the necessary **apparatus** includes a cuff with a smooth, wrinkle-free surface that is a proper size. Select a tourniquet so that the width of the cuff covers approximately one third of the patient's arm length. Check the tubing for leaks. The tourniquet gauge should have a safety valve release because excessively high pressures can cause paralysis. The inflating device must allow rapid attainment of desired pressure.
   b. Plan surgery to **minimize** the **operative time** and, as a consequence, the **tourniquet time.** The conventional safe maximum inflation time of the tourniquet is 2 hours. The cuff may be applied about the arm or thigh but generally not about the forearm or leg. There is no evidence that padding between the cuff and the skin is of any value, and such padding can cause skin wrinkles. Apply a plastic sheet with the adhesive edge placed on the skin distal to the tourniquet and cover the tourniquet with the plastic sheet as shown in **Fig. 10-1**, thereby preventing skin preparation solutions from getting underneath the cuff. Exsanguinate the limb with an Esmarch rubber bandage or with elevation of the limb above the patient's heart for 60 seconds before inflating the tourniquet. An Esmarch bandage should not be used in cases of tumors or infection. Flexing the knee or elbow before inflating the tourniquet makes positioning and closure easier and prevents the possible complication of a ruptured muscle, which can occur by forced flexion of a tourniquet-fixed muscle. Rapidly inflate to the desired pressure. This is 175 to 250 mm Hg in the upper extremity, depending on the arm circumference and the patient's systolic blood pressure, and 250 to 350 mm Hg in the lower extremity, depending on thigh circumference (9,12). Tissue pressure is always somewhat lower than tourniquet pressure, but at 30-cm circumference, it is close to 100%, declining to 70% at

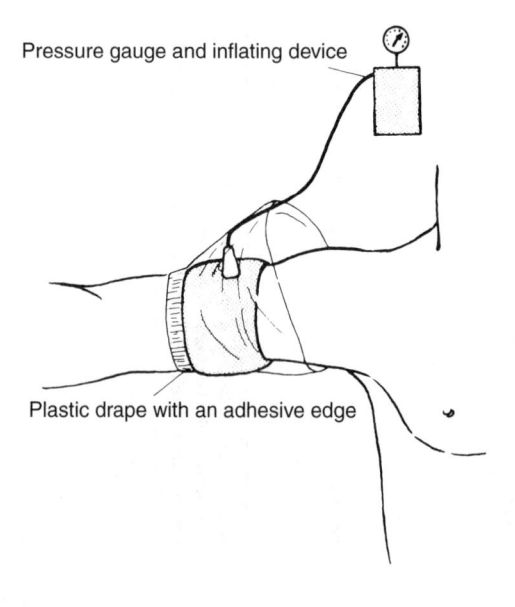

Figure 10-1. Application of a pneumatic tourniquet.

60 cm circumference (9,12–14). The pressures should be decreased for infants and small children. Immediately after deflation, remove or loosen the cuff to prevent a venous congestion from proximal constriction of the extremity. If the tourniquet is deflated and reinflated during surgery, the time for reversal of the tourniquet-produced ischemia is proportional to the tourniquet time; that is, approximately 20 minutes is required for reversal after 2 hours of tourniquet time. In addition, tourniquet effects occur more rapidly after repeated use, and there is probably some summation of these effects. Double tourniquets are used for IV-required anesthesia (Bier blocks) (15). Individual variations such as age, vascular supply of the limb, condition of the tissues, and vascular diseases all influence the patient's tolerance to tourniquet usage. In general, avoid using tourniquets in trauma cases except where dissection around major nerves is required.
  c. **Complications** of tourniquets include blisters and chemical burns (from "prep" solutions that leak under the tourniquet) of the skin, swelling, stiffness, and paralysis. Electromyographic changes have been demonstrated following the use of a tourniquet even within the approved time ranges.
3. The following is a **summary of Occupational Safety and Health Administration (OSHA) regulation No. 1920, "Bloodborne Pathogens,"** emphasizing staff and surgeon responsibilities.
  a. **Wash hands immediately after removing gloves.**
  b. **Wash** (with soap and water) **any exposed skin** (or flush mucous membranes) **immediately** (or as soon as feasible) **after contact with blood or potentially infectious materials.**
  c. **Do not bend, cut, recap, or remove needles or other sharps.** If recapping is the only feasible method, then it must be done by using a mechanical device or the one-handed method.
  d. **Do not eat, drink, smoke, apply cosmetics or lip balm, or handle contact lenses** in work areas where there is a reasonable likelihood of occupational exposure.
  e. **Perform all procedures involving blood or potentially infectious material to minimize spraying and splattering.**
  f. If **outside contamination of transport containers** is possible (or there is a potential for puncture), place potentially infectious material in a second container to **prevent leakage during handling.**
  g. **Use personal protective equipment** such as gloves, face shields, masks, gowns, shoe covers, and so on in situations in which there is risk of exposure to blood or potentially infectious material.
  h. **Following an exposure, complete an incident report identifying the route of exposure and source individual.** A tube of the patient's blood should be drawn, labeled "spin" and held until the patient's consent can be obtained. The employee health nurse is to be contacted for testing as indicated.
  i. **Hepatitis B virus (HBV) immunization is recommended for all employees** and is usually available by contacting the employee health nurse. The authors believe that every surgeon is responsible for knowing his or her own human immunodeficiency virus, hepatitis B, and hepatitis C serologic status.
4. **Prevention of surgical wound infections** (16)
  a. Operating room rituals are designed to **decrease infection**. Despite the best designs, wound contamination and subsequent wound infection continue. It is generally conceded that most wounds become contaminated; however, usually only those with devitalized tissue, large dead spaced with accumulating hematoma, or foreign bodies become frankly infected. A study of the possible sources of coagulase-positive staphylococci that contaminated surgical wounds during 50 operations revealed that bacteria of bacteriophage types that were present only in the air were found in 68% of the wounds; 50% of wounds contained bacteria of bacteriophage types

that were found in the patient's nose, throat, or skin; 14% had bacteriophage types found in the noses and throats of members of the scrubbed surgical team; and 6% of the wounds had bacteriophage types found on the hands of the scrubbed surgical team. Maximum contamination occurs early in the operative procedure when there is a considerable amount of air circulation caused by individuals moving about the room. After the air quiets, the rate of contamination is less, but an increased exposure time allows increased contamination. It is important to keep traffic in the operating room to an absolute minimum, to walk slowly, and to avoid fanning the air with quick opening of the doors, drapes, and towels.

b. Studies show considerable variation in the **filtration efficiency of different masks**. Cloth masks are only about 50% efficient in filtering bacterial organisms and are rarely used. Numerous disposable masks have a bacterial filtration efficiency greater than 94% according to the manufacturers. Fiberglass-free masks are probably safer. Prolonged use (averaging 4 1/2 hours of operation time) and the use of moist masks do not impair ability to filter, except in the case of cloth masks. Since the surgical masks work on a filtration principle, double masking can actually increase the air contamination with bacteria because double masking makes transportation of air through the mask pores more difficult and forces more unfiltered air to escape along the sides of the mask.

c. Although airborne contamination is by far the most important source of contamination, **skin contamination** does occur. Even with the use of 1% or 2% tincture of iodine, the deeper areas of the epidermis are not bacteria free. With a 1% concentration, no cases of skin irritation have occurred. If a higher concentration is used, however, then the excess iodine should be removed with alcohol after 30 seconds. One 5-minute scrub with povidone-iodine is as effective as a 10-minute scrub in reducing bacterial counts on the skin and keeping them down for as long as 8 hours. A 7.5% povidone-iodine (Betadine) skin disinfectant yields 0.75% available iodine. More recent work shows that **chlorhexidine gluconate** (Hibiclens) may be the scrub detergent of choice for both the surgeon and the patient (17). A comparative study between hexachlorophene (pHisoHex), povidone-iodine, and chlorhexidine showed the latter to be probably the most effective. There was a 99.9% reduction in resident bacterial flora after a single 6-minute chlorhexidine scrub. The reduction of flora on surgically gloved hands was maintained over the 6-hour test period. In addition, the pharmacology of chlorhexidine is reportedly more effective against gram-positive and gram-negative organisms, including *Pseudomonas aeruginosa*.

d. **Extremity draping.** Adhesive plastic drapes do not totally eliminate the patient's skin as a possible source of infection. Drape the extremities as described in **App. E**.

e. **Intraoperative procedures** to prevent postoperative wound infection include the elimination of any large collection of blood. A hematoma is an excellent potential culture medium. Wound suction is used whenever one anticipates continued bleeding into the wound; however, their use in fracture, joint replacement, and spine surgery has not been proven to decrease the incidence of wound infection. Surgical wounds are carefully irrigated to remove any potential contaminated residue before closing. *In vitro* experiments using bacitracin 50,000 units plus polymyxin B sulfate (Aerosporin) 50 mg in a liter of saline or lactated Ringer solution have shown that 100% of *Staphylococcus aureus, Escherichia coli,* the *Klebsiella* organisms, and *P. aeruginosa* bacteria were killed by a 1-minute exposure to the antibiotic solution (18). *Staphylococcus epidermidis* organisms were also killed. Only the *Proteus* organisms showed significant resistance to this antibiotic irrigation (only 3%–22% were killed). *Proteus* organisms are uncommon as a cause of immediate postoperative infections in musculoskeletal surgery, however, when the wounds are not previously contaminated or infected. Data indicate that irrigation of surgical wounds with a solution containing bacitracin and polymyxin B sulfate or bacitracin and neomycin could potentially lower the incidence of postoperative infections (19). A large number of patients are sensitive to neomycin, so its use is generally discouraged. Polymyxin B is sometimes difficult to obtain from the manufacturer. In this situation, some surgeons use a dilute Betadine solution as a topical antibiotic irrigant; however, this solution is toxic to tissue. Data confirming that antibiotic irrigants are superior to sterile saline in preventing surgical wound infection are generally lacking in orthopaedic surgery. Splash basins are a source of bacterial contamination and should not be used.

   f. The incidence of infection increases in wounds open for longer than 2 hours. Whether this is a result of the increased exposure to the air, failure of masks, skin contaminants, or more trauma in the wound is not certain. Even with lengthy surgical cases, with good surgical technique the rate of deep wound infection on "clean" orthopaedic cases should not exceed 1%.

   g. Laminar air flow systems appear to be an effective means of reducing postoperative infection rates as long as the flow of air is kept laminar or streamlined across the operative area (e.g., during hip surgeries). These systems are not effective if the air becomes turbulent across the operative area because, for example, of the position of people in the operating room (e.g., during knee replacement surgery) (20).

   h. Hooded surgical exhaust systems are effective but cumbersome and costly. They are often used to protect the operating team from infection by high-risk patients.

   i. Whenever a subsequent surgical wound infection occurs in a clean, uneventful surgical case, consider a **nasal culture** from all those present at the time of the operation.

5. Malignant hyperthermia

   a. Pathophysiology. The target organ in malignant hyperthermia is skeletal muscle. Certain triggering events, such as the administration of halothane or succinylcholine, precipitate release of calcium from the calcium-storing membrane (sarcoplasmic reticulum) of the muscle cell. The abnormal transport of calcium results in recurrent sarcomeric contractions and consequent muscle rigidity. The metabolic rate is accelerated, causing heat and increased carbon dioxide production with accelerated oxygen consumption. Core body temperature increases.

   b. History. The potentially fatal syndrome is an autosomal dominant metabolic disease. In 40% of reported cases, an orthopaedist is the first to encounter this disorder. The incidence in the United States is approximately 1:1,000. The syndrome is associated more frequently with patients having congenital and musculoskeletal abnormalities: kyphosis, scoliosis, hernia, recurrent joint dislocations, club foot, ptosis, or strabismus. Malignant hyperthermia can occur at any age but is most likely to occur in a young individual with a large muscle mass. After exposure to an anesthetic (or other stress), body temperature rapidly increases.

   c. Examination. A rapid elevation in body temperature is noted early. Cardiac arrhythmias usually are concurrent, can progress to ventricular tachycardia, and may end in ventricular fibrillation with subsequent death. The soda lime canister may turn blue and become palpably hot. Tetanic muscle contractions occur in approximately 60% of cases. Like so many conditions in orthopaedics, early recognition is crucial. Temperature and electrocardiographic monitoring during surgery is mandatory. A rapid temperature elevation (even from an initial subnormal temperature), tachycardia, hypertonia of skeletal muscle, unexplained hyperventilation, overheated soda lime canister, dark blood, sweating, and blotchy cyanosis are all indicative of possible malignant hyperthermia.

d. **Treatment**
   i. **Prevention**
      (a) Obtain a **careful past history and family history**, inquiring especially about fatal or near-fatal experiences following emotional, physical, traumatic, or surgical stress or about a relative who died of an obscure cause in the perioperative period.
      (b) Administer prophylactic **dantrolene (Dantrium) orally** in doses of 2.2 mg/kg body weight (range of 2–4 mg/kg body weight) at 12 and 4 hours before the induction of anesthesia when the history is positive.
      (c) **Avoid** the use of **halothane (Fluothane)** and **succinylcholine (Anectine)** in high-risk patients.
   ii. **Management** of an evolving malignant hyperthermia syndrome
      (a) Immediately **discontinue all anesthetic agents and muscle relaxants** and terminate the surgical procedure as quickly as possible.
      (b) **Hyperventilate with oxygen.**
      (c) **Use IV sodium bicarbonate**, 4 mL/kg body weight, and repeat as necessary until blood gases approach normal.
      (d) Administer **mannitol**, 1 g/kg body weight and **furosemide** (Lasix), 1 mg/kg body weight, which help maintain urine output to clear myoglobin and excessive sodium.
      (e) Treat hyperkalemia with approximately 50 mg of **IV glucose** with 50 units of **insulin.**
      (f) Control arrhythmias with procainamide (Pronestyl).
      (g) **Cool the patient** with immersion in ice water and expose to an electric fan to facilitate evaporation. Refrigerated saline or Ringer's lactate administered intravenously is helpful. Maintain cooling procedures until the body temperature is less than 38°C.
      (h) **Dantrolene** (approximately 12 mg/kg body weight) used intravenously **is one of the mainstays of treatment** and probably works by reducing calcium outflow from the sarcoplasmic reticulum into the myoplasm.
      (i) **Physiologic monitoring** by electrocardiography and measurement of the central venous pressure, blood gases every 10 minutes, volume and quality of renal output, serum electrolytes, glucose, serum glutamic oxaloacetic transaminase (SGOT), creatine phosphokinase (CPK), and blood urea nitrogen (BUN) is important.
      (j) Good **prognostic signs** are lightening of the coma (often heralded by restlessness), return of reflexes, return to normal temperature, reduced heart rate, improved renal output, and return of consciousness.
e. **Complications**
   i. **Weakness and easy fatigability** persist for several months.
   ii. **Death** owing to ventricular fibrillation can occur within 1 or 2 hours from the onset of the condition. If death occurs later, then it is usually a result of pulmonary edema, coagulopathy, or massive electrolyte and acid-base imbalance. If the patient dies after several days in a coma, then the cause is usually renal failure or brain damage.

II. **ORTHOPAEDIC OPERATING ROOM INSTRUMENTS AND THEIR USAGE**
   A. **Introduction.** Much of the remaining discussion is modified from a psychomotor skills course originally organized for the University of Washington Department of Orthopaedic Surgery residents by F. G. Lippert III, M.D., in the 1980s.
   B. **Techniques for checking the function of grasping type surgical instruments** (21). The breakdown of high-quality instruments is often the direct result of their misuse. Forceps, hemostats, needle holders, and clamps frequently are misused in orthopaedic surgery. They can be misapplied to various pins, nails, screws, and

plates when pliers are not readily available. They are also misused to clamp large sponges, tubing, and needles.

1. It is annoying to a surgeon and hazardous to the patient when **forceps or a hemostat** springs open. This mishap is caused by forceps malalignment, worn ratchet teeth, or lack of tension at the shanks.
    a. Start the equipment check by visually checking **jaw alignment** by closing the jaws of the forceps lightly. If the jaws overlap, they are out of alignment. Then, determine whether the teeth are meshing properly on forceps with serrated jaws. In addition, try to wiggle the instrument with the forceps open and holding one shank in each hand. If the box has considerable play or is very loose, then the jaws are usually malaligned and the forceps need repair.
    b. To check the **ratchet teeth** on instruments, clamp the forceps to the first tooth only. A resounding snap should be produced. Then hold the instrument by the box lock and tap the ratchet teeth portion of the instrument lightly against a solid object. If the instrument springs open, then it is faulty and needs repair.
    c. Test the **tension between the shanks** by closing the jaws of the forceps lightly until they barely touch. At this point there should be clearance of 1/16 or 1/8 inch between the ratchet teeth on each shank.
2. To test the function of the **needle holder**, first clamp the needle in the jaws of the holder, then lock the instrument on the second ratchet tooth. If the needle can be turned easily by hand, then set aside the instrument for repair. When the instrument is new, it holds a needle securely on the first ratchet tooth for a considerable time. Needle holders such as a Crile, Wood, Derf, or Halsey, used in plastic surgery, should hold at least a 6-0 suture. Needle holders such as Castroviejo or Kalt should hold a 7-0 suture.

C. **Surgical exposure instruments.** There are various methods for testing the efficiency of **surgical scissors**. The Mayo and Metzenbaum dissecting scissors should cut four layers of gauze with the tips of their blades. Smaller scissors (less than 4 in. long) should be able to cut two layers of gauze at the tips. All scissors should have a fine, smooth feel and require only minimum pressure by the blades to cut properly. The scissors action should not be too loose or too tight. Check the tips of the scissors for burrs or for excessive sharpness. Closed tips of the scissors should not be separated or loose. The precise setting of the blade is very important. Sharpening surgical scissors is a skilled procedure, usually requiring an exceptional craftsman to properly grind and set the blades.

1. **Periosteal elevators**
    a. Periosteal elevators are instruments designed to **strip (or elevate) periosteum from bone**. As the instrument is pushed along the surface of the bone, the soft tissue is lifted from the underlying bone. Periosteal elevators are thus instruments for blunt dissection and are designed to follow bony surfaces without gouging into the bone or wandering off into the soft tissues. They are also useful in blunt separation of other tissue planes such as in the exposure of the hip joint capsule. The use of periosteal elevators is most satisfactory in areas where tissue planes are not too firmly adherent. At bony attachments of a ligament or capsule, collagen fibers plunge deeply into the bone so that the elevator does not slide within a tissue interspace; sharp dissection with a scalpel is more appropriate here. In fracture fixation, periosteal stripping, which can adversely affect blood supply and bone healing, should be minimized where ever possible.
    b. Elevators are made in **different sizes and shapes**. They may be narrow or wide. Sharp corners allow insertion of the instrument into a tissue plane or beneath the periosteum. On the other hand, most blade corners are rounded to avoid producing damage when pressure is applied to the central portion of the blade.
    c. The **technique** of making a periosteal incision with a scalpel before the elevator is used helps form well-defined edges. When periosteum is being

elevated from bone, the first rule of safety is to always keep the blade against bone. If the instrument is allowed to slip off into the soft tissues, then vessels and nerves can be damaged. It is important to use two hands whenever possible to have a stable grasp on the instrument and to maintain fine control. A gentle rocking motion while advancing the blade produces more even results (**Fig. 10-2**). Although periosteal elevators need not be honed to the same sharp edge required for bone-cutting osteotomes, they do require some tissue-penetrating ability to be most effective. Nevertheless, they should not be so sharp as to incise soft tissue instead of stripping it.

- **d. Important guidelines for tool selection and usage**
    - **i.** Select the **correct size**. Generally, use a small elevator for small bones and a large elevator for large bones.
    - **ii.** Select the **correct shape**. Usually, a sharp elevator is used to elevate periosteum and a rounded elevator to dissect soft tissue.
    - **iii.** The **periosteum is incised with a scalpel.**
    - **iv.** The **corner of the elevator** is used to reflect a periosteal edge.
    - **v.** The **periosteum is elevated evenly** without tearing.
    - **vi.** The elevator is **kept on the bone.**
    - **vii.** The **bone is not engaged** by the elevator.
    - **viii.** A **rocking motion** is used while advancing the elevator.
    - **ix.** **Two hands** are used, one for power and one for stability and dissecting.
    - **x.** **Overpenetration** into the soft tissues by the elevator **should be avoided.**
    - **xi.** A **gentle technique** must be used.

D. Bone cutting instruments: osteotomes, gouges, and mallets
1. The **major difference** between an osteotome and a chisel is that an osteotome bevels on both sides to a point, whereas the chisel has a bevel on only one side (**Fig. 10-3**). The term **osteotome** is made up of **osteo**, which means "bone," and **tome**, which means "to cut;" the purpose of the tool is to cut bone. The cut should be produced under excellent control; otherwise, the bone can be split. Osteotomes come in different shapes and sizes. There are different types of handles that make for differences in holding and striking surface capabilities.

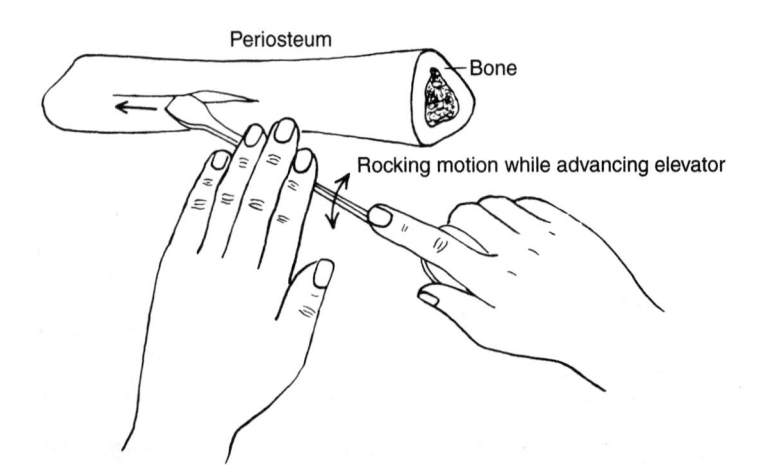

Figure 10-2. Proper use of a sharp-edged periosteal elevator. (From G. Spolek, unpublished data, 1974, with permission.)

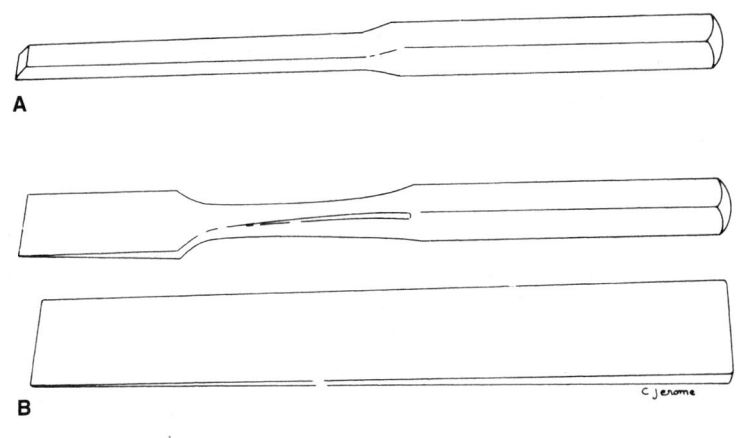

Figure 10-3. Differences between an osteotome and a chisel. **A:** A chisel. **B:** Two types of osteotome.

2. **Selection of instruments**
    a. **Chisels** are used to remove bone from around screws and plates instead of osteotomes because they can be easily sharpened when the edges are nicked from being hit against the metal. It is better to keep a set of chisels specifically for removing metal implants.
    b. **Osteotomes** are used to cut bone and to shave off osteoperiosteal grafts. In fusion procedures, they are used to remove the cartilage and subchondral bone as well as to perform "fish scaling" of the surface of bone for bone graft union.
    c. **Gouges** are used to provide strips of cancellous bone graft from the iliac crest. They are also used to clean out the cartilage and subchondral bone from concave joint surfaces.
    d. **Mallets** are used to produce power to drive the aforementioned tools through bone and cartilage.
3. **Proper technique**
    a. The dominant hand is used to grasp the mallet, which strikes the back of the instrument and drives it through bone. **While hitting the osteotome through bone of increasing density**, notice that the sound becomes high pitched and the osteotome moves a shorter distance with each blow. In addition, there is a tightening or holding quality about the osteotome so that it moves less freely. This tightness is an indication that bone is coming under more tension and that a split of the bone is about to occur. Decrease the tension by working the osteotome back and forth through the bone. Occasionally, it is necessary to remove the osteotome to take a different direction or a slightly different angle. It is frequently important to prescore the bone so that the cutting goes directly toward it instead of splitting the bone in an unwanted area.
    b. **Precautions** include preventing the osteotome from sliding off the bone or from cutting through the bone rapidly and then plunging into soft tissue. The nondominant hand merely supports and directs the osteotome against bone until it gets started but does not apply any major pressure on the tool. Starting the cut is best accomplished by placing the osteotome at right angles to the bone, then angling the tool only after the initial score and cut have begun. These precautions protect both the patient and the hands of the assistant.
4. Specific **maintenance** is necessary in the handling and sharpening of the tools. The sharpening of an osteotome or a gouge is a difficult and critical

procedure that must be undertaken with great caution. If the tool is overheated during sharpening, then the temper is lost. The loss can be recognized by the bluish-gray color of the metal in contrast to the silvery color usually associated with stainless steel. In addition, care must be taken in cleaning and handling the tools while they are on a surgical table so that the ends do not become damaged by other instruments. Keep them in a rack during the sterilization process, not in a basin with other tools.

E. **Bone saws and files.** In general, the operator must control the amplitude, direction, and length of force applied to the saw. The use of lactated Ringer (or saline) irrigation to disperse heat is always recommended.
   1. The proper use of **Gigli saw** includes making a scribe mark at the start of the technique if possible. The surgeon must be careful not to drop or tangle the saw cable, to keep the cable at approximately 90 degrees, and to use the middle two thirds of the saw while applying a constant, steady tension. Excess body movement should be avoided to produce a straight bone cut. The use of saline coolant is recommended.
   2. A **bone file** or rasp is usually used to round the edge of a bone cut. Both hands should be used to control the direction of the tool and only a forward force should be applied.

F. **General bone screw biomechanics**
   1. **Holes** are generally drilled in bone for the purpose of inserting screws to hold orthopaedic implants. Careful, even compulsive, attention to detail in selecting equipment and in drilling holes properly is vital to the performance of an implanted fixation device. The interlocking threads of screw and bone overlap by less than 0.02 inch. Any failure of equipment or technique that decreases this margin drastically reduces the holding power of the screw. Given the severe loading environment in which most orthopaedic implants operate, the holding power of a screw is an important matter. Force concentrations that occur when a screw fails to hold properly can result in a rapid failure of the implant.
   2. **Drill bits** (1)
      a. **Common defects in equipment.** Since hole drilling is frequently taken for granted (the major attention being paid to the implant itself), drill bits come to the operating room in various stages of disrepair.
         i. A **dull point** is one of the most serious and least noticed defects. When the point is sharp, virtually all heat generated in drilling is carried away in the bone chips that are formed. Even slight dullness drastically increases friction between the point and the bone. This friction causes excessive heating and can affect the strength of the bone around the hole as well as cause inefficient cutting, which results in an oversized hole.
         ii. The flutes should be examined for **nicks and gouges** that score the walls of the hole, causing excessive heating and oversized holes; if identified, the drill bit should be discarded.
         iii. A drill with a **scored shank** does not sit straight in the chuck and causes the same trouble as a drill sharpened off center.
         iv. Drill bits of the **wrong size** are sometimes selected. A difference of just 1/100th of an inch is enough to diminish the holding power of a screw severely, even though insertion of the screw appears normal.
         v. A **bent drill bit** causes the same difficulty as a drill bit sharpened off center. One cannot tell whether a drill bit is bent by simply looking at it; it must be rotated in the fingers. Even small **bends** create holes that are irregular, and the drill bit is very susceptible to breakage.
      b. **Technique**
         i. Prevent the drill point from **wandering off center.**
            (a) To keep the point from **wandering on penetration** and to protect surrounding soft tissues, use an appropriate-sized **drill guide.** Start the hole perpendicular to the surface. When bone

penetration begins, shift to the desired direction. Always use saline to cool the drill bit.
- **(b)** Thin surgical drill bits are flexible, and if the drill is inadvertently held **slightly off perpendicular** when starting the hole, the point may bend the opposite way, making the point wander.
- **(c)** If the drill bit is **not positioned properly in the chuck** or if debris is present in the chuck or on the shank, then the drill bit may wander off center. Another error involves insertion of the drill bit too deeply into the chuck, which causes damage to the flutes when the drill is tightened. Check the drill for these problems before proceeding.
  ii. **Tighten the chuck down.** If the chuck is loose, then it can rotate relative to the drill and score the shank.
  iii. **Too little force** (not too much force) is a common defect in technique. Push hard enough to cause a constant progression of the drill bit; otherwise, too much energy is being dissipated as friction rather than as cutting, causing excessive heating.
  iv. **Avoid overpenetration.** Slow the drill motor when the drill bit tip begins penetrating (noted by a change in resistance) and finish with care. With care, the surgeon will note that the pitch of the sound made by the drill drops just before penetration of the cortex. The tip should not penetrate more than one eighth of an inch through the opposite cortex.
  v. When the drill bit breaks through the opposite cortex, **keep it rotating in the same direction as you back it out.** The chips are thus carried out with the drill bit instead of being left in the hole.
  vi. Drill motors should be **lubricated frequently**. Special surgical lubricants are available. Do not use mineral oil or ordinary oil because they are not permeable by steam and can harbor bacteria and spores even after autoclaving.
  vii. Battery packs for power equipment should be kept charged with backups available.
- **c. Adhere to the following points when using drills:**
  i. **Choose the correct drill bit.** Reject dull, scored, bent, oversized, and incorrectly pointed drill bits. In general, use new drill bits for each case.
  ii. **Insert the drill bit correctly in the chuck** with the drill bit centered and the chuck tightened on the shank only. Use quick release systems whenever possible to avoid potential problems.
  iii. **Tighten the chuck sufficiently.**
  iv. **Start the drill hole perpendicular to the surface**; then change to the desired direction.
  v. **Maintain adequate pressure** on the drill to promote cutting and lessen heat production.
  vi. **Maintain the proper direction** of the hole and penetrate the far cortical wall carefully, with the drill bit minimally penetrating.
  vii. **Keep the drill rotating while backing it out** in order to clear the hole of bone chips.
3. **Screws** (1)
   a. **Cortical bone screws** are fully threaded and come in a variety of sizes for different sized bones. Non–self-tapping screws require a tap to cut the threads into the bone before insertion (**Fig. 10-4**).
   b. **Cancellous bone screws** have a thinner core diameter plus wider and deeper threads to better grip the "spongy" bone. They are fully or partially threaded. Tapping is required only through the cortical surface.
   c. **Lag screw fixation** can be achieved with either a partially threaded cancellous screw or by drilling a "gliding hole" (of the same size as the outer thread diameter) for the near cortex, allowing a cortical screw to produce lag compression.
   d. Large, medium and small **cannulated cancellous bone screws** are designed to pass over a guidewire. With this type of system the surgeon can

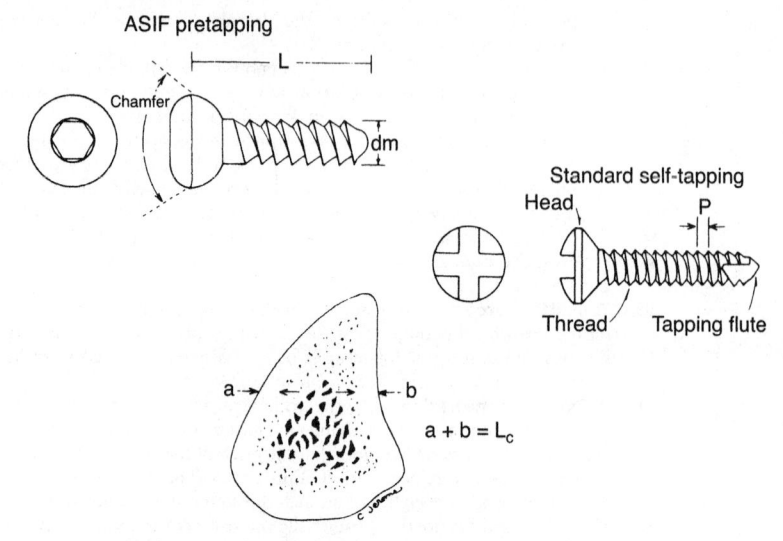

Figure 10-4. Comparison between Association for the Study of Internal Fixation (ASIF) and standard cortical bone screws.

place a guidewire exactly where desired so that the cannulated drill, tap, and screw passes over this wire for precise placement.
   e. **Length of screw.** Drilling the proper hole is only the first step in firmly fixing the screw into the bone. The second part is selecting a screw that is of adequate length (22).
      i. To use a **depth gauge** properly, do not insert the gauge any farther than necessary. Be sure to have hooked the far end of the hole and not an intermediate point. Consider allowing additional length (usually 2 mm) over the scale reading on the depth gauge when choosing the screw length.
      ii. A **self-tapping screw** has a tapered point whose holding power is further reduced by the flutes cut for tapping purposes. The **distal 2 mm of the self-tapping screw has no holding power at all, and the next 2 mm has very little. Screw lengths are measured from the proximal edge of the chamfered head to the distal point of the screw** (**Fig. 10-4**). If a screw is installed in a plate, then additional length must be allowed. Given the fact that bone screws hold principally in cortical bone, a screw that is short by 4 mm may lose 50% of its holding power.
      iii. When a screw is inserted on a **subcutaneous border of bone**, the hole should be **countersunk** before the depth is measured and the screw inserted.
      iv. **Tighten the screw snugly and no more**, so as not to strip the threads of the bone when inserting the screw. Retighten cortical screws three times to allow for the obligate loss of strain between screw and bone resulting from loss of fluid in the bone and stress relaxation.
G. **General principles of plating** are described in the following paragraphs and generally follow the concepts and techniques advocated by the Association for the Study of Internal Fixation (AO/ASIF) group, which supplies the most widely used fracture fixation implants in use. The plates are listed by their general biomechanical functions (11).
   1. Protection or **neutralization plates** are used in combination with lag or other screws and protect the screw fixation in diaphyseal fractures. Without the

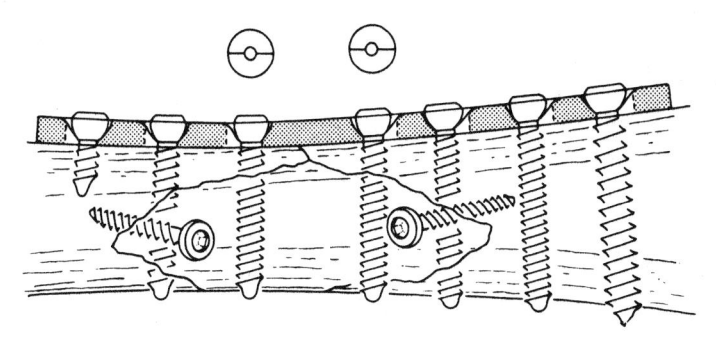

Figure 10-5. Application of a conventional or neutralization internal fixation plate. The neutral drill guide is used. Neutralization plate allows for more loading of the fracture than simple lag screw fixation.

plates, the screw fixation by itself does not withstand much loading and does not allow for early range of motion. The lag screws provide for most of the interfragmental compression and the plate protects the screws from torsion, bending, and shearing forces (**Fig. 10-5**).
2. The dynamic compression plate (DCP) brings compression to the fracture site by its design. Recently, low-contact dynamic compression plates (LCDCPs) and point contact plates (PCPs) have been developed that allow greater freedom in screw insertion through the plate and also limit the pressure necrosis effect of the plate on the cortical bone surface (1) (**Figs. 10-6, 10-7, 10-8**).

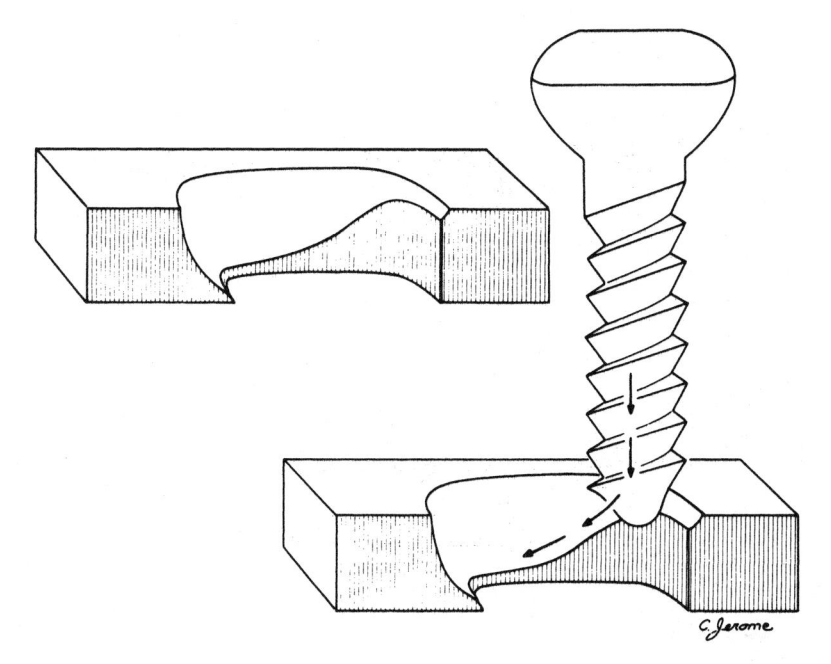

Figure 10-6. A longitudinal section of the dynamic compression plate (DCP) screw hole. Insertion of the Association for the Study of Internal Fixation (AO/ASIF) screw causes self-compression of the fracture site by the plate by sliding down an inclined cylinder to a horizontal one. (From Mueller ME, et al. *Manual of internal fixation,* 2nd ed. Berlin: Springer-Verlag, 1979:71, with permission.)

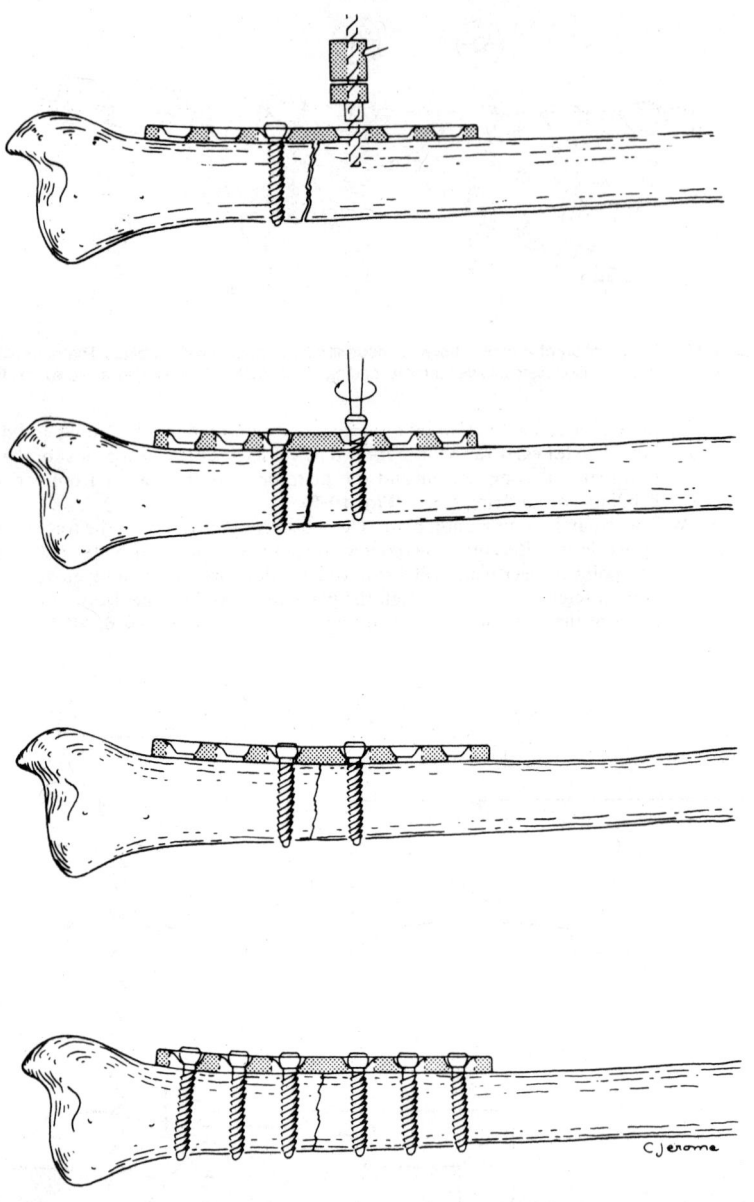

Figure 10-7. Application of self-compression plate. The load drill guide is used for placement of the second drill as shown in the top illustration. The other holes are drilled with the neutral drill guide. (From Mueller ME, et al. *Manual of internal fixation,* 2nd ed. Berlin: Springer-Verlag, 1979: 67,75.)

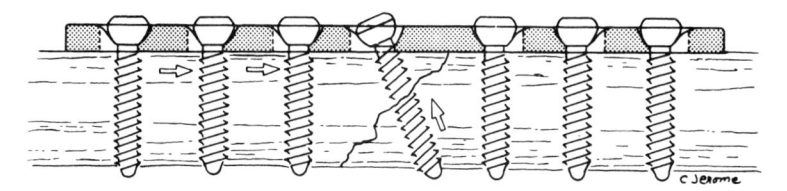

Figure 10-8. Dynamic compression plate with lag screw. The compression through the plate is applied first; then the lag screw is added to prevent a shear force on the lag screw.

3. By their nature, many epiphyseal and metaphyseal fractures are subject to compression and shearing forces. Lag screws are used to reconstruct the normal anatomy, but they cannot overcome the forces of shear and bending because of the thin cortical shells in these areas, especially in comminuted fractures. The fixation is supplemented with supporting or buttress plates to prevent subsequent fracture displacement from shear or bending stresses. Specially designed buttress plates include the T plate, the T **buttress plate**, the L buttress plate, the lateral tibial head plate, the spoon plate, the cloverleaf plate, and the condylar buttress plate. Additional plates for special locations (e.g., proximal and distal tibia, calcaneous) have recently been marketed.
4. To restore the load-bearing capacity of an eccentrically loaded fractured bone and minimize the forces borne by the fixation device, it is necessary to absorb the tensile forces (the result of a bending movement) and convert them into compressive forces. This requires **tension band fixation**, which exerts a force equal in magnitude but opposite in direction to the bending force (assuming the bone is able to withstand compression) (1). Therefore, comminuted fractures should be treated with other fixation devices or protected longer from bending moments.
   a. Ideally, **tension band plating** techniques are used on the femur, humerus, radius, and ulna (1).
   b. **Tension band wire internal fixation**
      i. The **purpose** of tension band wire internal fixation is to secure the fragments of fractures in such a way that the application of normal forces (muscle forces, loads generated by walking) produces a compression of the fragments at the fracture site instead of pulling the fragments apart. The advantage of this technique is that the fixation is secure enough to allow early (if not immediate) use of the limb. Indications for tension band wiring are generally in the treatment of avulsion fractures at the insertion of muscles, tendons, or ligaments. If one has to deal with a rotational component or when accurate reduction of the fragments is vital, then introduce two parallel Kirschner wires before the insertion of the tension band. The tension band then is passed around the wire ends.
      ii. The tension band **principle** works only when there are applied natural forces that tend to bend the bone at the fracture site. The olecranon, patella, and tip of the fibula are examples of such sites. **Fig. 10-9** describes the principles of tension band wire internal fixation for the treatment of a transverse fracture of the olecranon.
      iii. As shown on **Fig. 10-9, a single-screw fixation without a tension wire loop is not adequate** because the screw bends with triceps activity and only half the fracture site is placed in compression.
      iv. It is evident that the wire is pulled in tension by the bending effect of the muscle force. Therefore, whatever force is exerted across the bony interface must be **compressive and equal** in magnitude to the force carried by the wire.

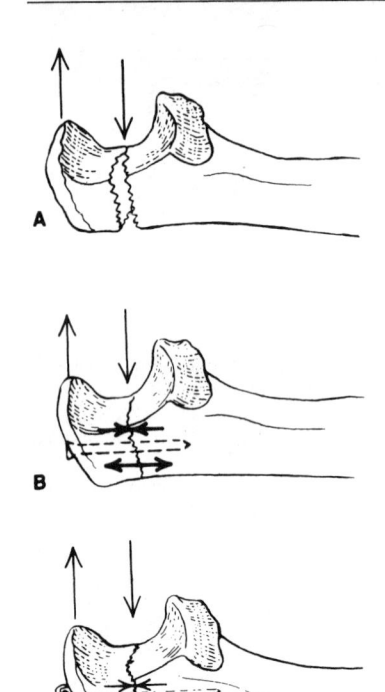

Figure 10-9. The principles of tension band wire internal fixation as applied to a transverse fracture of the olecranon. Forces on an intact olecranon cause a bending moment. **A:** Same forces on a transverse fracture of the olecranon cause the fracture to open. **B:** Screw fixation provides only partial compression of fracture. **C:** Fixation of the cortex under tension creates equal compressive forces across the fracture site.

- v. Note that the tension band wiring **does not provide the desired rigidity for loading from all directions**. It is intended to resist only the strong tension forces applied through the action of specific muscles or through loading.
- vi. The **application** of tension band wire fixation is discussed in the treatment of olecranon fractures in **Chap. 18, III.B** and of patellar fractures in **Chap. 24, III.A.3**.
5. **Numerous other plates and screws** serve the aforementioned functions with various shapes and sizes to adapt to the local anatomy. They include straight and offset condylar blade plates, reconstruction plates (more easily contoured in all three planes, which make them optimum for use in the pelvis and distal humerus), dynamic hip screws, dynamic condylar screws, and specialized locking plates where the screw head is threaded into the plate. These are especially useful in osteoporotic bone.
6. **Contouring internal fixation plates.** Internal fixation plates may be contoured to fit the bone before application. Such contouring increases the bone-plate interface area so that the loads normally carried by the bone can be transferred to the plate by friction rather than pure shearing on the bone screws. To contour a plate template, press the aluminum template of the proper length against the bone, then bend the plate to match. Plate benders may be handheld singular, handheld pliers, and table-mounted bending presses. Locking plates in general should not be contoured, as the hole configuration will be distorted.
    a. The **bending press** gets the most use because most contouring is two-dimensional. The anvil is adjustable so that the handle can be used in the position with the best control (near the end of its travel). The **hand press**

is used mainly for small plates, for plates with a semitubular cross section, and reconstruction picks. There are three different anvils (straight, convex, and concave) to prevent squashing of the semitubular plates. The **bending irons** are for applying twists and are most conveniently used when the jaws are opened upward to prevent the plate from falling out and when the handles are on the same side of the plate. Theoretically, uniform twist occurs between the irons, so start with them at the ends of the desired twist length. Once the twist is started, move the irons closer together to get localized contours. DCPs are weakest through the holes, where most of the twist occurs, so try to position the irons to prevent excessive bends at any one hole. Use the press first because the plate does not fit the anvil if the bending irons are used to twist beforehand. LCDCPs have more uniform characteristics and do not bend at the holes. **Fig. 10-10** illustrates the three types of instruments.
  b. **Important guidelines in usage**
      i. Bend the plate to form a **smooth, continuous contour.** Because the press causes a single, rather abrupt bend directly beneath the plunger, a long continuous curve is best formed by several small bends rather than a few sharp bends.
      ii. **Avoid bends through screw holes** because they alter the shape of the countersunk surface of the hole so that the screw does not seat properly. If a bend must be made through a screw hole, go easy on the press handle because the plate is weaker at a hole and less force is required to bend it.
      iii. If the required contour contains a series of **shallow and sharp bends,** do the shallow ones (greatest radius of curvature) first and progressively work toward the sharper bends, as shown in **Fig. 10-11**. This procedure tends to produce smooth contours and allows easier template matching. Contouring to fit a bump or knoll on the bone surface requires three bends: two convex and one concave.
      iv. **Do not overbend but ease into a contour** (see **Fig. 10-11**). Overbending requires straightening, which, besides being time-consuming work, hardens the plate in that area and thus reduces the strength of the plate.
      v. When contouring the plate, do not match the template exactly, but rather alter (underbend or overbend) the shape so that there is a **1- to 2-mm clearance between the plate and the bone at the site of a transverse fracture.** This technique causes compression of the cortex opposite the plate when the screws are tightened.
      vi. **Minimize scratching or marking of the plate surface.** If the surface is scratched, then a potential corrosion site is created. Therefore, use the proper bending irons with smooth jaws rather than vise grips.
H. **Cerclage** is a technique of encircling a fractured bone with Parham-Martin band, stainless steel or titanium wire, Dahl-Miles cable, or other nonabsorbable material to hold the fracture in reduction in conjunction with stronger, more permanent fixation. Cerclage is not recommended as a primary method of internal fixation of fractures. There are many techniques for applying cerclage wire.
  1. **General rules of wire cerclage**
      a. **Avoid putting kinks in the wire.** Kinking is easy, particularly if the wire is coiled. Kinks result in stress concentrations that drastically reduce the fatigue strength of the wire.
      b. **Be sure the loop around the bone is perpendicular to the long axis of the bone.** Otherwise, the loop may appear tight, but any slight movement causes it to shift and loosen.
      c. Use the cerclage wire only to hold the fracture site in reduction, not to apply compression. The wire is not strong enough to apply useful compression.

Bench press

Hand press

Bending irons

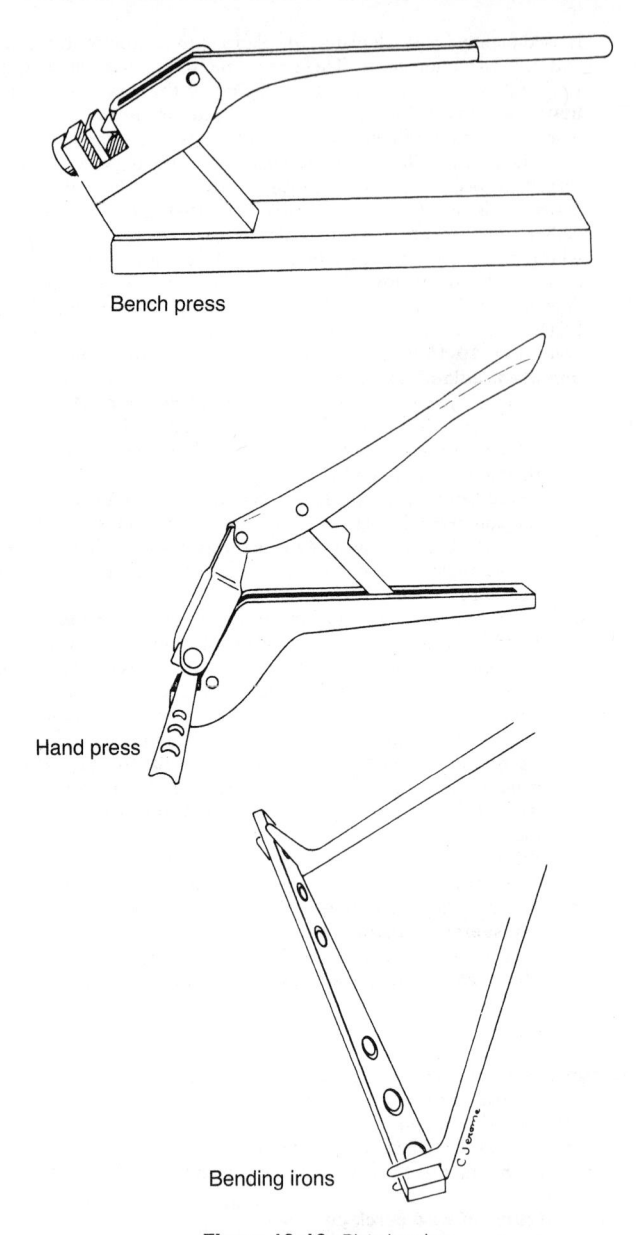

Figure 10-10. Plate benders.

Tighten the wire only until it is snug; be careful not to overtighten while making the knot.
   d. Use the **proper-sized wire**; 18-gauge is common and has sufficient strength. The area of the wire is a measure of its load-carrying capacity, which depends on the square of the diameter. Thus, the load-carrying capacity decreases considerably with even moderate decreases in radius.

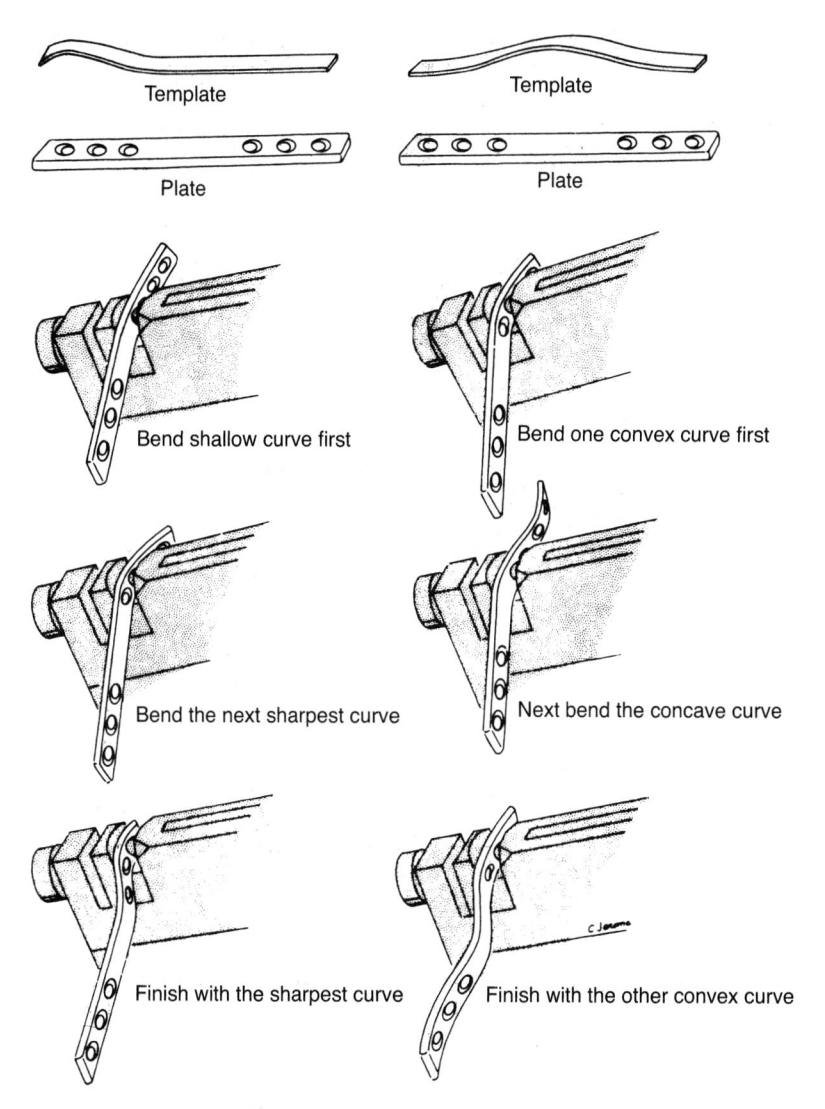

Figure 10-11. Steps in plate contouring.

2. **Wire tighteners**
   a. The **Bowen wire tightener is an excellent tightener (Fig. 10-12)**. Both wires are passed into the nose of the appliance and out the side. The outer wheel is turned to secure the wire against the inside cylinder. By turning the inside wheel, the inside cylinder is pulled up the handle of the device, effectively tightening the wire to the desired tension. The whole instrument is rotated to twist the wire, and the wires are then easily cut just distal to the last twist.
   b. The **Kirschner wire traction bows** (see **Fig. 9-1**) have a mechanical advantage that varies with the jaw opening. The lowest mechanical advantage

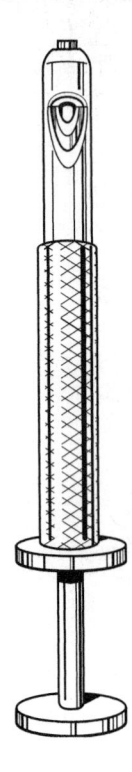

Figure 10-12. The Bowen wire tightener.

is in the fully closed position; this increases gradually with increasing jaw width. The average mechanical advantage for both the large and small bows is 30:1. The last one fourth inch of jaw opening coincides with a sudden increase in mechanical advantage of greater than 400:1, but this last one fourth inch rarely is used.

    c. Comparison of knot strength. The types of knots described here were tied in 20-gauge steel wire and pulled apart in a tension test machine:
        i. Type of knot/maximum force before failure
- **(a)** ASIF loop/15.8 lb
- **(b)** Twist (one turn)/23.2 lb
- **(c)** Twist (three turns)/24.2 lb
- **(d)** Square knot/59.0 lb

        ii. These results are preliminary, but they do afford some conclusions. An ASIF loop is the weakest and is heavily dependent on careful knot formation for its strength. The twist is 47% stronger, but additional turns beyond the first 360-degree turn do not significantly increase the strength of the knot. The reason for using several twists is to provide some residual resistance after untwisting begins, although whether this resistance actually occurs has not been determined. The square knot is the strongest of all. Failure occurs by wire fracture just below the knot.

I. Principles of intramedullary nailing
    1. An intramedullary nail allows for internal splinting with a fixation device in the medullary canal. The **possibility of gliding along the dynamically locked nail promotes compression forces at the fracture site, and the stability from the long working length of the nail provides stiffness.**
    2. This necessary reaming of the canal and resulting disruption of the endosteal blood supply in a severely open fracture that already has disruption of the

periosteal blood supply may increase the chance for a nonunion or infection. In these situations, the use of a smaller **unreamed nail** seems to provide satisfactory results. Because these smaller unreamed nails have less mechanical stability, they generally require interlocking (placing one or two screws across the cortex and nail superiorly and inferiorly) (1). The incidence of implant failure by fatigue fracture is much greater than the larger diameter implants inserted with reaming.

3. In addition to the aforementioned indications, the treatment of complex fractures requires an **interlocking nail** to prevent excessive shortening and rotation. It is recommended to always statically lock the nail to avoid malrotation and shortening, which can occur related to unrecognized minimally displaced cracks.

J. **External skeletal fixation**
   1. The **use of external fixation**, particularly in the treatment of comminuted or open fractures, **has regained popularity**. Lambotte (1902) is generally given credit for the first use of external pin fixation. Anderson (1934), Stader (1937), and Hoffman (1938) all popularized a technique of external skeletal fixation. Vidal and Adrey, using the Hoffman approach, further refined the technique. Most recently, Ilizarov developed and popularized the ring fixator with small wire transfixion for use in limb lengthening, bone transport, and fracture fixation.
   2. Multiple external fixators are currently on the market. Regardless of which technique is used, certain **basic principles** must be followed.
      a. The insertion of the pins and the attachment of the external skeletal fixation is a major procedure performed in the operating room **following all normal operating room procedures**.
      b. The skin and fascia must be incised so that there is **no shear stress on these structures** that could result in necrosis.
      c. The **pins** must be **inserted slowly** with a hand chuck after predrilling with a saline-cooled drill bit to avoid heat necrosis of bone.
      d. There must be a **minimum of two pins above and two pins below the fracture**. Three pins add a small amount of stability in some systems. Maximal fracture stability is achieved by using half pins separately within each bone segment and by placing the connecting bar as close to the skin as possible. Additional stability is attained by stacking a second bar (this must be done by planning ahead because parallel pins are required in some systems) or using a second row of pins and connecting bar.
      e. **Terminally threaded half pins** are used to prevent loosening and sliding of the unit in the bone.
      f. Avoid motion of skin and fascia against the pins.
      g. Use **strict aseptic techniques** when dressing the pin sites.
      h. **Avoid distraction.** Make adjustments to ensure coaptation or impaction of the fracture fragments during the course of healing.
      i. Studies have clearly shown that **external fixation devices can be used to treat fractures to union**. It was previously thought that the devices should be removed as soon as fractures are stabilized and be replaced by casts or cast-braces, if necessary, to allow weight bearing across the fracture to stimulate healing.
      j. External pin fixation is a complex procedure that **requires skill and attention to detail**.
   3. Possible **indications** for external skeletal fixation include the comminuted Colles' fracture and comminuted or open fractures of the tibia, particularly in the proximal and distal ends where intramedullary nailing is not feasible and the risk of infection from the more extensive soft-tissue stripping required for plating is significant. The apparatus should be used with caution for fractures in the humerus, femur, and pelvis because of the higher incidence of pin tract infection and pin loosening. Patient acceptance is also higher with other devices. The thin wire fixator technique developed by

Ilizarov has made application in the metaphyseal region more secure, but because of the use of these "through" pins, the anatomic knowledge required in inserting them is greater. The Ilizarov frames are useful for fracture management, bone transport, and limb lengthening.

K. **Obtaining bone graft material** is a common procedure in orthopaedics. On most occasions, the iliac crest is used for the graft, although various bone grafts are available. After closure of the wound, installation of 0.5% bupivacaine without epinephrine reduces the postoperative pain. The following is the recommended surgical technique:
   1. **For removal of a small amount of bone**, tension the skin over the iliac bone and cut to the ilium without entering muscle or fascial planes. A small periosteal flap is excised with sharp dissection from the superior aspect of the crest. A window then is cut through the cortical bone between the inner and outer tables. The periosteum is not stripped from the bone so pain is less.
   2. **For removal of sizable grafts**, the surgeon must decide whether to use the anterior or posterior part of the iliac crest. Often, the choice is dictated by the position of the patient during operation. Anticipating the possible need for iliac bone grafting for proper positioning, prepping, and draping is required for the smooth flow of the operation. Whenever possible, the patient should be positioned so that the area of the posterior superior iliac spine can be used.
      a. **Removal of bone from the anterior part of the iliac crest.** The skin incision must be long enough to allow a comfortable exposure of the anterior 4 to 5 in. of the iliac crest. Sharp dissection is used to expose the crest. A periosteal elevator is used to expose the inner or outer surface of the ilium. The bone may then be removed by an osteotome or gouge. Care should be taken not to involve both tables of the ilium to minimize hematoma formation and postoperative pain and deformity. One should also be careful to avoid the anterior superior spine for reasons of cosmesis as well as to prevent injury to the lateral femoral cutaneous nerve. Absorbable gelatin sponges (Gelfoam) may be used to help control bleeding. The wound may be closed over suction drainage.
      b. **Removal of bone from the posterior iliac crest.** An oblique incision is made over the iliac crest approximately 1 to 2 in. lateral to the midline. The incision is not extended far enough over the crest to involve the superior cluneal nerves. The periosteum from the outer table is lifted with the periosteal elevator, and the detached muscles are protected with warm, moist lap sponges. Cancellous strips are then removed, and care should be taken not to enter the sacroiliac joint. Excessive bleeding is helped by absorbable gelatin sponges. The wound may be closed over suction drainage.
      c. **Removal of bicortical grafts.** These are wafers of bone taken from the iliac crest with the bone removed as a single block with both cortices. Generally, bicortical grafts are used in vertebral body fusions and in situations in which a structural graft is required. The same surgical techniques described in the preceding sections (**J.2.a** and **b**) are used, except that the incision and the donor site is between the anterior (or posterior) superior iliac spine and the most cephalad portion of the iliac crest. Bicortical graft donor sites are nearly always symptomatic for a significant postoperative period and often are deforming cosmetically.

L. **Basic skin suture techniques**
   1. **General principles**
      a. Do not close the wound **if it may possibly be contaminated** (as in many open fractures). Delayed closure 3 to 5 days later is always preferable in doubtful cases.
      b. If skin edges are battered and ragged, debride them so that healthy tissues are brought together.

    c. Good **closure of subcutaneous tissues** is the key to good skin closure.
    d. **Approximate**, do not strangulate.
    e. **Cutting needles with monofilament suture or thin wire** are used for skin. Skin staples are also used frequently. Cotton and silk sutures are not recommended for skin closure because of the increased inflammatory response to these materials and because of the wick effect that can draw organisms into the wound.
    f. Before making a long incision, **mark it out with a surgical marking pen and make a crosshatch every 2 cm**. Then, when closing, make sure the crosshatches match up. Never make skin marks with a knife or needle because scarring results.
    g. **Steri-Strips** are useful adjuncts for skin closure, but they should never be applied when the skin is under significant tension. They also can impede drainage because they provide a fairly watertight closure.
    h. Consider placing a film of Polysporin ointment or a Betadine nonadherent dressing over the closed incision before applying outer dressings.
    i. Use **pickups,** rather than pincers, **as skin hooks**.
2. **Types of skin suture.** All types of skin closure rely on good subcutaneous suturing to provide strength and to relieve some of the tension from the skin edges.
    a. The needle path with a **box** or simple suture is perpendicular to the dermis. The depth of each half of the suture is equal. When tying the knot, have the edges just touch, as shown in **Fig. 10-13**. Never tie the knot so tightly that the skin bunches up.
    b. Start the **everting** suture as for a large box-type closure, then reverse the direction, thus making a minibox suture of just the dermis. Match the depth in the opposite side, as shown in **Fig. 10-14**. Tie the knot so that the slightest skin pucker results.
    c. An **intradermal** (or subcuticular) suture is entirely in the dermis and does not hold together with appreciable skin tension. Begin the closure several centimeters from the end of the wound and pass the needle from the starting point to the dermis at the apex of the wound. Obtain a secure amount of dermis on one side and then the other. Match the exit point on one side of the dermis with the entrance point on the other side, that is, directly opposite and of equal depth, as shown in **Fig. 10-15**. Occasionally pull the ends of the suture back and forth so that it slides well. End

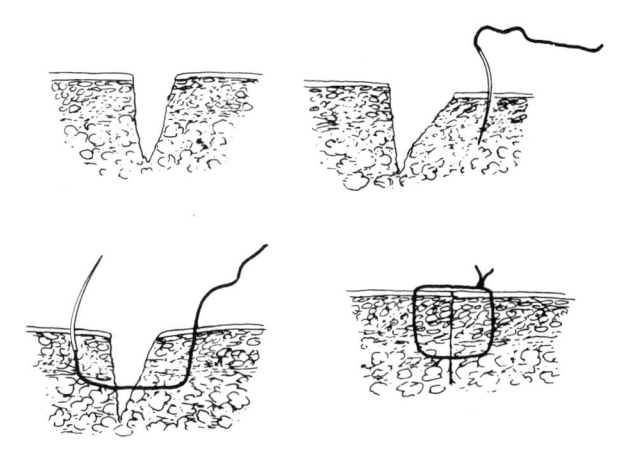

Figure 10-13. Technique for a box suture.

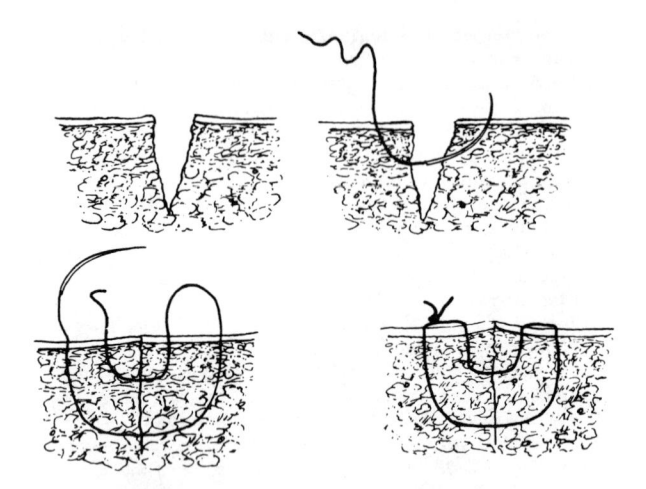

178 Chapter 10: Operating Room Equipment and Techniques

Figure 10-14. Technique for an everting suture.

the suture as it was begun. The ends of the suture may be knotted or taped to the skin to prevent them from pulling out. The suture line is then splinted with Steri-Strips.

  d. The **"near-far/far-near"** suture may be used when the skin must be closed under some tension. Begin with a deep box-type suture that is near the wound edge on one side and far from it on the other. Complete the technique

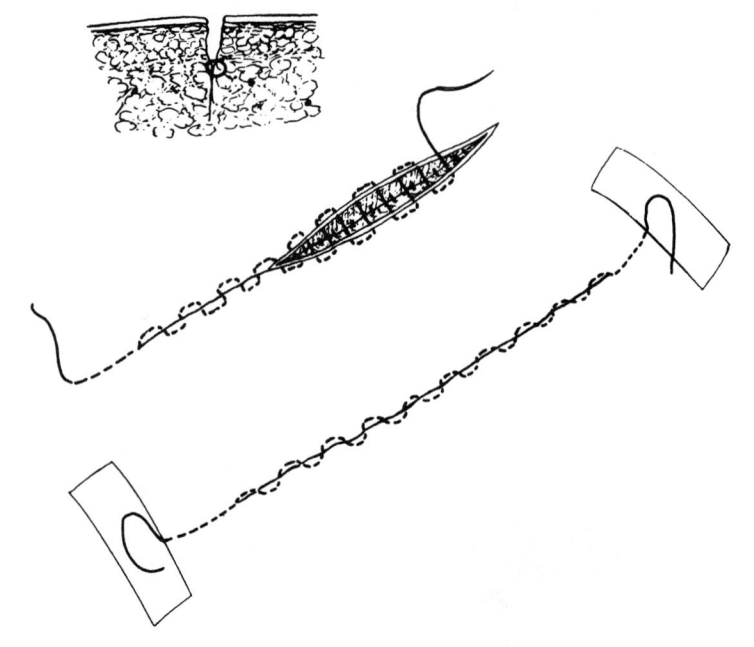

Figure 10-15. Technique for an intradermal (subcuticular) suture.

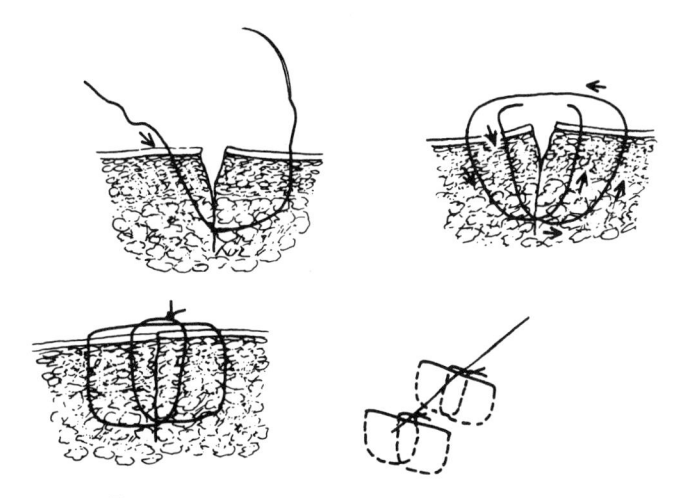

Figure 10-16. Technique for a "near-far/far-near" suture.

with a box-type suture with the near and far sides reversed. Tie the suture so the skin edges are approximated (**Fig. 10-16**).

e. The **Donati skin suture** technique, which was popularized by the AO/ASIF group, is another modified mattress suture technique. It is useful when closing skin under tension. The suture courses deeply across the wound and then goes through the subdermal area without exiting the skin on the second side. Begin with a deep box-type suture on the first side of the wound. Pass back into the original side and exit between the wound and the original entrance site (**Fig. 10-17**).

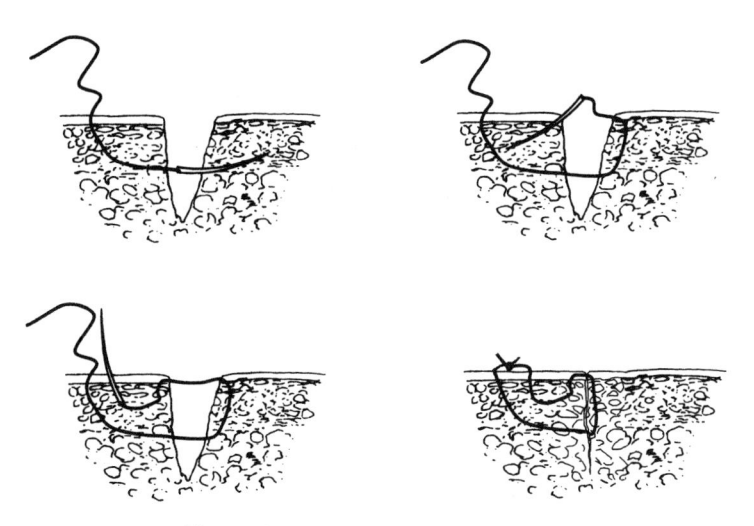

Figure 10-17. Technique for a Donati suture.

References

1. Mueller ME, Allgower M, Schneider R, et al. *Manual of internal fixation*, 3rd ed. New York: Springer-Verlag, 1990.
2. Abramowicz M. *Med Lett Drugs Ther* 1992;34:5.
3. Neu HC. Cephalosporin antibiotics as applied in surgery of bones and joints. *Clin Orthop* 1984;190:50–64.
4. Williams DN, Gustilo RB. The use of preventive antibiotics in orthopaedic surgery. *Clin Orthop* 1984;190:83–88.
5. Castles JJ. Clinical pharmacology of glucocorticoids. In: McCarty DJ, ed. *Arthritis and allied conditions*, 9th ed. Philadelphia, PA: Lea & Febiger, 1979:399.
6. McKenzie PJ, Loach AB. Local anaesthesia for orthopaedic surgery. *Br J Anaesth* 1986;58:779–789.
7. Raj PR, Cacodney A, Cannella J. Useful nerve blocks for pain relief and surgery. In: Browner B, ed. *Skeletal trauma*. Philadelphia, PA: WB Saunders, 1992.
8. Martin JT. Complications associated with patient positioning. *Anesth Analg* 1988;67(Suppl 4S):1.
9. Reid HS, Camp RA, Jacob WH. Tourniquet hemostasis: a clinical study. *Clin Orthop* 1983;177:230–234.
10. Sapega AA, Heppenstall RB, Chance B, et al. Optimizing tourniquet application and release times in extremity surgery: a biochemical and ultrastructural study. *J Bone Joint Surg (Am)* 1985;67:303–314.
11. Shaw JA, Murray DG. The relationship between tourniquet pressure and underlying soft-tissue pressure in the thigh. *J Bone Joint Surg (Am)* 1982;64:1148–1152.
12. Moore MR, Garfin SR, Hargens AR. Wide tourniquets eliminate blood flow at low inflation pressures. *J Hand Surg (Am)* 1987;12:1006–1011.
13. McLaren AC, Rorabeck CH. The pressure distribution under tourniquets. *J Bone Joint Surg (Am)* 1985;67:433–438.
14. Van Roekel HE, Thurston AJ. Tourniquet pressure: the effect of limb circumference and systolic pressure. *J Hand Surg (Br)* 1985;10:142–144.
15. Neimkin RJ, Smith RJ. Double tourniquet with linked mercury manometers for hand surgery. *J Hand Surg (Am)* 1983;8:938–941.
16. Nelson JP, Glassburn AR Jr, Talbott RD, et al. The effect of previous surgery, operating room environment, and preventive antibiotics on postoperative infection following total hip arthroplasty. *Clin Orthop* 1980;147:167–169.
17. Peterson AF, Rosenberg A, Alatary SD. Comparative evaluations of surgical scrub preparations. *Surg Gynecol Obstet* 1978;146:63–65.
18. Scherr DD, Dodd TA, Buckingham WW Jr. Prophylactic use of topical antibiotic irrigation in uninfected surgical wounds. *J Bone Joint Surg (Am)* 1972;54: 634–640.
19. Benjamin JB, Volz RG. Efficacy of a topical antibiotic irrigant in decreasing or eliminating bacterial contamination in surgical wounds. *Clin Orthop* 1984;184: 114–117.
20. Lidwell OM. Clean air at operation and subsequent sepsis in the joint. *Clin Orthop* 1986;211:91–102.
21. Pencer G. What you should know about surgical instruments. *Surg Team* 1974;3:39.
22. Brod JJ. The concepts and terms of mechanics. *Clin Orthop* 1980;146:9–17.

Selected Historical Readings

Anderson R. An ambulatory method of treatment of the tibia and fibula. *Surg Gynecol Obstet* 1934;58:639.

Arnold WD, Hilgartner MW. Hemophiliac arthropathy. *J Bone Joint Surg (Am)* 1977;59:287–305.

Bagby GW. Compression bone-plating. *J Bone Joint Burg (Am)* 1977;59:625–631.

Bechtol CO, Ferguson AB, Laign PG. *Metals and engineering in bone and joint surgery*. Baltimore, MD: Williams & Wilkins, 1959.

Bowers WH, Wilson FC, Green WB. Antibiotic prophylaxis in experimental bone infections. *J Bone Joint Surg (Am)* 1973;55:795–807.

Boyd KS, Burke JF, Colton T. A double-blind clinical trial of prophylactic antibiotics in hip fractures. *J Bone Joint Surg (Am)* 1973;55:1251–1258.

Burke JF. Sources of wound contamination. *Ann Surg* 1963;158:898.

Cooney WP, Linscheid RL, Dobyns JH. External pin fixation for unstable colles' fractures. *J Bone Joint Surg (Am)* 1979;61:840–845.

Dineen P. Clinical research in skin disinfection. *AORN J* 1971;14:73–78.

Dineen P. Microbial filtration by surgical masks. *Surg Gynecol Obstet* 1971;133:812–814.

Ha'eri GB, Wiley AM. The efficacy of standard surgical face masks: an investigation using tracer particles. *Clin Orthop* 1980;148:160–162.

Ha'eri GB, Wiley AM. Wound contamination through drapes and gowns: a study using tracer particles. *Clin Orthop* 1981;154:181–184.

Hamilton HW, Booth AD, Lone FJ, et al. Penetration of gown material by organisms from the surgical team. *Clin Orthop* 1979;141:237–246.

Hargens AR, McClure AG, Skyhar MJ, et al. Local compression patterns beneath pneumatic tourniquets applied to arms and thighs of human cadaver. *J Orthop Res* 1987;2:247–252.

Heppenstall RB, Scott R, Sapega A, et al. A comparative study of the tolerance of skeletal muscle in ischemia: tourniquet application compared with acute compartment syndrome. *J Bone Joint Surg (Am)* 1986;68:820–828.

Hoffmann R. Rotules á os pour la reduction dirigé, non sanglante, des fractures (ostéotaxis). *Helv Med Acta* 1938;5:844–856.

Jacobs JR, et al. Evaluation of draping techniques in prevention of surgical wound contamination. *JAMA* 1963;184:293.

Jardon OMl. Malignant hyperthermia. *J Bone Joint Surg (Am)* 1979;61:1064–1070.

Katz JF, Siffert RS. Tissue antibiotic levels with tourniquet use in orthopedic surgery. *Clin Orthop* 1982;165:261–264.

Matthews LS, Hirsch C. Temperatures measured in human cortical bone drilling. *J Bone Joint Surg (Am)* 1972;54:297–308.

Post M, Telfer MC. Surgery in hemophilia patients. *J Bone Joint Surg (Am)* 1975;57:1136–1145.

Whiteside LA, Lesker PA. The effects of extraperiosteal and subperiosteal dissection. *J Bone Joint Surg (Am)* 1978;60:26–30.

ACUTE SPINAL INJURY   11

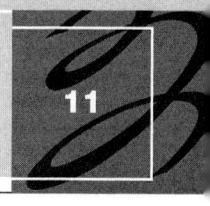

I. **INTRODUCTION**
   A. **Initial evaluation and management.** Optimal outcome following acute spinal injury depends upon early recognition of the injury and appropriate management to prevent further injury. Adherence to the principles of advanced trauma life support (ATLS) is mandatory. All patients with a mechanism of injury compatible with spinal injury should be assumed to have a spinal injury until proven otherwise.
   B. **Clearance of spine in trauma patients.** While protection of the spine is mandatory at all stages of managing the traumatized patient, "clearance" of the spine should take place only after potentially life-threatening injuries have been stabilized.
      1. In the cognitively intact patient (including the absence of drugs or alcohol) and cooperative patient, clinical clearance of the spine may be possible. While case reports have documented bony and ligamentous spinal injuries in such patients, unstable spinal injuries or neurologic deterioration in these patients have not been reported. Accordingly, routine radiographic evaluation in such cases is not indicated. However, the physical examination findings of neck or back pain, neurologic abnormalities, bruising, spinal deformity, pain with active range of motion, or significant "distracting" nonspinal injury should prompt further investigation.
      2. Obtunded or uncooperative patients, as well as alert patients with physical examination findings consistent with spinal injury, should be maintained on spinal precautions until thorough clinical and radiographic evaluation of the spine has been completed.
   C. **Studies**
      1. **Roentgenograms.** The standard radiographic evaluation of the cervical spine includes the lateral, open-mouth (odontoid), and anteroposterior plain films. The lateral view will detect up to 85% of significant cervical spine injuries provided that the occiput-C1 and C7–T1 junctions are visualized. Despite normal x-rays of the upper cervical spine and the absence of clinical findings suggestive of a lower-cervical injury, one study has detected a 3.1% incidence of occult fractures at the C7–T1 level on computed tomographic (CT) scanning (1). CT scanning of the upper cervical spine has become the method of initial evaluation in many trauma centers. While the addition of orthogonal oblique views does not increase the sensitivity of plain film evaluation, these views provide excellent visualization of the cervical posterior elements and foramina. Anteroposterior and lateral images of the thoracic and lumbar segments are indicated in the presence of pain or abnormal physical examination findings in these regions and in cognitively impaired patients who cannot cooperate with the physical examination. Additionally, because up to 6% of spinal injuries have a noncontiguous injury elsewhere in the spine, the presence of an injury anywhere in the spine should prompt radiographic evaluation of the entire spine.
      2. Important points to consider in interpreting plain radiographs include (**Fig. 11-1**):
         a. Any alteration in the **alignment** of the bodies. Straightening of the cervical spine can result from muscle spasms or from positioning the patient's head in slight flexion.

183

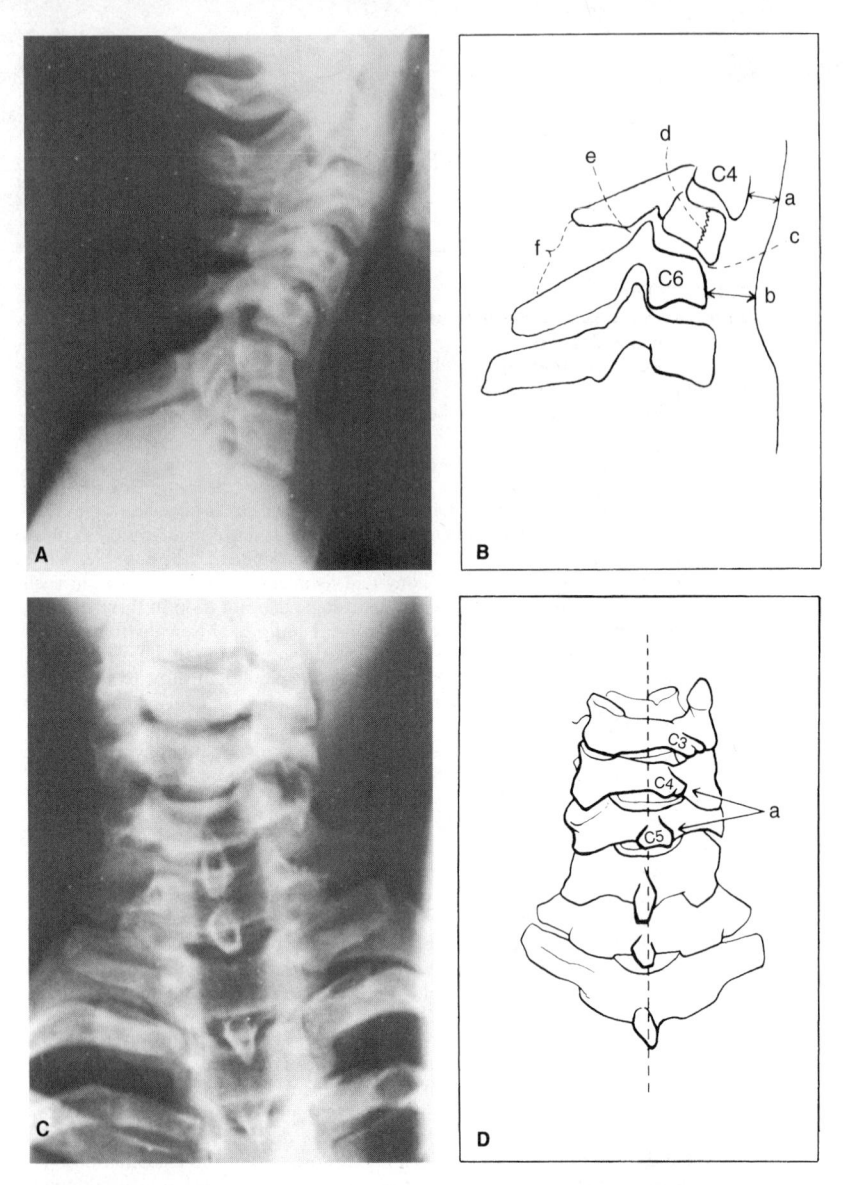

Figure 11-1. Important roentgenographic signs of a cervical spine injury. **A** and **B:** (a) Normal width of the retropharyngeal space at C4 is 4 to 6 mm. (b) Normal width of the retropharyngeal space at C6 is 8 to 10 mm. (c) An alteration in the alignment of the bodies. (d) Look for fracture lines in the bodies or in the posterior elements. (e) A step-off in the line of the posterior intervertebral facet joint. (f) An increased distance between two spinous processes. **C** and **D:** The C4 spinous process is displaced laterally in relation to C5, demonstrating facet disruption.

b. Any **step-off** in the line of the posterior intervertebral **facet joints**.
c. Any increase in the **width of the retropharyngeal space** in front of the vertebral bodies (normal is 4–6 mm at C3 and 15–20 mm at C6). This rule does not apply in a crying child.
d. Any **fracture lines** in the bodies or in the posterior elements.
e. Any **increase of distance between two spinous processes**.
f. Any **displacement of the spinous process** on the cephalad side, which is toward the side of any unilateral dislocation on the anteroposterior film.
g. Any **indication that the body of one vertebra has moved forward in relation to another on the lateral roentgenogram because such movement usually indicates a dislocation or fracture-dislocation of one or both joint facets at that level.** If the amount of displacement is more than half the width of the vertebral body, the dislocation is bilateral and the spine is extremely unstable.

3. **CT scanning** can provide rapid and detailed assessment of the spine. This should include high-resolution imaging (2- to 3-mm collimation and 1.5-mm pitch) from the occiput to T1 with sagittal and coronal reconstructions. Several studies have demonstrated high levels of sensitivity (90%) and specificity (100%) of screening CT scanning in polytrauma patients (2–4). While CT appears to be a cost-effective primary screening tool in patients at high or moderate risk for cervical injuries (5), CT scanning represents the standard of care in all patients when:
   a. poorly visualized areas are encountered on plain films
   b. visualization of T1 is not improved with gentle downward traction on the arms, swimmer's views, or oblique views
   c. fractures or dislocations are identified elsewhere in the spine
   d. in patients who are intubated, as plain films will miss up to 17% of injuries to the upper cervical spine in the presence of an endotracheal tube

4. Magnetic resonance imaging (MRI) is less sensitive, less specific, and less cost effective than the plain film series or screening CT for the identification and evaluation of cervical fractures (6). However, MRI is extremely sensitive and specific for evaluation of the paravertebral soft tissues, including the spinal cord, intervertebral discs, and ligamentous structures. Patients with abnormal neurologic findings, particularly incomplete injuries, should undergo MRI scanning of the relevant spinal segment(s) to visualize the spinal cord and nerve roots.

5. **Dynamic fluoroscopy.** Passive flexion and extension stressing of the cervical spine, performed by an experienced physician under fluoroscopy, has a reported sensitivity of 92.3% and specificity of 98.8% for detecting significant ligamentous injuries and instability of the cervical spine (7). While some centers support the use of this technique in clearing the spine of unconscious patients, the risk of neurologic deterioration may outweigh its benefits, especially given the widespread availability of CT and MRI imaging (7).

II. **SPINAL CORD INJURY.** Spinal cord injuries may be **classified** as complete or incomplete neurologic injuries; patients with **complete spinal cord injuries** have no motor or sensory function distal to the level of cord injury and patients with **incomplete spinal cord injuries** have some function, whether motor or sensory, distal to the lesion.

A. The **ASIA (American Spinal Injury Association) classification** is a modification of the Frankel scale and is the most commonly used classification of spinal cord injuries. The ASIA classification grades spinal cord injuries from A through E, where **ASIA A** represents complete loss of motor and sensory function below the level of the lesion and **ASIA E** represents normal sensory and motor function. Incomplete spinal cord injuries are classified as **ASIA B** (preserved sensation but no motor function below the level of the injury), **ASIA C** (motor function less than or equal to grade 3 distal to the level of the injury), or **ASIA D** (motor function greater than grade 3 but less than normal distal to the level of the injury).

B. **Partial cord syndromes.** Incomplete spinal cord injury may involve discrete anatomical zones of the spinal cord, resulting in characteristic patterns of neurologic deficits.
   1. The **anterior cord syndrome** involves loss of neural function in the anterior two thirds of the spinal cord. Patients with these injuries experience complete loss of motor function and of pain and temperature sensation but retain sensations of vibration, proprioception, and light touch. These preserved functions result in an improved prognosis.
   2. The **posterior cord syndrome** is characterized by loss of proprioception and vibrational sensation. Motor function and gross touch sensation typically are spared due to the ventral location of the descending motor tracts and spinothalamic tracts, respectively. The prognosis in posterior cord syndrome is fair.
   3. The **central cord syndrome** is typically associated with a cervical hyperextension injury, often in older patients. This syndrome consists of a disproportionately greater weakness in the upper extremities compared with lower extremities, various sensory changes at or below the site of the lesion, and urinary bladder dysfunction. Proposed causes include hematomyelia, contusion, cord swelling, and ischemia of the cervical spinal cord. The anterior horn cells at the level of injury may also be involved. The prognosis depends on the amount of initial neurologic involvement and the rapidity of subsequent recovery. The signs of neurologic damage tend to disappear in reverse order of their appearance.
   4. A penetrating injury or unilateral facet dislocation can result in unilateral injury to the spinal cord: the **Brown-Séquard syndrome**. Patients experience loss of ipsilateral motor and dorsal column function and contralateral pain and temperature sensation.
C. **Pharmacologic management of spinal cord injuries.** Pharmacologic agents thought to mitigate the secondary effects of spinal cord injury have been extensively studied and widely debated in recent years. These agents include opiate antagonists, calcium channel blockers, free radical scavengers, neurotropic compounds, and, most notably, steroids (8) and gangliosides (9).
   1. **Methylprednisolone.** The National Acute Spinal Cord Injury Studies (NASCIS I, II, and III) have studied the use of parenteral methylprednisolone following spinal injury. NASCIS I detected no benefit in the treatment group, but the steroid dose used was found to be below the therapeutic threshold in subsequent animal experimentation (10). In NASCIS II, patients were randomly assigned to receive a higher loading dose of methylprednisolone, naloxone (an opiate antagonist), or placebo within 12 hours of acute spinal cord injury (11). While investigators found no overall benefit in the methylprednisolone group, post hoc analysis of the data suggested small gains in total sensory and motor scores in a subgroup of patients who had received drugs within 8 hours of the injury. Naxolone was less effective than methylprednisolone. Despite the weakness of the data, high-dose methylprednisolone infusion over 24 hours became the standard of care in patients treated within 8 hours of acute spinal cord injury. NASCIS III compared 48-hour infusion with 24-hour infusion and found no benefit to extending the treatment beyond 24 hours (12). Again, in post hoc analysis of the data, there appeared to be a benefit from extending the infusion to 48 hours when treatment began between 3 and 8 hours after the injury. While no other study has verified the results of the NASCIS conclusions, most centers have adopted the following protocol:
      a. An initial loading dose of **30 mg/kg of methylprednisolone intravenous (IV)**, given over one hour, followed by:
         i. a **23-hour infusion** of **5.4 mg/kg** of the same drug if administered **within 3 hours of injury** or
         ii. a **47-hour infusion** of **5.4 mg/kg** of the same drug if administered **within 3 to 8 hours after injury**
      b. Newer pharmacologic regimens are being studied to clarify their role in improving outcomes (9,12).

III. FRACTURES, DISLOCATIONS, AND FRACTURE-DISLOCATIONS IN ADULTS
A. Fracture of the C1 vertebra (Jefferson fracture)
1. **Mechanism of injury.** The superior articular processes of the atlas face upward, inward, and slightly backward. A vertical compression force can thrust the articular facets of the occipital condyles of the skull downward, push the lateral masses outward, and disrupt the ring of the atlas producing a C1 ring fracture, as shown in **Fig. 11-2** (13). Less commonly, this same mechanism can produce an occipital condylar fracture, which can be isolated or associated with a basilar skull fracture (14).
2. **Anatomic considerations.** The anteroposterior diameter of the ring of the atlas is approximately 3 cm. The spinal cord and the odontoid process each are approximately 1 cm in diameter, approximately one third the diameter of the ring. According to **Steel rule of thirds**, the remaining centimeter of free space allows for some degree of pathologic displacement. Therefore, anterior displacement of the atlas exceeding 1 cm (the thickness of the odontoid process) threatens the adjacent segment of cord. This usually occurs with disruption of the transverse ligament of C1. This ligament maintains the proper relationship of the dens to C1 and is often ruptured as a pure ligamentous disruption from a flexion injury. Because the cardiac and respiratory centers lie at this level, displacement of the atlas threatens the life of the patient. If the ring of the atlas is capacious (greater than 3 cm in diameter either as an anatomic feature or as a result of a C1 ring fracture), there is less danger, whereas if it is narrow and unfractured, there is more (13).
3. **History.** If consciousness is not lost as a result of a concurrent head injury, the history should suggest a mechanism for a vertical compression injury. The injury often results from a diving accident or any mechanism that applies axial force to the head.
4. **Examination.** Clinical symptoms and signs vary from minimal complaints to severe pain and gross limitation of movement. Extension usually produces some pain, but rotation may be relatively pain free. Because the suboccipital nerve crosses the ring posterior to each lateral mass and the greater occipital nerve emerges just below the posterior ring of the atlas to supply the skin over the occiput, testing of sensation can show involvement of the suboccipital or, more commonly, the greater occipital nerve. Damage to the spinal cord is uncommon because a significant cord injury at this level causes immediate death.
5. **Roentgenograms.** Anteroposterior films, including an open-mouth view and a lateral view, are routine and CT scanning may be indicated. The common fracture sites are the anterior arch, either midline or just lateral to the midline, and the posterior arch at its narrowest portion just posterior to each lateral mass. Displacement of the fracture can be minimal. In an open-mouth roentgenogram of the odontoid process, when a comminuted fracture of C1

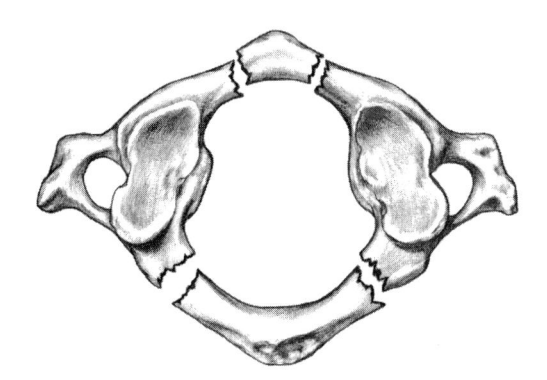

Figure 11-2. Jefferson fracture.

X + Y ≥7 mm

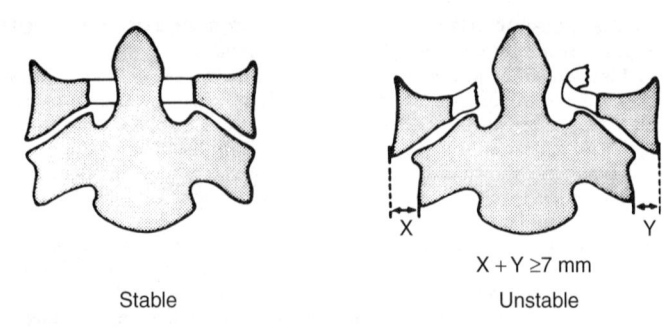

Stable　　　Unstable

Figure 11-3. Jefferson fractures. When a comminuted fracture of C1 shows bilateral overhang of the lateral masses that total 7 mm or more, rupture of the transverse ligament has probably occurred, rendering the spine unstable. (From White AA III, Panjabi MM. *Clinical biomechanics of the spine.* Philadelphia, PA: JB Lippincott, 1978:203, with permission.)

shows bilateral overhang of the lateral masses totaling 7 mm or more, a rupture of the transverse ligament may have occurred, rendering the spine unstable (**Fig. 11-3**).

6. **Treatment.** Treat by immobilization in a cervicothoracic orthosis or halo vest until healing occurs, usually in 2 to 3 months. Initially, use 5 to 8 lb of tong traction in bed while the extent of the injury is assessed. Reduction of the fracture is best accomplished by adjusting the relative position of the head to the thorax. Head extension is required when the transverse ligament is ruptured (14,15).

B. **Fracture of the odontoid process** (15,16)
 1. **Mechanism of injury.** The C1 vertebra and the odontoid process of C2 are a single functional unit. The apical/alar and transverse ligaments on the posterior aspect of the odontoid process can remain intact following an injury, producing a fracture of the base of the process. The skull, the C1 vertebra, and the odontoid process of the C2 vertebra then move relatively independently of the body of the C2 vertebra.
 2. **History.** Symptoms can be minimal, but severe pain behind the ears and stiffness following a flexion or extension injury are frequent. The patients often report a feeling of instability at the base of the skull and present themselves by holding their head with both hands. There is seldom any suggestion of weakness or numbness of the limbs following an acute injury.
 3. **Examination.** Tenderness in the suboccipital region may be present. The neurologic examination is generally normal.
 4. **Roentgenograms.** A lateral roentgenogram demonstrates that the C1 vertebra has moved in relation to C2, and it is also usually seen that the anterior arch of the C1 vertebra and the odontoid process are in their normal relationship; that is, the odontoid process has been carried with the arch of the C1 vertebra (16). Translation of C1 or C2 of 3.0 to 4.5 mm, with neurologic symptoms or signs, can indicate clinical instability. Normally, the position of the posterior part of the C1 ring is equidistant between the base of the skull and the spinous process of C2. An open-mouth anteroposterior roentgenogram usually shows a fracture line at the base of the odontoid process, and this fracture line may run inferiorly, possibly involving the upper part of the vertebral body. The fracture must be differentiated from congenital etiologies such as a secondary ossification center with an open apophyseal plate, which may be seen in younger patients, or from a failure of segments of the odontoid process to fuse to the body of C2, which may be seen in older patients. With a congenital etiology, the radiolucency usually is situated more cephalad and is less irregular than that seen with an acute fracture. In addition, an increased incidence of

anomalies of the anterior arch of C1 and of the atlanto-occipital articulation is seen with congenital abnormalities of the odontoid process (15–17). CT scans are usually helpful.

5. **Treatment** (15,16)
   a. **Type I** is a fracture through the upper portion of the odontoid process. Treatment with a cervical orthosis is satisfactory. Nonunion usually presents few problems because the fracture is too far above the level of the transverse ligament to cause instability. These fractures are rare.
   b. **Type II** is a fracture at the junction of the dens with the vertebral body of C2. Reduction of an anteriorly displaced C1 with a fractured odontoid process can often be achieved by allowing the head to sink into extension with the patient in a supine position in traction. This reduction is more easily done by sedating the patient adequately and inserting a pillow behind the shoulder to allow extension of the head and neck. Light traction in Gardner-Wells tongs should be applied. Lateral roentgenograms should be obtained at frequent intervals until the reduction has been confirmed. Then the head and neck should be immobilized with the fracture reduced and held in a halo vest without distraction of the fracture. Apply the orthosis as soon as is feasible so the patient can sit up and become ambulatory. Immobilization of the fracture should be continued until the fracture is healed, usually 3 to 4 months; then progressive mobilization of the neck should be initiated. A soft collar is used until muscle strength has returned. This fracture is associated with a 15% to 85% incidence of nonunion (15–17).
   c. **Type III** is really a fracture through the body of the atlas at the base of the dens. Treat with very light traction for 2 to 3 days to provide reduction of the fracture. Follow this with a halo vest that controls the spine effectively for an additional 12 to 14 weeks.
   d. Increasingly displaced type II fractures are treated with anterior screw fixation (1). Although technically demanding, the results are predictable in terms of fracture union, with rates in the range of 90%. Alternatively, posterior fusion of C1–C2 with iliac grafting and wiring or screw-based instrumentation may be considered. *In situ* fusion is appropriate if the patient is neurologically intact. Rarely, a fusion of occiput to C2 is indicated if the fracture is associated with a C1 ring fracture (unless screw-based instrumentation is utilized).

6. **Complications.** As revealed by roentgenography, union of the fracture may not be achieved in all cases. In a review of 60 odontoid fractures, it was found that fractures at the junction of the odontoid process with the body of C2 had a nonunion rate of 36%, which is the usual rate given to type II fractures (see Anderson and D'Alonzo in Selected Historical Readings). With type III fractures, only 10% went on to nonunion. It was theorized that the vertebral body consisted of more cancellous bone, which is associated with a higher union rate. The use of traction beyond the first few days is contraindicated because it may produce distraction and it does not immobilize the fracture. This common practice may account for the high incidence of nonunion. At 4 months after injury, flexion and extension films should be obtained. If there is instability, a posterior C1-C2 fusion should be recommended, although 10% to 15% of neck rotation will be lost (15–17).

C. **Fracture of C2 vertebra (hangman fracture)**
   1. **Mechanism of injury.** Although the hangman causes this injury by distraction and extension, the other mechanisms of injury that produce the same fracture seem to be confusing and indefinite. Patients have remembered "hanging" their chins on the steering wheel or dashboard or striking their foreheads on the sun visor of cars involved in accidents. The classic injury is a bilateral fracture passing through the posterior part of the lateral masses or pars interarticularis of the axis and into the intervertebral notch (13). The body of the

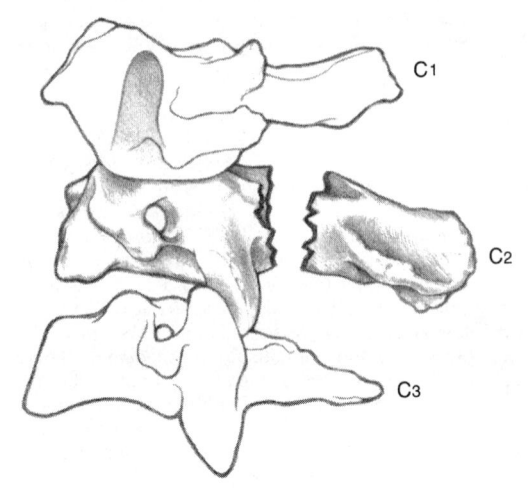

Figure 11-4. Classic hangman fracture.

axis is then subluxated or dislocated in relation to the body of C3. The skull and C1 move as a unit with the body of C2, while the posterior elements of C2 remain as a unit with the posterior elements of C3, as shown in **Fig. 11-4**.
2. **Examination.** Involvement of the spinal cord in patients who survive the initial trauma is relatively uncommon, so the patient may complain of little more than local pain and stiffness. There is, however, tenderness over the spinous process of C2.
3. **Roentgenograms.** Anteroposterior and lateral roentgenograms and tomograms or CT scans are essential. The retropharyngeal space may be widened on the lateral view (normal is 4–6 mm at C3). The injury is occasionally accompanied by other injuries in the lower part of the cervical spine, and these must be carefully excluded.
4. **Treatment.** The fracture tends to be reduced with the neck in a neutral position, but the most appropriate position should be adopted. Halo vest immobilization should follow a brief 1- to 2-day period of tong traction and must often continue for 3 months. Traction can produce distraction and subsequent nonunion or ligamentous instability. If minimally displaced, a cervical brace (such as a Philadelphia collar) may be used. The fracture usually heals and primary operative treatment is unwarranted.
5. **Complications.** Patients rarely require intubation or tracheotomy because of initial severe retropharyngeal swelling.

D. **Fractures and dislocations of the lower cervical spine** (18,19). In this region of the spine, dislocations without fractures are common, but fractures and fracture-dislocations do occur. The spinal cord and nerve roots frequently are involved; in addition to displaced bony elements, the intervertebral disc can become displaced and function as the leading "impact force" against the spinal cord (19,20). Injury to the vertebral arteries is not uncommon, particularly with injuries that produce quadriparesis (21).
   1. **Mechanisms of injury**
      a. Although the effects of a **vertical compression** or bursting injury are seen in C1, vertical compression can also produce injuries lower in the cervical spine. C5 is most commonly involved with this mechanism.
      b. An **extension injury** produces tearing of the anterior longitudinal ligament with or without an avulsion fracture of the anterior aspect of one of the vertebral bodies. Fractures of the pedicles or facets and posterior

subluxation can occur. This injury commonly is associated with a rear-end automobile accident. Subsequent symptoms may last for a prolonged period of time without objective documentation of any osseous or soft-tissue abnormalities (see Spence et al. in Selected Historical Readings).
   c. **Flexion injuries**
      i. A **unilateral dislocation** or **fracture-dislocation** occurs with a dislocation of the facets on one side, with the facets on the other side remaining intact and in normal relationship to one another (18). This phenomenon generally occurs in the lower cervical spine, C5–C7.
      ii. **Bilateral dislocations** or **fracture-dislocations** involve the facet joint on both sides. This diagnosis is easier to make on the lateral cervical roentgenogram because it is associated with more marked posterior displacement of the upper segment relative to the lower segment. Because displacement of disc material is common (20), neurologically intact patients and patients with incomplete spinal cord injuries should undergo emergent MRI imaging to rule out displacement of disc material ventral to the spinal cord.
2. **Examination.** Carefully search for bruising, lacerations, or abrasions in the region of the face, forehead, and occiput (22). Presence and distribution of such lesions often gives an indication of the mechanism of injury. Assume that any patient with facial or forehead lacerations who has been involved in a high-speed impact has a cervical spine fracture until proven otherwise. Local examination of the neck reveals tenderness over one or more spinous processes, and there is limitation of movement and muscle spasm. The examination must include a careful neurologic assessment. It is not enough to decide whether there is evidence of cord damage. The level of a neurologic lesion must be accurately defined by both motor and sensory examinations as well as pathologic reflexes and must be recorded with the time and date, preferably in a flow-sheet format. Patients must be reexamined frequently in the first 24 hours after injury, especially those with incomplete spinal cord injury (19,22,23).
3. **Initial treatment.** Whether or not neurologic damage is present, reduction of any displacement should be undertaken. To reduce and treat the fracture properly, however, the fracture pattern must be understood. This usually is best assessed by attempting to understand the mechanism of injury as well as through high-quality roentgenograms. The suggested method for reduction of dislocations or fracture–dislocations, whether unilateral or bilateral, is with skull tongs inserted as described in **Chap. 9, V.B**. It is prudent to be sure that disc material has not been displaced into the spinal canal with a prereduction MRI, especially with bilateral facet dislocations in a neurologically intact individual. While awake closed reduction despite disc herniation has been successful in certain cases (24); some patients may require anterior decompression surgery prior to reduction.
4. The patient is placed in skull tong traction, usually with 15 lb of weight. **Use traction in the direction of the deformity**, not in line with the patient's body. The weight may be gradually increased by 5 lb every hour. Obtain lateral roentgenograms every 30 to 60 minutes. Record a neurologic examination at 30-minute intervals. With a unilateral facet dislocation, after 60 lb (or one third of body weight) of traction force has been applied, then consider bending the head away while rotating the upper neck toward the side of the dislocation. Reduction should be achieved rapidly by this method; then the weight may be decreased to 5 lb. If reduction is not achieved rapidly or if the dislocation is old, then consultation with an experienced spinal surgeon is important because it may be necessary to proceed with an operation to achieve reduction. Reduction of the fracture or fracture-dislocation is the best and safest method of achieving decompression of the spinal cord or roots (19). Laminectomy is contraindicated because it may produce increased instability while adding surgical trauma.

5. **Management after reduction** is through immobilization by light tong traction for several days with the neck in the optimum position as demonstrated by lateral roentgenograms. In the absence of significant neurologic deficit, the patient may then be placed in a halo vest. If extensive neurologic deficit is present, then immobilization in bed may be necessary. To avoid the complications of bed rest (e.g., pneumonia, urinary stasis, and bed sores), operative stabilization is frequently indicated. Deep venous thrombosis prophylaxis must be used because of the very high rates of this complication in spinal cord–injured patients (25). In unstable injuries, it is wise to use a halo apparatus. Other types of cervical orthoses occasionally are used but are not as effective as the halo apparatus and are reserved for stable injuries. For unstable injuries, surgical stabilization and early mobilization of the patient is almost always indicated (19).
    a. Posterior cervical fusion is recommended for most patients with **bilateral facet dislocations**. If reduction has been achieved by tong traction, then surgery is usually delayed 5 to 7 days to avoid the neurologic deterioration that can occasionally occur in quadriplegic patients. As noted earlier, before reduction and before surgery, the location of the intervertebral disc must be determined by CT scanning, myelography, or MRI. If the disc is retropulsed into the canal, then anterior decompression may be required prior to posterior surgery.
    b. The treatment of a **unilateral facet dislocation** is controversial (17). Many consultants recommend treatment in a halo vest following reduction in tong traction. Other authors recommend posterior cervical fusion for this condition because anatomic alignment can then be maintained.
E. The **hyperextension whiplash injury**
    1. The **mechanism of injury** is similar to that for the cervical spine extension injuries described in **D.1.b.**
    2. Likewise, the **history** is similar; for example, the patient was an occupant in a car that was suddenly struck in the rear by another automobile.
    3. The **examination** shows tenderness along the scalene muscles and within the body of the trapezius muscle.
    4. In a pure soft-tissue injury without tearing of the anterior longitudinal ligament, the **roentgenograms are normal.**
    5. **Recommended treatment** for the first 10 to 14 days includes a properly sized soft collar to immobilize the neck, sufficient analgesics for pain relief, and rest. Soft collars are preferable to rigid collars for comfort. Collars should be high posteriorly and low under the chin to keep the cervical spine in a neutral or slightly flexed position. Avoid hyperextension in whiplash injuries and cervical radiculopathy. Cold packs may be used for the first 24 hours, followed by warm packs. A folded towel can be used as a neck collar. Ice may be placed within the towel initially; then a damp warm towel may be used. Corticosteroid injection of the facet joints has not been proven to be effective in a randomized controlled trial (26).
    6. The long-term **prognosis** for these injuries was reported as follows: 43% of the patients had residual symptoms 5 years after injury (see Hohl in Selected Historical Readings). There were degenerative changes in 39% of the patients. A poorer prognosis was predicted if shortly after injury the following findings were present:
        a. **Pain or numbness in an upper extremity**
        b. Sharp **reversal of the cervical lordosis** as seen on the roentgenograms. This is not a completely reliable sign.
        c. **Restricted motion** at one interspace as seen in flexion-extension roentgenograms; these should not be obtained until 3 weeks after injury to improve their sensitivity in detecting instability.
        d. **Need for a cervical collar for more than 12 weeks or for home traction.**
        e. **Need to resume physical therapy** more than once because of recurrence of symptoms.

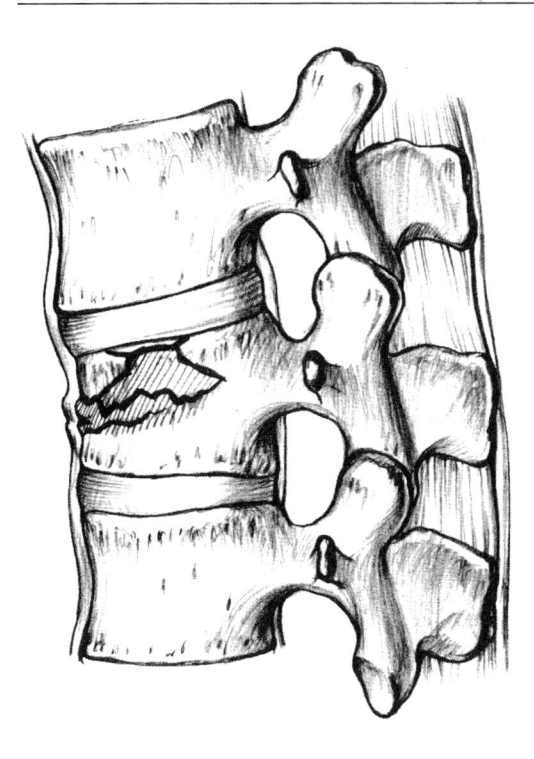

Figure 11-5. Compression fracture of the thoracolumbar spine. (From Hansen ST, Swiontkowski MF. *Orthopaedic trauma protocols.* New York: Raven, 1993:216, with permission.)

F. **Fractures and fracture-dislocations of the thoracic, thoracolumbar, and lumbar spine.** Denis improved upon Holdsworth concepts to develop the three-column theory for thoracolumbar fractures (27). McAfee has shown the utility of using CT to classify fractures to aid in treatment decisions (28).
   1. **Types of injury** (28)
      a. **Compression fracture (Fig. 11-5).** A wedge compression fracture of the vertebral body is produced by a flexion force, but the posterior ligament complex (i.e., supraspinous ligaments, interspinous ligaments, ligamenta flava, and capsules of the intervertebral joint) remains intact. There is no fracture of the posterior elements. Kyphotic angulation (as measured by the angle between lines drawn from the end plates of the injured vertebrae to those of the adjacent uninjured vertebra) is usually less than 10 degrees, and loss of anterior vertebral height is no greater than 40%. Therefore, this injury is classified as relatively stable but requires close observation for progressive kyphotic deformity.
      b. **Stable burst fracture (Fig. 11-6).** Burst fractures of the thoracolumbar spine are generally stable. By reviewing the plain roentgenograms and CT scan, the anterior and middle columns are parted with bone retropulsed into the spinal cord, but the posterior column is uninjured (the facet joints and ligaments are intact). Kyphosis is limited to 15 degrees and loss of vertebral height is less than 50%. These patients are neurologically intact.
      c. **Unstable burst fracture (Fig. 11-7).** In these injuries, the posterior column is disrupted as well. The hallmark is pedicle widening on the anteroposterior roentgenogram. The amount of neurologic injury varies based more on the level of the injury than the degree of canal compromise by bone fragments. One must remember that the spinal cord ends at L2, and

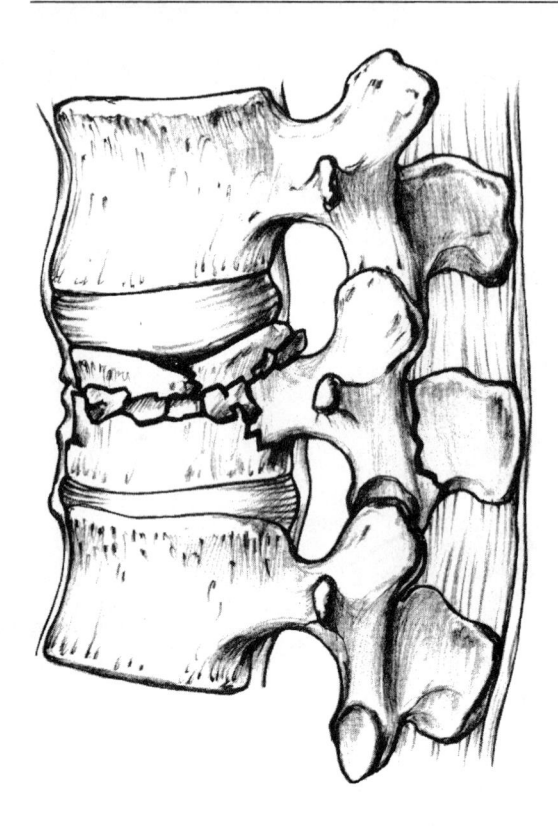

Figure 11-6. Stable burst fracture. (From Hansen ST, Swiontkowski MF. *Orthopaedic trauma protocols.* New York: Raven, 1993: 217, with permission.)

fractures above this level have greater neurologic involvement. Stenosis of 80% is tolerated well below this level, whereas stenosis of 30% in the thoracic spine may be associated with paraplegia.

  d. **Flexion-distraction injury (Fig. 11-8).** These injuries result from failure of the posterior elements in tension while the anterior and middle columns are compressed. The most common mechanism is a lap belt in a motor vehicle accident. On the lateral roentgenogram, widening of the spinous processes is seen. The vertebral body is wedged anteriorly and occasionally a small fragment of bone is retropulsed into the canal. The neurologic injury is variable.

  e. **Chance fracture (Fig. 11-9).** Generally, these fractures result from tension failure of all spinal bony elements as a result of hyperflexion over a secured lap belt. These injuries, which commonly occur in back seat passengers, are seen frequently in children. Bowel injuries occur in up to 65% of these patients because the lap belt provides the fulcrum against the abdominal wall (29). The injury can be ligamentous, bony, or both, but there is no compromise of the anterior elements if the injury is primarily ligamentous. Most often surgery is indicated.

  f. **Translational injuries (Fig. 11-10)** are caused by shear forces that fracture or dislocate the facets. Paraplegia is generally the result. Anteroposterior translation of the vertebral bodies is present on the roentgenograms. Surgical stabilization is generally advisable.

2. **Diagnosis.** The diagnosis is suspected from the mechanism of injury or, in the elderly patient, following a sudden jolt or fall. Tenderness to palpation or

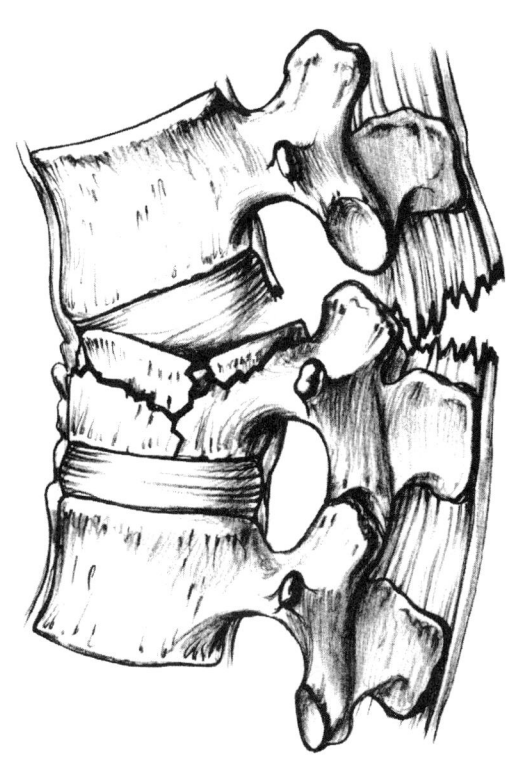

Figure 11-7. Unstable burst fracture. (From Hansen ST, Swiontkowski MF. *Orthopaedic trauma protocols.* New York: Raven, 1993:218, with permission.)

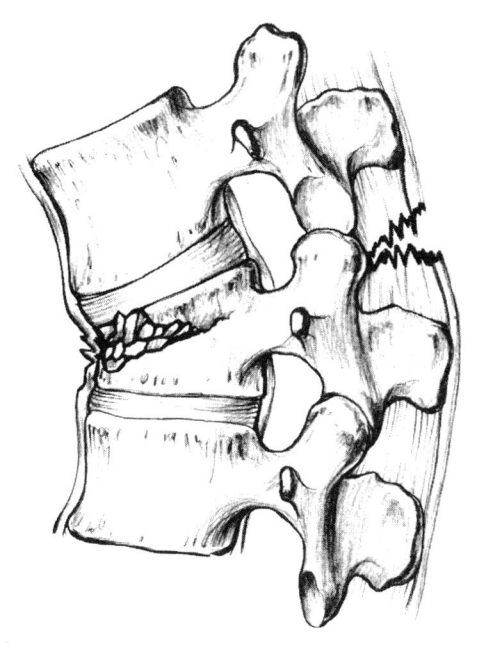

Figure 11-8. Flexion-distraction injury. (From Hansen ST, Swiontkowski MF. *Orthopaedic trauma protocols.* New York: Raven, 1993:219, with permission.)

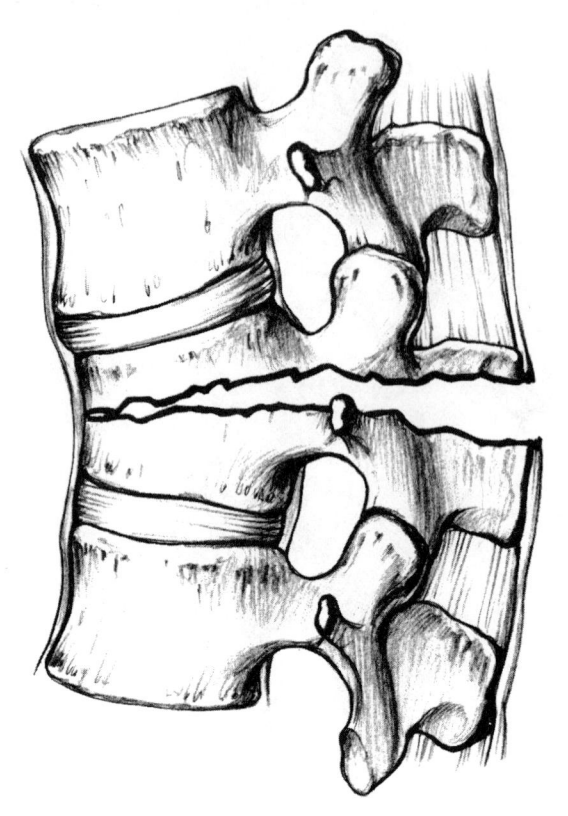

Figure 11-9. Chance fracture. (From Hansen ST, Swiontkowski MF. *Orthopaedic trauma protocols.* New York: Raven, 1993:221, with permission.)

      percussion over the involved segment is common. Hematomas and gaps between spinous processes may be palpable.
  3. **Examination.** On initial examination, a neurologic assessment must be completed. If a sensory level is detected, mark it on the chart and on the trunk with the time and date of examination. If there is any motor deficit, then record it on a simple muscle chart. It is sufficient to record function of muscle groups rather than of individual muscles. A drawing of the patient can be helpful to illustrate pertinent neurologic findings. A flow sheet is another useful device to document changes in the neurologic status over time.
  4. **Roentgenograms.** Excellent quality anteroposterior and lateral films are required, and CT scans often are indicated to evaluate the posterior elements and to assess stability (28). The pattern of injury must be accurately determined. If there is neurologic involvement and the roentgenograms and CT scans do not reveal a fracture, MRI is indicated. This study identifies herniated disc material or hematoma as the cause of the deteriorating neurologic examination (30,31).
  5. **Treatment.** Logroll the patient on a firm mattress until stability of the fracture is assessed.
    a. **Minor fractures**
      i. **Bed rest** on a firm bed for a few days with light analgesia is usually all that is required. Patients may be turned in a logrolling fashion

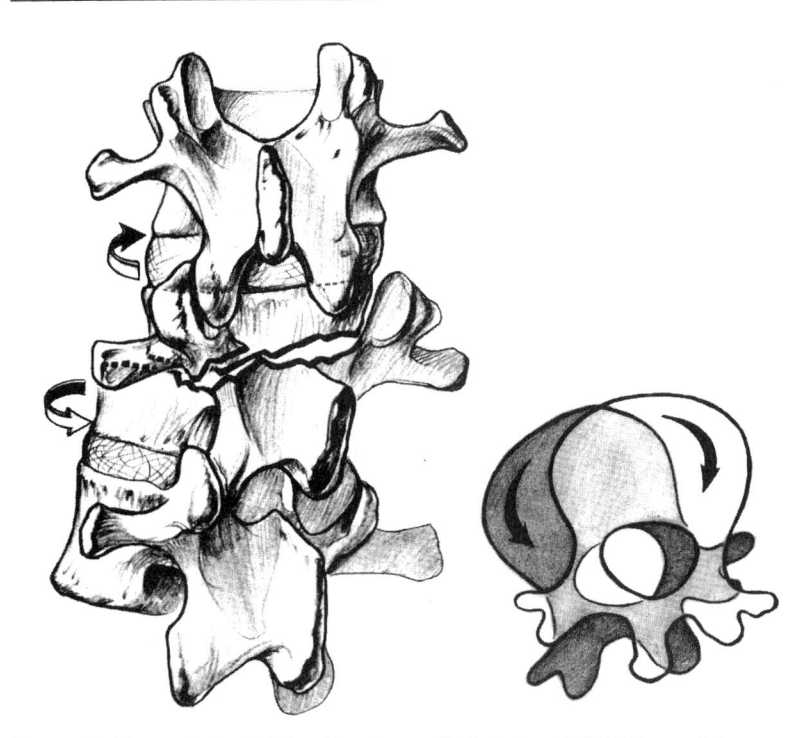

Figure 11-10. Translational injuries. (From Hansen ST, Swiontkowski MF. *Orthopaedic trauma protocols.* New York: Raven, 1993:222, with permission.)

      every 2 to 4 hours. An off-the-shelf Jewett brace or Risser cast is generally used for 12 to 16 weeks.

  ii. Paralytic **ileus** tends to develop, particularly in patients with lumbar compression fractures. This development should be anticipated and the patient should take nothing by mouth until normal bowel activity is ensured; IV fluid maintenance is required.

  iii. As soon as the patient is comfortable in a cast or brace, start **extension exercises** to strengthen the thoracic and lumbar spinal extensor muscles. As soon as good muscle control is obtained, the patient may be allowed to ambulate.

  iv. **Lifting or flexion activities should be avoided** for 3 months.

b. **Major fractures or fracture-dislocations.** Spinal fractures can be missed in unconscious obtunded patients; complete spine films must be obtained and carefully scrutinized (32). In a severe anterior compression fracture with a marked kyphosis, reduction with some type of posterior instrumentation such as a rod/hook or rod/pedicle screw construct may be indicated. Otherwise, **stable fractures** rarely require operative intervention. In a prospective, randomized study comparing operative and nonoperative treatment of stable thoracolumbar burst fractures in patients without neurologic deficits, investigators found no significant difference between the two groups with respect to return to work, pain scores, spinal deformity, or health-related quality of life, although complications were more frequent in the operative group (29). Accordingly, most of these patients should be managed in a well-fitting hyperextension cast or suitable orthosis. **Unstable fractures** should be evaluated for stabilization with appropriate instrumentation by a spine surgeon trained in the use of these devices (27,31,33).

  i. **Stable fractures without neurologic deficit** include most compression injuries and burst fractures resulting from vertical compression forces. Place the patient on strict bed rest until the pain is reduced sufficiently to allow an active exercise program. When good muscle function has been restored, the patient can be mobilized in a plaster or plastic body jacket or a suitable brace. Minor degrees of compression should be treated as are compression fractures elsewhere (see **F.5.a**).
  ii. **Unstable injuries without neurologic involvement.** The most common of these injuries is the unstable burst type. If nonoperative treatment is selected, then provide external immobilization for 12 to 16 weeks, depending on the fracture pattern and physical build of the patient (29,34). Mild paresthesias or dysesthesias can be seen in this type of injury without other neurologic symptoms or signs; these do not constitute an indication for immediate operation. Consider operative intervention if motor, reflex, or sensory deficits develop. If significant deformity is likely, then surgery is generally recommended.
  iii. **Unstable injuries with progressive neurologic damage.** This is one condition for which surgeons agree that reduction, decompression of the neural elements, and internal stabilization is required (31). Methylprednisolone therapy is recommended (12,35).
  iv. **Unstable injuries with incomplete neurologic deficit.** Treat these cases with a logrolling frame while the neurologic lesion is assessed. If it worsens or remains the same, then consider treatment as noted in the preceding paragraph. If it is improving, then no operative intervention for the lesion is needed, but the fracture instability should be evaluated to determine whether operative stabilization or early mobilization in a cast or custom plastic body jacket is the method of choice. Parenteral steroid therapy may also be indicated.
  v. **Unstable fractures with complete neurologic deficit.** If paraplegia is immediate and complete and there is no evidence of return of function within 48 hours, then early operative stabilization should be considered to allow earlier rehabilitation.
  c. **Indications for immediate operation**
     i. **An advancing or progressive neurologic deficit**
     ii. **Paraplegia in the absence of bony injury and in the presence of a complete block as revealed by MRI or myelography**, which may indicate an acute traumatic disc prolapse or hematoma
     iii. **Severe root pain** from root compression at the level of the injury—another indication for exploration but seldom requiring immediate operation
  G. **Fractures of the transverse process in the lumbar spine.** These fractures can result from different mechanisms of injury and should be treated symptomatically. Patients tend to have significant pain and require heavier analgesia. Consider and rule out associated renal injury with screening urinalysis and CT scan if indicated.

IV. **SPECIAL CONSIDERATIONS IN CHILDREN**
  A. **Pseudosubluxation.** Subluxation of the vertebral body of C2 on C3 may be difficult to evaluate in a child who has sustained neck trauma because this may present as a normal variant. Careful evaluation of the posterior intralaminar line (the line of Swischuk) may help differentiate physiologic subluxation from pathologic subluxation. An intact posterior intralaminar line is characteristic of pseudosubluxation.
  B. **Disproportionate head-to-torso ratio.** Because children up to 6 years of age have a disproportionately larger head size than older children and adults, supine

positioning on a firm surface results in a slightly flexed position of the cervical spine. To lessen the potential for associated neurologic injury or difficulties in interpretation of imaging studies, the torso should be elevated on padding in order to produce a neutral position of the cervical spine.

C. **Spinal cord injury without radiographic abnormality (SCIWORA).** Due to the relative elasticity of the bone and soft tissues in children, significant disruption and displacement of the soft tissues can occur at the time of injury, without bony injury. An MRI scan identifies the soft tissue or hematoma associated with the injury. In a review of 159 pediatric patients with acute spinal cord or vertebral injuries, 26 (16%) sustained SCIWORA (36). The mechanism of injury, its severity, and the prognosis for recovery were related to the patient's age. In young children, SCIWORA accounted for 32% of all spinal injuries and tended to be severe, while in older children, SCIWORA accounted for only 12% of the spinal injuries and had an excellent prognosis for complete recovery of neurologic function.

References

1. Tan E, Schweitzer ME, Vaccaro L, AR, Spettel C, et al. Is computed tomography of nonvisualized C7-T1 cost-effective?. *J Spinal Disord* 1999;12:472–476.
2. Blackmore CC, Mann FA, Wilson AJ. Helical CT in the primary trauma evaluation of the cervical spine: an evidence-based approach. *Skeletal Radiol* 2000;29: 632–639.
3. Nunez DB. Jr. Helical CT for the evaluation of cervical vertebral injuries. *Semin Musculoskelet Radiol* 1998;2:19–26.
4. Nunez DB Jr, Zuluaga A, Fuentes-Bernardo DA, et al. Cervical spine trauma: how much more do we learn by routinely using helical CT? *Radiographics* 1996;16:1307–1318; discussion 18–21.
5. Blackmore CC, Ramsey SD, Mann FA, et al. Cervical spine screening with CT in trauma patients: a cost-effectiveness analysis. *Radiology* 1999;212:117–125.
6. Vaccaro AR, Kreidl KO, Pan W, et al. Usefulness of MRI in isolated upper cervical spine fractures in adults. *J Spinal Disord* 1998;11:289–293; discussion 94.
7. Davis JW, Kaups KL, Cunningham MA, et al. Routine evaluation of the cervical spine in head-injured patients with dynamic fluoroscopy: a reappraisal. *J Trauma* 2001;50:1044–1047.
8. Bracken MB. Methylprednisolone and acute spinal cord injury: an update of the randomized evidence. *Spine* 2001;26:S47–S54.
9. Geisler FH, Dorsey FC, Coleman WP. Recovery of motor function after spinal-cord injury—a randomized, placebo-controlled trial with GM-1 ganglioside. *N Engl J Med* 1991;324:1829–1838.
10. Bracken MB. Methylprednisolone in the management of acute spinal cord injuries. *Med J Aust* 1990;153:368.
11. Bracken MB, Shepard MJ, Collins WF Jr, et al. Methylprednisolone or naloxone treatment after acute spinal cord injury: 1-year follow-up data. Results of the second national acute spinal cord injury study. *J Neurosurg* 1992;76:23–31.
12. Bracken MB, Shepard MJ, Holford TR, et al. Administration of methylprednisolone for 24 or 48 hours or tirilazad mesylate for 48 hours in the treatment of acute spinal cord injury. Results of the third national acute spinal cord injury randomized controlled trial. National acute spinal cord injury study. *JAMA* 1997;277: 1597–1604.
13. Levine AM, Edwards CC. The management of traumatic spondylolisthesis of the axis. *J Bone Joint Surg Am* 1985;67:217–226.
14. Anderson PA, Montesano PX. Morphology and treatment of occipital condyle fractures. *Spine* 1988;13:731–736.
15. Aebi M, Etter C, Coscia M. Fractures of the odontoid process. Treatment with anterior screw fixation. *Spine* 1989;14:1065–1070.
16. Clark CR, White AA III. Fractures of the dens. A multicenter study. *J Bone Joint Surg Am* 1985;67:1340–1348.
17. Ryan MD, Taylor TK. Odontoid fractures. A rational approach to treatment. *J Bone Joint Surg Br* 1982;64:416–421.

18. Beyer CA, Cabanela ME, Berquist TH. Unilateral facet dislocations and fracture-dislocations of the cervical spine. *J Bone Joint Surg Br* 1991;73:977–981.
19. Bohlman HH, Anderson PA. Anterior decompression and arthrodesis of the cervical spine: long-term motor improvement. Part I—Improvement in incomplete traumatic quadriparesis. *J Bone Joint Surg Am* 1992;74:671–682.
20. Rizzolo SJ, Piazza MR, Cotler JM, et al. Intervertebral disc injury complicating cervical spine trauma. *Spine* 1991;16:S187–S189.
21. Williams N, Ratliff DA. Gastrointestinal disruption and vertebral fracture associated with the use of seat belts. *Ann R Coll Surg Engl* 1993;75:129–132.
22. Mermelstein L. Initial evaluation and emergency treatment of the spine-injured patient. In: Browner B, Jupiter JB, Levine AM, eds. *Skeletal trauma*, 2nd ed. Philadelphia, PA: WB Saunders, 1992:745–768.
23. Marshall LF, Knowlton S, Garfin SR, et al. Deterioration following spinal cord injury. A multicenter study. *J Neurosurg* 1987;66:400–404.
24. Vaccaro AR, Falatyn SP, Flanders AE, et al. Magnetic resonance evaluation of the intervertebral disc, spinal ligaments, and spinal cord before and after closed traction reduction of cervical spine dislocations. *Spine* 1999;24:1210–1217.
25. Gunduz S, Ogur E, Mohur H, et al. Deep vein thrombosis in spinal cord injured patients. *Paraplegia* 1993;31:606–610.
26. Barnsley L, Lord SM, Wallis BJ, et al. Lack of effect of intraarticular corticosteroids for chronic pain in the cervical zygapophyseal joints. *N Engl J Med* 1994;330:1047–1050.
27. Denis F. The three column spine and its significance in the classification of acute thoracolumbar spinal injuries. *Spine* 1983;8:817–831.
28. McAfee PC, Yuan HA, Fredrickson BE, et al. The value of computed tomography in thoracolumbar fractures. An analysis of one hundred consecutive cases and a new classification. *J Bone Joint Surg Am* 1983;65:461–473.
29. Wood K, Buttermann G, Mehbod A, et al. Operative compared with nonoperative treatment of a thoracolumbar burst fracture without neurological deficit. A prospective, randomized study. *J Bone Joint Surg Am* 2003;85-A:773–781.
30. Delamarter RB, Sherman JE, Carr JB. 1991 Volvo Award in experimental studies. Cauda equina syndrome: neurologic recovery following immediate, early, or late decompression. *Spine* 1991;16:1022–1029.
31. Gertzbein SD. Neurologic deterioration in patients with thoracic and lumbar fractures after admission to the hospital. *Spine* 1994;19:1723–1725.
32. Born CT, Ross SE, Iannacone WM, et al. Delayed identification of skeletal injury in multisystem trauma: the 'missed' fracture. *J Trauma* 1989;29:1643–1646.
33. Gumley G, Taylor TK, Ryan MD. Distraction fractures of the lumbar spine. *J Bone Joint Surg Br* 1982;64:520–525.
34. Limb D, Shaw DL, Dickson RA. Neurological injury in thoracolumbar burst fractures. *J Bone Joint Surg Br* 1995;77:774–777.
35. Bracken MB, Shepard MJ, Collins WF, et al. A randomized, controlled trial of methylprednisolone or naloxone in the treatment of acute spinal-cord injury. Results of the second national acute spinal cord injury study. *N Engl J Med* 1990;322:1405–1411.
36. Dickman CA, Zabramski JM, Hadley MN, et al. Pediatric spinal cord injury without radiographic abnormalities: report of 26 cases and review of the literature. *J Spinal Disord* 1991;4:296–305.

Selected Historical Readings

Anderson LD, D'Alonzo RT. Fracture of the odontoid process of the axis. *J Bone Joint Surg (Am)* 1974;56:1663.

Bohler L. Fracture and dislocation of the spine. In: Bohler L, Bohler J, eds. *The treatment of fractures*, 5th ed. New York: Grune & Stratton, 1956.

Bohlman HH. Acute fractures and dislocations of the cervical spine. *J Bone Joint Surg (Am)* 1979;61:1119.

Braakman R, Vinken PJ. Unilateral facet interlocking in the lower cervical spine. *J Bone Joint Surg (Br)* 1967;49:249.

Chance GQ. Note on a type of flexion fracture of the spine. *Br J Radiol* 1948;21:452.

Clawson DK. Low back pain. *Northwest Med* 1970;69:686.

Dawson EG, Smith L. Atlanto-axial subluxation in children due to vertebral anomalies. *J Bone Joint Surg (Am)* 1979;61:582.

Dickson JH, Harrington PR, Erwin WD. Results of reduction and stabilization of the severely fractured thoracic and lumbar spine. *J Bone Joint Surg (Am)* 1978;60:799.

Fielding JW, et al. Tears of the transverse ligament of the atlas. *J Bone Joint Surg (Am)* 1974;56:1683.

Fielding JW, Hensinger RN, Hawkins RJ. Os odontoideum. *J Bone Joint Surg (Am)* 1980;62:376.

Griswold DM, et al. Atlanto-axial fusion for instability. *J Bone Joint Surg (Am)* 1978;60: 285.

Holdsworth F. Fractures, dislocations, and fracture-dislocations of the spine. *J Bone Joint Surg (Am)* 1970;52:1534.

Hohl M. Soft-tissue injuries of the neck in automobile accidents. Factors influencing prognosis. *J Bone Joint Surg (Am)* 1974;56:1675.

Johnson RM, et al. Cervical orthoses. *J Bone Joint Surg (Am)* 1977;59:322.

Rand RW, Crandall PH. Central spinal cord syndrome in hyperextension injuries of the cervical spine. *J Bone Joint Surg (Am)* 1962;44:1415.

Schatzker JE, Cecil H, Waddell JP. Fractures of the dens (odontoid process), an analysis of thirty-seven cases. *J Bone Joint Surg (Br)* 1971;53:392.

Schneider RC, et al. "Hangman's fracture" of the cervical spine. *J Neurosurg* 1965;22: 141.

Spence KF Jr, Decker S, Sell KW. Bursting atlantal fracture associated with rupture of the transverse ligament. *J Bone Joint Surg Am* 1970;52:543–9.

Stauffer ES. Current concepts review: internal fixation of fractures of the thoracolumbar spine. *J Bone Joint Surg (Am)* 1984;76A:1136.

White AA III, Panjabi MM. *Clinical biomechanics of the spine.* Philadelphia, PA: JB Lippincott, 1978.

DISORDERS AND DISEASES OF THE SPINE   12

I. **LOW BACK PAIN AND SCIATICA.** The lifetime incidence of low back pain is 50% to 70% and of sciatica is 30% to 40%. The cause of the low back pain in approximately 90% of the patients is related to disc degeneration.

   A. **History taking in the patient with low back pain.** Low back pain is common and the most frequent causes are benign and self-limiting. Still, it is extremely important to "rule out" the dangerous causes. Generally this can be accomplished with a thorough history. The common patient with back pain is between the ages of 20 and 50 and has no signs or symptoms of systemic illness. Be on the alert for back pain in the young and the old. A thorough review of systems should include questions about associated fever, sweats, weight loss, or change in bowel or bladder.

   B. **Physical examination.** The physical examination begins with observing the body position chosen by the patient (patients with acute sciatica may choose to avoid sitting in a slouched position as this places extra pressure on the impinged nerve root). The back should be exposed and one should note if there is any redness or warmth. Note range of motion of the spine. A straight leg raise is generally performed with the patient in the supine position, but can be done first with the patient in the seated position when the patient's physical symptoms seem disingenuous. The lower legs and feet should be exposed in order to test distal strength, sensation, and reflexes.

   C. **Causes of low back pain.** Low back pain is a symptom, not a disease, and the pathologic basis of the pain frequently lies outside the spine. There are many causes, which are classified in **Table 12-1**.

      1. **Vascular back pain.** Aneurysms or peripheral vascular disease may give rise to backache or symptoms resembling sciatica.
      2. **Neurogenic back pain.** Tension, irritation, and compression of lumbar nerves and roots may cause pain down one or both legs. Lesions anywhere along the central nervous system, particularly of the spine, may present with back and leg pain.
      3. **Viscerogenic back pain** may be derived from disorders of the organs in the lesser abdominal sac, the pelvis, or the retroperitoneal structures such as the pancreas and kidneys.
      4. **Psychogenic back pain.** Clouding and confusion of the clinical picture by emotional overtones may be seen. A pure psychogenic component is rare.
      5. **Spondylogenic back pain.** Common conditions causing spondylogenic back pain are outlined in **Table 12-2**.

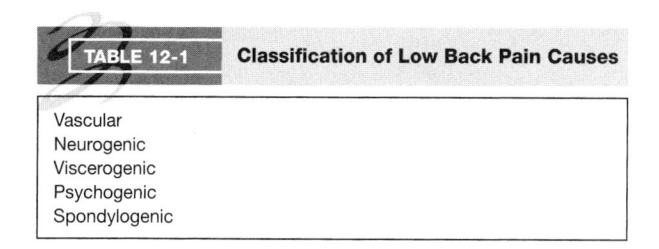

TABLE 12-1 Classification of Low Back Pain Causes

Vascular
Neurogenic
Viscerogenic
Psychogenic
Spondylogenic

TABLE 12-2	Common Conditions Causing Spondylogenic Back Pain

1. Disc degeneration
2. Spondylolisthesis
3. Trauma
    Myofascial sprains/strains
    Fractures
4. Infection (bacterial tuberculosis)
5. Tumor (benign, malignant, metastatic)
6. Rheumatologic
    Ankylosing spondylitis/spondyloarthropathy
    Fibrositis/fibromyalgia
7. Metabolic
    Osteoporosis
    Osteomalacia
    Paget disease

a. **Disc degeneration** is by far the most common cause of back pain. Disc degeneration may occur anywhere along the spine and produce neck pain, thoracic spine pain, or lumbar or low back pain. Disc degeneration may be associated with nerve root irritation, which would then result in radicular leg pain. The nerve root irritation or compression may be due to an acute disc herniation or impingement by bony stenosis or a combination of soft-tissue and bony impingement.
   i. **Anatomy.** The spine provides stability and a central axis for the limbs that are attached. The spine has to move, to transmit weight, and to protect the spinal cord. When the spine is viewed from the side, the thoracic spine is concave forward (kyphosis) and the cervical and lumbar regions are concave backward (lordosis).
   ii. **Vertebral components**
       (a) Each segment of the vertebral column transmits weight through the vertebral body anteriorly and the facet joints posteriorly. Between adjacent bodies are the intervertebral discs, which are firmly attached to the vertebrae. The disc consists of an outer annulus fibrosis, which is made up of concentric layers of fibrous tissue. It surrounds and contains a central avascular nucleus pulposus, which consists of a hydrophilic gel made of protein, polysaccharide, collagen fibrils, sparsely chondroid cells, and water (88%). The spinal cord and caudal equina are found within the spinal canal. At each intervertebral level, nerve roots leave the canal through the intervertebral foramina.
       (b) A functional spinal unit or motion segment consists of two adjacent vertebrae and the intervertebral disc. It forms a three-joint complex with the disc in front and two facet joints posteriorly. The facet joints, like other joints in the body, have capsules, ligaments, muscles, nerves, and vessels. Changes in one joint affect the other two. Narrowing of the disc space, therefore, may result in malalignment of the facet joints and, with time, lead to wear-and-tear degenerative arthritic changes in those joints.
   iii. **Pathology.** Normal aging is associated with a gradual dehydration of the disc. The nucleus pulposus becomes desiccated and the annulus fibrosus develops fissures parallel to the vertebral end plates running mainly posteriorly. Small herniations of nuclear material may squeeze through the annular fissures and may also penetrate the vertebral end plates to produce Schmorl nodes. If the nuclear material squeezes

against the nerve, it may produce nerve root irritation. The flattening and collapse of the disc results in osteophytes along the vertebral bodies. Malalignment and displacement of the facet joints is an inevitable consequence of disc space collapse, leading to osteophytes that may narrow the lateral or subarticular recess of the spinal canal or the intervertebral foramina. This narrowing of the spinal canal or of the intervertebral neural foramina is called spinal stenosis.

iv. **Disc degeneration without nerve root irritation.** There are three patterns of low back pain associated with disc degeneration: **acute incapacitating backache**, which may occur a few times in a person's life and not be a regular problem; **recurrent aggravating backache**, which is the most common type and is associated with regular periods of recurrence and remission of back pain; and **chronic persisting backache**, which is the most difficult to treat and the patients have constant disabling back pain.

   (a) The back pain associated with disc degeneration is mechanical in nature. It is aggravated or brought on by activity and relieved by rest. There may be a referred component of back pain into the legs, but this is usually down the back of the legs and rarely goes beyond the knee. The low back pain may be due to periods of hard work, prolonged standing or walking, or prolonged sitting in one position. The peak incidence of back pain in the general population is in the 40s and 50s. This is the time when the discs have collapsed and there is relative instability at the motion segment. The natural history, however, is for the spine to stiffen up with increased fibrosus around the facet joints and the discs. As the patient gets older, the physical demands become less and the spine becomes stiffer; the incidence of back pain, therefore, declines beyond the 60s.

   (b) Patients who give a history of fever, weight loss, malaise, night and rest pain, morning stiffness, and colicky pain should be carefully evaluated for the possibilities of infection, tumor, spondyloarthropathy, or viscerogenic back pain.

v. **Disc degeneration with root irritation**

   (a) Nerve root irritation and compression may be due to an **acute disc herniation** or may be associated with **spinal stenosis**. Acute disc herniation results in "sciatica." Essentially, this involves severe, incapacitating pain that radiates from the back down the leg. It may be associated with paresthesia, neurologic symptoms, or motor sensory or reflex changes. The pain may be constant and is frequently aggravated by coughing, sneezing, and straining. Intradiscal pressure is increased in a bending and sitting position, especially if lifting is performed, therefore increasing the amount of pain. The pain may be lessened by lying down.

   (b) The **most frequent sites of disc herniation** are in the spinal canal, resulting in impingement of the traversing nerve root. Less common disc herniation may be laterally in the foramen, resulting in impingement of the existing nerve root. The leg pain or sciatica is accompanied by signs of nerve root tension, which can be diagnosed by a straight-leg raising test, bowstring sign, or Lasegue's test.

   (c) In **spinal stenosis**, the leg pain or radicular pain is brought on by prolonged walking or standing (neurogenic claudication). The pain may be associated with paresthesia and is relieved by sitting or stooping. There are few physical findings or neurologic deficits unless the condition has been present for a long time and is advanced. Neurogenic claudication associated with spinal stenosis should be distinguished from vascular claudication caused by peripheral vascular disease.

TABLE 12-3 Neurology of the Lower Extremity

Root	Muscles	Sensation	Reflex
L2	Hip flexion	Anterior thigh (proximal)	None
L3	Knee extension (quadriceps)	Anterior thigh (distal)	Patellar
L4	Anterior tibialis	Medial leg	Patellar
L5	Extensor hallucis longus	Lateral leg and dorsum of foot	None
S1	Gastrocsoleus peroneus longus and brevis	Lateral foot	Achilles

vi. **Neurology of the lower extremities.** The nerve roots leaving the spine at each segmental level may be affected by acute disc herniations, bony foraminal stenosis, or a stenosis associated with both soft-tissue and bony compression. The nerve root may be affected within the central spinal canal, in the subarticular recess, or in the intervertebral foramen. The nerve root traversing the motion segment or the exiting nerve root may be affected. It is important to correlate the patient's symptoms and physical findings with the abnormalities seen on radiographs, magnetic resonance imaging (MRI) scans, and computed tomography (CT) studies. It is important, therefore, to have knowledge of the nerve roots and their distal enervation. The main nerve roots are listed in **Table 12-3**.

vii. **Imaging studies (Table 12-4)**
  (a) **Radiographs** may appear normal or demonstrate disc space narrowing, osteophyte formation, or instability on lateral flexion and extension views. There is no clear-cut correlation between low back pain and the presence of disc space narrowing on plain radiographs (1).

TABLE 12-4 "Red Flags" in Patients Presenting with Back Pain (Typically Indications for Imaging)

Concern for malignancy
    Age >50
    Previous history of cancer
    Unexplained weight loss
    Pain unrelieved by bed rest
    Pain lasting >1 mo
    Failure to improve within 1 mo
    Acute trauma
Concern for Infection
    Erythrocyte sedimentation rate >20 mm
    Intravenous (IV) drug abuse
    Urinary tract infection
    Skin infection
    Fever
Concern for compression fracture
    Corticosteroid use
    Age >70
    Age >50
Concern for neurologic problem
    Sciatica
New bowel or bladder incontinence

- **(b) Myelograms** are invasive and are less commonly used. They may be used in combination with CT scans in patients who have complex problems or who have had multiple surgeries. Myelograms should be ordered either by or with direct consultation of the treating surgeon.
- **(c) CT scans** are generally helpful when MRI scans cannot be obtained. They give better detail of the bone.
- **(d) MRI scans** of the lumbar spine are noninvasive and an excellent way to evaluate the compromise of neural structures.
- **(e) Bone scans** of the spine and pelvis are useful if tumor and infection are suspected, although these abnormalities can also be picked up easily on an MRI scan.
- **(f) Indications for imaging acutely in low back pain.** Acute imaging is indicated only if there is a history of trauma, concern for infection or tumor, presence of a neurologic deficit, suspicion for osteoporosis, and acute fracture.

b. **Spondylolisthesis.** Spondylolisthesis is the forward slippage of one vertebra on another. Spondylolysis is the presence of a bony defect of the pars interarticularis, which may result in spondylolisthesis. The incidence of spondylolysis/spondylolisthesis in the asymptomatic population is 3% to 5%. It is unclear how common this entity results in back pain in adult patients. What is clear is that adolescents who present with back pain are suffering from this entity at a much higher level and they must be followed much more closely due to the fear of the slippage progressing. This is especially true if they are gymnasts or performing other activities which place extra stress upon their posterior-lateral elements.

   i. **Classification**
      - (a) Congenital
      - (b) Isthmic
      - (c) Traumatic
      - (d) Pathologic
      - (e) Degenerative

   ii. **Congenital spondylolisthesis** is a congenital deficiency of the facets. Isthmic spondylolisthesis is the typical defect in the pars interarticularis allowing forward slippage of the vertebrae. It may be related to an acute fracture, a fatigue fracture, or an elongation or attenuation of an intact pars interarticularis. Traumatic spondylolisthesis is an acute fracture of the pedicle, lamina, or facet. Pathologic spondylolisthesis is an attenuation of the pedicle caused by weakness of bone (e.g., osteogenesis imperfecta). The most common type of spondylolisthesis is **degenerative spondylolisthesis**.

   iii. The **Meyerding grading system** is used to indicate the percentage of displacement of the superior vertebral body on the inferior vertebral body as follows: grade I, 0% to 25%; grade II, 25% to 50%; grade III, 50% to 75%; grade IV, 75% to 100%; grade V, greater than 100% spondyloloptosis.

   iv. **Etiology.** The initial onset of a lesion occurs at approximately 8 years of age. History of minor trauma may exist. The onset of symptoms coincides closely with either the adolescent growth spurt or repetitive athletic activity. It is thought to originate in a stress or fatigue fracture. The shear stresses are greater on the pars interarticularis when the spine is extended. Such stresses are seen with certain activities (e.g., back walkovers in gymnastics, carrying heavy backpacks, heavy lifting).

   v. **Clinical findings in isthmic spondylolisthesis.** Patients may be asymptomatic, but most patients have low back pain during the adolescent growth spurt. A few patients do have nerve root or radicular pain in the lower extremities. Hamstring tightness or spasm is

commonly found in symptomatic patients. A palpable step-off may be felt at the level of the slip.
  vi. Anteroposterior and lateral radiographs are helpful in making the diagnosis to demonstrate the slip of spondylolisthesis. An undisplaced spondylolysis is best seen on the oblique views of the lumbar spine. The "Scottie dog" sign describes the appearance of the facet joints and pars interarticularis on the oblique radiographs. The "Scottie dog's" neck representing the pars is broken in isthmic spondylolysis. For the young patient with back pain felt to be due to spondylolisthesis, it is important to institute activity modification and follow closely. If symptoms persist, then consultation is advised. There is no urgency about surgical treatment of spondylolisthesis unless serial radiographs have demonstrated progression of the slip or if there is significant neurologic impairment.

D. **Treatment of acute, nonradicular low back pain**
  1. Initial treatment includes activity modification. This includes bed rest not to exceed 2 days, although activity as tolerated appears equally efficacious (2,3). Also, use of nonsteroidal anti-inflammatory drugs (NSAIDs) has demonstrated benefit (4). The addition of short duration treatment (several days) with muscle spasm medication appears beneficial (5). The exact role for physical therapy is unclear although aerobic exercise has a positive correlation with spine health (6). Manual therapy (such as chiropractic, osteopathic, or physical therapy applied manual techniques) appears to shorten the duration and intensity of symptoms (7). There is no role for surgery in the treatment of acute, low back pain. The use of guidelines appears to have some benefit, but has had variable use to date (8).
  2. **Treatment of acute sciatica.** Initial treatment is directed at making the symptoms tolerable for the patient until the natural history of improvement occurs. This involves use of NSAIDs or other medications as necessary. The exception to this approach is cauda equina syndrome (CES) with bowel and/or bladder dysfunction where surgical decompression is required within 24 to 48 hours of onset or there is low probability of neurologic recovery (9,10). Progressive neurologic deterioration without CES is a relative indication for expedited surgery. There is recent evidence that transforaminal epidural steroid injections (ESI) may avoid surgery in a number of patients (11). If unacceptable pain persists at 6 to 12 weeks, then surgical treatment is of benefit. Previously the Weber study has been misquoted as indicating that there are no differences between surgical and nonsurgical management, yet appropriate analysis of this classic study demonstrates the benefit of surgery (12,13).
  3. **Treatment of lumbar spinal stenosis.** Neurogenic claudication is a chronic disease that appears to be slowly but irregularly progressive (14). Treatment modalities used have included NSAIDs, physical therapy, epidural steroids, and decompression. The data to support the efficacy of nonoperative treatment is limited. The benefit of lumbar decompression appears sound (15). In the particular circumstance of lumbar stenosis due to single level degenerative spondylolisthesis, there is good data indicating the benefit of decompression and fusion (16). There is much debate about the benefit of spinal instrumentation in combination with fusion. Successful fusion provides better clinical results than pseudarthrosis (17). Spinal instrumentation increases the fusion rate.
  4. **Treatment of chronic low back pain.** This is a very controversial subject (18). The first difficulty is diagnosis of the pain generator. There are many confounding variables such as workers compensation, smoking (19), litigation, diabetes, and psychological issues. The pain generator could be disk degeneration, facet degeneration, chemically mediated nerve irritation, or other as yet undefined mechanisms (20). Since these patients are such a variable cohort, conflicting data arise form studies with highly variable entry criteria. There is great variability in recommended nonoperative treatment with highly variable results. There is also variability in surgical treatment recommendations ranging from uninstrumented

posterior fusion, instrumented posterior fusion, various interbody fusion techniques, and minimally invasive techniques using these same strategies to the newest technologies for motion preservation such as artificial disc replacement or posterior ligamentous tethering devices. There is a prospective randomized trial from Sweden demonstrating the benefit of surgery compared to nonoperative treatment (21). The benefit of spinal instrumentation in this study was not profound. The availability of rhBMP-2 has led to excellent results and avoided harvesting autogenous iliac crest bone graft, when used in anterior stand alone one level fusion (22). So controversy remains and will persist.

II. **DEFORMITIES OF THE SPINE.** There are three basic types of spinal deformity: **scoliosis, kyphosis,** and **lordosis.**
  A. Scoliosis
    1. Scoliosis is a side to side curvature when the spine is viewed in the coronal plane. This deformity may be flexible and reactive or fixed and structural. In the former, there is no structural change and the deformity is correctable. There are three causes: **postural, compensatory** (to another curve, pelvic tilt, or short leg), and **sciatic.** In structural scoliosis, there is a three-dimensional deformity. The vertebrae are deformed and are rotated toward each other. The resulting rotation of all the attachments and appendages of the vertebrae, such as ribs and processes, results in asymmetry of the body, waistline, and paravertebral prominences, as well as shoulder elevation.
    2. The broad **categories of structural scoliosis** are as follows:
      a. Idiopathic (infantile, juvenile and adolescent)
      b. Osteopathic (congenital)
      c. Neuropathic (cerebral palsy, poliomyelitis)
      d. Myopathic (muscular dystrophies)
      e. Connective tissue (Marfan's, Ehlers Danlos)
      f. Neurofibromatosis
    3. Scoliosis is also seen in other disease processes such as spinal cord injuries, infections, metabolic disorders, and tumors.
    4. Curve types
      a. A **structural curve** is a segment of the spine with lateral curvature lacking normal flexibility.
      b. A **primary curve** is the first or earliest of several curves to appear. A compensatory curve is a curve above or below a major curve. It may progress to be a fixed or secondary curve.
    5. **Adolescent idiopathic scoliosis.** This is the most common type and has no known cause. It presents around puberty and may progress until skeletal maturity has been reached. There may be one, two, or three curves occurring most frequently in the thoracic and lumbar spine.
      a. **Risk factors for progression of adolescent idiopathic scoliosis.** Progression is related to the size of the curve, the area of the spine involved, and the physiologic age of a patient. Large thoracic curves progress to a greater degree than single lumbar or thoracolumbar curves. The younger the skeletal age, the more likely the curve progression. Progression is less likely to progress in boys than in girls.
    6. **Clinical findings.** Presentation of a painless deformity occurs between 10 and 15 years of age. If severe and persistent pain is present, the possibility of a tumor (most commonly osteoid osteoma), sciatic scoliosis, or spondylolysis should be considered. The rotational deformity is more noticeable on forward flexion, creating a paravertebral prominence. Other clinical features include shoulder elevation, neckline prominence on side asymmetric waistline, or prominent hip. The term **spinal imbalance** refers to the head or the trunk being off center with respect to the pelvis. Clinically, this can best be measured by dropping a plumb line from the base of the skull. Any deviation of the line from the gluteal cleft measures the amount of spinal imbalance to the left or right. A complete history and physical examination is performed to exclude other causes of scoliosis.

a. The **history** of a patient with spinal deformity should include age when the deformity was first noted, the perinatal history, and the family history of scoliosis. In children and adolescents, scoliosis is generally not painful. If persistent pain is present, appropriate diagnostic tests should be performed to exclude bony or spinal tumor, herniated discs, or other abnormalities. The patient is examined, undraped, except for undershorts, and asymmetries in the shoulder, scapular, waistline, and pelvic region are identified. The balance of the thoracic area over the pelvis is assessed. The C7 plumb line test is used to evaluate the balance of the head over the pelvis and the range of motion of the spine in flexion and extension. Side bending is also noted. The patient should also be observed from the side for evaluation of kyphosis or lordosis. The forward bend test is useful to identify areas of asymmetry in the paravertebral areas. Prominence of the scapula or rib on one side is called a "rib hump." A complete neurologic examination should be performed. Pubertal stages in girls and boys are assessed. Leg length from the anterior-superior iliac spine to the medial malleoli is measured. The lower extremities are evaluated for deformities or contractures.
7. **Radiographic evaluation** includes full length views of the entire spine in a standing position. The angle of curvature is measured. The size of the curve is measured by the **COBB method**. The upper and lower end vertebrae are identified, and perpendicular lines are erected to their transverse axis. The intersection of the perpendicular lines is the COBB angle. Radiographs are also used to evaluate the degree of skeletal maturity. The **Risser classification** evaluates the degree of ossification of the iliac epiphysis. This measures the degree of skeletal maturity. There are five grades.
8. **Treatment.** The natural history of these curves varies. Some curves remain the same, others progress, and yet others progress relentlessly. The goal of treatment is to prevent curve progression. Serial radiographs are obtained every 4 months until skeletal maturity. Risk of curve progression is greatest in younger patients with larger curves.
   a. **Braces** are indicated in the growing patient with curves of 20 to 40 degrees. Braces have distinct limitations. They brace the body and torso and indirectly exert forces on the spine (e.g., pressure pads on ribs attached to convex vertebrae) and are used to prevent further curve progression rather than straighten the curvature.
   b. **Surgery** is indicated for curves greater than 40 degrees in the skeletally immature patient who has failed conservative treatment. Anterior or posterior instrumentation is performed to correct the curvature and stabilize the spine. Bone grafting is added to achieve spinal fusion.

B. **Kyphosis**
1. The gentle posterior curvature of the normal thoracic spine when viewed from the side (sagittal plane) is kyphosis. The normal range is 20 to 40 degrees. Excessive posterior curvature beyond normal is also referred to as kyphosis.
2. **Adolescent round back** (postural kyphosis) is a flexible deformity evenly distributed throughout the thoracic spine and without any structural changes. It may be due to lax ligaments or poor muscle tone and is associated with other postural defects such as flat feet. Treatment is the same as for Scheuermann kyphosis.
3. **Structural kyphosis** refers to stiff curves with vertebral wedging. It is seen in Scheuermann disease and osteoporosis (round back of old age). Congenital kyphosis has underlying structural change and usually has a local sharp posterior angulation, also termed kyphus, which may also be seen in fracture or infection.
4. **Classification**
   a. Postural kyphosis
   b. Scheuermann disease
   c. Myelomeningocele
   d. Traumatic kyphosis

e. Postsurgical kyphosis
   f. Postradiation kyphosis
   g. Metabolic disorders
   h. Skeletal dysplasia
   i. Tumors
5. **Scheuermann disease** (adolescent kyphosis). This is a growth disorder of uncertain etiology involving the vertebral growth plates.
   a. Clinical findings
      i. There are two types based on location. The **classic form** of Scheuermann disease occurs in the thoracic spine. Criteria for diagnosis include wedging of at least 5 degrees of three adjacent vertebrae. End plates are irregular. This type is twice as common in girls as boys. The painless deformity is usually first noticed by parents. Pain may occur but is a rare symptom. Onset is usually around 10 years of age. A distinct hump at the apex of the kyphosis is frequently noted. The deformity is accentuated on forward flexion and its rigidity prevents correction on extension.
      ii. The **lumbar form** of Scheuermann disease occurs more commonly in teenaged males. They present with chronic mechanical lumbar pain, which may improve with maturation.
      iii. Kyphosis is a change in the alignment of a segment of the spine in the sagittal (side view) plane that increases the normal posterior convex angulation. The COBB method of measuring kyphosis is used to measure angulation greater than 45 to 50 degrees in the thoracic spine.
6. **Treatment.** A progressive kyphosis of the thoracic spine in a skeletally immature patient is treated in a **Milwaukee brace** until maturity. Surgery is reserved for select cases with curves greater than 75 degrees that have pain or are unresponsive to bracing. Lumbar Scheuermann disease is not responsive to bracing. It is treated by exercises and anti-inflammatories if painful.

References

1. Boden SD. Current concepts review—the use of radiographic imaging studies in the evaluation of patients who have degenerative disorders of the lumbar spine. *J Bone Joint Surg (Am)* 1996;78(1):114–124.
2. Malmivaara A, Häkkinen U, Aro T, et al. The treatment of acute low back pain: bed rest, exercises, or ordinary activity? *N Engl J Med* 1995;332:351–355.
3. Hagen KB, Hilde G, Jamtvedt G, et al. The cochrane review of bed rest for acute low back pain and sciatica. *Spine* 2000;25(22):2932–2939.
4. van Tulder MW, Scholten RJPM, Koes BW, et al. Nonsteroidal anti-inflammatory drugs for low back pain: a systematic review within the framework of the cochrane collaboration back review group. *Spine* 2000;25(19):2501–2513.
5. van Tulder MW, Touray T, Furlan AD, et al. Muscle relaxants for nonspecific low back pain: a systematic review within the framework of the cochrane collaboration. *Spine* 2003;28(17):1978–1992.
6. van Tulder MW, Malmivaara A, Esmail R, et al. Exercise therapy for low back pain: a systematic review within the framework of the cochrane collaboration back review group. *Spine* 2000;25(21):2784–2796.
7. Cherkin DC, Deyo RA, Battie M, et al. A comparison of physical therapy, chiropractic manipulation, and provision of an educational booklet for the treatment of patients with low back pain. *N Engl J Med* 1998;339:1021–1029.
8. McGuirk B, King W, Govind J, et al. Safety, efficacy, and cost effectiveness of evidence-based guidelines for the management of acute low back pain in primary care. *Spine* 2001;26(23):2615–2622.
9. Ahn UM, Ahn NU, Buchowski JM, et al. Cauda equina syndrome secondary to lumbar disc herniation: a meta-analysis of surgical outcomes. *Spine* 2000;25(12):1515–1522.

10. Kohles SS, Kohles DA, Karp AP, et al. Time-dependent surgical outcomes following cauda equina syndrome diagnosis: comments on a meta-analysis. *Spine* 2004; 29(11):1281–1287.
11. Riew KD, Yin Y, Gilula L, et al. The effect of nerve-root injections on the need for operative treatment of lumbar radicular pain: a prospective, randomized, controlled, double-blind study. *J Bone Joint Surg (Am)* 2000;82:1589–1593.
12. Weber H. Lumbar disc herniation: a controlled, prospective study with ten years of observation. *Spine* 1983;8:131–140.
13. Bessette L, Liang M, Lew RA, et al. Classics in spine: surgery literature revisited. *Spine* 1996;21(3):259–263.
14. Spivak JM. Current concepts review: degenerative lumbar spinal stenosis. *J Bone Joint Surg (Am)* 1998;80:1053–1066.
15. Amundsen T, Weber H, Nordal HJ, et al. Lumbar spinal stenosis: conservative or surgical management? A prospective 10-year study. *Spine* 2000;25(11):1424–1436.
16. Herkowitz HN, Kurz LT. Degenerative lumbar spondylolisthesis with spinal stenosis. A prospective study comparing decompression with decompression and intertransverse process arthrodesis. *J Bone Joint Surg (Am)* 1991;73:802–808.
17. Kornblum MB, Fischgrund JS, Herkowitz HN, et al. Degenerative lumbar spondylolisthesis with spinal stenosis: a prospective long-term study comparing fusion and pseudarthrosis. *Spine* 2004;29(7):726–733.
18. Hanley EN, David SM. Current concepts review: lumbar arthrodesis for the treatment of low back pain. *J Bone Joint Surg (Am)* 1999;81:716–730.
19. Feldman DE, Rossignol M, Shrier I, et al. A risk factor for development of low back pain in adolescents. *Spine* 1999;24(23):2492–2496.
20. Luoma K, Riihimaki H, Luukkonen R, et al. Low back pain in relation to lumbar disc degeneration. *Spine* 2000;25(4):487–492.
21. Fritzell P, Hagg O, Wessberg P, et al. The swedish lumbar spine study group. Chronic low back pain and fusion: a comparison of three surgical techniques: a prospective multicenter randomized study from the swedish lumbar spine study group. *Spine* 2002;27(11):1131–1141.
22. Burkus JK, Heim SE, Gornet MF, et al. Is INFUSE bone graft superior to autograft bone? An integrated analysis of clinical trials using the LT-CAGE lumbar tapered fusion device. *J Spinal Disord Tech* 2003;16(2):113–122.

FRACTURES OF THE CLAVICLE 13

I. **GENERAL INFORMATION**
   A. **Anatomy and mechanism.** The clavicle, otherwise known as the collarbone, is the main stabilizer between the axial (via the sternoclavicular joint) and the appendicular (via the acromioclavicular joint) skeleton. Any force absorbed by the upper extremity transmits to the thorax through the clavicle. This fact, in addition to its superficial location, explains why it is vulnerable to injury. In fact, it has been estimated to be the most commonly fractured bone (1,2).

   Most frequently, clavicle fractures result from a blow to the shoulder region such as during a fall to the turf, though they also may result from a direct hit to the collarbone. These fractures are most commonly seen in children and young adults (1), although they are diagnosed with increasing frequency in later decades where more active lifestyles are taking place in the context of epidemic osteoporosis.

   B. **Classification.** Allman classified these fractures according to whether they were proximal, middle, or distal one third injuries and noted that the middle one-third fracture was by far the most common (3). The distal one-third clavicle fracture should be distinguished further as to whether it is intraarticular or extraarticular and whether or not it is displaced, which would imply disruption of the coracoclavicular ligaments (4).

II. **DIAGNOSIS**
   A. **History and physical exam.** Pain and deformity localized to the clavicle provide the most typical presentation. Frequently, ecchymosis and tenting of the skin are recognized. The typical deformity in the common middle third fracture is caused by the proximal (medial) fragment bone spike being pulled by the sternocleidomastoid muscle, which inserts on the proximal clavicle. The deformity is accentuated by the weight of gravity on the upper extremity pulling downward on the distal (lateral) fragment.

   Physical exam will frequently detect bony crepitance and should include inspection of the skin for punctures or lacerations consistent with an open fracture. As the clavicle is directly anterior to the brachial plexus and the subclavian artery, exam should also include neurovascular assessment, particularly in injuries associated with high-energy mechanisms.

   B. **Radiographs.** A standard anteroposterior view of the clavicle usually confirms the diagnosis of a fracture. Comminution and displacement should be described. The degree of overriding of the fracture fragments should be noted as well since impaction forces to the lateral forequarter can cause medialization of the shoulder. This is an important variable in deciding on treatment. Oftentimes, in the setting of polytrauma, a chest x-ray provides the initial radiographic diagnosis. Surrounding structures such as the scapula and ribs should be inspected for injury as well.

III. **TREATMENT**
   A. **Nonoperative.** The vast majority of clavicle fractures should be treated nonoperativley. Extraarticular fractures displaced less than 1 cm are treated with a simple sling or sling-and-swathe immobilizer for comfort. A figure-of-8 strap may be used to maintain the shoulder in a retracted position to theoretically improve alignment. This technique may be most useful for children, in which case care must be

taken not to snug it too tightly, which can compromise skin and compress the brachial plexus. Studies do not seem to suggest, however, that there is any difference in shoulder function, range of motion, or residual deformity between the use of a sling or a figure-of-8 strap (5).

Intraarticular distal clavicle fractures most often also warrant nonoperative treatment if the coracoclavicular ligaments are intact and there is not much displacement of the proximal clavicular shaft. In the case of intraarticular clavicle fractures, the patient should be warned of the possibility of arthritic symptoms if there is stepoff or comminution at the acromioclavicular joint. This outcome can be treated on a delayed basis with distal clavicle resection. In children, a couple of weeks of relative immobilization is all it takes before calus begins to provide the splinting necessary for healing of the bone ends. In adults, a month of such immobilization will provide the same relief.

B. Operative. There are several indications for operative management of clavicle fractures.

1. The clearest indication is the case of an open fracture which requires irrigation, debridement, and stabilization. The most common form of internal fixation is with plate and screws.
2. Fractures lateral to the coracoid may be associated with torn coracoclavicular ligaments, in which case the shaft of the clavicle tends to displace proximally. This injury variant is associated with a higher rate of nonunion. Conservative management should be discussed with the patient and placed in the context of the patient's activity level, hand dominance, age, and co-morbidities. If this lateral fracture variant is displaced more than 1 cm, strong consideration should be given to openly reduce and fix the fracture. A method similar to fixation of an acromioclavicular dislocation as described in **Chap. 14** should be used.
3. Another relative indication for surgery is medialization more than 2 cm as determined by the amount of overriding of the clavicle shaft fragments. McKee et al. documented poorer performance on endurance testing, as well as on a validated outcome test, in patients with more than 2 cm of shortening (6) and showed that malunions of this type can improve function and strength with operative correction (7).
4. If the neck of the scapula (glenoid) is fractured along with the clavicle, this is also a relative indication for surgery. In such a circumstance, a displaced clavicle fracture should be fixed to stabilize the "floating shoulder." This injury complex implies that the glenohumeral joint has no support and is one type of a double disruption of the superior shoulder suspensory complex (8). Other authors have suggested the alternative of scapula fixation in that setting instead, and yet others have advocated fixation of both injuries (9).

C. Follow-up. Patients should be followed up in the office at 2 and 4 weeks after the injury to check radiographs to make sure that further displacment has not occurred. They need reassurance that discomfort, crepitance, and deformity are expected during this phase of healing. After this juncture, passive and gentle active range of motion should be encouraged, as well as light lifting, guided by the patient's symptoms. Most often, good function has been restored by 3 months post injury, at which time restrictions can usually be lifted. Radiographic healing should be nearly complete by this juncture but can take months, particularly in the elderly.

D. Complications. Patients should be counseled from the beginning that they should anticipate a lump in the region of the fracture if treated nonoperatively. Reported nonunion rates are in the range of 0.1% to 0.8% (2,6,10), though certain risk factors such as displaced distal fractures and clavicle fractures in the elderly have been identified (10).

> **HCMC Treatment Recommendations**
> *Clavicle Fractures*
>   *Diagnosis:* Anteroposterior shoulder radiograph, 15-degree cephalad oblique view, clinical examination
>   *Treatment:* Sling and/or figure-of-8 bandage for comfort: 2–4 weeks, institute range-of-motion exercises at 2 weeks
>   *Indications for surgery:* Open fractures, vascular injuries, non-unions, or initial displacement of greater than 2 cm
>   *Recommended technique:* 3.5-mm reconstruction plate or low contact dynamic compression plate (LCDCP) applied to anteroinferior surface of the clavicle

References

1. Robinson CM, Cairns DA. Primary nonoperative treatment of displaced lateral fractures of the clavicle. *J Bone Joint Surg (Am)* 2004;86:778–782.
2. Wilkins RM, Johnston RM. Ununited fractures of the clavicle. *J Bone Joint Surg. (Am)* 1983;65:773–778.
3. Allman FL. Fractures and ligamentous injuries of the clavicle and its articulation. *J Bone Joint Surg (Am)* 1967;9A:774–784.
4. Robinson CM. Fractures of the clavicle in the adult: epidemiology and classification. *J Bone Joint Surg (Br)* 1988;70:461–464.
5. Andersen K, Jensen PO, Lauritzen J. Treatment of clavicular fractures figure-of-eight bandage versus a simple sling. *Acta Orthop Scand* 1987;57:71–75.
6. McKee MD, Pederson EM, Wild LM, et al. Previously unrecognized deficits after nonoperative treatment of displaced midshaft fracture of the clavicle detected by patient based outcome measures and objective muscle strength testing. Conference Proceedings, Defining Indications for New Techniques in Fracture Fixation, OTA Specialty Day, San Fransisco, CA 2003.
7. McKee MD, Wild LM, Schemitsch EH. Midshaft malunions of the clavicle. *J Bone Joint Surg (Am)* 2003;85A:790–797.
8. Goss TP. Double disruptions of the superior shoulder suspensory complex. *J Orthop Trauma* 1993;7:99–106.
9. Lenny KS, Lam TP. Open reduction and internal fixation of ipsilateral fractures of the scapular neck and clavicle. *J Bone Joint Surg (Am)* 1993;75:1015–1018.
10. Robinson, CM, Court-Brown CM, McQueen MM. Estimation of the risk of nonunion after a fracture of the clavicle. Paper Presented at: Defining Indications for New Techniques in Fracture Fixation, OTA Specialty Day, San Fransisco, CA, 2003.

Selected Historical Readings

Allman FL. Fractures and ligamentous injuries of the clavicle and its articulation. *J Bone Joint Surg (Am)* 1967;49:774–784.
Neer CS. Fractures of the distal third of the clavicle. *Clin Orthop* 1968;58:43–50.
Neer CS. Nonunion of the clavicle. *JAMA* 1960;172:1006–1011.
Rowe CR. An atlas of anatomy and treatment of midclavicular fractures. *Clin Orthop* 1968;58:29–42.

STERNOCLAVICULAR AND ACROMIOCLAVICULAR JOINT INJURIES

14

I. **STERNOCLAVICULAR INJURIES**
   A. **General information**
      1. **Anatomy and mechanism.** The sternoclavicular joint is a diarthroidal joint between the medial clavicle and the clavicular notch of the sternum. Though there is little intrinsic osseous stability, the sternoclavicular ligaments are reinforced by the costoclavicular ligaments, disc ligament, interclavicular ligament, and joint capsule; thus explaining the rarity of this injury.

      The sternoclavicular joint is the major articulation between the axial and appendicular skeleton. The majority of scapulothoracic motion occurs through the sternoclavicular joint, which allows approximately 45 degrees of rotation around its long axis. Injuries to the sternoclavicular joint represent only 3% of shoulder girdle injuries (1).

      A sternoclavicular injury is always a high-energy event, and, therefore, other injuries should be expected. Due to the posterior proximity of critical structures such as the great vessels, phrenic nerve, trachea, and esophagus, associated injuries should be diagnosed promptly.

      The mechanism of injury can either be from a direct blow to the anterior clavicle causing a posterior dislocation or an indirect medial force vector to the shoulder. If the medial force drives the scapula posteriorly (retracted) along the thorax, the sternoclavicular joint dislocates anteriorly, and if driven anteriorly (protracted), the sternoclavicular joint dislocates posteriorly.
      2. **Classification.** The joint may sustain a simple strain (**Type I**) which is not dislocated but painful, have subluxation (**Type II**), or frank dislocation (**Type III**), depending on the degree of ligament disruption (2). More importantly, sternoclavicular dislocations are described according to the direction of dislocation, **anterior or posterior** dislocation.

      An important point to distinguish is the possibility of a medial clavicular physeal fracture which can displace anteriorly or posteriorly as well, thus mimicking a dislocation. This physis does not close until the early 20s and should be suspected under the age of 25.

      As an aside, there is an atraumatic type of dislocation due to ligamentous laxity, but emphasis in this chapter will remain on the traumatic variety.
   B. **Diagnosis**
      1. **History and physical exam.** The history always is significant for a high-energy mechanism, usually a motor vehicle collision. The patient should be asked about the presence of shortness of breath and difficulty breathing or swallowing. Hoarseness and stridor should be documented. Pain is well localized and associated with swelling and ecchymosis. There is usually a palpable and mobile prominence just anterior and lateral to the sternal notch in the case of the more common anterior dislocation, or perhaps a puckering of the skin with a sense of fluctuance due to a posterior dislocation. Chest auscultation and a thorough neurovascular exam to the ipsilateral extremity is important to document early.
      2. **Radiographs.** A **serendipity** x-ray view of the shoulder is a 40-degree cephalic tilt view centered on the manubrium (3). In this view, an anterior dislocation will be manifested with a superior appearing clavicular head.

      Once suspected, a computed tomography (CT) examination with 2-mm cut intervals should also be obtained to visualize the location and extent of

dislocation, evaluate the retrosternal region for soft tissue injury, differentiate between medial clavicle fractures, or possibly elucidate a physis (when it appears above the age of 18) injury.

C. Treatment

1. **Nonoperative.** The majority of sternoclavicular injuries are anterior dislocations, and these should be treated nonoperativley with the expectation of good functional results and usually with complete resolution of pain (3). Cosmetic asymmetry will remain, closed reduction will not remain reduced, and no brace has been proven to be efficacious in this regard. This expectant result also holds true for the growth plate injuries which are displaced anteriorly.

2. **Operative.** An acute posterior dislocation should undergo a manipulative reduction to unlock the retrosternal clavicular head. The rationale for the need for closed reduction relates to the concern that impingement on critical structures may yield late sequelae from erosion or irritation (4).

    A pointed bone tenaculum may be useful to grab the head of the clavicle and pull it back to its proper relation to the manubrium. A roll between the shoulder blades while the patient is supine, in combination with lateral traction of the abducted arm, is a helpful adjunctive maneuver. Due to possible violation of critical structures in the mediastinum, anesthesia should always be on hand to manage the airway, and a thoracic surgeon should always be on standby during the procedure. Performing the reduction maneuver under general anesthesia with optimum airway control should be considered.

    Many authors have described techniques for stabilization of the unstable sternoclavicular joint using various tendon reconstructions and/or Kirschner wires with mixed results (5). A warning against the use of smooth wires is restated throughout the literature due to the problem of migration.

3. **Follow-up.** A sling may be used for 1 month to support the extremity during the acute phase of pain during a period of relative immobility. Motion and function should be allowed to advance as discomfort allows. Shorter or longer periods with relative rest are required according to which type (I, II, or III) dislocation is present. The patient may need reassurance for months during a period of gradually resolving symptoms.

4. **Complications.** Retrosternal dislocations are frequently missed, likely due to the lack of physical exam findings in the context of a multiply injured patient (6). Missed or late diagnosis of associated injuries of the mediastinum and brachial plexus are well documented. Failure of fixation, hardware migration, and redislocation have also been reported after operative stabilization and are likely due to the high forces acting on this main articulation between the upper extremity and the axial skeleton (7). Lastly, arthritic symptoms of the sternoclavicular joint are not uncommon, and many authors have described resection of the clavicular head to address refractory pain (8).

II. ACROMIOCLAVICULAR INJURIES

A. General information

1. **Anatomy and mechanism.** The acromioclavicular joint is a synovial, diarthroidal joint that contains a small, round meniscus composed of fibrocartilage much like the knee. The static linkage of the lateral clavicle to the upper extremity is via the coracoclavicular and acromioclavicular ligaments as well as the joint capsule. The acromioclavicular AC joint capsule is strongest at its superior and posterior margin (9). The scapula is suspended from the clavicle via the coracoclavicular ligaments, which run from the base of the coracoid to the undersurface of the clavicle (**Fig. 14-1**).

    The acromioclavicular dislocation, commonly referred to as a shoulder separation, is a much more common injury, likely due to its more vulnerable position on the lateral aspect of the shoulder. The joint absorbs direct force with any blow to the shoulder such as the most common mechanism of a fall on the shoulder.

2. **Classification (Fig. 14-2).** The Tossy classification was the first to grade acromioclavicular dislocations (Types I–III). Rockwood modified this classification by

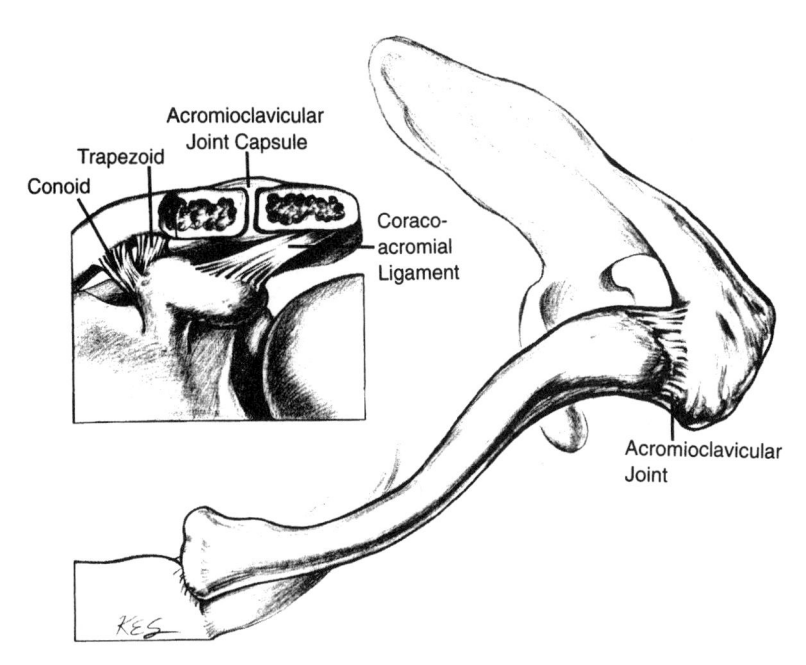

Figure 14-1. This illustration highlights the anatomy of the acromioclavicular joint. The joint capsule as well as the conoid and trapezoid portions of the coracoclavicular ligament are the static stabilizers of the the acromioclavicular joint. (From Hansen ST, Swiontkowski MF. *Orthopaedic trauma protocols.* New York: Raven Press, 1993:80, with permission.)

adding three more types (IV, V, and VI), based on directions of displacement (10). The joint may sustain a simple strain with minimal displacement referred to as a **Type I**. The **Type II** injury is described as being displaced superiorly less than one half the diameter of the clavicle and is thought to be associated with complete tearing of the acromioclavicular ligaments but relative sparing of the coracoclavicular ligaments. The **Type III** dislocation represents complete disruption of the coracoclavicular and acromioclavicular ligaments with superior displacement. A **Type IV** acromioclavicular dislocation is complete and displaced posteriorly; whereas a **Type V** is an extreme variation of Type III, where the clavicle buttonholes through the trapezius into the subcutaneous tissue and thus is associated with much more stripping of trapezius and deltoid. The **Type VI** dislocation is an inferior dislocation under the coracoid process.

B. Diagnosis
  1. **History and physical exam.** The history usually details a fall to the shoulder, and it is associated with well-localized pain. The acromioclavicular joint is typically swollen and point tender. If a visual or palpable stepoff exists, or the distal clavicle feels reducible, then there is at least a Type II injury. In Types III to VI, the physical findings are dramatic.
  2. **Radiographs.** Typically, an anteroposterior x-ray of the shoulder reveals the injury, though imaging of the joint can be enhanced with a 10-degree cephalic tilt view. Visualization of both acromioclavicular joints on the same large x-ray cassette helps to understand relative displacement. Such a radiograph taken with the patient hanging weights in each hand was a popular study but has fallen into disfavor because it is painful and does not change management. The examiner looks for increased distance between the coracoid and the clavicle.

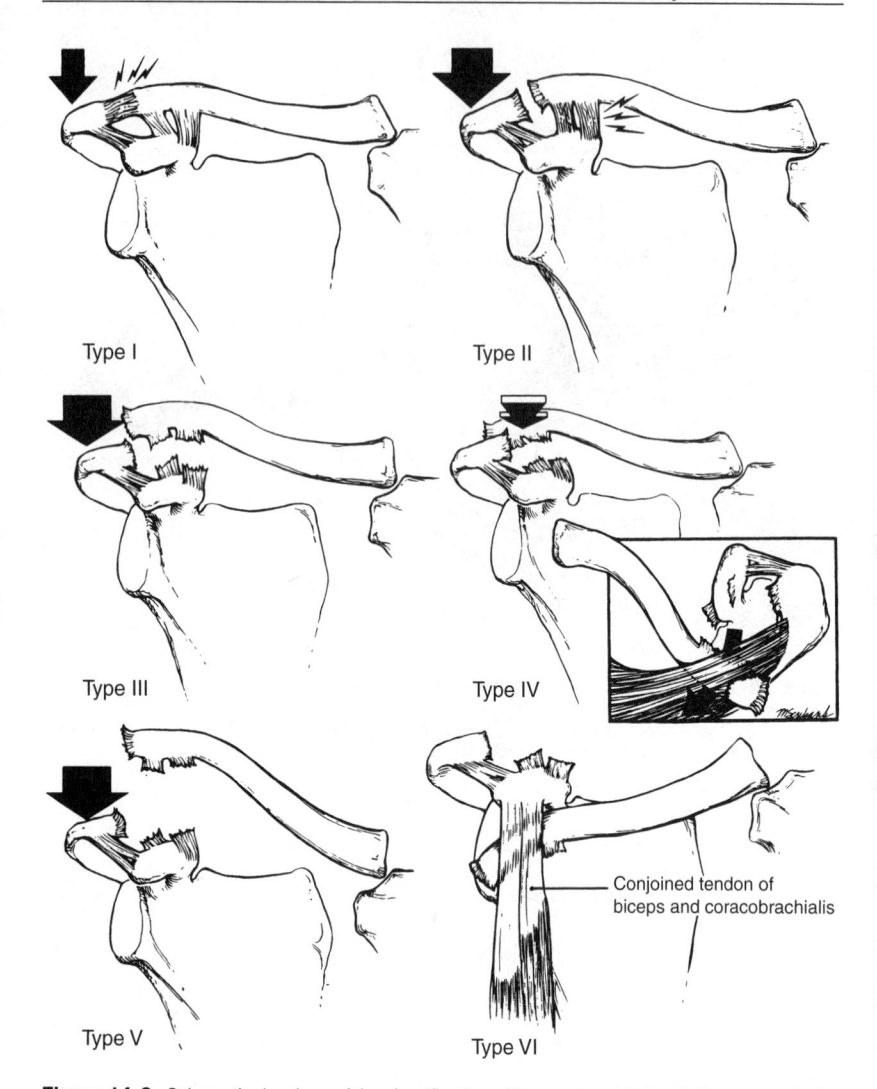

Figure 14-2. Schematic drawings of the classification of ligamentous injuries that can occur to the acromioclavicular ligament. **Type I:** A mild force applied to the point of the shoulder does not disrupt either the acromioclavicular or the coracoclavicular ligaments. **Type II:** A moderate to heavy force applied to the point of the shoulder will disrupt the acromioclavicular ligaments, but the coracoclavicular ligaments remain intact. **Type III:** When a severe force is applied to the point of the shoulder, both the acromioclavicular and coracoclavicular ligaments are disrupted. **Type IV:** In this major injury, not only are the acromioclavicular and coracoclavicular ligaments disrupted but also the distal end of the clavicle is displaced posteriorly into or through the trapezius muscle. **Type V:** A violent force has been applied to the point of the shoulder, not only rupturing the acromioclavicular and coracoclavicular ligaments but also disrupting the deltoid and trapezius muscle attachments and creating a major separation between the clavicle and the acromion. **Type VI:** Another major injury is an inferior dislocation of the distal end of the clavicle to the subcoracoid position. The acromioclavicular and coracoclavicular ligaments are disrupted. (From Rockwood CA, Williams GR, Young DC. Injuries to the acromioclavicular joint. In: Rockwood CR, Green DP, Bucholz RW, et al., eds. *Fractures in adults,* 4th ed. Philadelphia, PA: Lippincott-Raven, 1996:1354, with permission.)

C. Treatment

1. **Nonoperative.** Type I and II acromioclavicular injuries should be treated nonoperativley with the expectation of good functional results and usually with complete resolution of pain (11). Ice should be provided in the acute setting to relieve swelling, as welll as to support the arm against gravity. As is the case for the sternoclavicular dislocation, a closed reduction will not remain reduced, and no brace has been proven to be efficacious in this regard.

   As for Type III dislocations, clinical studies comparing operative versus nonoperative treatment seem to indicate that there is no benefit from surgical treatment (11–14), though some experts believe that the overhead throwing athlete and manual laborer should undergo reconstruction (10).

2. **Operative.** Many surgical procedures have been described to repair an acromioclavicular dislocation with the goal of preventing superior migration. The strategy is either to fix the distal clavicle directly to the acromion or to augment the coracoclavicular ligaments to maintain a reduced joint. Some surgeons advocate a combination of these two strategies to maintain the reduction against the great forces acting to displace the clavicle. Though each strategy can be employed in the acute or delayed setting, if a reconstruction is done late, it is usually combined with a distal clavicle resection.

   The most widely known procedure is the Weaver-Dunn (15), and most surgeons augment some variation of this repair with fixation across the acromioclavicular joint, into the coracoid, or around the base of the coracoid and clavicle like a sling. The Weaver-Dunn itself involves bringing up the coracoclavicular ligament through the end of a resected distal clavicle.

   A new device called the hook plate is gaining popularity. The plate is fixed to the cephalad border of the distal clavicle, and a terminal hook sweeps under the acromion so the clavicle is restrained from springing superiorly.

3. **Follow-up.** As is the case with the sternoclavicular dislocation, a sling may be used for a few weeks to support the extremity during the acute phase of pain. A period of relative immobility is instituted, but motion is advanced as discomfort allows. Shorter or longer periods with relative rest are required according to which Type (I–III) of injury is present. Often the Type I and II injuries hurt for a longer period of time than the Type III injuries due to partial communication of the joint surfaces and tethering of partially torn ligamentous structures. The patient may need reassurance for months during a period of gradually resolving symptoms.

4. **Complications.** Occasionaly, symptomatic posttraumatic osteolysis or arthritis of the acromioclavicular joint develops. An arthroscopic or open resection of the distal clavicle can be done to resect the distal 1.5 to 2.0 cm of bone, and results have generally been favorable (16).

   Most of the complications related to surgery relate to failure of fixation causing chronic symptomatic instability. Hardware failure such as slippage of Kirschner wires or cutout of coracoclavicular screws, as well as graft or suture cutting through the distal clavicle, are not uncommon events and underscore the technically demanding nature of the reconstruction.

HCMC Treatment Recommendations
AC injuries

- *Diagnosis:* Anteroposterior shoulder radiograph, 15-degree cephalad oblique radiograph, clinical examination
- *Treatment:* Grades I–III, sling for comfort for 7–10 days, then range-of-motion exercises
- *Indications for surgery:* Grade IV, V, or VI injuries
- *Recommended technique:* Subcoracoid suture loop with coracoclavicular (CC) ligament and deltotrapezial fascial repair

References

1. Yeh GL, Williams GR Jr. Conservative management of sternoclavicular injuries. *Orthop Clin North Am* 2000;31:189–203.
2. Wirth MA, Rockwood CA Jr. Acute and chronic traumatic injuries to the shoulder joint. *J Am Acad Orthop Surg* 1996;4:268–278.
3. Rockwood CA Jr., Wirth MA. Disorders of the sternoclavicular joint. In: Rockwood CA Jr, Matsen FA III, eds. *The shoulder*. Philadelphia, PA: WB Saunders, 1990: 477–525.
4. Sclamberg S, Visotsky J. Sternoclavicular Injuries. In: Mirzayan R, Itamura JM. eds. *Shoulder and elbow trauma*, New York: Thieme Medical Publishers, 2004:135–146.
5. Spencer EE, Kuhn JE. Biomechanical analysis of reconstructions for sternoclavicular joint instability. *J Bone Joint Surg (Am)* 2004;86:98–105.
6. Thomas DP, Davies A, Hoddinott HC. Posterior sternoclavicular dislocations—a diagnosis easily missed. *Ann R Coll Surg Engl* 1999;81:201–204.
7. Flatow EL. The biomechanics of the acromioclavicular, sternoclavicular, and scapulothoracic joints. In: Heckman JD. ed. *Instructional course lectures 42*, Rosemont, IL: American Academy of Orthopaedic Surgeons, 1993:237–245.
8. Rockwood CA, Groh GI, Wirth MA, et al. Resection arthroplasty of the sternoclavicular joint. *J Bone Joint Surg (Am)* 1997;79:387–393.
9. Fukuda K, Craig EV, An KN, et al. Biomechanical study of the ligamentous system of the acromioclavicular joint. *J Bone Joint Surg* 1986;68A:434–439.
10. Rockwood CA Jr. Disorders of the acromioclavicular joint. In: Rockwood CA Jr, Matsen FA III, eds. *The shoulder*. Philadelphia, PA: WB Saunders, 1985:413–476.
11. Taft TN, Wilson FC, Oglesby LW. Dislocation of the acromioclavicular joint—an end result study. *J Bone Joint Surg (Am)* 1987;69:1045–1051.
12. Bannister GC, Wallace WA, Stablforth PG, et al. The management of acute acromioclavicular dislocation: a randomized prospective controlled trial. *J Bone Joint Surg (Br)* 1989;71:848–850.
13. Galpin RD, Hawkins RJ, Grainger RW. A comparative analysis of operative versus non-operative treatment of grade III acromioclavicular separations. *Clin Orthop* 1985;193:150–155.
14. Smith MJ, Stewart MJ. Acute acromioclavicular separations: a 20-year study. *Am J Sports Med* 1979;7:62.
15. Weaver JK, Dunn HK. Treatment of acromioclavicular injuries, especially complete acromioclavicular separation. *J Bone Joint Surg (Am)* 1972;54:1187–1194.
16. Martin SD, Baumgarten TE, Andrews JR. Arthroscopic resection of the distal aspect of the clavicle with concomitant subacromial decompression. *J Bone Joint Surg (Am)* 2001;83:328.

Selected Historical Readings

Allman FL. Fractures and ligamentous injuries of the clavicle and its articulations. *J Bone Joint Surg (Am)* 1967;49:774.

Tossy JD, Mead NC, Sigmond HM. Acromioclavicular separations: useful and practical classification for treatment. *Clin Orthop* 1963;28:111–119.

Urist MR. Complete dislocation of the acromioclavicular joint: the nature of the traumatic lesion and effective methods of treatment with an analysis of 41 cases. *J Bone Joint Surg (Am)* 1946;28:813–837.

Weaver JK, Dunn HK. Treatment of acromioclavicular injuries, especially complete acromioclavicular separation. *J Bone Joint Surg (Am)* 1972;54(A):1187–1194.

ACUTE SHOULDER INJURIES   15

I. **GENERAL PRINCIPLES**
   A. **Anatomy.** The ability to place your hand functionally above your head, behind your back, and at all points in between is largely dependent on the shoulder's extreme range of motion. This degree of flexibility defines it as an unconstrained joint. The stability can be divided into static and dynamic constraints. Statically, there is a small flat glenoid surface articulating with the large humeral head. The depth of the glenoid cavity is augmented by the labrum, which also serves as the anchor point for the capsular ligaments to the glenoid and the origin of the biceps. The glenoid articulation and the labrum in themselves have little constraint to the glenoid humeral joint. The ligaments serve as additional static restraints at the extreme range of motion. The dynamic component of stability for the glenohumeral joint comes from the surrounding musculature. The rotator cuff muscles (supraspinatus, infraspinatus, and teres minor) plus the subscapularis and the long head of the biceps are very important dynamic stabilizers (3). Another degree of dynamic stability comes through the scapulothoracic articulation which provides one third of the total active motion of the shoulder girdle. The position of the scapula is the foundation off which the glenohumeral joint functions. The periscapular muscles are extremely important in positioning the glenoid cavity correctly as well as providing a stable platform from which the glenohumeral joint functions. The neurovascular bundle lies directly anterior and inferior to the glenohumeral joint, which accounts for the frequency of neurovascular injuries, especially with anterior dislocations that are associated with shoulder trauma.
   B. **Differential diagnosis.** The majority of patients presenting with acute shoulder pain are suffering from either a dislocation, fracture, or muscle rupture. Still, it is important to consider that a variety of other entities may cause acute shoulder pain including:
      1. Cervical disc disease (C5 nerve root)
      2. Thoracic outlet
      3. Brachial neuritis
      4. Diaphragmatic irritation
      5. Pleural irritation
      6. Superior sulcus tumors (Pancoast tumor or metastatic disease)
      7. Cholecystitis (right shoulder)
      8. Cardiac symptoms (typically left shoulder)
   C. The majority of shoulder disorders can be managed and produce a good outcome by nonsurgical treatment which centers around physical therapy to regain the strength of muscles around the joint and range-of-motion exercises to maintain flexibility.
II. **SHOULDER DISLOCATIONS**
   A. **Classification.** Approximately 50% of all major joint dislocations involve the glenohumeral joint. Dislocations are commonly classified by direction (anterior, inferior, posterior, or multidirectional), onset (acute, recurrent, chronic), and by etiology (traumatic, minimally traumatic, atraumatic, microanterior instability). Anterior dislocations are the most common. Dislocations that occur in patients younger than 20 years old typically involve an avulsion of the ligaments and labrum from the glenoid. Dislocations that occur in patients older than 30 years of age tend to involve interligamentous tears. Dislocations in patients older than 50

are often associated with rotator cuff tears and/or greater tuberosity fractures. The older the patient, the lower the rate of recurrence of dislocations, but older patients also have a higher rate of posttraumatic shoulder stiffness (13).

B. Anterior dislocations
  1. **Mechanism of injury.** The injury usually results from a traumatic event in which the position of the arm is in an externally rotated and forward-flexed or an abducted position.
     a. In patients younger than 20 years of age, the anterior capsule and labrum are avulsed from the glenoid, occasionally with a small fragment of bone (Bankart lesion). The humeral head dislocates anterior to the glenoid fossa and under the coracoid process. A compression fracture may occur on the posterolateral humeral head (Hill-Sachs lesion) from impaction of the head on the anterior edge of the glenoid (2).
     b. In patients older than 40 years of age, intrasubstance failure of the anterior capsule and an acute rotator cuff tear can occur. An acute rotator cuff tear can be difficult to repair if not detected within the first 6 weeks postinjury.
     c. Recent basic science studies have shown that sectioning of the anterior capsule alone does not cause gross anterior instability. Damage to the posterior or superior capsule must also occur for a complete anterior dislocation to occur.
  2. **Examination.** Individuals with an acute dislocation hold their arm in an adducted position. There is a loss of symmetry of their shoulders and the humeral head can be palpated anterior and inferior to the coracoid process. Any attempt at range of motion of the shoulder is extremely painful. A thorough neurovascular check of the upper extremity is necessary before any attempt is made to reduce the dislocation. Attention to checking the sensory function of the axillary nerve over the lateral aspect of the shoulder is important.
  3. **Roentgenograms.** In all patients with a suspected initial dislocation of the shoulder, a standard trauma series should be obtained (10). This series includes an anteroposterior and a transscapular lateral ("Y") view. If the presence and direction of the dislocation are not clearly evident, an axillary view is obtained. This view is difficult to obtain and painful for the patient; it may require physician assistance to position the patient's shoulder. Any associated tuberosity fractures or epiphyseal injuries should be clearly visualized.
  4. **Treatment of the first dislocation**
     a. **Reduction without general anesthesia.** Prompt reduction of the dislocation provides a great deal of pain relief. To achieve a gentle and pain-free reduction, muscle relaxation and pain relief are required. Multiple methods of reduction have been described, but the author prefers one of the following methods:
        i. **Prone reduction** under lidocaine block (14). The patient is allowed to remain sitting on the examination table, and the posterior aspect of the shoulder is sterilely prepped. Ten to 20 mL of 1% lidocaine are injected into the glenohumeral joint posteriorly. The patient is then placed prone on the examination table with the involved arm and shoulder hanging in a dependent position over the edge of the table. A 10-lb weight is suspended from the patient's wrist. After 10 to 15 minutes, good analgesia and relaxation are present and the shoulder can be reduced by elevation and forward rotation of the medial border of the scapula.
        ii. **Reduction by traction.** If the first method fails, the patient is repositioned supine and additional intravenous (IV) sedation is administered. A sheet is placed around the patient centered in the axillary region. An assistant holds the two ends of the sheet above the patient and provides countertraction while the physician grasps the forearm of the involved shoulder and gently pulls in a line of 30 degrees of abduction and 20 to 30 degrees of forward flexion. Sustained traction for 5 minutes may be necessary. Vigorous and forceful attempts

at reduction are to be avoided since this may result in a fracture, especially in older osteopenic patients.
- b. **Reduction under anesthesia.** If the aforementioned methods fail or if a significant fracture is present, a reduction under general anesthetic with complete muscle relaxation is indicated. The shoulder typically reduces easily with little risk of further damage to the glenohumeral joint or its surrounding structures.
5. **Postreduction treatment.** The length of immobilization has no effect on the incidence of redislocations (12). The shoulder should be immobilized for a brief period as needed for pain control after a dislocation or subluxation episode. A range-of-motion and rotator cuff strengthening program is initiated early, but the extremes of range of motion for forward flexion or external rotation are avoided. Patients are allowed to return to sports and other activities when the shoulder has good strength and minimal apprehension in an abducted, externally rotated position (1, 6). A general rule is the younger the patient, the higher the possibility of recurrent instability (9).
6. **Recurrent dislocations or subluxations.** If necessary, the shoulder is reduced as in **B.4** (above). Occasionally, if witnessed "on the field" and the evaluation suggests a recurrent dislocation without fracture, then an attempt for reduction can be made prior to radiographic imaging. If anesthesia is not available, reduction is the best pain relief. A postreduction, physical therapy program is prescribed as in **B.5** (above). Recurrent instability episodes may be painful and disabling. Many different types of surgical repairs have been described (12,15,16,19). The author prefers either an open or arthroscopic Bankart repair or capsular shift reconstruction (15,17). The open type of repair has been associated with success rates of 97% with few significant complications. Arthroscopically assisted repairs are technically possible but have not yet achieved success rates comparable to open capsular repairs, especially in athletes in high contact sports.
7. **Complications**
   - a. **Damage to the nerves** originating with the brachial plexus occurs in 5% to 14% of shoulder dislocations. The axillary nerve and musculocutaneous nerve are most commonly injured. Most injuries are a neuropraxia, and a full recovery is typical. The same is true with postoperative neurologic injuries. While the injured nerve is recovering, it is important not to allow any secondary contractures of the joint to develop.
   - b. **Rotator cuff tears** are common in patients older than 40 years with an anterior dislocation. If good range of motion and strength have not returned within 3 to 4 weeks after the injury, visualization of the rotator cuff with magnetic resonance imaging (MRI) or ultrasound is indicated.

C. Posterior dislocations
1. **Mechanism of injury.** Posterior instability results from a fall on an adducted and forward flexed arm, which drives the head of the humerus posterior to the glenoid fossa. A compression fracture of the anterolateral aspect of the humeral head may develop (reverse Hill-Sachs lesion). In younger individuals, an avulsion of the posterior labrum with a small fragment of the posterior glenoid rim (reverse Bankart lesion) may occur. Seizures or electrocution are other mechanisms that often produce posterior instability (7).
2. **Examination.** An obvious clinical deformity is typically not present and the patient may be complaining of only minimal symptoms. Many posterior dislocations are not diagnosed and reduced in the emergency department. External rotation of the shoulder is limited and painful, and is the hallmark of a posterior shoulder dislocation.
3. **Roentgenograms.** Anteroposterior views often are normal and misleading except that the arm is positioned in a markedly internally rotated position, which produces a "light bulb sign" with the proximal humerus. A transscapular "Y" view and an axillary view show the posterior position of the humeral head.

4. **Treatments.** Muscle relaxation via IV sedation is recommended. Reductions can usually be obtained by gentle traction on the arm with an additional anterior and laterally directed force applied to the posterior aspect of the humeral head. Postreduction treatment is similar to that for anterior dislocation (**B.5.**) except internal rotation and adduction extremes are avoided. If the shoulder dislocates immediately after being reduced, the arm should be braced in a neutral rotation and an abducted position for 4 weeks to maintain stability. Posterior dislocations that result from seizures or electrocutions may have large or reverse Hill-Sachs lesions that lead to further instability episodes.
5. **Recurrent dislocations** that occur as a result of traumatic events and have evidence of ligament damage may be treated with a reverse capsular shift. Many patients with posterior instability do not have a history of a significant traumatic event that initiated the instability and may be able to **voluntarily dislocate** or sublux their shoulder. These patients have poor operative results and should undergo treatment with physical therapy and activity or lifestyle restrictions (5).

D. **Multidirectional instability (MDI)**
1. **Mechanism of injury.** MDI is diagnosed when there is clinical evidence that the shoulder is unstable in two or more directions. There is often no history of significant trauma and the patient may be able to voluntarily dislocate the shoulder.
2. **Examination.** The typical patient is a "double-jointed" adolescent female. A sulcus sign is present and the patient is apprehensive with the arm in positions that stress both the anterior and posterior capsule.
3. **Roentgenograms.** Often, radiographs are normal. The presence of a Hill-Sachs or a reverse Hill-Sachs lesion is detected on a Stryker notch view but often is not in fact present.
4. **Treatment.** Nonoperative treatment is strongly advised because operative management has a high failure rate (18). A procedure using thermal energy to arthroscopically "shrink" the redundant capsule has not proven successful and has been associated with significant complications including capsular necrosis and chondrolysis (8).

E. **Inferior dislocations.** Inferior dislocations are rare. The patient's arm is locked in an overhead position. Reduction is obtained by IV sedation and relaxation. The arm is then reduced with lateral distraction while the arm is brought out of an abducted position.

III. **ACUTE TEARS OF THE ROTATOR CUFF**
A. **Mechanism of injury.** Acute tears of the rotator cuff are rare and occur mainly in individuals younger than 40 years old who have a history of significant trauma. Attritional tears of the rotator cuff are more common and occur in older individuals (see **Chap. 16**).
B. **Examination** (see **Chap. 16**).
C. **Roentgenograms.** Damage to the glenohumeral joint, including the greater tuberosity, is best assessed on an anteroposterior view, obtained with the arm in 30 degrees of external rotation. An outlet view and an axillary view should also be obtained. Young individuals who are suspected of having a rotator cuff tear on history or examination should undergo an MRI scan or an ultrasound evaluation to assess the status of their rotator cuff.
D. **Treatment.** In young or active patients with a true acute rotator cuff tear, early (within 3 months) operative repair is indicated. Early repair is also indicated in those cases associated with a displaced avulsion fracture of the greater tuberosity (4). Displacement of a greater tuberosity fragment by more than 1 cm correlates highly with an acute rotator cuff tear.

IV. **RUPTURES OF THE LONG HEAD OF THE BICEPS BRACHII**
A. **Mechanism of injury.** Injuries of the long head of the biceps (LHB) tendon may occur with forceful elbow flexion or hand supination. Eighty percent of the cases are associated with ongoing rotator cuff problems and shoulder impingement syndrome. Steroid use for body conditioning is an increasingly common etiology.

B. **Examination.** A visible asymmetry of the injured versus noninjured upper arm is evident when the patient is asked to "make a biceps" muscle. This deformity is called a "Popeye" sign.
C. **Treatment.** Ruptures of the LHB tendon are treated nonoperatively. The indications for repair are mainly cosmetic in nature because little functional disability results. In patients with evidence of impingement syndrome, an appropriate workup of the rotator cuff is indicated, particularly in active patients or those under 60 years of age.
V. **RUPTURE OF THE PECTORALIS MAJOR.** The pectoralis major muscle or tendon typically ruptures with a bench press lift, a seated fly lift, or a similar functional maneuver. The patient has pain and an ecchymosis in the anterior shoulder. On examination, there is a loss or defect in the anterior axillary line. Treatment is usually symptomatic except in the heavy laborer or athlete in whom early operative repair is indicated. Ruptures at the muscle tendon junction are difficult to repair and have a worse outcome than tears at the bone/tendon or tendon/tendon interface. A preoperative MRI scan is indicated in those individuals for whom operative repair is being considered to determine at what level the defect has occurred.
VI. **SCAPULAR FRACTURES.** These injuries are frequently treated **nonoperatively**, with early range of motion of the shoulder girdle. Displaced fractures involving greater than 25% percent of the articular surface of the glenoid or glenoid neck fractures with medial displacement are generally treated operatively to reduce the risk of glenohumeral instability or arthritis (11).

HCMC Treatment Recommendations

Diagnosis: Anteroposterior, transscapular lateral, axillary lateral radiographs, clinical examination

Treatment: Reduction in emergency department under analgesia or intraarticular lidocaine, sling for comfort followed by assisted range-of-motion exercises beginning at 2 to 3 weeks after injury

Indications for surgery: Recurrent dislocation

Recommended technique: Bankart repair, open or arthroscopic depending on activity level, dominant or nondominant shoulder, and cosmetic concerns

---

References

1. Arciero RA, Wheeler JH, Ryan JB, et al. Arthroscopic bankart repair vs. non-operative treatment for acute, initial, anterior shoulder dislocations. *Am J Sports Med* 1994;22:589–594.
2. Baker CL, Uribe JW, Whitman C. Arthroscopic evaluation of acute initial anterior shoulder dislocations. *Am J Sports Med* 1990;28:25–28.
3. Bassett RW, Browne AO, Morrey BF, et al. Glenohumeral muscle force and moment mechanics in a position of shoulder instability. *J Biomech* 1990;23:405–415.
4. Bassett RW, Cofield RH. Acute tears of the rotator cuff: the timing of surgical repair. *Clin Orthop* 1983;175:18–24.
5. Bigliani LU, Pollock RG, McIlveen SJ, et al. Shift of the posteroinferior aspect of the capsule for recurrent posterior glenohumeral instability. *J Bone Joint Surg (Am)* 1995;77:1011–1020.
6. Bottoni CR, Wilckens JH, DeBeradino TM, et al. A prospective, randomized evaluation of arthroscopic stabilization versus nonoperative treatment in patients with acute, traumatic, first-time shoulder dislocations. *Am J Sports Med* 2002;30:576–580.
7. Buhler M, Gerber C. Shoulder instability related to epileptic seizures. *J Shoulder Elbow Surg* 2002;11:339–344.
8. Burkhead WZ, Rockwood CA. Treatment of instability of the shoulder with an exercise program. *J Bone Joint Surg (Am)* 1992;74:890–896.
9. Deitch J, Mehlman CT, Obbehat A, et al. Traumatic anterior shoulder dislocation in adolescents. *Am J Sports Med* 2003;31:758–763.

10. Engebretsen L, Craig EV. Radiologic features of shoulder instability. *Clin Orthop* 1993;291:29–44.
11. Hardegger FH, Simpson L, Weber BG. The operative treatment of scapular fractures. *J Bone Joint Surg (Br)* 1984;66:725–731.
12. Hovelius L. Anterior dislocation of the shoulder in teenagers and young adults: five-year prognosis. *J Bone Joint Surg (Am)* 1987;69:393–399.
13. Johnson JR, Bayley JI. Early complications of acute anterior dislocation of the shoulder in the middle-aged and elderly patient. *Injury* 1982;13:431–434.
14. Lippitt SB, Kennedy JP, Thompson TR. Intraarticular lidocaine verses intravenous analgesia in the reduction of dislocated shoulders. *Orthop Trans* 1992;16:230.
15. Morgan CD, Bodenstab AB. Arthroscopic bankart suture repair: technique and early results. *Arthroscopy* 1987;3:111–122.
16. Morrey BF, James JM. Recurrent anterior dislocation of the shoulder: long-term follow up of the putti-platt and bankart procedures. *J Bone Joint Surg (Am)* 1976;58:252–256.
17. Rowe CR, Pierce DS, Clark JG. Voluntary dislocation of the shoulder. *J Bone Joint Surg (Am)* 1973;55:445–460.
18. Rowe CR. Acute and recurrent dislocations of the shoulder. *J Bone Joint Surg (Am)* 1962;44:998–1008.
19. Torg JS, Balduini FC, Bonci C, et al. A modified Bristow-Helfet-May procedure for recurrent dislocation and subluxation of the shoulder: report of two hundred and twelve cases. *J Bone Joint Surg (Am)* 1987;69:904–913.

Selected Historical Readings

Bankart ASB. Recurrent or habitual dislocation of the shoulder joint. *BMJ* 1923;2:1132.

Mosley HF. The basic lesions of recurrent anterior dislocation of the shoulder. *Surg Clin North Am* 1963;43:631.

NONACUTE SHOULDER DISORDERS   16

I. **ROTATOR CUFF DISORDERS**
   A. **Anatomy.** The muscle tendon units of the supraspinatus, infraspinatus, and teres minor compose the rotator cuff. Each has its own specific muscle body but they coalesce together into one tendon as they pass through the subacromial space. The borders of the subacromial space are as follows: superiorly, the undersurface of the acromion and the acromioclavicular (AC) joint; anteriorly, the coracoacromial ligament and coracoid; inferiorly, the humeral head. The subacromial bursa also exists in the subacromial space above the rotator cuff but underneath the acromion. The long head of the bicep tendon and the subscapularis muscles are important anterior stabilizers of the glenohumeral joint.
   B. **Mechanism of injury.** Any anatomic influences that narrow the already confining subacromial space have the potential to compromise, in particularly, the superspinatus tendon and irritate the SA bursa. Thickening of the bursa, undersurface spurring of the AC joint, instability of the glenohumeral joint, or changes in the shape of the acromion (**Fig. 16-1**) are the most common reasons for rotator cuff compromise. This process of rotator cuff attrition is manifested as **impingement syndrome**. The process of cuff disease begins with bursitis and reversible tendinosis and gradually progresses to full-thickness cuff pathology over time.
   C. **History.** The typical patient with impingement syndrome is older than age 40 and complains of anterolateral shoulder pain, which is worse with overhead activities and positionally at night.
   D. **Examination.** Examination begins by general inspection of the anterior and posterior shoulder. Clearly visible atrophy of the posterior shoulder in the region of the supraspinatus and/or infraspinatus muscle belly is an indicator of a large rotator cuff tear. The differential diagnosis for this atrophy would include suprascapular nerve entrapment. Shoulder motion is often symmetric except for a loss of internal rotation. Special tests include those for rotator cuff strength, impingement, and instability. Supraspinatus weakness and pain is usually present to strength testing. Tenderness is present over the anterior rotator cuff and SA bursa. Significant weakness to external rotation strength testing often indicates that a large rotator cuff tear is present.
   E. **Roentgenograms.** Plain roentgenograms should be obtained in patients with a history of acute trauma or in those who do not improve with standard nonoperative treatment. Sclerosis of the greater tuberosity, narrowing of the acromiohumeral distance, or spur formation at the AC joint or the anterior acromion are all evidence of ongoing impingement syndrome. An acromion that has an inferiorly directed hook at its anterior edge is classified as a type III acromion (1) (**Fig. 16-1**). This hooked acromion may predispose some patients to developing anterior rotator cuff pathology by narrowing the SA space. Usually the supraspinatus tendon is affected first. With patients in whom operative intervention is indicated, further imaging studies may be obtained. Arthrograms are widely available and easily used to detect the presence of a rotator cuff tear. However, they do not give reliable information regarding tear location, size, atrophy, or other associated subacromial pathology. A magnetic resonance imaging (MRI) scan, gives more detailed information regarding pathology in the SA space. It is more expensive and may be susceptible to technical problems and misinterpretation. An MRI

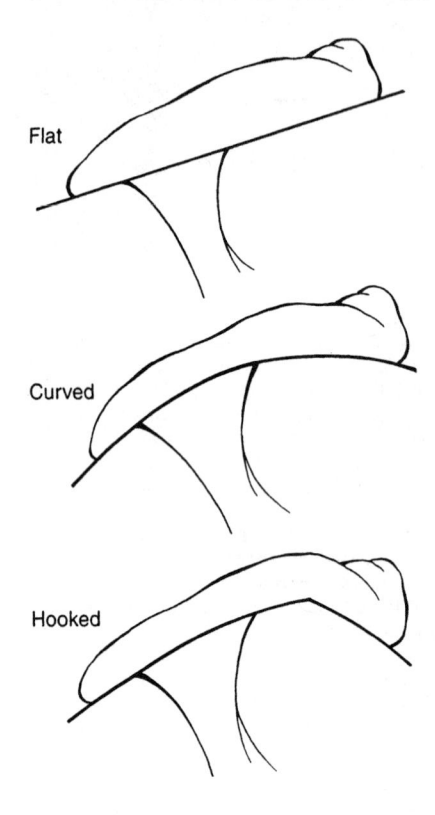

Figure 16-1. Bigliani classification of acromial morphology: type I, flat; type II, curved; type III, hooked. (From Bigliani LU, Morrison DS, April EW. The morphology of the acromion and rotator cuff impingement. *Orthop Trans* 1986; 10:288.)

should only be ordered if it will change treatment recommendation (**Table 16-1**). Physicians without adequate experience in the shoulder exam may wish to refer prior to ordering the MRI. Ultrasonagraphy is another diagnostic test that can, in the hands of an experienced ultrasonagrapher, give good visualization of rotator cuff pathology.

F. **Diagnosis.** The topic of nonacute shoulder disorders often falls into the broad categories of impingement and instability. While the former tends to affect people older than age 30, and instability tends to affect those younger than age 30, there is a large overlap. Additionally, both may occur in the same patient. Impingement is generally the result of either some bursitis, tendinopathy, or rotator cuff tears. These issues will be addressed below. Instability, or a hyper-mobile glenohumeral joint was addressed under the topic of shoulder dislocations in **Chap. 15, II.C.** Additional categories of

---

TABLE 16-1 MRI Scan Indications

1. Shoulder dislocation over age 40.
2. Significant rotator cuff weakness.
3. Family history of rotator cuff disease.
4. Failure to respond to nonsurgical measures (physical therapy, injection).

AC joint arthritis, adhesive capsulitis, arthritis, and scapulothoracic disorders are causes of non-acute shoulder disorders and will be discussed below.

G. Treatment

1. **Bursitis/tendinopathy/impingement (Fig. 16-2).** The focus of treatment for chronic shoulder disorders is physical therapy (PT). PT forms the basis for recovery for those who suffer from impingement-type symptoms (e.g., with bursitis or rotator cuff tendinopathy), instability, adhesive capulitis, scapulothoracic dysfunction, and other nonacute shoulder pathology. The current

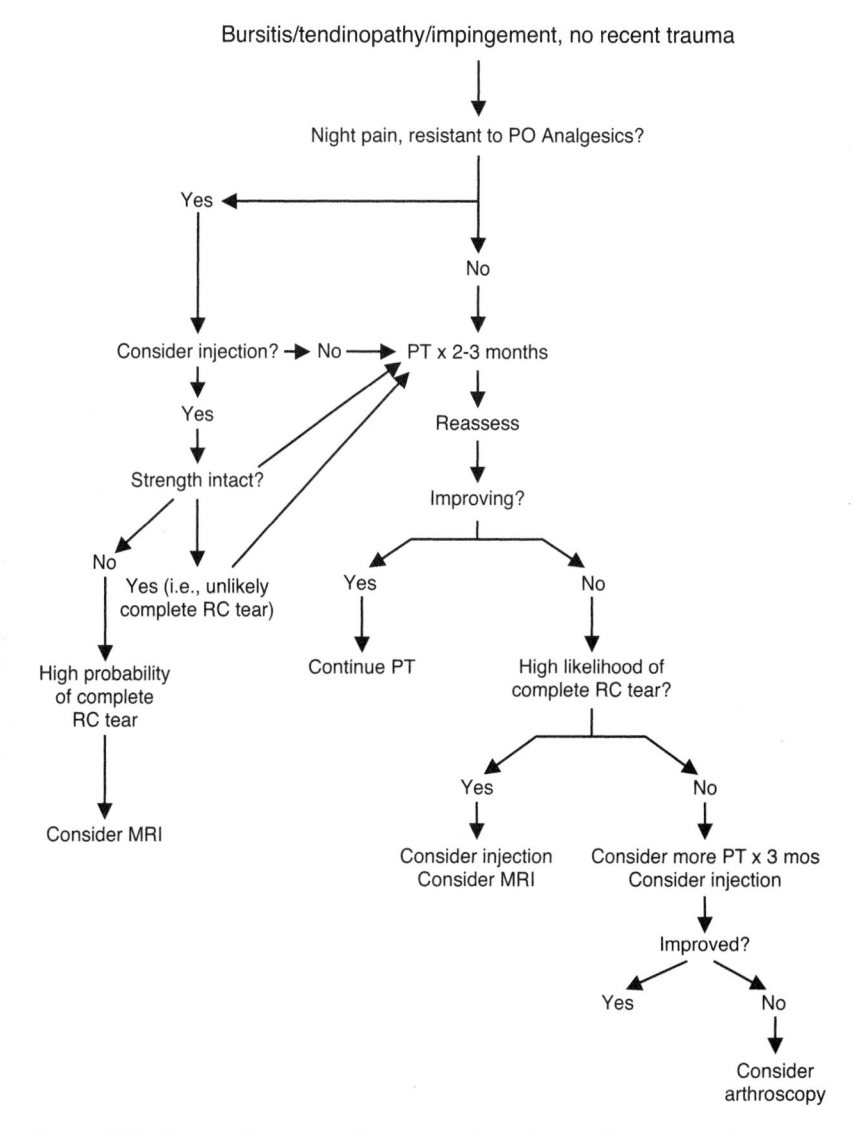

Figure 16-2. Diagram of treatment pathway for bursitis/tendinopathy/impingement with no recent trauma. PT, physical therapy; RC, rotator cuff.

standard for successful treatment is on returning the patient to his or her full range of motion prior to focusing on strength. Poor posture associated with our increasingly inactive lifestyles seems to be cause of poor scapulothoracic stability and subsequent shoulder pain. It is important to ask your physical therapists to address scapular stabilization in the rehabilitation of most patients with chronic shoulder problems. The scapula forms the starting point of the rotator cuff muscles (thus important in rotator cuff tendinopathy), the origin of the acromion (thus important in other causes of impingement), and of the glenoid (thus important in shoulder instability). Our personal preference is for the patient to have at least 6 to12 months of concentrated PT prior to surgery unless otherwise indicated (e.g., if there is a complete, acute rotator cuff tear).

Injections provide another important component in the treatment of nonacute shoulder problems (**Table 16-2**). The most common is an SA injection, for which we prefer a posterolateral approach due to its ease and avoidance of major neurovascular structures (see chapter on injections for details). The SA shoulder injection can be done with either diagnostic or therapeutic goals. Diagnostically, one can theoretically "rule out" a complete rotator cuff tear if a patient who had pain and weakness demonstrates normal strength after an anesthetic injection. Therapeutically, pain relief from an injection is for those who have pain that cannot be treated adequately with oral medications (either due to a lack of efficacy or side effects), those who are unable to perform PT due to pain, and those with night pain that interrupts their sleep.

a. **Nonoperative** treatment is successful in the majority of patients. The cornerstone of treatment is **Physical therapy** to rehabilitate the rotator cuff muscles (especially the supraspinatus), to regain scapulothoracic stability, and to correct any contractures (typically loss of internal rotation). If physical therapy alone is not successful, an **injection** of corticosteroid and lidocaine into the SA space often brings the patient's symptoms under control. If the diagnosis of impingement syndrome is correct, the lidocaine should give an excellent relief of pain for 2 to 3 hours. If no lidocaine effect is obtained, alternative diagnoses should be considered. The steroid typically takes 2 to 4 days to take effect. The indications for an SA injection at the initial visit include significant night pain or symptoms severe enough to make progress in PT difficult.

b. **Operative treatment** is indicated in individuals who fail a minimum 6-month course of nonoperative treatment. The goal of surgery is to open the SA space. This is typically accomplished by excision of the thickened and

TABLE 16-2 Anterior Shoulder Pain

Diagnosis	Initial visit (6–8 weeks)	Second visit (if not improved)	Third visit (6–8 weeks after 2nd visit)
Anterior/lateral pain Posterior/lateral pain Mild restriction of ROM Weakened to rotator cuff strength testing	Physical therapy • Low weight • Free weight SA injection if night pain significant	SA injection Continue PT	X-ray • AP in ER • Outlet • Axillary Consider MRI[a]

[a]See MRI scan indications.
SA, subacromial; PT, physical therapy; AP, anteroposterior; ER, external rotator; ROM, range of motion; MRI, magenetic resonance imaging.

scarred bursa, recession of the coracoacromial ligament, and an anterior acromioplasty. Any other factors (AC joint hypertrophy or glenohumeral instability) that may predispose the patient to impingement syndrome should also be addressed. This opening of the SA space is termed a **decompression**. A decompression may be completed through either open or arthroscopic techniques. Arthroscopic techniques allow an evaluation of the glenohumeral joint for any concomitant pathology. In addition, a patient with an arthroscopic SA decompression recovers approximately 1 month sooner than an open SA decompression.

2. **Rotator cuff tears**
   a. **Younger patients** (younger than 55 years old) or those with true acute tears typically undergo surgical repair. Repairs for complete tears are best done if within 3 months of injury when possible.
   b. **Older patients** often do well with physical therapy and nonoperative treatment. MRI studies of asymptomatic patients older than 60 years of age have shown that 50% have some form of rotator cuff pathology. An SA decompression and rotator cuff repair are indicated only after nonoperative measures have failed. In older, low functional demand patients with large rotator cuff tears, an SA decompression alone often yields good pain relief, but only limited improvement in function. Patients with a massive, irreparable rotator cuff tear and glenohumeral arthritis often respond well to physical therapy and an SA injection. If nonoperative treatment fails, arthoscopic glenohumeral joint debridment and limited SA decompression may be indicated. A hemi-arthroplasty is another acceptable form of operative intervention.

3. **Calcific bursitis.** involves deposition of a calcium salt into the substance of the rotator cuff tendon. This paste-like material may escape into the SA bursa, causing an acute inflammatory bursitis. Severe symptoms of impingement syndrome result. An SA injection with corticosteroids with lidocaine and PT are effective in controlling acute symptoms. If repetitive episodes of pain occur, an arthroscopic excision of the calcific deposit is indicated.

4. **Long head of biceps tendinitis** (see **Chap. 15, IV**) often occurs as part of impingement syndrome and is treated with the same program.

II. **GLENOHUMERAL DISORDERS.** Patients who present with severely limited shoulder range of motion may have a problem with their glenohumral joint, either a bony obstruction (arthritis) or a capsular adhesion (adhesive capsulitis or "frozen shoulder"). Note that these two problems can be distinguished from a rotator cuff tear by noting differences between active and passive range of motion. A patient with a rotator cuff tear may have more passive than active range of motion, whereas, one with true glenohumeral pathology will have equal passive and active range of motion (**Table 16-3**).

A. **Arthritis**
   1. **Etiology.** Arthritis of the glenohumeral joint may be idiopathic (osteoarthritis), secondary to inflammatory disease (rheumatoid or psoriatic arthritis), or posttraumatic. Given that the shoulder is not a weight-bearing joint, symptomatic arthritis of the glenohumeral joint is not as common as arthritis of the knee and hip.

TABLE 16-3   **Diagnostic Range of Motion**

Etiology	Range of motion
Full thickness rotator cuff tear	Passive may be greater than active
Osteoarthritis	Passive = Active
Adhesion capsulitis	Passive = Active

2. **History.** Nonspecific lateral shoulder pain is present, which is made worse with increased activities. Stiffness is also a frequent complaint. Polyarticular complaints should arouse the suspicion of an inflammatory disorder.
3. **Examination** reveals loss of active and passive range of motion, crepitus on joint motion, and mild diffuse muscle atrophy. Strength is usually not significantly affected. Distal neurovascular changes are rare.
4. **Roentgenographic** studies should include an anteroposterior view of the shoulder in 30 degrees of external rotation and an axillary view. Narrowing of the glenohumeral joint space and inferior spur formation on the humeral head is an indication of osteoarthritis. Periarticular erosions are suspicious for inflammatory disease. A computed tomography scan to exactly determine glenoid version or an MRI scan to assess rotator cuff status and glenoid version may be indicated preoperatively.
5. **Treatment**
   a. **Nonoperative treatment** is directed toward controlling the pain with analgesics, injections of the glenohumeral joint with anesthetics and corticosteroids, and improvement of joint mechanics (especially range of motion) with PT and lifestyle modification.
   b. **Operative treatment.** In early cases of inflammatory arthritis, an arthroscopic synovectomy may yield improvement of symptoms. Once the articular surface is eroded to bone, either a hemiarthroplasty, a total shoulder replacement, or an arthrodesis is indicated. A total shoulder replacement results in the best function of the glenohumeral joint and pain relief (2) but may not be indicated in young patients or patients with heavy occupational demands.

B. **Adhesive capsulitis** (frozen shoulder)
1. **Etiology**
   a. Idiopathic adhesive capsulitis results from capsular fibrosis. The pathologic mechanism for this fibrosis is not well understood (3).
   b. Adhesive capsulitis may result from capsular fibrosis from a traumatic or surgical event or may be associated with a systemic disease such as diabetes, thyroid disorders, cervical disc disease, or neoplastic disorders of the thorax.
2. **History.** The patient complains of a deep, achy pain in the shoulder that is present at rest as well as with activities. Complaints of loss of motion follow the onset of the pain by several weeks. A careful past medical history and review of systems is necessary to rule out any systemic causes. Diabetes mellitus and thyroid abnormalities often predispose people to adhesive capsulitis. Distal neurovascular complaints are rare.
3. **Examination.** A global loss of active and passive range of motion is noted. Internal and external rotation are typically affected first. Nonspecific tenderness is usually present early in the disease process. Rotator cuff strength is often normal but may be difficult to assess secondary to the limited and painful range of motion.
4. **Roentgenographs** are typically unremarkable.
5. **Treatment**
   a. **Nonoperative** management with a home-based stretching program as well as pain medication if necessary is successful in 90% of patients. Symptoms may take up to 18 months to resolve. Occasionally, an injection of the glenohumeral joint with corticosteroid is necessary to control pain (4).
   b. **Operative treatment** is directed at releasing the contracted capsule in a sequential fashion to improve range of motion. This may be accomplished either closed or arthroscopically. Any associated pathology (especially in the SA space) should also be addressed (5). Operative intervention typically not indicated until the patient fails 12–18 months of nonoperative care.

III. **ACROMIOCLAVICULAR JOINT DISORDERS**
A. **Arthritis**
1. **Etiology.** Osteoarthritis of the AC joint is extremely common in individuals older than 50 years of age and most are asymptomatic (6). Inflammatory

processes such as rheumatoid arthritis or fractures of the distal clavicle can also cause AC joint symptoms. Younger patients may develop nonacute AC joint pain from activities such as weight lifting.
2. **History.** Pain is localized to the superior aspect of the AC joint. Symptoms are worse when sleeping on the affected side. Overlap symptoms with impingement syndrome are common.
3. **Examination.** Tenderness over the subcutaneous aspect of the AC joint is present. The extreme motions of forward flexion and cross body adduction are limited and painful. Frequently, coexisting rotator cuff findings are present.
4. **Roentgenograms** are similar to those obtained for patients with impingement syndrome. A Zanca view is helpful.
5. **Treatment** is directed at controlling local symptoms with PT, analgesics, and, if necessary, a corticosteroid and lidocaine injection into the AC joint. A typical AC joint will accept 1 to 2 cc of volume. If nonoperative treatment fails, a distal clavicle resection is indicated. This may be completed either via arthroscopic or open techniques (7).
B. **Osteolysis** of the clavicle may occur following a traumatic injury to the AC joint or in individuals who place repeated unusual stress on the AC joint, such as weight lifters. Radiographic changes consist of osteopenia and erosive changes in the articular surface. Treatment is similar to that described for arthritic conditions.

IV. **SCAPULOTHORACIC DISORDERS**
A. **Scapulothoracic bursitis** (snapping scapula)
1. **Etiology.** The scapula has a significant excursion across the chest wall with range of motion of the shoulder girdle. This motion requires the presence of a large bursa between the scapula and the thorax. Inflammation of this bursa can be caused by overuse of the shoulder, serratus anterior contracture, or a bony deformity on the undersurface of the scapula (8).
2. **History.** Patients complain of pain deep and medial to the scapula on the thorax posteriorly. The hallmark symptoms of this disorder are catching or crepitus with motion of the scapula.
3. **Examination.** Scapulothoracic motion may be limited. The patient can usually reproduce a palpable sensation of crepitus under the scapula.
4. **Imaging studies** are not typically useful unless there is a history of trauma or there is suspicion of an osteochondroma under the scapula.
5. **Treatment** is directed at increasing motion of the superior medial angle of the scapula away from the thorax and strengthening the periscapular muscles, or noninvasive techniques may include deep friction massage and ultrasound. Occasionally, a corticosteroid injection into the scapulothoracic bursa is necessary. If nonoperative methods fail, an arthroscopic or open excision of the bursa and the superior medial angle of the scapula is indicated (9).
B. **Winging of the scapula**
1. **Etiology.** The scapula is held against the thorax by the serratus anterior muscle, which is innervated by the long thoracic nerve. Anything that disrupts either of these two structures results in winging of the scapula. Pseudo-winging of the scapula (scapular dyskinesia) is far more common than true winging and develops when the periscapular muscles do not work in a synchronized manner.
2. **History.** Weakness and loss of active motion of the shoulder is noticed first. Secondary symptoms of rotator cuff inflammation (secondary impingement syndrome) may develop. A history of trauma to the chest wall in the location of the long thoracic nerve may be present. Most patients do not have a readily identifiable cause for their serratus anterior dysfunction (10). Fascioscapulohumeral muscular dystrophy often initially presents with isolated winging of one or both scapulae.
3. **Examination.** Winging of the scapula occurs when the medial border of the scapula is rotated outward and laterally, causing the scapula to give the appearance of "wings" on the patient's back (**Fig. 16-3**).

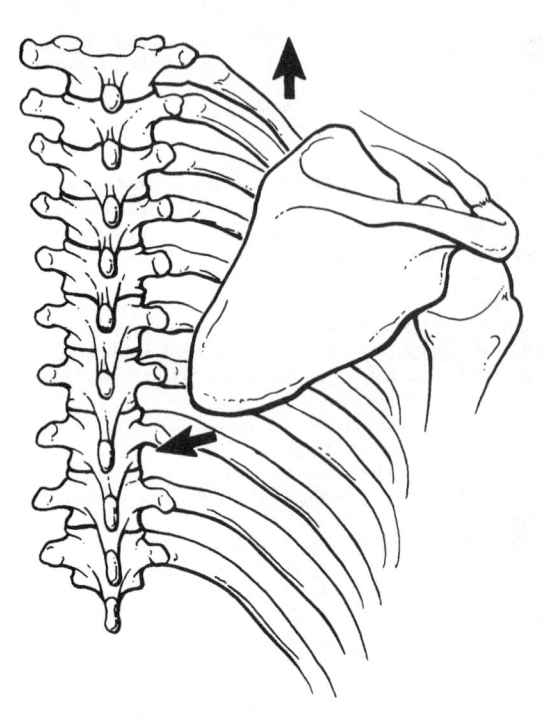

Figure 16-3. Position of the scapula with primary scapular winging due to serratus anterior palsy. The scapula pulls away from the back and does not protract on arm elevation. (From Kuhn JE, Hawkins, RJ. Evaluation and treatment of scapular disorders. In: Warner JJP, Iannotti JP, Gerber C, eds. *Complex and revision problems in shoulder surgery*. Philadelphia, PA: Lippincott-Raven, 1997: 357–375.)

  4. **Treatment** is directed at strengthening the periscapular muscles and observation to determine whether the long thoracic nerve will recover. If after 18 months no recovery is present, either a pectoralis major tendon transfer or a scapulothoracic fusion is indicated.

References
1. Bigliani LU, Morrison DS, April EW. The morphology of the acromion and its relationship to rotator cuff tears. *Orthop Trans* 1983;175:18.
2. Cofield RH. Uncemented total shoulder arthroplasty: a review. *Clin Orthop* 1994;66(A):899–906.
3. Bunker TD, Anthony PP. The pathology of frozen shoulder. A Dupuytren-like disease. *J Bone Joint Surg (Br)* 1995;77:677–683.
4. Dacre JE, Beeney N, Scott DL. Injections and physiotherapy for the painful stiff shoulder. *Ann Rheum Dis* 1989;48:322–325.
5. Harryman DT II, Sidles JA, Matsen FA III. Arthroscopic management of refractory shoulder stiffness. *Arthroscopy* 1997;13:133–147.
6. Grimes DW, Garner RW. The degeneration of the acromioclavicular joint. *Orthop Rev* 1980;9:41–44.
7. Peterson CJ. Resection of the lateral end of the clavicle: a 3 to 30-year follow-up. *Acta Orthop Scand* 1983;54:900–907.
8. Edelson JG. Variations in the anatomy of the scapula with reference to the snapping scapula. *Clin Orthop* 1996;322:111–115.

9. Strizak AM, Cowen MH. The snapping scapula syndrome. *J Bone Joint Surg* 1982;64A:941–942.
10. Foo CL, Swann M. Isolated paralysis of the serratus anterior: a report of 20 cases. *J Bone Joint Surg (Br)* 1983;65:552–556.

Selected Historical Readings

Neer CS II. Anterior acromioplasty for the chronic impingement syndrome in the shoulder. *J Bone Joint Surg* 1972;54A:41–50.

FRACTURES OF THE HUMERUS 17

I. **FRACTURES OF THE PROXIMAL HUMERUS**
   A. **General principles.** Epiphyseal fractures are considered separately. Fractures of the proximal humerus are seen in all age groups but are more common in older patients. In young adults, they are a result of high-energy trauma. In older patients, treatment is designed to maintain glenohumeral motion. Considerable angulation at the fracture site may be accepted; motion is begun early to avoid shoulder stiffness.
   B. **Classification and treatment.** Neer divides proximal humeral fractures into six groups, as shown in **Fig. 17-1**, and this concept is useful in considering the management of the injury. There is lack of reliability in interpreting radiographs to accurately classify proximal humerus fractures. Elderly patients who are too ill to be considered for surgery are treated as described for the first group.
      1. **Fractures with minimal displacement and displaced anatomic neck fractures.** Approximately 85% of all fractures of the proximal humerus are in this category. Any fracture pattern can be seen, but the displacement of all components must be less than 1 cm, except anatomic neck fractures, to be considered in this group according to Neer's concept. Angulatory or rotatory deformity should not exceed 45 degrees. Stability is usually afforded by some impaction and the preservation of soft-tissue attachments. A sling is the preferred treatment. Wrist and hand exercises are begun immediately. Circumduction exercises should be started as soon as they can be tolerated, generally within 5 to 7 days. The patient is instructed to bend to 90 degrees at the waist, allowing the arm to either hang or swing in a gentle circle and avoid active contraction of the shoulder muscles (1). Assisted forward elevation and assisted external rotation exercises in the supine position can generally be started approximately 10 to 14 days after injury. The fracture site is often completely pain free after 2 to 3 weeks, and full range of motion is possible in 4 to 6 weeks. Some form of protection may be needed for 6 to 8 weeks; then more vigorous physical therapy may be prescribed, including wall climbing, overhead rope-and-pulley, passive range of motion, and rotator cuff strengthening exercises (2).
      2. **Displaced surgical neck fractures.** The fracture generally occurs with the arm in abduction. The rotator cuff is usually intact. Undisplaced linear fractures that extend into the humeral head can occur. The fracture site is often angulated more than 45 degrees or malrotated. Neurovascular injury can occur in this type of fracture because the shaft may be displaced into the axilla. This is more common in elderly patients with atherosclerotic (less compliant) arteries.
         a. **Treatment is by closed reduction** under general or supraclavicular regional anesthesia. Align the distal fragment to the proximal one. This alignment usually requires abduction and flexion. Reduction of the fracture depends on an intact posteromedial periosteal sleeve in younger patients. The fracture may be stable enough to permit immobilization of the arm at the side in a sling-and-swathe but may require a spica cast or abduction pillow splint to hold the arm in the reduced position. Fixation can be added percutaneously to maintain the reduction; this is generally advised in younger patients. This treatment should be chosen with caution in patients with significant osteoporosis. As soon as the immobilization is

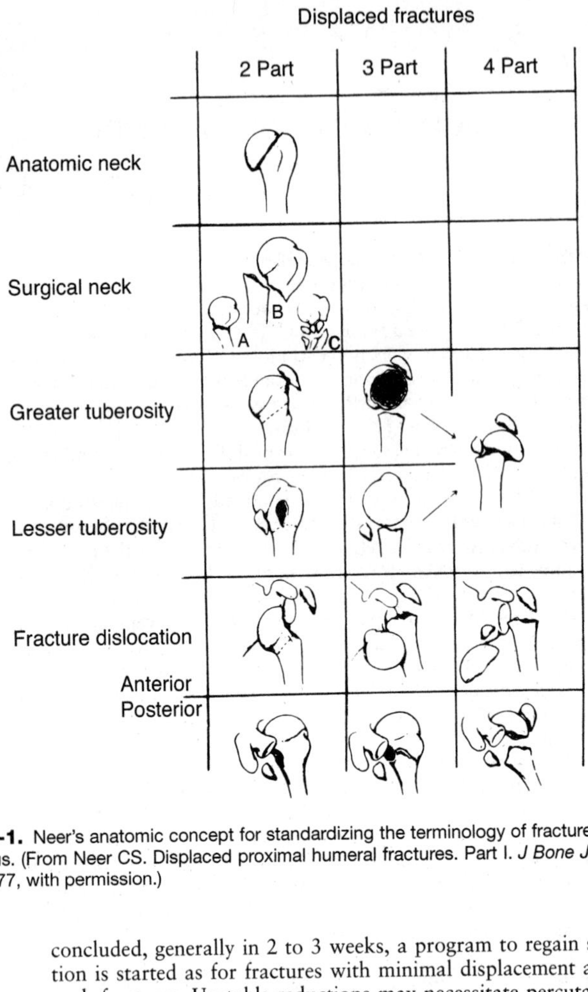

Figure 17-1. Neer's anatomic concept for standardizing the terminology of fractures of the proximal humerus. (From Neer CS. Displaced proximal humeral fractures. Part I. *J Bone Joint Surg (Am)* 1970;52:1077, with permission.)

concluded, generally in 2 to 3 weeks, a program to regain shoulder motion is started as for fractures with minimal displacement and anatomic neck fractures. Unstable reductions may necessitate percutaneous pin or screw fixation. In unreliable patients, the fixation may need to be protected with a shoulder spica cast for 3 weeks. With reliable patients, gentle circumduction exercises can be started immediately after pinning and the exercise program advanced as described at 4 to 6 weeks after surgery for pin removal.

    b. If closed reduction is impossible, then consideration is given to open reduction and plate fixation or tension band wiring. A low profile plate such as the AO/ASIF (Association for the Study of Internal Fixation) cloverleaf small fragment plate or proximal humeral locking plate is preferred. The locking plates are particularly useful in patients with osteopenia.

3. Displaced greater or lesser tuberosity fracture, or both. Rarely, a three-part fracture is encountered involving the lesser or greater tuberosity as well as the surgical neck. If the fracture is displaced, then the rotator cuff function is compromised and open reduction of the fracture is indicated. The fracture should be anatomically reduced and held firmly with tension band wiring or screw fixation. It is also possible to fix these fractures percutaneously, but this

will not address a rotator cuff tear. The rotator cuff tear can be addressed later if pain and weakness remain after the rehabilitation program is implemented.
4. **A fracture-dislocation of the shoulder**, whether anterior or posterior, may be reduced by a closed method under general anesthesia. If closed reduction fails, then open reduction with internal fixation or prosthetic replacement (in older patients) is indicated.
5. Neer (see Selected Historical Readings) states that open reduction is indicated for any displaced **three-part fracture** and that prosthetic replacement is preferable treatment for any displaced **four-part fracture**. This is because of the high rate of posttraumatic humeral head osteonecrosis in four-part fractures. We believe that, at best, these are difficult fractures to treat and that operative treatment should be undertaken only by surgeons with special expertise in managing shoulder trauma.

C. Complications
1. The most common complication is **loss of some glenohumeral motion**, especially of internal rotation and abduction. This often occurs as a result of malposition of the greater tuberosity. The best way to rehabilitate the glenohumeral joint is to start motion early and to achieve primary fracture union. Careful attention to starting an early physical therapy program can markedly improve the end result. Home programs where exercises are performed by a motivated patient two to three times per day with weekly physical therapy monitoring seems to produce the best results. Open treatment may be indicated to achieve adequate stability of displaced fractures to allow early motion.
2. **Delayed union or nonunion** is not uncommon with displaced fractures, especially surgical neck fractures. When it occurs, some loss of joint motion generally results, regardless of subsequent treatment. If the patient experiences pain and loss of motion in association with the nonunion, then the treatment is either replacement arthroplasty or internal fixation with bone grafting.
3. **Associated nerve and vascular damage** is not rare with displaced fractures and should be identified early so that prompt, effective treatment can be instituted. Involvement of the axillary, median, radial, and ulnar nerves is reported with nearly equal frequency.

II. PROXIMAL HUMERAL EPIPHYSEAL SEPARATION
A. Examination.
The injury is most often seen in children 8 to 14 years of age. On examination, the shoulder usually is deformed. Roentgenograms reveal the correct diagnosis. The epiphyseal fracture is usually a Salter class 2 or, less commonly, a class 1 fracture (see **Chap. 1, VII.B**).
B. Treatment.
The fracture may usually be reduced by closed methods after appropriate anesthesia. Reduction requires aligning the distal fragment to the proximal one, usually by abduction and external rotation of the distal fragment. Up to the age of 9 years in a girl and 10 years in a boy, remodeling produces a normal shoulder as long as the rotation of the two fragments relative to one another is correct. Up to 11 years in a girl and 12 in a boy, 50% apposition is acceptable, but varus malalignment should not exceed 45 degrees and rotary deformity must be minimal. The younger child is placed in a shoulder spica cast with the arm in the reduced (abducted) position. The cast is maintained for 4 to 6 weeks, at which time it may be removed and the arm brought to the side. Treatment is then carried out in a sling with circumduction exercises. Open reduction rarely is indicated, but closed manipulation and percutaneous pin fixation should be considered if closed reduction fails to achieve an acceptable degree of correction and stability. The mature adolescent should be treated as an adult.

III. DIAPHYSEAL FRACTURES
A.
The **diagnosis** is usually self-evident, and the exact fracture pattern is confirmed by anteroposterior and lateral roentgenographic examination. The incidence of this fracture is bimodal occurring at the highest rate in young adults and individuals 60 years of age and older (9). Although the fracture may occur in any part of the diaphyseal bone, the middle third is most commonly involved.

B. Physical examination should be thorough to rule out any nerve or vascular damage. Radial nerve injury is common with this fracture. The time of onset of any nerve involvement must be accurately documented. There are three separate mechanisms by which the nerve may be involved.
   1. **Damage at the time of injury** usually produces a neurapraxia, less commonly an axonotmesis or traction injury, and rarely a neurotmesis. Neurotmesis is most commonly associated with open fractures (4).
   2. **During the process of manipulation and immobilization**, neurapraxia can occur, and if the pressure is not relieved, then it can become an axonotmesis. This usually is a result of the nerve's becoming trapped between the fracture fragments.
   3. **During the process of internal fixation**, neurapraxia or axonotmesis can develop from manipulation of the nerve.

C. Treatment (4–10)
   1. The **fracture** should be treated by placing the forearm in a collar and cuff by immobilizing the arm against the thorax with plaster coaptation splints, as shown in **Fig. 17-2**. The splint can be removed and the patient placed into a snug-fitting commercial or custom fracture orthoses at 2 to 3 weeks after injury (10,11). Shoulder and elbow motion is then initiated. Bayonet apposition is acceptable as long as alignment is good. Distraction should be avoided and is generally a harbinger of nonunion. Open reduction is indicated for a vascular injury, for Holstein fracture (an oblique distal third fracture with radial nerve injury where the nerve can be trapped in the fracture), for an open fracture (where the nerve should be explored), for bilateral fractures, for massive obesity (where closed reduction and orthotic treatment is not possible), and for patients with polytrauma (3,5). Plates and screws, reamed intramedullary nails, and flexible intramedullary nails seem to be equally efficacious. Intramedullary nails can be placed without opening the fracture site, but they do result in a 20% to 30% incidence of postoperative shoulder pain (4–8). For

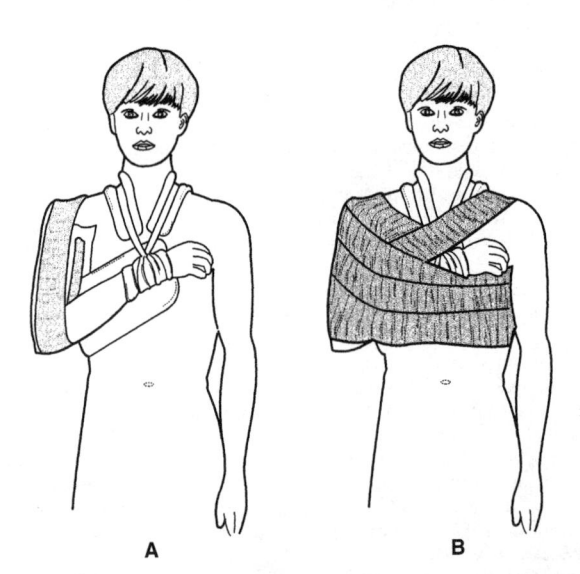

Figure 17-2. Treatment of the humeral shaft fractures. **A:** The first step is to apply coaptation splints to the arm and then to apply a commercial collar and cuff or one made of muslin. Stockinet should not be used because it stretches. The neck and wrist are padded beneath the collar and cuff with felt. **B:** After adequate padding in the axilla and beneath the forearm, the arm and forearm can be immobilized against the thorax with a swathe.

this reason, plate fixation is the preferred method of operative stabilization in most settings.
2. Treatment of an associated **radial nerve injury**
   a. **Nerve involvement at the time of injury** calls for passive range-of-motion exercises of the wrist and fingers and for use of a **radial nerve splint for the wrist and fingers** if return of function is not beginning at 2 to 3 weeks. Follow up the patient for nerve recovery as outlined in **Chap. 1, V.E** for nerve injuries. The prognosis for recovery is excellent, with 90% or more patients regaining full function.
   b. **Nerve involvement at the time of closed reduction** should be treated with nerve exploration and fixation as soon as possible.
   c. **Late nerve involvement** is also an indication for exploration and neurolysis.
D. **Complications.** Delayed unions and nonunions do occur. They are best treated with compression plating and a cancellous bone graft. Longer plates and the use of methyl methacrylate in screw holes may be necessary in osteoporotic patients. If nonunion occurs after intramedullary nailing, plate fixation with bone grafting results in healing in approximately 90% of cases; repeat IM nailing is generally not advisable.

IV. SUPRACONDYLAR FRACTURES

A. A supracondylar fracture is most common in children and elderly patients, but it may occur at any age (12). The **mechanism of injury** is extension or flexion, or a direct blow as a result of high-energy trauma. The extension type of injury is produced by a fall on the extended arm and is stable only in significant flexion. Such a fracture may have an intracondylar or intracapsular component. The flexion type is produced by a fall on the flexed elbow and is relatively stable in extension.
B. **Examination.** The elbow injury is obvious clinically, but the full extent of the damage must be demonstrated with good roentgenograms. Because of the potential for associated vascular and nerve injury, it is essential to conduct a careful assessment for such injuries. Vascular damage, nerve damage, or marked displacement constitutes a surgical emergency. At times, it is possible to bring about relief by reducing the fracture with sedation and applying a splint.
C. **Treatment**
  1. **Children**
     a. Because of the seriousness of the potential complication of Volkmann's contracture with a **supracondylar fracture**, nearly all children with a displaced fracture are admitted to the hospital as close monitoring of the neurovascular status is required. As soon as the condition of the patient allows, a definitive reduction under general anesthesia is attempted. The technique of reduction is illustrated in **Figs. 17-3 and 17-4**. The authors prefer percutaneous or open cross–Kirschner-wire fixation after reduction. If the patient is seen late and the swelling is massive, an alternative is the use of Dunlop traction until the swelling resolves (see **Fig. 9-5**). In the younger child, there is some latitude in anteroposterior angulation or displacement. The direction of the initial displacement provides a clue for the proper forearm position after reduction. If the initial displacement is medial, then placing the forearm into pronation tightens the medial hinge, closes any lateral gap in the fracture line, and helps prevent subsequent cubitus varus. If the initial displacement is lateral, then placing the forearm in supination tightens the lateral soft-tissue hinge, closes the medial aspect of the fracture line, and helps prevent cubitus deformity. The use of **Baumann angle** to guide treatment was described in the German literature in 1929. To use this technique, bilateral roentgenograms of the distal humerus are necessary. A line is drawn down the center of the diaphysis of the humerus, and another is drawn across the epiphyseal plate of the capitellum. If the angle is 5 degrees different from the unaffected side, the reduction is not complete and a significant abnormality in the carrying angle, such as cubitus varus, may result. The reduction is generally off in rotation. On the lateral radiograph, the anterior humeral line must pass through the capitellum to ensure that there is not a malreduction with rotation or extension.

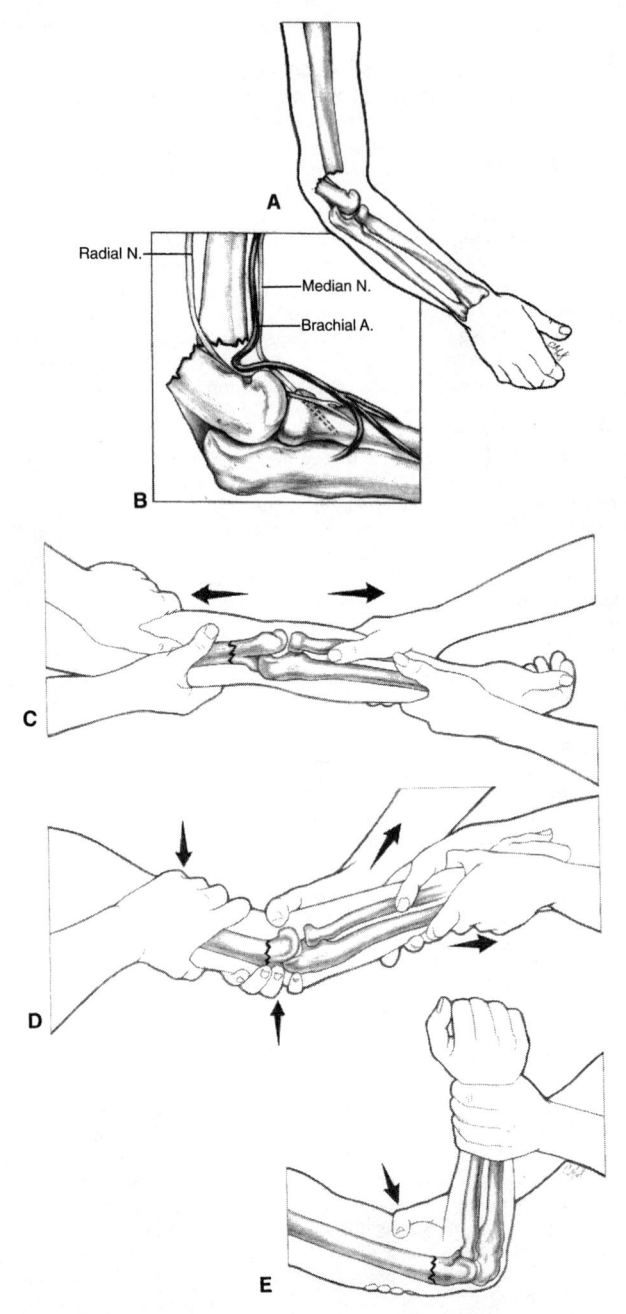

Figure 17-3. Reduction technique for supracondylar humeral fractures that occur with the elbow in flexion. **A:** Distal fragment is displaced posteriorly. **B:** The brachial artery may become entrapped at the fracture site. **C:** Restore length by applying traction against countertraction. **D:** With pressure directed anteriorly on the distal fragment, provide reduction. **E:** The reduction is generally stable with the elbow in flexion with the forearm pronated.

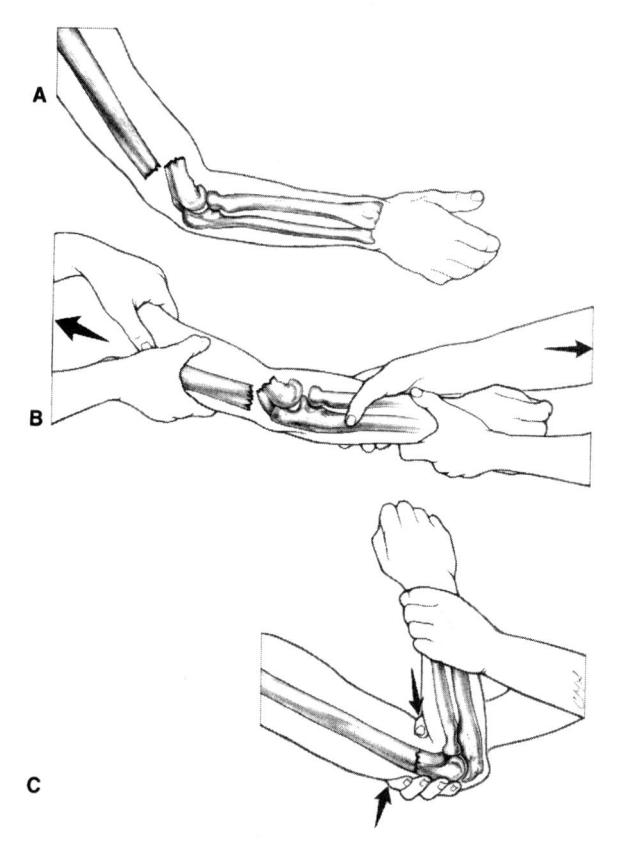

Figure 17-4. Reduction technique for supracondylar fractures that occur with the elbow in extension. **A:** The distal fragment is displaced anteriorly relative to the proximal fragment. **B:** Restore length by applying traction against countertraction. **C:** With pressure directed posteriorly on the distal fragment, the fracture is reduced. The elbow is then extended to enhance stability of the reduction in most circumstances.

Open reduction may be necessary if repeated attempts at closed reduction fail. Small incisions are recommended to place the pin starting from the medial side to be sure the ulnar nerve is not injured (12). An anterior or lateral incision may be used to expose the fracture. The anterior incision may provide the easiest direct exposure because of the generally extensive damage to the brachial muscle by the fracture displacement. Internal fixation or percutaneous smooth pins are often required to maintain a satisfactory reduction. Because there is the serious possibility of causing nerve and vascular damage in this region, repeated manipulation should be infrequent and the rule "one doctor, one manipulation" applies. Splint the elbow in 20 to 30 degrees of flexion after pinning the fracture to allow for swelling. This is only possible when the fracture has been stabilized by pin fixation. The patient must be observed for at least 24 hours for the signs and symptoms of compartment syndrome. Frequent checks of the radial pulse by palpation and Doppler are recorded in the chart, and the patient is closely observed for the signs of compartmental syndrome (see **Chap. 2, III**). The pins are removed after 3 to 4 weeks, and intermittent active motion is started out of cast or splint. The splint is discarded 6 weeks after the

injury. Stiffness may result from overzealous attempts of family, friends, and therapists to aid the child in regaining motion quickly. The child should be allowed to use the elbow, and the family should be reassured that he or she will gain extension of the joint with time and growth.
- **b. Distal humeral epiphyseal slips** in younger children are rare, but when they occur, they should be treated as supracondylar fractures.

2. **Adults.** These injuries occur rarely and generally in elderly individuals. Stiffness in the elbow develops rapidly in the older patient when the elbow is immobilized for any length of time. One of the requirements for any method of treatment is to allow early mobilization. Therefore, treatment should be as follows:
   - **a.** If the fracture is **minimally displaced and stable**, then supination-pronation exercises are begun within 2 to 3 days without removal of the posterior splint. After 2 weeks, the splint may be removed during these sessions to allow some active flexion and extension.
   - **b.** If the fracture is displaced, the **percutaneous pins** may be used for stability to allow early motion as outlined in **1.a** (above).
   - **c. Open reduction and internal fixation** should be considered if steps **a** and **b** do not produce satisfactory alignment and stability (13,14).
   - **d.** If the elbow is grossly swollen and difficult to treat by the aforementioned methods or if marked comminution precludes stable fixation, then **olecranon pin traction** with early movement is an option; it is rarely indicated.

D. **Complications**
1. **Cubitus varus and valgus (varus is far more common)**
2. **Loss of elbow motion**
3. **Tardy ulnar nerve palsy**

V. **INTERCONDYLAR FRACTURES**
A. **Type of injury.** "T" and "Y" fractures are typically supracondylar fractures of the lower end of the humerus with a vertical component running into the elbow joint, but any combination of fractures in this area (e.g., comminuted fractures, fractures of the capitulum) are included in this category. Some comminution usually is present.
B. **Roentgenograms.** Films must be of excellent quality to assess the fracture pattern adequately. Intraoperative traction films may be helpful in defining the fracture pattern.
C. **Treatment.** If the fracture is one in which reduction and firm fixation can be achieved by open reduction and internal fixation, then this is performed (14). Highly comminuted fractures should be referred to experienced fracture surgeons to prevent the situation of open reduction and unstable fixation. Optimum exposure for anatomic reduction of the joint surface often requires an olecranon osteotomy; patients undergoing internal fixation should be started on active range-of-motion exercises within 3 to 5 days of the procedure. If the degree of comminution is so great that the internal fixation cannot be satisfactorily achieved and referral is not an option, then the fracture may rarely be treated by olecranon pin traction and early motion. Begin movement of the hand and fingers, and commence shoulder movements after 2 weeks. If traction is not used, active flexion from the position of immobilization is encouraged if it does not cause pain. Tenderness usually disappears in 4 to 6 weeks; the splint is then discarded, and further active elbow movement is encouraged. This injury commonly results in significant loss of elbow extension. In the most comminuted fractures in elderly individuals, total elbow replacement is an excellent option. This requires referral to an experienced elbow surgeon.

VI. **LATERAL CONDYLE FRACTURES**
A. **Type of injury.** These are nearly always seen in children and are a serious injury type of the disruption of the joint surface.
B. **Roentgenograms.** Routine anteroposterior and lateral films are obtained, but oblique films and films of the uninjured elbow often are needed to define the injury accurately.
C. **Treatment.** If displacement is present, then open reduction and pin (two small Kirschner wires) fixation are essential. If no displacement is evident, then additional

roentgenograms should be obtained in 5 to 7 days to check position. Open reduction is done through a lateral approach with minimal stripping of the bony fragment. Rotation of the fragment must be accurately assessed. The pins are removed at 3 weeks; gentle exercises are started at 6 weeks.
   D. Complications
      1. **Failure to achieve accurate reduction of the fracture** results in cubitus valgus, late arthritic changes, nonunion, or a tardy ulnar nerve palsy.
      2. When the epiphysis is open, **overgrowth of the lateral condyle** occasionally occurs, with a resulting cubitus varus.
VII. **MEDIAL EPICONDYLE FRACTURES**
   A. **Mechanism of injury.** The center of ossification of the medial epicondyle of the humerus appears at 5 to 7 years of age. Displacement of the medial epicondyle as an isolated injury is uncommon. The common mechanism is the result of an elbow dislocation with avulsion of the fragment. This is most common in children but can occur in adults. The medial ligament of the elbow maintains its inferior attachment and pulls the medial epicondyle from the humerus.
   B. The **diagnosis** may be made clinically in a great majority of cases. When the medial epicondyle has been avulsed, there is a surprisingly large defect, which is easily palpated even in a swollen elbow.
   C. **Roentgenograms** are used to identify the position of the medial epicondyle. Roentgenograms of the normal elbow are helpful.
   D. **Treatment.** Reduce any elbow dislocation by linear traction with sedation and assess the position of the fragment roentgenographically. The medial epicondyle may be trapped within the joint, causing incomplete motion. If the epicondyle is in the joint, then open reduction is required. The medial epicondyle fracture can be reduced and held by pin fixation. In adults, consider small fragment screws. If open reduction is undertaken, the ulnar nerve must be protected but need **not** be transpositioned anteriorly.
   E. **Complications** are largely those of an elbow dislocation. If the medial epicondyle remains displaced, ulnar nerve problems are not uncommon. If the epicondyle is anatomically reduced and the elbow joint space is roentgenographically sound, then the injury can be treated by splinting for 7 to 10 days followed by early active motion exercises (earlier in adults).

HCMC Treatment Recommendations
Proximal Humerus Fractures

Diagnosis: Anteroposterior shoulder radiograph with axillary view and transscapular lateral (shoulder trauma series) view. Consider computed tomography scan with reconstructions if a displaced three- or four-part fracture is noted on plain radiographs and the patient is a surgical candidate.

Treatment: Be sure the humeral head is located. If the fracture is impacted or minimally displaced, apply sling for comfort and begin assisted range-of-motion exercises at 7–14 days.

Indications for surgery: Marked (greater than 1 cm) displacement of tuberosity fragments, varus angulation of head, dislocated humeral head, head-splitting fracture, or open fractures.

Technical options: Based on age of the patient, type of fracture, and bone quality:

- Greater tuberosity fractures: open reduction and screw or tension band fixation
- Two-part surgical neck fractures: closed reduction and percutaneous pinning. In pediatric fractures, plate or intramedullary nail fixation in adults
- Three-part fractures: closed reduction and pinning versus open reduction with internal fixation with tension band technique
- Four-part fractures, head-splitting fractures: prosthetic replacement is advisable for elderly patients with markedly comminuted fractures or those associated with humeral head dislocation.

HCMC Treatment Recommendations
Humeral Shaft Fractures
  Diagnosis: Anteroposterior and lateral radiographs, physical examination. Be sure to check radial nerve function.
  Treatment: Closed reduction and application of coaptation splints—convert splints to functional brace and begin range-of-motion exercises for shoulder and elbow 2 weeks following injury.
  Indications for surgery: Multiply injured patient or extremity, open fractures, non-union.
  Recommended technique: 4.5-mm large fragment low contact dynamic compression plate (LCDCP), explore and protect radial nerve. Alternatively, use an antegrade interlocking humeral nail but expect shoulder pain in 20% to 30% of individuals.

HCMC Treatment Recommendations
Distal Humerus Fractures
  Diagnosis: Anteroposterior and lateral elbow radiographs and physical examinations.
  Treatment: Initial long arm splint after documenting neurocirculatory status.
  Indications for surgery: Any displacement of the joint surface greater than 2 mm, open fractures.
  Recommended technique: Posterior approach with olecranon osteotomy where articular displacement is severe. Fixation with two 3.5-mm reconstruction plates at right angles. Olecranon osteotomy fixed with 6.5-mm cancellous screws with tension band wire.

References

1. Wijgman AJ, Roolker W, Patt TW, et al. Open reduction and internal fixation of three and four part fractures of the promimal part of the humerus. *J Bone Joint Surg (Am)* 2002;84:1919–1925.
2. Young TB, Wallace WA. Conservative treatment of fractures and fracture-dislocations of the upper end of the humerus. *J Bone Joint Surg (Br)* 1985;68:373–377.
3. Tytherleigh-Strong G, Walls N, McQueen MM. The epidemiology of humeral shaft fractures. *J Bone Joint Surg (Br)* 1997;80:249–253.
4. Foster RJ, Dixon GL, Bach AW, et al. Internal fixation of fractures and nonunions of the humeral shaft. *J Bone Joint Surg (Am)* 1985;67:857–864.
5. Bell MJ, Beauchamp CG, Kellam JK, et al. The results of plating humeral shaft fractures in patients with multiple injuries: the sunnybrook experience. *J Bone Joint Surg (Br)* 1985;67:293–296.
6. Brumback RJ, Bosse MJ, Poka A, et al. Intramedullary stabilization of humeral shaft fractures in patients with multiple trauma. *J Bone Joint Surg (Am)* 1986;68:960–970.
7. Dabezies EL, Banta CJ, Murphy CP, et al. Plate fixation of the humeral shaft with and without nerve injuries. *J Orthop Trauma* 1992;6:10–13.
8. John H, Rosso R, Neff U, et al. Operative treatment of distal humerus fractures in the elderly. *J Bone Joint Surg (Br)* 1994;76:793–796.
9. Vandergriend R, Tomasin L, Ward EF. Open reduction and internal fixation of humeral shaft fractures. *J Bone Joint Surg (Am)* 1986;68:430–433.
10. Wallny T, Westermann K, Sagebiel C, et al. Functional treatment of humeral shaft fractures: indications and results. *J Orthop Trauma* 1997;11:283–287.
11. Zagorski JB, Latta LL, Zych GA, et al. Diaphyseal fractures of the humerus. Treatment with prefabricated braces. *J Bone Joint Surg (Am)* 1988;70:607–610.
12. Skaggs DL, Hale JM, Bassett J, et al. Operative treatment of supracondylar fractures of the humerus in children. The consequences of pin placement. *J Bone Joint Surg (Am)* 2001;83:735–740.

13. Pereles TR, Koval ICJ, Gallagher M, et al. Open reduction and internal fixation of the distal humerus. Functional outcome in the elderly. *J Trauma* 1997;43:578–584.
14. Ring D, Jupiter JB, Gulotta L. Articular fractures of the distal part of the humerus. *J Bone Joint Surg (Am)* 2003;85:232–238.

Selected Historical Readings

Baumann, E. Beiträge zur Kenntnis der Frakturen an Ellbogengellenk unter besonderer Berücksichtigung der Spätfolgen. I. Allgemeines und Fractura supra condylica. *Beitr f Klin Chir* 1929;146:1–50.

Brown RF, Morgan RG. Intercondylar T-shaped fractures of the humerus. *J Bone Joint Surg (Br)* 1971;53:425–428.

Hardacre JA, Nahigian SH, Froimson AI, et al. Fractures of the lateral condyle of the humerus in children. *J Bone Joint Surg (Am)* 1971;53:1083–1095.

Holstein A, Lewis GB. Fractures of the humerus with radial nerve paralysis. *J Bone Joint Surg (Am)* 1963;45:1382–1388.

Nacht JL, Ecker ML, Chung SM, et al. Supracondylar fractures of the humerus in children treated by closed reduction and percutaneous pinning. *Clin Orthop* 1983;177:203–209.

Neer CS II. Displaced proximal humeral fractures. Part I. *J Bone Joint Surg (Am)* 1970;52:1077–1089.

Neer CS II. Displaced proximal humeral fractures. Part II. *J Bone Joint Surg (Am)* 1970;52:1090–1103.

Riseborough EJ, Radin EL. Intercondylar T fractures of the humerus in the adult. A comparison of operative and nonoperative treatment in twenty-nine cases. *J Bone Joint Surg (Am)* 1969;51:130–131.

Sarmiento A, Kinman PB, Galvin EG, et al. Functional bracing of fractures of the shaft of the humerus. *J Bone Joint Surg (Am)* 1977;59:596–601.

Weiland AJ, Meyer S, Tolo VT, et al. Surgical treatment of displaced supracondylar fractures of the humerus in children. *J Bone Joint Surg (Am)* 1978;60:657–661.

ELBOW AND FOREARM INJURIES   18

I. **RUPTURES OF THE DISTAL BICEPS BRACHII**
   A. **Location.** Rupture of the distal biceps may occur at the muscle tendon junction or more commonly at its tendinous insertion into the radial tuberosity.
   B. **Mechanism of injury.** Often a chronic case of distal biceps tendinitis has been present, making the tendon susceptible to failure with forceful supination of the hand or elbow flexion.
   C. **Examination.** A palpable defect is present at the elbow and the bulk of the biceps muscle is retracted proximally. Often, this shortened muscle is prone to spasm for several weeks after the injury occurs. The patient has minimal weakness to elbow flexion but does have weakness to hand supination.
   D. **Treatment.** If the rupture occurs at the muscle tendon junction, nonoperative care with early range-of-motion (ROM) exercises are indicated (1). Treatment of distal tendon tears is controversial. The biceps functions as a weak elbow flexor, but it is a strong supinator of the hand. Individuals who do not like the cosmetic deformity or are involved in activities that require supination strength should undergo operative repair. A single curvilinear incision is made that allows exposure to locate the retracted tendon proximally, and the original biceps tunnel to the radial tuberosity is used. A repair of the tendon to the tuberosity with suture anchors is completed. A sling is used for 4 weeks postoperatively with an active assisted ROM program initiated immediately postoperatively.

II. **DISLOCATION OF THE ELBOW JOINT** accounts for 20% of all dislocations, second only to glenohumeral and interphalangeal joints.
   A. The **mechanism of injury** is usually a fall on an hyperextended arm.
   B. The **history** of an elbow injury must document, if possible, the mechanism of injury; type and location of pain; amount of immediate sensory, motor, and circulatory dysfunction; treatment before examination; time when swelling began; and any history of elbow injuries.
   C. The **examination** of an injured elbow must document, if possible, the degree of effusion, location of any ecchymosis, ROM, and stability of the joint when compared with that of the opposite side. In the examination of an injured elbow, there may be confusion about whether the deformity arises from a dislocation of the elbow or from a supracondylar fracture, but this can be resolved clinically by comparing the relative positions of the two epicondyles and the tip of the olecranon by palpation. These **three bony points** form an isosceles triangle. The two sides remain equal in length in a supracondylar fracture. If the elbow is dislocated, however, the two sides become unequal (**Fig. 18-1**). The position of the proximal radius should also be palpated on the lateral surface of the elbow to rule out a radial head dislocation. The function of the peripheral nerves and the state of the circulation to the hand, including capillary refill and presence of radial pulse, should be carefully noted. The anterior interosseous branch of the median nerve and the radial nerve are most frequently involved.
   D. **Roentgenograms** demonstrate whether the displacement is directly posterior (most common), posterolateral, or posteromedial. Roentgenograms should include a lateral view of the elbow, an anteroposterior view of the humerus, and an anteroposterior view of the forearm. Fractures of the coranoid process have been identified in 10% to 15% of elbow dislocations.

251

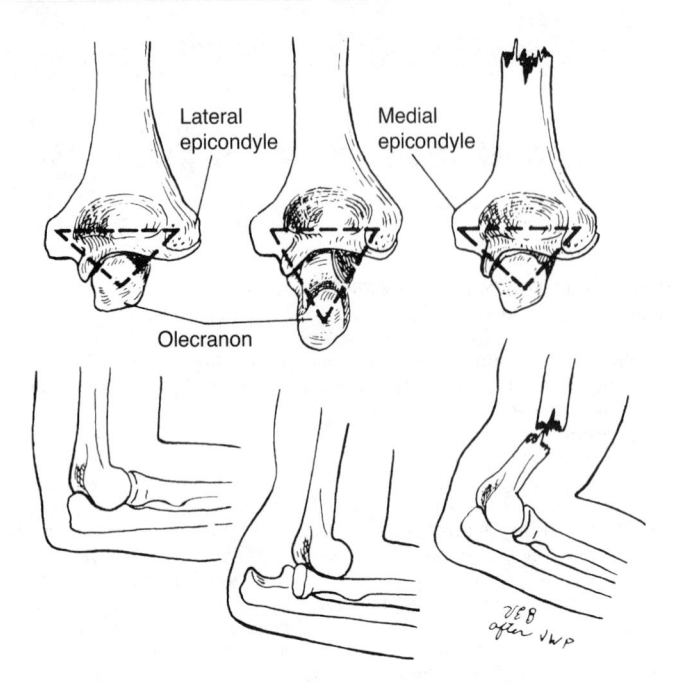

Figure 18-1. The two epicondyles and the tip of the olecranon form an isosceles triangle. This triangle is maintained with a supracondylar humeral fracture, but with an elbow dislocation, the two sides of the triangle become unequal or distorted.

E. **Treatment** consists of immediate closed reduction, which is essential, and may require anesthesia for proper muscle relaxation. Reduction can usually be achieved by gentle traction on the slightly flexed elbow, applying countertraction to the humeral shaft. After reduction, motion should be nearly full, and medial and lateral stability should be assessed. With a simple posterior elbow dislocation, a portion of the collateral ligaments are generally intact so the joint is fairly stable and early motion may be instituted after 3 to 5 days of splinting (2). With other dislocations, the collateral ligaments may be completely disrupted, creating an unstable joint and necessitating longer immobilization before active exercises are started. Postreduction roentgenograms are mandatory because they, too, help determine postreduction treatment. If the joint space is not congruent, generally cartilage fragments, bony debris, or ligament is in the joint, and open reduction and collateral ligament repair are indicated. If significant articular fragments are displaced, they should be internally fixed with recessed small or "minifragment" implants at the same time. Coranoid fractures, unless involving more than 50% of the length, do not require internal fixation (3). If the elbow is stable after collateral ligament repair, motion should be initiated as with stable reductions treated in a closed manner. For an unstable elbow, following operative repair external fixators, which allow active ROM, are useful (4).

F. **Postreduction treatment**
   1. If the medial and lateral ligaments are intact and are providing a **stable elbow joint**, the elbow is placed in a padded posterior splint in 90 degrees of flexion that extends far enough to support the wrist. The elbow is kept elevated above the heart until the swelling recedes. Active flexion is begun in 3 to 5 days to achieve as much ROM as possible. Passive ROM is contraindicated. Repeat radiographs should be obtained within 3 to 5 days to make certain the

joint remains congruent. The elbow is kept in the posterior splint when not being exercised. As soon as the patient can achieve near full extension, use of the splint may be discontinued.
2. If the **elbow is unstable** and the joint is congruent on roentgenograms, it is splinted in 90 degrees of flexion for 2 to 3 weeks with initial elevation to help control swelling. Radiographs must be obtained in the splint initially and at 3 to 5 days to ensure that the elbow is congruous. An active exercise program is then begun to regain ROM. Open reduction is generally not necessary; there is no documented advantage to open reduction over closed reduction (2,5,6).

G. Complications
1. **Up to 15 degrees limitation of full extension** as well as some limitation of flexion is common unless an intensive rehabilitation program is instituted.
2. Traumatic **peripheral nerve injuries** may occur: Ulnar, median, combined ulnar and median, and brachial plexus injury have all been reported.
3. **Compromise of circulation** can occur as a result of posttraumatic swelling or injury to the brachial artery. See **Chap. 2, III,** for a discussion of compartmental syndromes.
4. **Myositis ossificans** can develop, and its treatment should follow the guidelines in **Chap. 2, V.** Posttraumatic elbow stiffness can be successfully treated by open release (7). If associated with postresection instability, a hinged external fixator distractor can be used with good results in motivated patients (8).
5. **Chronic instability** can be difficult to diagnose; when recognized, surgical reconstruction is generally successful (6).

III. **FRACTURES OF THE OLECRANON**
A. **Fractures of the olecranon may be divided into four groups:**
1. **Transverse and undisplaced**
2. **Transverse and displaced**
3. **Comminuted and minimally displaced** with clinical findings suggesting an intact triceps aponeurosis
4. **Comminuted and displaced,** indicating a disrupted extensor mechanism

B. **Treatment**
1. Undisplaced fractures should be treated in a posterior splint with the elbow flexed 90 degrees. Pronation and supination movements are started in 2 to 3 days, and flexion-extension movements are started at 2 weeks. Protective splinting or a sling is used until there is evidence of union (usually approximately 6 weeks). Closed clinical and roentgenographic follow-up is essential to ensure full ROM and to identify any displacement.
2. Displaced fractures should be reduced anatomically and fixed internally with tension band wiring technique or by tension band plating via a posterior approach. An olecranon lag screw should not be used without tension band wire. If used alone, the screw does not provide maximum stabilization when the elbow flexes because half of the fracture is placed in compression and the other half is placed in tension, as shown in **Fig. 10-9**. Regardless of the type of internal fixation used, motion should be started within the first few days postoperatively.
    a. The **tension band wiring technique for a transverse displaced fracture** of the olecranon begins with reduction without devitalization of the fragments. Stabilization of the fragments is accomplished by two Kirschner wires introduced parallel to each other and to the anterior cortex of the ulna. Place the drill hole just distal to the fracture, transversely through the posterior cortex of the ulna. Thread the 1.2-mm (or 16 to 18 gauge) wire through the drill hole, cross the ends in a figure-8 style, pass the wire around the protruding ends of the Kirschner wires, and tie the wire under tension, providing two twists, one on each side of the ulna. This makes the tension even across the fracture site. The result should be a figure-8 tension band wire with the crossover point lying over the fracture. Finally, shorten the projecting ends of the Kirschner wires and bend them to form U-shaped hooks that are then impacted gently into the bone over the tension wire (**Fig. 18-2**) and

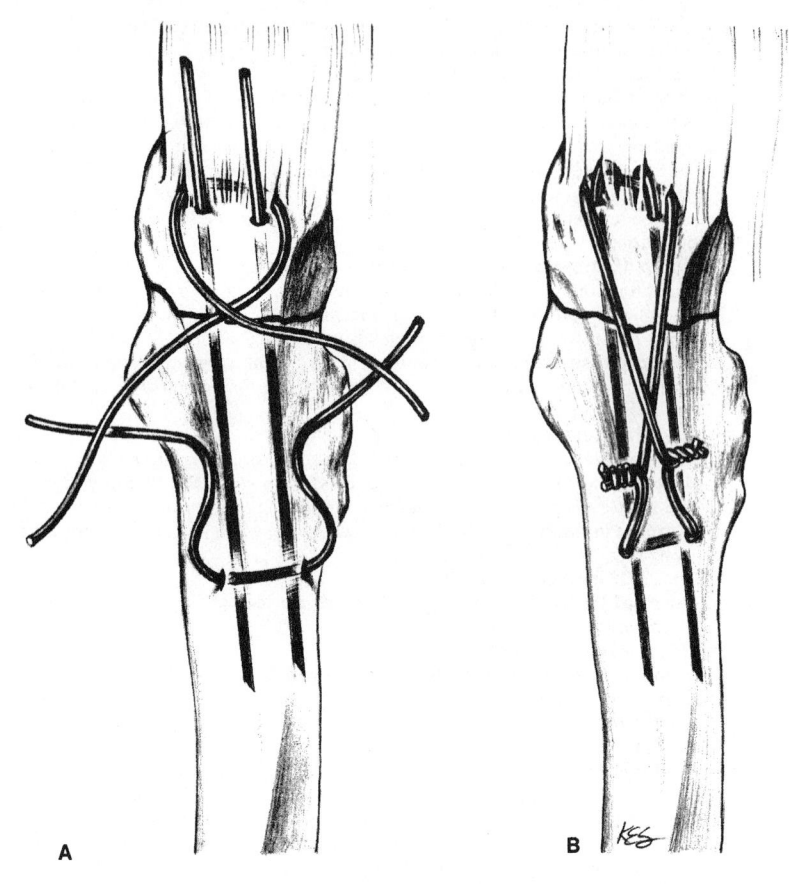

Figure 18-2. The tension band wiring technique. Two parallel Kirschner wires cross an olecranon fracture at right angles. One strand of 18-gauge wire has been inserted within the triceps tendon anterior to the Kirschner wires. The second wire is inserted through the dorsal ulnar cortex of the ulna **(A)**. The fixation is secured **(B)**. (JB Lippincott From Hansen ST, Swiontkowski MF. *Orthopaedic trauma protocols.* New York: Raven Press, 1993:112, with permission).

reconstruct the triceps incision over the bent wires. Similar results can be obtained by inserting a 6.5-mm cancellous screw (with or without a large washer) across the fracture and using the same figure-8 technique.
   b. **The tension-band wiring technique for comminuted displaced fractures** of the olecranon is much the same except that an anatomic reduction is more difficult to achieve and small Kirschner wires may be required for stabilization of minor fracture fragments.
IV. **EPIPHYSEAL FRACTURES OF THE PROXIMAL RADIUS**
   A. **Mechanism of injury.** These pediatric injuries occur from a fall on the outstretched hand.
   B. **Examination.** Pain, occasionally swelling, and tenderness are usually present over the upper end of the radius. There is also limitation of motion.
   C. **Treatment**
      1. **Fractures with less than 15 degrees of angulation** are immobilized in a long-arm splint for 2 weeks. Active exercise is then initiated while the arm is protected in a sling.

2. **Angulation of greater then 15 degrees** calls for manipulation under anesthesia. If this fails, operative reduction is required. After reduction, the fracture is usually stable. If not, internal fixation is used with a fine, smooth Kirschner wire introduced from distal to proximal, stopping short of the articular surface of the radial head. The pin can be removed at 3 weeks and active motion initiated. The radial head should never be removed in children.

V. **FRACTURES OF THE HEAD AND NECK OF THE RADIUS**
   A. **Mechanism of injury.** This injury should be suspected following a fall on the outstretched hand whenever there is swelling of the elbow joint, tenderness over the head of the radius, and limitation of elbow function (especially painful pronation and supination).
   B. **Roentgenograms.** If the fracture is not apparent on the anteroposterior and lateral roentgenograms, films obtained with the head of the radius in varying degrees of rotation are helpful. An anterior fat pad sign, indicative of an elbow effusion, should alert the treating physician to order these special roentgenograms.
   C. **Treatment**
      1. **Minimally displaced (less than 1 mm) fractures of the head (Mason 1) or impacted fractures of the radial neck** are treated with a posterior splint with active motion exercises beginning in the first 3 to 5 days. This treatment is followed by the wearing of a sling and active movement of the elbow. Acutely, it is helpful to aspirate the elbow effusion and inject 5 mL of 1% lidocaine to be sure that elbow motion is full and unimpeded.
      2. Displaced fractures involving less than one third of the articular surface (Mason 2) are treated by early motion if the postaspiration and lidocaine injection examination reveals a full ROM. If motion is blocked or if there is an associated elbow fracture or dislocation, the fracture is treated by open reduction with minimal fragment screws and early motion (9,10). The radial head should not be excised.
      3. Comminuted or displaced fractures of the head that involve more than one third of the articular surface and displaced or unstable fractures of the neck are treated by early excision of the radial head with or without placement of a metal prosthesis if it is anticipated that after 4 to 5 days pain will restrict active exercises (5,11). If adequate movement can be achieved before the fifth day after injury, excision may be avoided. The end result of excision of the radial head is good, but a normal elbow motion is generally not achieved. Fifty percent of the patients have a late complication of subluxation and pain at the distal radioulnar joint (12,13). Insertion of a Silastic prosthesis to prevent late complication appears warranted, but complications from the prosthesis itself are not uncommon (synovitis, prosthesis fracture); therefore, the authors recommend a metal prosthesis when indicated (11).

VI. **MONTEGGIA FRACTURE-DISLOCATION OF THE ELBOW**
   A. This is a dislocation of the radial head and a fracture of the proximal ulna. There are **four types**, as described by Bado (see Selected Historical Readings), depending on the direction of radial head dislocation and associated radial fracture.
   B. The **mechanism of injury** may be a "failed" posterior dislocation of the elbow, that is, the ulna fractures instead of dislocating because of an axial loading force. Alternatively, the injury may occur as a result of an anteriorly or posteriorly directed blow.
   C. **Treatment**
      1. **Children.** Closed reduction of the ulna is carried out. If the radial head has not been indirectly reduced by realigning the ulna, reduction of the radial head is attempted by supination of the forearm and direct pressure on the radial head, which usually is successful. When the radial head cannot be anatomically reduced, removal of the interposing joint capsule with repair of the anular ligament is advisable.
      2. **Adults.** Operative treatment is recommended (14–16). Open reduction with compression plate fixation of the ulna is generally followed by indirect reduction of the radius. If reduction of the radius is not obtained, an open reduction

must be done. If the radial head is unstable, cast for approximately 6 weeks in supination, then start active exercises. If the radial head is stable after closed reduction or open repair, start early active motion with a hinged elbow orthosis, maintaining the forearm in supination. Protect the arm until the fracture is healed. With anterior dislocation and an unstable closed reduction, the arm may be immobilized in 100 degrees to 110 degrees of elbow flexion, which relaxes the biceps and helps maintain reduction of the radial head. If the radial head remains subluxed after ulnar fixation, the forearm should be supinated while applying pressure over the radial head.

VII. **DIAPHYSEAL FRACTURES OF THE RADIUS AND ULNA** (3,10,15–23)
   A. **Roentgenograms.** Of all fractures, this type best exemplifies the need for visualizing the joint above and below fractures of long bones (elbow and wrist).
   B. **Treatment**
   1. **Children.** The fractures are usually of the greenstick type, and even with considerable displacement, a dense periosteal sleeve ordinarily remains. This sleeve is usually sufficient to make satisfactory closed reduction possible. Greenstick fractures tend to redisplace unless the fracture is overreduced, that is, unless the opposite cortex has been fractured with the reduction. For the closed reduction in which angulation is the only deformity to be corrected, conscious sedation and hematoma block may be adequate. Where there is total displacement with shortening of either of both bones, a brief general anesthetic enhances a traumatic reduction. In the child, operative treatment is generally unnecessary because remodeling with growth is excellent and there is an increased likelihood that cross-union will develop after operative treatment. In the mature adolescent, failure to obtain a satisfactory closed reduction is an indication for open reduction and treatment as for the adult. Bone grafting of operatively reduced fractures in the adolescent is not necessary.
   2. **Adults.** (16,17,20–22)
      a. **Principles.** It is difficult to achieve a satisfactory closed reduction of displaced fractures of the forearm bones, and, if achieved, it is hard to maintain. Unsatisfactory results of closed treatment have been reported to range from 38% to 74% (19). For this reason, open reduction with internal fixation is routine except in cases of undisplaced fractures.
      b. **Undisplaced single bone fractures** should be treated in a long-arm cast until there is roentgenographic evidence of union or definitive evidence or delayed union.
      c. **Fractures of both bones or a displaced isolated fracture** of the radius or ulna should be treated by open reduction, plate fixation, and cancellous bone grafting whenever there is bone loss. Bone grafting should not be performed routinely (21,22). This treatment is carried out as a semielective procedure as soon as the patient's condition warrants; reduction is easiest when the fracture is treated within the first 48 hours. At a minimum, there must be screws engaging six cortices above and below the fracture site. Great care must be exercised to restore the length and curvature of the radius relative to the ulna to prevent loss of pronation and supination (19,20). The use of a 3.5-mm plate system has nearly eliminated the problem of refracture after plate removal (16,24). Previously, this problem was thought to be related to "stress-protection" of the underlying cortical bone but is now understood to be related to cortical bone ischemia (16). Plates should not be routinely removed from healed adult diaphyseal forearm fractures. Eight-hole plates are used most often. If bone grafting is indicated because of significant bone loss, the graft should be taken without disturbing either table of iliac bone or its muscle attachments, as described in **Chap. 10, II.K;** postoperatively, morbidity from the graft site is minimized. Reliable patients may be placed in a removable splint and early motion started as soon as wound healing is complete.

VIII. GALEAZZI FRACTURE OF THE RADIUS (25)
A. Description. This fracture is at the junction of the middle and distal third of the radius and is combined with a subluxation of the distal radioulnar joint (said to represent approximately 5% of forearm fractures).

B. Treatment. The treatment of choice is the same as for an isolated displaced fracture of the radius with forearm immobilization in supination for 6 weeks. The radius is fixed anatomically with a volar approach and plate fixation as for bone forearm fractures. If the distal radioulnar joint remains stable in supination as documented radiographically, a long-arm splint is applied to this position. In a reliable patient, elbow motion can be started with the forearm in supination using a hinged orthoses or Munster cast as soon as wound healing is confirmed. Occasionally, an open reduction of the distal radioulnar joint is necessary because of inability to reduce the joint. If the reduction is unstable, fixation with two Kirschner wires from the ulna to the radius is advisable; the wires are removed in 4 weeks. The Kirschner wire should be a minimum size of .062 in. or larger to avoid breaking. The distal radioulnar joint must be confirmed to be reduced by roentgenograms during the immobilization period.

IX. ISOLATED ULNA FRACTURES
A. Mechanism. This fracture frequently occurs as the result of a blow across the subcutaneous surface of the bone, thus the term "nightstick fracture."

B. Treatment. If the fracture is displaced and not associated with radial head subluxation, it can be well treated conservatively. Functional bracing or treatment with casting yields 95% to 98% union rates with good fixation (26–28).

X. COLLES' FRACTURE (29)
A. This extraarticular fracture of the distal radius was first described by Abraham Colles in 1814. In this important paper, he differentiated this injury from the rare dislocation of the wrist on clinical grounds without the aid of roentgenograms.

B. Examination. The wrist and hand are displaced dorsally in relation to the shaft of the radius (**Fig. 18-3**) to form the classic silver-fork deformity. Tenderness is found over the distal radius and over the ulnar styloid.

C. Roentgenograms. Anteroposterior and lateral films are essential and often show the following:
  1. **Comminution of the dorsal cortex**
  2. The following **displacements,** in varying degrees, of the distal fragments:
     a. **Dorsal displacement**
     b. **Dorsal angulation**

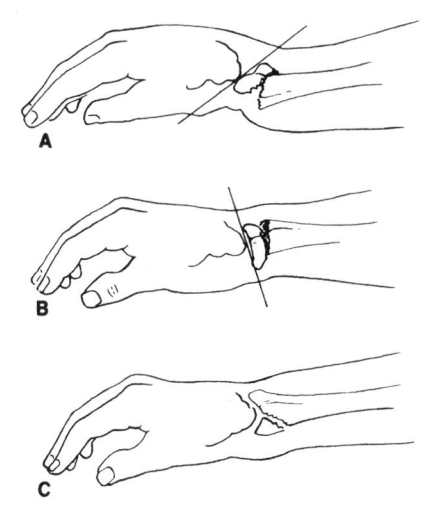

Figure 18-3. A: Colles' fracture. **B:** Smith fracture (reversed Colles' fracture). **C:** Barton fracture (causes displacement of the anterior portion of the articular surface).

c. **Proximal displacement**
d. **Radial displacement**
e. **Articular extension.** If the articular fractures are displaced, treatment is different.

D. **Treatment** must be directed as vigorously toward maintaining hand, elbow, and shoulder function as toward obtaining an acceptable cosmetic result.
1. The **radiocarpal joint normally faces palmarward** anywhere from 0 degrees to 18 degrees, so any amount of dorsal angulation is usually unacceptable, and better alignment should be attempted. Reduction of extraarticular fractures that are angulated palmarward between 1 degrees and 15 degrees depends on the age of the patient and the activity level desired; ordinarily, no reduction is necessary. If the palmar tilt is between 10 degrees and 20 degrees, the fracture should be immobilized with no attempt at reduction. The normal radial deviation of the radiocarpal joint ranges from 16 degrees to 28 degrees.
2. **Reduction** of this fracture usually is easy to achieve but difficult to maintain. It may be performed under a hematoma block, a Bier block (intravenous regional anesthetic), or an axillary block. Reducing the deformities that have been described previously involves the following steps:
   a. Fingertrap traction with a 10-lb weight hung from a strap across the arm is used, and the elbow is flexed 90 degrees in the line of the forearm to **disimpact the fracture**. Manual traction is an equally effective alternative.
   b. While traction is maintained, pressure is applied to the dorsal aspect of the distal fragment and to the palmar aspect of the proximal fragment to **correct dorsal displacement and rotation**.
   c. Pressure is applied on the radial aspect of the distal fragment to **correct radial deviation**.
3. The following are useful clinical **tests of reduction**:
   a. **Palpation** of the normal wrist shows that the radial styloid lies 1 cm distal to the ulnar styloid, and this relationship should be restored on the injured side.
   b. There should be **no tendency toward recurrence of the deformity**; that is, when one holds the elbow with the forearm parallel to the ground, the wrist contour appears normal. This may be difficult to assess with severe swelling.
4. **Methods of immobilization**
   a. The **wrist usually is immobilized** with the hand in ulnar deviation, the wrist neutral to no more than 15 degrees of volar flexion, and the anterior splints or single posterior splint extending over the first and second metacarpals to maintain the full ulnar deviation. Splints should be placed over a single layer of Webril applied with an adherent. Splints are wrapped in place by bias-cut stockinet or by an elastic bandage. Because of the potential for swelling, a circular cast is not advisable as initial treatment. The splints may be incorporated into a circular cast after all adjustments for swelling have been made. It is essential to allow full (90-degree) flexion of all metacarpophalangeal joints.
   b. **Short-arm versus long-arm casting.** If the surgeon wishes to maintain an accurate reduction, the elbow joint should be immobilized. A forearm splint-cast is appropriate, however, in the following situations:
      i. When the individual is **debilitated or elderly**
      ii. When an **incomplete reduction is to be accepted**
      iii. When **no reduction is attempted,** and the **impacted position of the fragments is accepted**
   c. In the younger individual with a severely comminuted and displaced extraarticular fracture, consider **external skeletal fixation** through the radius and the second metacarpal to maintain proper position and length (21). Immobilization in the fixator for at least 6 weeks is usually necessary, followed by mobilization of the wrist. In the older patient with badly comminuted fractures, early excision of the distal ulna and acceptance of radial

shortening may also be considered (29). See **Chap. 10, II.J,** for a discussion of external skeletal fixation.
    d. The presence of **intraarticular extension** changes the treatment paradigm in all but the most debilitated patients. A displacement of more than 3 to 4 mm mandates an attempt at closed reduction. Displacement of more than 2 mm warrants reduction in an adult because of the association of residual displacement with degenerative joint disease of the radiocarpal joint (30). Closed reduction of articular displacement is rarely successful. Therefore, an open reduction through a dorsal approach; Kirschner wire fixation; bone graft for the dorsal defect; and pins, external fixation, or small fragment plates for neutralization are generally recommended. There has been increased interest in open reduction in the internal fixation over the last decade to improve functional outcomes of these fractures in adults younger than 65 to 70 years of age where functional decrease is high (18,31).

E. **Aftercare**
   1. Frequent **active movements of the fingers and elevation of the hand** are both essential to reduce swelling and relieve pain. **Full movement of the shoulder joint also must be maintained.**
   2. Within 1 week of treatment, the following criteria should be met:
      a. There is **full, active movement of the fingers and the shoulder.**
      b. **Pain is minimal** and readily controlled with minimal analgesics.
      c. The **immobilization is satisfactory and comfortable.**
   3. **Follow-up roentgenograms** obtained through the splint should be obtained:
      a. After reduction
      b. On the **third day or when the swelling subsides**
      c. After **10 to 14 days**
      d. At **6 and 12 weeks after injury**
   4. **Duration of immobilization.** If the fracture is unreduced, it should be immobilized for 4 to 6 weeks. If the fracture is reduced, it should be immobilized for 6 to 8 weeks. Diminishing of tenderness over the site of fracture is evidence of progressive union. The wearing of a removable dorsal splint for several weeks after cast removal can improve patient comfort while allowing mobilization of the extremity.

F. **Complications**
   1. The most frequent complication is **stiffness of the finger joints and shoulder**.
   2. Pain with finger movement or numbness in the radial three digits often can signify a **carpal tunnel syndrome**. The pain usually is associated with complaints or abnormal neurologic findings in the median nerve distribution. If the abnormal findings persist for 3 days or increase in severity over 4 to 12 weeks, the carpal tunnel should be surgically released. If the patient has severe median nerve deficit, carpal tunnel release should be part of the initial management, which generally involves percutaneous pinning, external fixation, or open reduction.
   3. **Pain over the distal radioulnar joint** on supination of the forearm is a common complaint when immobilization is discontinued. The symptoms usually disappear within 6 months. Warn the patient of this problem in advance; if symptoms persist after full mobilization of the hand, excision of the distal ulna should be considered.
   4. **Some recurrence of deformity** is common. It is rare for the fractured wrist to have the same appearance as a normal wrist. Give the patient advance warning about this discrepancy and stress the desirability of good function rather than cosmesis.
   5. If **rupture by attrition of the extensor pollicis longus** is diagnosed, early repair is indicated. This may occur even with nondisplaced fractures. This is thought to be due to damage to the blood supply to the paratenon.

XI. **DISTAL RADIAL AND ULNAR FRACTURES IN CHILDREN**
   A. **Description.** These fractures are often referred to incorrectly as Colles' fractures because the deformity of the wrist is similar.

B. Roentgenograms. Roentgenographic examination is diagnostic. Be certain that the fracture is not one of the types of epiphyseal slips described below in **XIII**.

C. Treatment. When completely displaced, these fractures can be difficult to reduce. Manipulation should be done with the patient anesthetized or under conscious sedation, and the rule "one doctor, one manipulation" applies. Direct traction alone is rarely successful and should not be attempted, especially without complete patient relaxation under an anesthetic.

1. **Manipulative reduction** consists of either
   a. **Traction in line with the deformity** until the bone ends can be "locked on," followed by correction of the deformity.
   b. **Increasing the angulation of the distal fragments by manipulation (re-creating the deformity)** until the bone ends can be "locked on," followed by alignment of the distal fragment to the proximal fragment to correct the deformity.
2. **If reduction can be achieved**, it is usually stable, and treatment then consists of immobilization as for a Colles' fracture in a long-arm splint with the elbow at 90 degrees.
3. The fracture infrequently requires **open reduction**.

XII. SMITH AND BARTON FRACTURES OF THE DISTAL RADIUS

A. Smith fracture is a fracture of the distal radius with the distal fragment and accompanying carpal row displaced volarly (reversed Colles' fracture; **Fig. 18-3B**). The articular surface of the radius is not involved. This injury is usually secondary to a blow on the dorsum of the wrist or distal radius with the forearm in pronation.

1. **Treatment** may initially consist of a closed reduction under anesthesia. Longitudinal treatment is applied in a line with the deformity (pronation and flexion) until the fragments are distracted. Supination and pushing dorsally on the distal fragment reduce the fracture. The fracture should be immobilized with the forearm positioned in supination and the wrist in extension. These fractures are highly unstable and the patient should be informed that this may occur and that open reduction with pins or small fragment plates is generally necessary.
2. **Postmanipulative care is the same as for a Colles' fracture.**

B. Barton fracture is a fracture-dislocation in that the triangular fragment of the volar surface of the distal radius is sheared off (**Fig. 18-3C**). This fragment along with the carpus is displaced volarly and proximally.

1. The **mechanism of injury** is usually forced pronation under the axial load.
2. **Treatment** of this fracture by closed methods is difficult. Unless there is significant comminution, open reduction and fixation with a volar buttress plate is recommended.

XIII. DISTAL RADIAL EPIPHYSEAL SEPARATION

A. The usual **mechanism of injury** is a fall on the outstretched hand with a forced rotation of the wrist into dorsiflexion, resulting in dorsal displacement of the distal radius through the epiphyseal plate.

B. This fracture follows the rule of epiphyseal injuries (see **Chap. 1, VIII.B**). It is usually a **Salter class 1 or 2 fracture of the epiphysis**; hence, growth arrests may occur. The parents of an injured child must be gently acquainted with this fact.

C. Good-quality roentgenograms are essential in determining the type of epiphyseal separation.

D. Treatment. The younger the child, the more angulation and displacement can be accepted with assurance of normal subsequent function and cosmesis. In a child of any age, **angulation exceeding 25 degrees or displacement exceeding 25% of the radial height should be reduced**. A less-than-automatic reduction is preferable to repeated manipulations. The reduction is accomplished after adequate anesthesia to ensure complete muscle relaxation. Traction is applied in the line of deformity. The manipulation and postreduction treatment are the same as for a Colles' fracture. The patient should be immobilized in a long-arm cast for 3 to 4 weeks, followed by a short-arm cast for 2 to 4 weeks. Parents should be reassured that remodeling of the plate and joint motion will occur.

HCMC Treatment Recommendations
Elbow Dislocations
   Diagnosis: Anteroposterior and lateral radiographs of the elbow, physical examination.
   Treatment: Reduction under sedation in the emergency department—longitudinal traction with the elbow slightly flexed—postreduction stability examination and radiographs are essential for planning. If the elbow has good stability, start ROM exercises at 7 to 10 days.
   Indications for surgery: Unstable elbow after reduction, intraarticular fragments, associated fractures, especially of the coronoid process or radial head/neck.
   Recommended technique: Repair of the collateral ligaments, joint irrigation, fixation of sassociated fractures, particularly coronoid fractures of any significant size. Splint for 7 to 10 days and then start active range-of-motion (AROM) exercises.

HCMC Treatment Recommendations
Proximal Ulna Fractures
   Diagnosis: Anteroposterior and lateral radiographs, physical examination.
   Treatment: Splint initially, then generally open reduction with internal fixation (ORIF).
   Indications for surgery: Displacement of fracture of more than 2 mm or any persistent angulation, especially when associated with radial head dislocation.
   Recommended technique: Posterior approach, ORIF with tension band wire loop (figure-8) around K wires. ORIF with small fragment plates for more complicated fractures.

HCMC Treatment Recommendations
Radial Head Fractures
   Diagnosis: Anteroposterior and lateral elbow radiographs, physical examination.
   Treatment: Aspiration of intraarticular hematoma, injection of lidocaine followed by ROM (especially pronation and supination) of the elbow.
   Indications for surgery: A markedly displaced (>3–4 mm) Mason 2 fracture that inhibits pronation and supination or a displaced type 3 fracture.
   Recommended technique: ORIF wherever technically possible using minifragment screws (or mini plates for Mason 3). Excision of radial head where reduction is not possible using metallic spacer where there is an ipsilateral wrist injury.

HCMC Treatment Recommendations
Forearm Shaft Fractures
   Diagnosis: Anteroposterior and lateral radiographs of the forearm, physical examination.
   Treatment: ORIF with 3.5-mm plates and screws for any displaced forearm shaft fracture in an adult. The exception is the isolated ulna fracture with minimal shortening (<1–2 mm) and at least 50% apposition of bone fragments. Generally use eight-hole plate length or longer; plates should be left in wherever possible.

- Galeazzi variant—fixation of radius as described, with examination of distal radioulnar joint. If stable in supinated position, hold forearm in supinated position for 6 weeks; if joint is unstable, apply temporary K wire fixation.
- Monteggia variant—fixation of ulna fracture as described, examination (radiographic and clinical) of radiocapitellar joint. If not reduced, check ulna reduction for anatomicity and, if perfect, undertake open reduction of radius.
- Isolated ulna—ORIF with technique described for fractures with significant displacement and shortening.
- Isolated radius—ORIF with technique described for fractures with significant displacement (>2–3 mm of shortening) or loss of radial bow.

HCMC Treatment Recommendations
Distal Radius Fractures
  Diagnosis: Anteroposterior and lateral radiographs of the forearm, physical examination. Computed tomography scan can be helpful for intraarticular fractures.
  Treatment:

- Extraarticular variant—closed reduction under intravenous regional or hematoma block. Follow up radiographs in 3 to 7 days to be sure that reduction is maintained. Comminution at the fracture site makes redisplacement likely. The reduction must be neutral on the lateral with >4 mm loss of radial length on anteroposterior view—this is age dependent. External fixation is also an option.
- ORIF or closed reduction with percutaneous pinning for intraarticular fractures with greater than 2-mm displacement.

  Recommended technique: ORIF with K wires or small fragment specialized plates. Volar approach with small T plate for Barton (volar, partial articular fractures).

References
1. Baker BE, Bierwagen D. Rupture of the distal tendon of the biceps brachii. Operative vs. nonoperative treatment. *J Bone Joint Surg (Am)* 1985;67:414–417.
2. Melhoff TL, Noble PC, Bennett LB, et al. Simple dislocation of the elbow in the adult. *J Bone Joint Surg (Am)* 1988;70:244–249.
3. Regan W, Morrey BF. Fractures of the coronoid process of the ulna. *J Bone Joint Surg (Am)* 1989;71:1348–1354.
4. Pugh DM, Wild LM, Schemitsch EH, et al. Standard surgical protocol to treat elbow dislocations with radial head and coronoid fractures. *J Bone Joint Surg (Am)* 2004;86:1122–1130.
5. Josefsson PO, Gentz CF, Johnell O, et al. Surgical versus nonsurgical treatment of ligamentous injuries following dislocations of the elbow. *J Bone Joint Surg (Am)* 1987;69:605–608.
6. O'Driscoll SW, Morrey BF, Korinek S, et al. Elbow subluxation and dislocation: a spectrum of instability. *Clin Orthop* 1992;280:17–28.
7. Husband JB, Hastings H II. The lateral approach for operative release of posttraumatic contracture of the elbow. *J Bone Joint Surg (Am)* 1990;72:1353–1358.
8. Morrey BF. Treatment of the contracted elbow: distraction arthroplasty. *J Bone Joint Surg (Am)* 1990;72:601–618.
9. King GJ, Evans DC, Kellom JF. Open reduction and internal fixation of radial head fractures. *J Orthop Trauma* 1991;5:21–28.
10. Ring D, Quintero J, Jupiter JB. Open reduction and internal fixation of fractures of the radial head. *J Bone Joint Surg (Am)* 2002;84:1811–1815.
11. Moro JP, Werier J, MacDermid JC, et al. Arthroplasty with a metal radial head for unreconstructible fractures of the radial head. *J Bone Joint Surg (Am)* 2001;83:1201–1211.
12. Broberg MA, Morrey BF. Results of delayed excision of the radial head after fracture. *J Bone Joint Surg (Am)* 1986;68:669–674.
13. Mikic ZD, Vukadinovic SM. Late results in fracture of the redial head treated by excision. *Clin Orthop* 1983;181:220–228.
14. Mih AD, Cooney WP, Idlers RS, et al. Long-term follow-up of forearm bone diaphyseal plating. *Clin Orthop* 1994;199:156–158.
15. Ring D, Jupiter J, Simpson HS. Montegoia fractures in adults. *J Bone Joint Surg (Am)* 1998;80:1733–1744.
16. Unthoff HK, Boiscert D, Finnegan M. Cortical porosis under plates, reaction to unloading of necrosis? *J Bone Joint Surg (Am)* 1994;76:1502–1512.
17. Chapman MW, Gordon JE, Zissimos AG. Compression plate fixation of acute fractures of the diaphysis of the radius and ulna. *J Bone Joint Surg (Am)* 1989;71:159–169.

18. Ring D, Prommersberger K, Jupiter JB. Combined dorsal and volar plate fixation of complex fractures of the distal part of the radius. *J Bone Joint Surg (Am)* 2004;86:1616–1652.
19. Sarmiento A, Ebramzaden R, Brys D, et al. Angular deformities and forearm function. *J Orthop Res* 1992;10:121–133.
20. Schemitsch EH, Richards RR. The effect of malunion on functional outcome after plate fixation of both bones of the forearm in adults. *J Bone Joint Surg (Am)* 1992;74:1068–1078.
21. Vaughan PA, Lui SM, Harrington IJ, et al. Treatment of unstable fractures of the distal radius by external fixation. *J Bone Joint Surg (Br)* 1985;67:385–389.
22. Wei SY, Born CT, Abene A, et al. Diaphyseal forearm fractures treated with and without bone graft. *J Trauma* 1999;46:1045–1048.
23. Wright RR, Schmeling GL, Schwab JP. The necessity of acute bone grafting in diaphyseal forearm fractures: a retrospective review. *J Orthop Trauma* 1997;11:288–294.
24. Beaupre GS, Csongrad LL. Refracture risk after plate removal in the forearm. *J Orthop Trauma* 1996;10:87–92.
25. Moore TM, Klein JP, Patzakis MJ, et al. Results of compression plating of closed Galeazzi fractures. *J Bone Joint Surg (Am)* 1985;67:1015–1021.
26. Atkin DM, Bohay DR, Slabangh P, et al. Treatment of ulnar shaft fractures: a prospective, randomized study. *Orthopedics* 1995;18:543–547.
27. Gebuhr P, Holmich P, Orsnes T, et al. Isolated ulnar shaft fractures: comparison of treatment by a functional brace and long-arm cast. *J Bone Joint Surg (Br)* 1992;74:757–759.
28. Sarmiento A, Lotta LL, Zych G, et al. Isolated ulnar shaft fractures treated with functional braces. *J Orthop Trauma* 1998;12:420–424.
29. Altissimi M, Antencci R, Fiacca Mancini GB. Long-term results of conservative treatment of fracture of the distal radius. *Clin Orthop* 1986;206:202.
30. Knirk JL, Jupiter JB. Intraarticular fractures of the distal end of the radius in young adults. *J Bone Joint Surg (Am)* 1986;68:647–659.
31. Simic PM, Weiland AJ. Fractures of the distal aspect of the radius: changes in treatment over the past two decades. *J Bone Joint Surg (Am)* 2003;85:552–564.

Selected Historical Readings

Bado JL. The Monteggia lesion. *Clin Orthop* 1967;50:71–86.
Burwell HN, Charnley AD. Treatment of forearm fractures in adults with reference to plate fixation. *J Bone Joint Surg (Br)* 1964;46:404–425.
Fowles JV, Sliman N, Kassab MT. The Monteggia lesion in children: fracture of the ulna and dislocation of the radial head. *J Bone Joint Surg (Am)* 1983;65:1276–1282.
Fuller DJ, McCullough CJ. Malunited fractures of the forearm in children. *J Bone Joint Surg (Br)* 1982;64:364–367.
Linscheid RL, Wheeler DK. Elbow dislocations. *JAMA* 1965;194:1171–1176.
Mason M. Some observations on fractures of the head of the radius with a review of 100 cases. *J Bone Joint Surg (Br)* 1954;42:123–132.
Monteggia GB. *Instituzione chirugiche*, 2nd. Milan: G. Maspero, 1814.
Morrey BF, Chao EY, Hui FC. Biomechanical study of the elbow following excision of the radial head. *J Bone Joint Surg (Am)* 1979;61:63–68.
Taylor TK, O'Connor BT. The effect upon the inferior radioulnar joint of excision of the end of the radius in adults. *J Bone Joint Surg (Br)* 1964;46:83–88.

ACUTE WRIST AND HAND INJURIES   19

I. **BASIC PRINCIPLES AND DATA.** Acute injuries to the hand and wrist are common. Obvious reasons for this fact stem from use of the hand as a working tool in sometimes dangerous environs (e.g., as an object holder immediately adjacent to a power tool) and the all too frequent use of the arm as brake (fall onto an outstretched arm). A patient's general health characteristics may play an important role in determining the frequency and outcome from such accidents (e.g., diabetics with originally reduced sensation and ongoing reduced blood supply/immune function and osteoporosis with reduced skeletal strength). There are several issues to be considered with all patients:

  A. **Date of last tetanus immunization.** One should consider the possibility of skin compromise with injuries to the hand and wrist. Even without obvious laceration, penetration of infectious organisms into the subcutaneous tissue has been known to occur. The effects of infection from one such organism (tetanus) are largely preventable. Consequently, whenever possible, verify the status of tetanus immunization in all patients whom you are treating for hand or wrist trauma.

  B. **Injury site characteristics.** These may alter your treatment choices. For example, a fracture with a nearby clean laceration from a sharp object can often be managed as though the skin had remained closed, whereas the same fracture associated with a minimal but contaminated (farmyard or sewage) puncture into the fracture hematoma must first be thoroughly irrigated. **Thus,** the first key characteristic is to establish the extent of the skin injury and to specifically determine if any external injection of organisms deep into the skin surface is likely to have occurred. In the case of burns (cold or hot), knowledge of the depth of the skin injury is important. It is important to be specific when describing wounds. Adjectives used to modify established terminology (e.g., severe "bad" or not bad) should be avoided. Use phrases or classification with known meaning whenever possible.

  Helpful adjectives used in characterizing a wound include:
   1. **Open or closed:** used most commonly in association with a fracture. **If** the skin is open to a fracture, it is considered open. This same phraseology is important in treating lacerations close to joints and some tendon injuries.
   2. **Clean or contaminated:** generally, a kitchen knife would be considered clean as compared to a saw blade picked up from a farmyard workbench.
   3. **Tidy or untidy:** the margin of a laceration can be so ragged as to prevent repair. In the hand (the same applies to the foot and face), this can preclude tensionless wound closure and thus necessitate advanced wound management methods.

  C. **Patient's habits and addictions.** Without doubt, the most important habit to be aware of is the patient's habit of following medical advice. This is particularly important in children, and the emergently consulted physician has a known responsibility to enable timely follow-up care. The majority of hand and wrist injuries requiring consultation from an orthopaedic specialist will need early (2–14 days) follow-up, and failure to ensure this care may result in disability. Other habits of importance include the following:
   1. **Tobacco use disorder.** In addition to being an established diagnosis (ICD-9 = 305.1), this problem will impact bone healing (known) as well as other tissues (skin, tendon, nerve) (suspected).
   2. **Recreational drug use.** Impaired patients will place stresses on casts and dressings such that the medical repairs may fail. In some circumstances, hospital admission with appropriate consults is required.

D. Systemic illness. Illness which compromises immune function is a common reason for delayed recovery after hand/wrist injury. Additionally, diseases such as rheumatoid arthritis or advanced osteoporosis will impact the result from injury and the type of treatment that can be chosen.

II. HISTORY

A. Where and how did the injury occur? As noted above, record the location of the injury and its mechanism. This is important for two basic reasons. First, you need to know the cleanliness of the wound and how much **energy** was applied to the tissues. Second, you need to record the where (work, home, motor vehicle accident, etc.) and how (an allegedly defective tool, a reported assailant, etc.) because the first examining document will be used henceforth as the "truth." Thus, your written history should contain few adjectives and only known facts.

B. How did the patient become aware of the injury? Some injuries will present after the suspected injury occurred. In these instances, recording additional facts related to the patient's presentation is important.

C. Pain
1. **Location.** Be specific. Use anatomic descriptors. Try to avoid use of "medial and lateral" and numbering the digits (due to misinterpretations). The second finger is not the index but the middle. Thus, do not use number references for fingers as too many physicians and most lay people mistake the index for the second finger (which it is not). Use the following terms: radial and ulnar; dorsal and volar; thumb, index, middle, ring, and small finger.
2. **Qualities.** Phrases such as "really bad pain" are meaningless. Words such as burning, radiating, and tingling may be helpful in detecting/isolating a nerve injury, whereas words such as deep, constant, and throbbing may be associated with an infection.

D. Numbness
1. **Location** (similar to **C.1**). Describe the anatomic location of the numbness using precise words (e.g., the radial border of the ring finger). These phrases will hopefully be anatomically possible and serve to isolate the nerve difference. Patients describing anatomically unlikely numbness are occasionally seeking secondary gain.
2. **Qualities.** As in **C.2**, specificity is important. In addition, record frequency and inciting factors (e.g., the numbness occurs when I am driving for 20 minutes or more).

E. Range of motion. Specific ranges to be recorded are demonstrated in **Fig. 19-1** and summarized in **Table 19-1**.

Idealized numbers are inserted. The key to a successful exam is to measure left and right in the affected areas.
1. **Active.** Active motion helps to document the integrity of tendons and the stability/congruity of joints.
2. **Passive.** Differences and similarities between active and passive motion can help to document/differentiate several conditions, for example, disrupted tendons (active will be low/absent and passive will be high/normal) and stiff joints (active will be low and passive will be low).

F. Strength. Generally, the international classification for muscle strength is used. Thus, a muscle can be graded from 0 (flaccid and no evidence of innervation) to 5 (normal). However, specific strengths are often measured in the hand and forearm and compared over time.
1. **Pinch strength.** Measured with a "pinch gauge" and recorded in pounds or kilograms.
   a. **Key.** Thumb to side of index or middle finger (strong, used for rotation)
   b. **Chuck.** Thumb to pulp of two fingers (strong and moderately precise)
   c. **Tip.** Thumb to one finger pulp (weakest and most precise)
2. **Grip strength.** Measured with a "dynomometer" and recorded in pounds or kilograms.
   a. Can be recorded in several diameters and useful to "quantify" malingering as well as recovery over time.

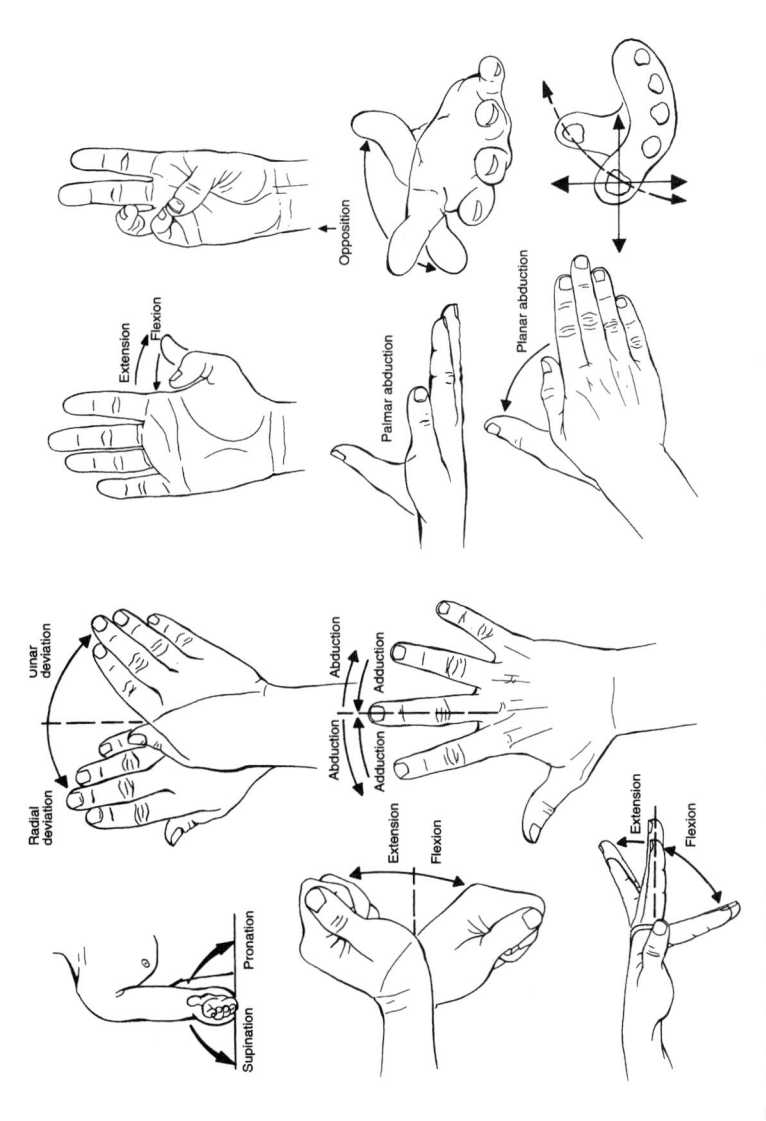

Figure 19-1. Terminology for describing forearm, hand, and digital motion. (From Seiler JG III. *Essentials of hand surgery*, Lippincott Williams & Wilkins, Philadelphia, PA, 2002, with permission.)

TABLE 19-1 Normal Hand and Wrist Motion

Motion: Active (passive)	Right	Left
Supination (occurs at distal radio-ulnar joint)	90 (90)	Same
Wrist flexion (occurs at radiocarpal and midcarpal joints)	70 (90)	Same
Wrist extension (occurs at radiocarpal and midcarpal joints)	70 (90)	Same
Wrist radial deviation (occurs at radiocarpal and midcarpal joints)	20 (30)	Same
Wrist ulnar deviation (occurs at radiocarpal and midcarpal joints)	40 (50)	Same
Finger abduction and adduction (occurs at metacarpalphalangeal joint (MCPJ), index to small)	20 (20)	Same
Finger base extension and flexion (occurs at MCPJ, index to small)	10 (30)	Same
Thumb and finger individual joint extension and flexion	0 to 90 (10, extension to 100, flexion)	Same
Thumb palmar abduction	45 (45)	Same
Thumb opposition (how close to small finger base)	0 cm; able to touch base of small finger	Same
Thumb radial (planar) abduction	45 (45)	Same

III. PHYSICAL EXAM

A. General. The hand and wrist are extensions of the extremity and, as such, depend upon an intact skin envelope to protect against systemic illness (e.g., septicemia).

Beyond skin, the hand has three primary functions: sensation, movement, and cosmesis. Nerves; bones and joints; and tendons and muscles all play an important role in determining the outcome after injury and care.

B. Region specific exam

  1. Distal radio-ulnar joint. This joint works in combination with the proximal radio-ulnar joint to guide the rotation of the distal radius around the ulnar head (distal portion of the ulna). **Fig. 19-2** demonstrates this important motion.

  a. Muscle. The pronator quadratus muscle originates immediately proximal to the distal radioulnar joint (DRUJ). It has a deep and superficial head and helps to stabilize and pronate the forearm. The muscle is innervated by the terminal branch of the anterior interosseous nerve. The muscle can be injured in conjunction with distal radius fractures.

  b. Tendon. The extensor carpi ulnaris and the extensor digiti minimi tendons run alongside and dorsal to the ulnar head. Occasionally, the tendon sheath will tear and the extensor carpi ulnaris (ECU) tendon can become unstable. Also, a lax or irregular DRUJ can damage the extensor digit minimi (EDM) tendons. Otherwise, no direct attachment of tendon to the joint occurs.

  c. Joint/bone. The DRUJ is interesting. It is a "roll and slide" joint. Considerable variance in design occurs. What is universally true is that an unstable DRUJ is uncomfortable or painful. When the joint does not work well, it usually results in a loss of supination. An unusual but possible injury to the joint would be dislocation without fracture in either the volar or dorsal direction.

  d. Triangular fibrocartilage complex (TFCC). First described in 1981, the TFCC is the major ligamentous stabilizer of the distal radio-ulnar joint and the ulnar-carpus joint. Within this triangular complex is cartilaginous material that may be injured either acutely (e.g., from a fall onto an outstretched hand) or chronically (e.g., from overuse with the wrist in an

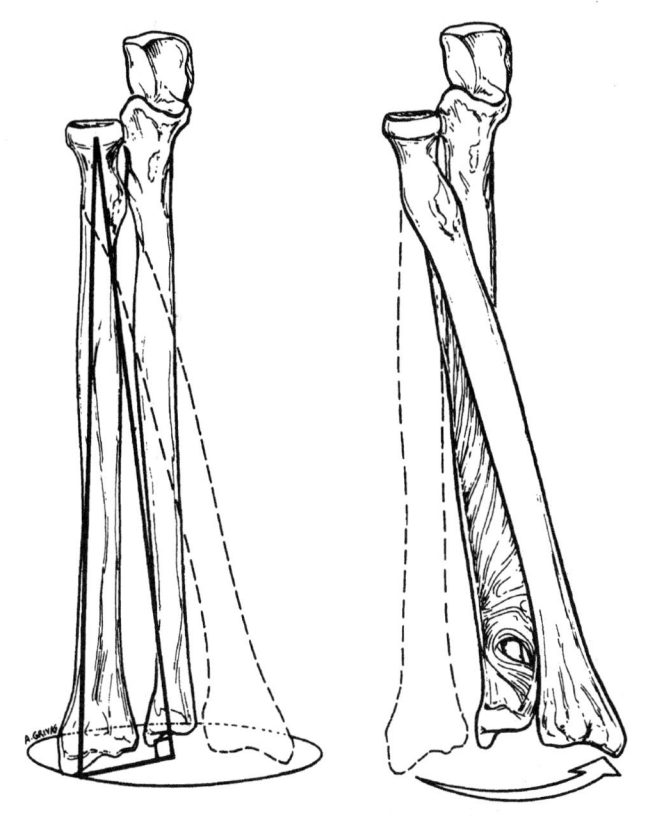

Figure 19-2. The axis of rotation of the radius with respect to the ulna, with the center of the axis of rotation being aligned beginning at the center of the radial head and ending near the center of the distal part of the ulna. Rotation is guided by the interosseous membrane and the triangular fibrocartilage. (From Peimer CA. *Surgery of the hand and upper extremity.* New York: McGraw-Hill, 1996, with permission.)

ulnar-deviated position such as with the use of a computer mouse). Patients with ulnar-sided wrist pain that is made worse with compression (analogous to hyperflexion of the knee when assessing for meniscal tears) may have a TFCC injury.

    e. Nerve and vessel. A rare but reported injury is entrapment of the ulnar nerve and/or ulnar artery following reduction of a completely dislocated DRUJ. This would generally require a complete separation to occur between the radius and ulnar head but could also occur in a young child who could fracture through the physeal plate and in combination with a fracture just proximal to the ulnar head. In any event, the important point is to carefully assess nerve function before and after reduction maneuvers and carefully account for any change in function after reduction.

2. Wrist

    a. Muscle. Indirectly and directly, muscles arise from the wrist. Specifically, the thenar and hypothenar muscles arise from the transverse carpal ligament (thenars) or the hook of hamate and the pisiform (hypothenars). Function of these muscles can be reduced in combination with injuries to their attachments. This would include an indirect injury to the attachments

of the transverse carpal ligament such as would occur with a trapezial fracture, scaphoid tubercle fracture, or pisiform fracture.
  b. **Tendon.** Tendons do not attach directly to any of the main seven carpal bones (the pisiform is a sesamoid and not a true carpal bone; the flexor carpi-ulnaris does surround the pisiform). However, the flexor carpi-radialis does appear to attach indirectly by way of a sheath to the scaphoid tubercle and consequently transfer a flexion vector to the scaphoid. Also, the wrist and its adjacent soft tissues act as a guide for both the flexor and extensor tendons. Specifically, the carpal canal guides the thumb and finger flexors as well as the median nerve. The extensor retinaculum (**Fig. 19-3**, the wrist extensor compartments 1 to 6) stabilizes the finger extensors immediately proximal to the radio-carpal joint and acts as both a pulley for these motors both in extension as well as radial and ulnar deviation. Fractures or lacerations affecting tendons in this area often result in significant stiffness. This may be the result of many structures being injured as well as a consequence of tendons in this area possessing a large excursion. Thus, any loss of tendon glide will be noticeable.
  c. **Joint/bone.** Motion of wrist depends upon ligament control of two rows of bones affected by muscles attaching to bones at varying distances distal to the wrist. This arrangement is similar to the ankle. However, nonobvious ligament tears [normal x-rays and nonspecific magnetic resonance imaging (MRI) scans] can significantly disable the normal wrist. This is often the result of a disconnection occurring between the proximal and distal carpal rows. This type of disconnection can occur without obvious bone

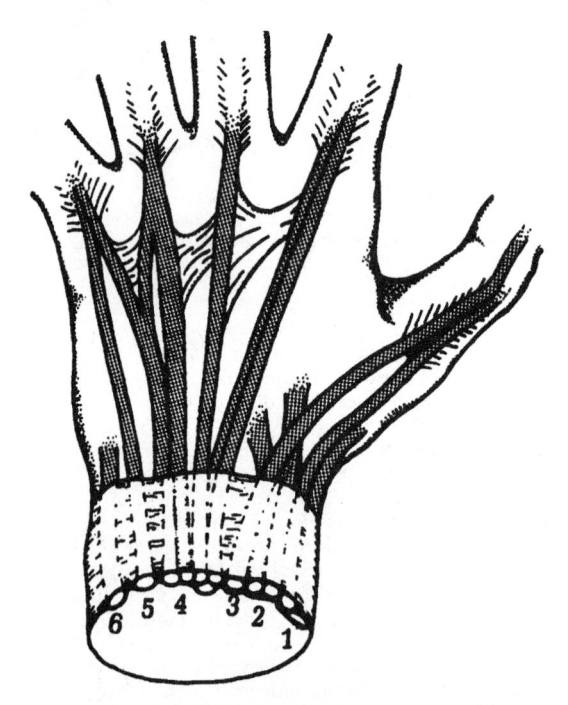

Figure 19-3. Arrangement of extensor tendons at the wrist into six compartments: dorsal and cross-sectional views. (From Seiler JG III. *Essentials of hand surgery*, Lippincott Williams & Wilkins, Philadelphia, PA, 2002, with permission.)

injury. Usually, injury to the scapho-lunate interosseous ligament (SLIL) is the cause of such a injury. However, bone injury can produce the same effect upon the wrist, and the most common fracture causing wrist instability is a scaphoid waist fracture. Finally, although not frequently causing wrist instability, distal radius fractures can cause ligament injury in addition to causing joint surface irregularity and/or poor fit with resultant joint capsular stiffness.

    d. Nerve and vessel. Close proximity of three sensory (radial, median, and ulnar) and two motor (median and ulnar) nerves can result in nerve compression symptoms. Actual direct injury to the nerves is rare.

3. Proximal hand
    a. Muscle. The base of the hand is the site of attachment for extrinsic (muscles originating from the forearm) wrist extensors, flexors, and deviators as well as the thumb abductor. Also, the hand base is the origin of the hand intrinsics. Destabilization by fracture of the hand base or metacarpal shafts can be made significantly worse by muscle tone. Splinting attempts to neutralize these forces.

    b. Tendon. The finger extensors are adjacent to the dorsal metacarpal bone surface. Thus, in addition to acting as a shortening force, the extensors can be injured or entrapped by displaced metacarpal fractures. Tendons overlying dorsally angulated mid-shaft fractures are most at risk.

    c. Joint/bone. Two joints are involved in the proximal hand separated by the metacarpal shaft. The proximal joint varies from the near universal thumb base to the effectively immobile second and third carpalmetacarpal (CMC) joints. The distal joint is remarkable for its unicondylar, multiaxial shape. Distally, the bone shape allows some radial-ulnar laxity which is reduced to none as the metacarpalphalangeal joint (MCPJ) moves into flexion and the collateral ligaments tighten. An interesting note: the metacarpal epiphyseal plate is distal in the second thru fifth fingers and proximal in the thumb.

    d. Nerve and vessel. Immediately distal to the volar aspect of CMC joints, the ulnar and median nerve splits into its common digital nerve components. In this same region, interconnections between the radial and ulnar artery via the deep and superficial arches occur. Significant swelling, displacement, or lacerations can result in loss of vascular injury.

4. Fingers
    a. Muscle. The fingers do not contain any muscle tissue.

    b. Tendon. The fingers are balanced by an intricate arrangement of flexor and extensor tendons. **Fig. 19-4** depicts the complex balance achieved by the extrinsic and intrinsic extensors. The apparent key finger extension occurs at the proximal interphalangeal joint (PIPJ). At this level, the intrinsic tendons transit from volar to dorsal and rely upon thin, easily injured, retinacular structures to maintain their position. Closed injury to these structures with progressive loss of PIPJ and increasing fixed extension at the distal interphalangeal joint are the hallmarks of the developing boutonierre deformity. **Fig. 19-5** illustrates the anatomy of the flexor pulleys. These pulleys guide the flexor tendon and its surrounding tenosynovial sheath during motion of the flexor tendons. Injuries involving the flexor pulleys can result in scarification to the tendons themselves even without tendon laceration. Perhaps more importantly, the pulleys enclose a space which is easily infected after a puncture wound and can serve as a path for infection into the palm and, in the case of the small finger and thumb, into the wrist and forearm (see **V.A**).

    c. Joint/bone. Unlike the more proximal unicondylar MCPJs, the finger interphalangeal joints are bicondylar and uniaxial. This configuration results in a joint which is stable throughout the axis of rotation. Theoretically, this results in a more stable arrangement for pinch and grip activities. However, this lack of rotational tolerance also means that small changes in rotation of

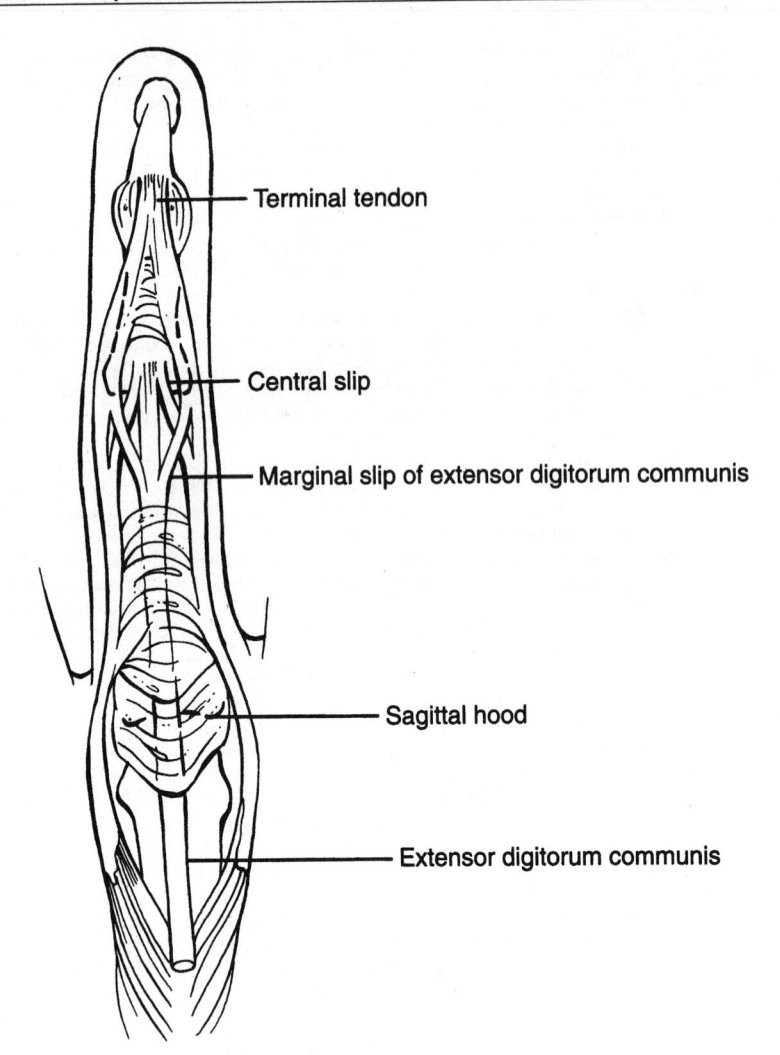

Figure 19-4. Extensor apparatus over the dorsum of the digits. (From Seiler JG III. *Essentials of hand surgery*, Lippincott Williams & Wilkins, Philadelphia, PA, 2002, with permission.)

a finger may be easily noticed and interfere with adjacent digit function. **Fig. 19-6** illustrates the problem associated with rotational deformity of a finger. Thus, the key deformity to rule out when evaluating a finger fracture is rotational over- or underlap. Because one role of the fingers is grasp/pinch and release, it is apparent that stable joints are essential. But, ligament injuries to the fingers and thumb are common. One such injury is a "gamekeepers's" thumb. As illustrated in **Fig. 19-7**, this injury may be a partial sprain or can result in complete disruption of the ulnar collateral ligament at the MCPJ and require surgical repair. Similar injures can occur at the PIPJ of the fingers and occasionally overlap with complete dislocations. In all such patients, an x-ray should be obtained and a congruent joint reduction should be present.

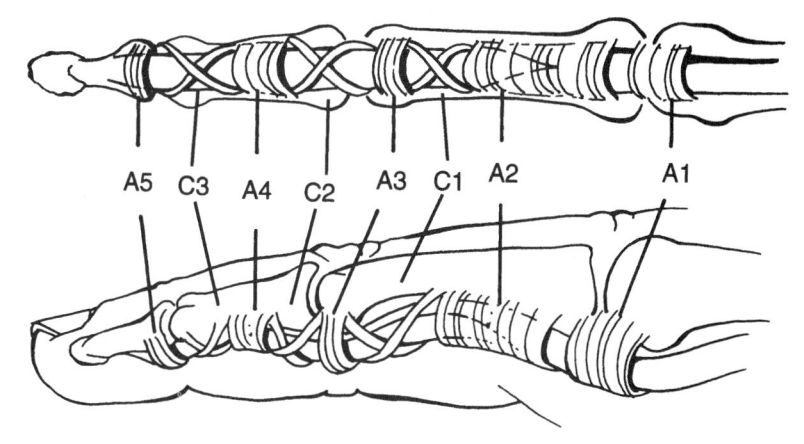

Figure 19-5. The annular and cruciate pulleys of the flexor tendon sheath. (From Seiler JG III. *Essentials of hand surgery*, Lippincott Williams & Wilkins, Philadelphia, PA, 2002, with permission.)

d. **Nerve and vessel.** The nerves and blood vessels are situated immediately adjacent to the flexor tendons and maintained in position by dorsal (Cleland's) and volar (Grayson's) fascial "ligament-like" tissue. Isolated injuries to the nerve and vessel do occur and are sometimes described as cuts with excessive bleeding. However, restoring blood flow is almost never an issue because of sufficient redundancy from the remaining blood vessel, whereas single nerve injuries can be problematic and require repair when the injury involves pinch surfaces and or border digits. For central digits, nerve repair is elective and oftentimes performed only to manage painful neuromas.

IV. **SPECIFIC INJURIES**
   A. **Wrist**
   1. **Tendon and nerve.** Nerve and tendon injuries in this region are uncommon (flexor zone 5). Some of the injuries in this region are self-inflicted and, for this reason, the patient's mental status should **always** be carefully evaluated. As long as blood flow to the hand is adequate, repair of nerve and tendon tissue in this region is urgent and not emergent. Thus, initial care should focus on wound/tetanus status, skin closure, medical care, and mental health status clearance.
   2. **Joint.** Patients with pain and a history of significant load (e.g., fall while rollerblading) whose x-ray are normal often have a **real** ligament injury. The most common of these is injury to the scapho-lunate ligament. Obtaining an x-ray with a "clenched fist" may demonstrate separation of these bones not seen on standard films. Close follow-up must be ensured. Early MRI might be valuable but should be ordered by the specialist. This is particularly true in light of the specialist's ability to "see" the ligament tear when completing fluoroscopic evaluation, whereas the same tear might not be visible in the MRI exam and, thus, ordering the MRI would be cost-inefficient.
   3. **Bone.** Three bone injuries occur commonly.
      a. **Dorsal triquetral avulsion fractures.** This may be the most common wrist fracture. Fortunately, treatment is symptomatic and fractures which have not healed and remain painful can be excised.
      b. **Scaphoid fractures.** Many scaphoid fractures are hard to "see" initially. Some of these fractures are actually serious ligament sprains. Regardless, **all high-energy** wrist injuries, without a clear diagnosis, should be

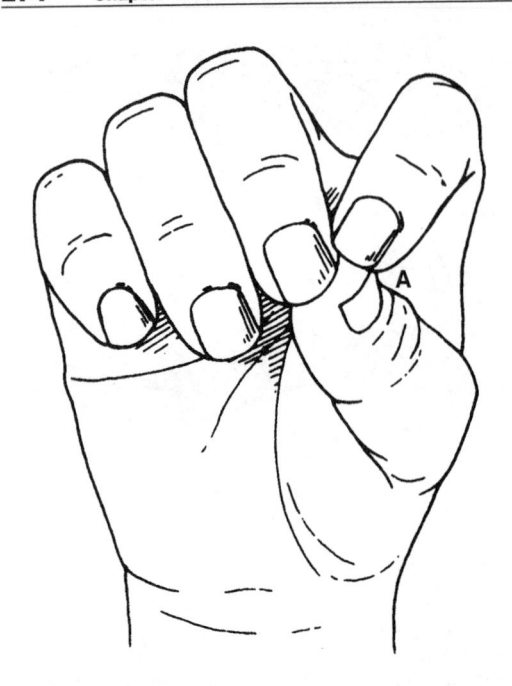

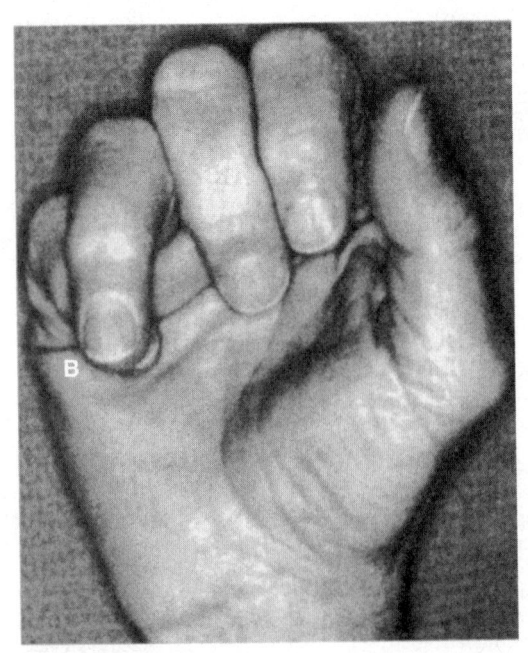

Figure 19-6. A: When the digit is flexed, the deformity is quite apparent. **B:** Active finger flexion generates malrotation of ring finger with digital overlapping. (From Seiler JG III. *Essentials of hand surgery*, Lippincott Williams & Wilkins, Philadelphia, PA, 2002, with permission.)

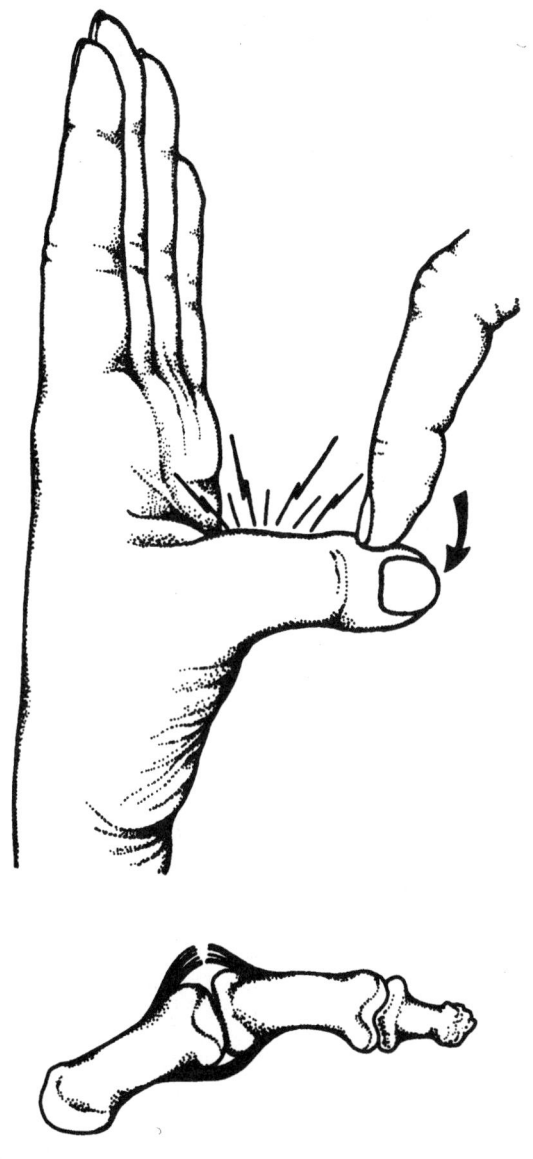

Figure 19-7. Rupture of ulnar collateral ligament of the metacarpophalangeal joint of the thumb. (From Seiler JG III. *Essentials of hand surgery*, Lippincott Williams & Wilkins, Philadelphia, PA, 2002, with permission.)

splinted and follow-up should be arranged with a physician in 10 to 14 days. Original x-rays should include four views of the scaphoid (including a specific "scaphoid view" with the wrist in ulnar deviation to elongate the view of the bone). Follow-up x-rays would be similar. Continued pain without diagnosis might warrant an MRI.

- c. **Distal radius fractures.** Most of these fractures are obvious. During initial evaluation, the function of the DRUJ and the median and ulnar nerve should be evaluated. Initial-care focus is to splint the fracture with sufficient alignment and stability so as to allow comfortable finger, elbow, and shoulder motion. The original splint should immobilize the wrist and the elbow with the forearm in neutral rotation and the wrist in neutral flexion/extension. The splint should not block finger or thumb flexion/extension. An ideal splint is the "sugar-tong" splint. This is a dorsal and volar splint with opening at the side to allow for swelling. Patients who cannot be pain stabilized so that home discharge (prior to more definite care) can be accomplished may be developing compartment syndrome or acute carpal tunnel syndrome. In either case, emergent specialty consultation is needed.

4. **Amputation.** Fortunately, traumatic amputation at this level is rare. Surprisingly, results of replantation at this level are better than those seen at the midpalm or with multiple digits. The keys to successful management are
   a. Cooling (floating) the injured part in ice water. **Do not place the part onto ice.**
   b. Antibiotics and tetanus administration
   c. Systemic fluid balance
   d. Transfer to a qualified specialist

B. **Hand**
1. **Skin.** Surface burns from cold or heat exposure require tetanus and antibiotic treatment. All blisters should be left intact. In addition to sterile dressings, the hand should be splinted in a functional position. In the case of frostbite, current guidelines recommend rapid rewarming. Evolving guidelines involve antithrombolytic agents, especially for frostbite.
2. **Nail plate and pulp.** Infections are common in the hand and fingernail. Do not confuse herpetic whitlow and its vesicles with actual paronychia and associated cellulitis. Drainage of a herpes infection can result in a super-infection with bacteria. When herpes is suspected in an individual in contact with others, the patient must be isolated until the lesions have resolved. Bacterial infection in this region either is around the nail or in the pulp tissues (felon). Felons are hardest to treat. **Fig. 19-8** depicts a felon. The need to drain the entire pulp is emphasized. Noninfectious problems in this area include simple subungual hematomas from trauma. Drainage of the hematoma through the nail plate usually results in complete and immediate relief of the pressure pain.
3. **Tendon**
   a. **Flexor.** Flexor tendon lacerations are surgical urgencies. Diagnosis should be made based upon functional loss after a trauma. Some important injuries (avulsion of the distal end of the flexor digitorum profundus) can occur without a laceration. This may occur when a grasping hand is suddenly pulled away from an object (jersey finger). Failure to make an early diagnosis of a flexor tendon injury may preclude a good result. **Thus, after a finger/hand laceration or a sudden pull-away injury, the key diagnostic step is an active motion exam at all joint levels and not wound exploration.** It is essential to test finger flexion with the nonaffected fingers in full extension. Then test the affected finger without further obstruction and with forced extension at the PIP in order to isolate both the profundus tendons and the superficialis tendon respectively. Once a flexor tendon laceration is diagnosed or suspected, immediate referral to a hand specialist is recommended. Almost never should a flexor repair be completed in the emergency department. Almost always, a skin laceration

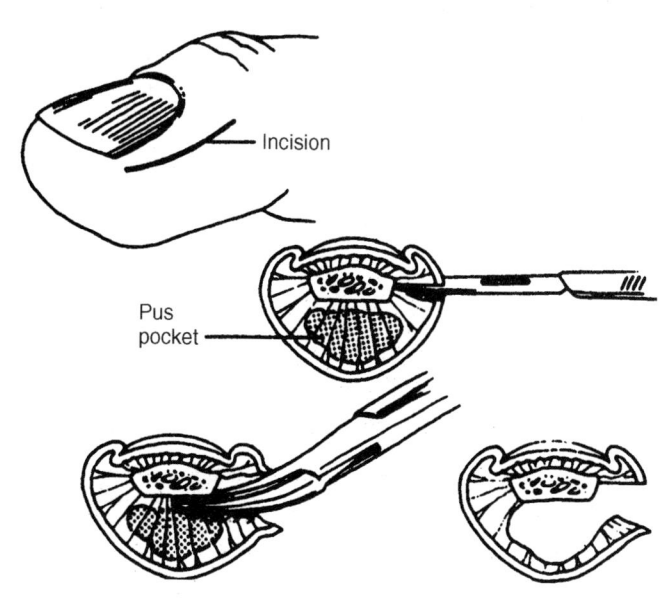

Figure 19-8. Drainage of a felon using a midlateral incision. Complete division of the vertical septae should be performed. (From Seiler JG III. *Essentials of hand surgery*, Lippincott William & Wilkins, Philadelphia, PA, 2002, with permission.)

over or near a suspected tendon laceration should be closed before the patient is discharged from the emergency department.

    b. Extensor. Extensor tendon lacerations must be urgently managed if they involve the joint. Because of the close proximity of the MCPJ, PIPJ, and DIPJ to the tendon, it is possible to contaminate the joint while only partially disrupting the tendon's function. Any laceration which may have contaminated the joint deserves a tourniquet-controlled exam and complete irrigation. Lacerations in the extensor region not involving the joint do not always require direct repair. **Occasionally**, an extensor repair can be completed in the emergency department. Lacerations which can be seen to involve extensor tendon but which do not alter active function (partial tendon lacerations) should be cleaned and closed without placement of sutures into tendon. If a definite (at least 10-degree) active extension loss distal to the observed laceration is documented, consultation with a specialist should be completed before discharge from the emergency department. Almost always, a skin laceration over or near a suspected tendon laceration should be closed before the patient is discharged from the emergency department.

4. Nerve. Nerve injuries in the distal arm region are common. Unless they are present in conjunction with a devascularized arm, nerve injuries can be managed on a delayed basis. The most common nerve injury by frequency is a digital nerve laceration. When these occur, the ipsilateral digital artery will often be damaged. In this situation, the volume of bleeding is often the concern. **Do not attempt to cauterize or "tie off" the bleeding vessel.** The close proximity of the artery to the nerve makes greater damage to the nerve almost a certainty. Thus, in the case of a finger laceration with bleeding uncontrolled by pressure and time, expert exploration of the wound with proper lighting, instruments, and magnification is appropriate. The keys to satisfactory outcome after nerve injury in the finger are more related to not missing any associated flexor tendon lacerations and not over-managing initial bleeding, thereby creating a larger nerve injury. Many digital nerve injuries are never repaired and yet the patient functions satisfactorily.

5. **Joint.** An overlap between ligament and joint injuries in the fingers exists. The small size of the joints accounts for this fact. **Fig. 19-9** depicts a common fracture pattern in the DIPJ of a finger. However, in this injury, the fracture fragment is large enough so as to destabilize the joint. This destabilization is obvious because a line drawn through the diaphyses of one phalanx no longer bisects the adjacent phalanx. In this example, the fragment must be reduced to achieve a congruent and stable joint. A simple and universal rule is that the joint surface must have equal space between the bony elements at any joint at any location in both a true anteroposterior and lateral x-ray. If the distance between bone elements is not equal, the joint is unstable. One common exception to this statement does exist: This is the bony mallet deformity. Such an injury is similar to **Fig. 19-9** in that a portion of the distal phalanx is fractured. However, mallet deformities (with or without a bony fragment) differ from **Fig. 19-9** because they do not result in volar or dorsal migration of the remainder of the phalanx. Initial treatment of all mallet deformities is a neutral extension splint (**Fig. 19-10**).

6. **Bone.** Overlap between bone and joint injuries is common as mentioned above. One further overlap is discussed below (fight bites in **V.B**). Four more common fracture conditions exist.

   a. **Boxer's fracture. Fig. 19-11** depicts a common result of pugilistic activity. The fracture shown is at the proximal margin of the metacarpal neck and is almost a diaphyseal fracture. This is an important point. Because boxer's fractures occur in the neck (immediately proximal to the metacarpal head/joint), significant flexion deformity can be accommodated. The exception to this is in the rare cases when the digits involved are the index or middle fingers (typically the small finger is affected). Thus, open operative treatment is rarely indicated. There are two keys for successful outcome when managing a boxer's fracture:

   i. Do not overlook a puncture wound/open fracture.
   ii. Do not miss a rotational deformity. In order to exclude rotational deformity, the finger must be gently flexed at the MCPJ, and grip flexion posture must be examined and compared to the adjacent digits.

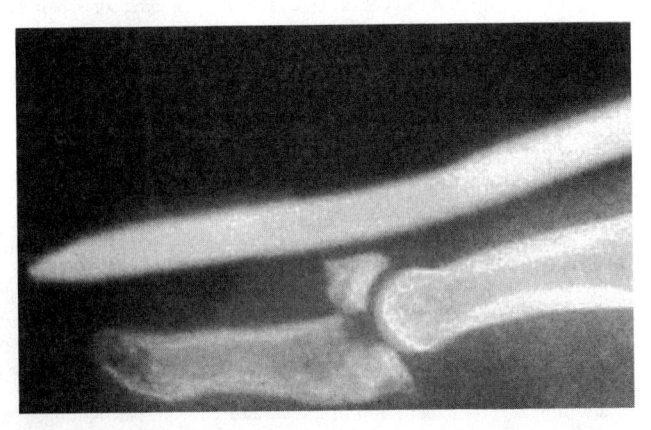

Figure 19-9. Bony mallet fracture with joint subluxation that will require reduction and stabilization. (From Seiler JG III. *Essentials of hand surgery*, Lippincott Williams & Wilkins, Philadelphia, PA, 2002, with permission.)

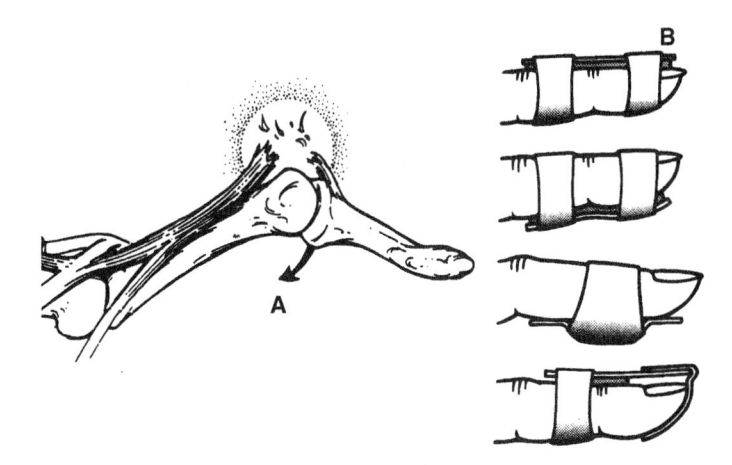

Figure 19-10. A: Mechanism. Due to the extensor apparatus lesion, the distal phalanx flexes by effect of the flexor profundus tendon. The proximal stump of the distal conjoined extensor tendon retracts in a proximal direction and consequently the lateral bands are slack initially and later contract and displace dorsally. Due to the concentration of the extension forces over the middle phalanx, the PIP joint is progressively set in hyperextension. **B:** Various splints (dorsal padded aluminum splint, volar padded aluminum splint, concave aluminum splint). Dorsal padded aluminum splint allows adjustable fixation of the DIP joint. (From Peimer CA. *Surgery of the hand and upper extremity.* New York: McGraw-Hill, 1996, with permission.)

- b. **Thumb base fracture and small finger base fracture.** Axial load applied to the border of the hand can result in fracture-subluxation at the finger base. Any such fracture is unstable. Almost all such fractures require operative stabilization. The key to successful treatment is early recognition. When treated early, a closed reduction and pinning is usually sufficient. Delay in treatment by as little as 1 week can necessitate open reduction and a more complicated management program. Thus, the first examiner's job is diagnosis. In the case of the thumb, it is easier to obtain a revealing x-ray. Along the ulnar border of the hand, it is usually necessary to obtain several oblique x-rays before a diagnosis can be made or excluded.
- c. **Phalangeal fractures.** Fractures at the base or in the mid-shaft of the phalanx are tricky. Many of these fractures have significant angular and/or rotational differences. Oblique films in combination with standard anteroposterior x-rays are often more helpful than lateral x-rays, which could be confusing because of overlapping digits. Regardless, measurement of rotational difference by clinical exam and shortening of the bony length by x-ray exam are the key facts to be considered when planning treatment. Unless, the fracture is essentially nondisplaced with **zero** rotational deformity, early referral to a hand specialist is warranted.
- d. **Splint placement.** One of the common problems seen after initial hand fracture care by specialist physicians is poor splint technique. The key to good splint placement is maintaining fully lengthened ligaments. In the hand, this is translated to 70 to 80 degrees of MCPJ flexion and no more than 10 degrees of PIPJ and DIPJ flexion. Such a splint is illustrated in **Fig. 19-12.** By maintaining fully lengthened ligaments, the physician reduces adjacent joint stiffness following fracture care.
7. **Amputation.** Thankfully, amputations have become less common in conjunction with enhanced product safety and public education. Nonetheless, they still do occur. Single digits cut in flexor zone 2 should almost never be replanted. A whole arm might be replanted but to do so is life threatening. Guidelines for replantation include:

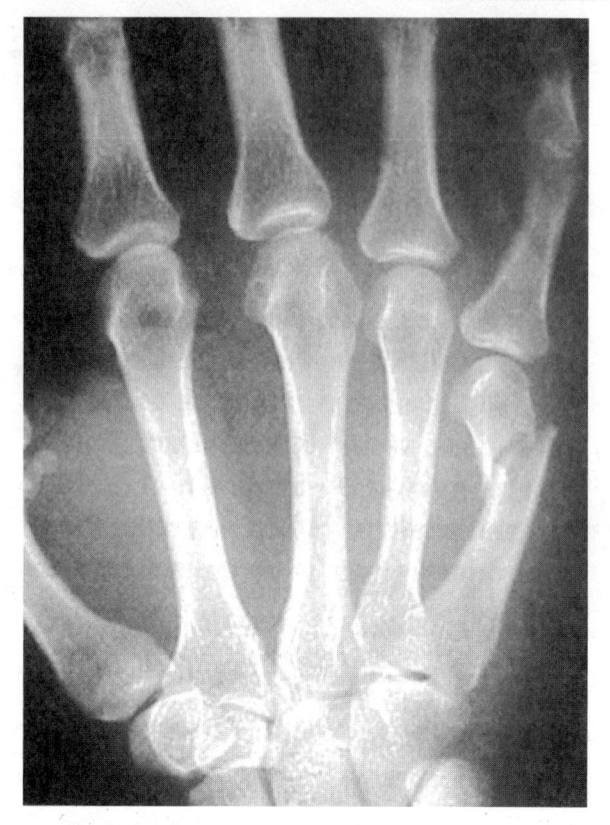

Figure 19-11. A "boxer's fracture" that can be treated with closed reduction and splinting in approximately 4 weeks. (From Seiler JG III. *Essentials of hand surgery*, Lippincott Williams & Wilkins, Philadelphia, PA, 2002, with permission.)

      a. Almost any child (not tip injuries as these seem to reform naturally); adolescents are adults
      b. Almost any thumb
      c. Multiple digits
      d. Whole hand
      e. Digit in flexor zone 1 with clean bony injury

V. PEARLS AND PITFALLS
  A. Injection injury. Fig. 19-13 depicts the mechanism of injection injury. This seemingly innocuous original injury should not be overlooked. Failure to treat can result in death and at least near loss of limb function. Even with emergent care, the outcome of treatment is uncertain. Emergent care by a specialist is mandatory. The keys to diagnosis are:
    1. Injury history. Use of a high pressure injector is often revealed.
    2. Exam. One or several small puncture wounds with more proximal tenderness or swelling is evident.
    3. Pain. The pain is seemingly greater than the wound would account for.
  B. Fight bites. This injury is often overlooked. Sometimes this will occur in conjunction with a boxer's fracture. The patient may not provide an accurate history, and substance misuse in this situation is common. Look for a small laceration

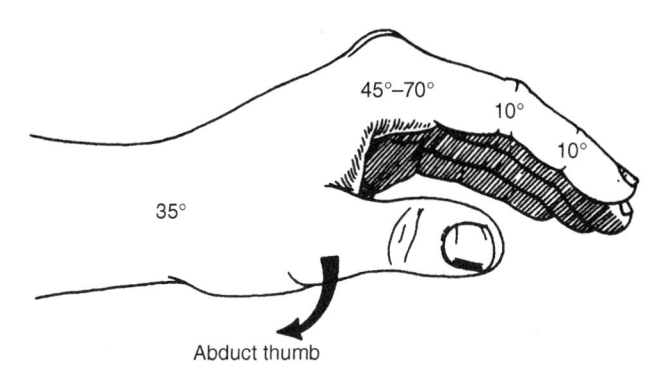

Figure 19-12. Hand dressing: "safe" position of fingers. (From Seiler JG III. *Essentials of hand surgery*, Lippincott Williams & Wilkins, Philadelphia, PA, 2002, with permission.)

overlying the joint which usually communicates to the joint if the finger is brought into a fist position. Flexing the fist during laceration exam is the key to identifying these patients. Treatment includes tetanus, antibiotics, complete wound cleansing, placement of a wound drain, and delayed closure.

C. **Compartment syndrome.** In addition to all the normal places, compartment syndrome can occur in the hand. Tight fascial compartments surrounding the hand's intrinsic musculature can swell after injury and cause muscle ischemia. Diagnosis is suspected when pain is increasing and passive motion is becoming more difficult. Sensory change may not occur because of nerve anatomy being outside of the pressurized area. Pressure monitoring and occasional surgical release may be needed.

D. **Scaphoid fracture and scapho-lunate ligament tears.** Often, these are diagnoses of suspicion. Almost no patient has been made worse by temporary splinting and early follow-up with a specialist. Whenever a patient presents after a significant injury mechanism (fall onto an outstretched arm), the patient should not be discharged without follow-up even in the face of normal x-rays. Appropriate follow-up does not require a specialist but does require a care provider familiar with the nuances of significant wrist sprains and scaphoid fractures mimicking a mild wrist contusion during the first 4 to 12 weeks of recovery.

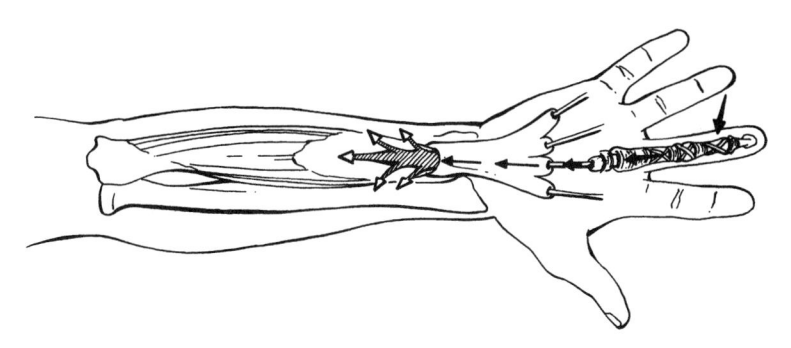

Figure 19-13. Palmar wounds at high pressure may spread into the proximal forearm. (From Seiler JG III. *Essentials of hand surgery*, Lippincott Williams & Wilkins, Philadelphia, PA, 2002, with permission.)

Selected Historical Readings

Peimer CA. *Surgery of the hand and upper extremity*. New York: McGraw-Hill, 1996:1–1336.

Seiler JG III. *Essentials of hand surgery*. Philadelphia, PA, Lippincott Williams & Wilkins, 2002:1–276.

Trumble, TE, ed. *Hand surgery update 3*, Rosemont, IL. Amer. Society for Surgery of the Hand, 2003: 1–776.

NONACUTE ELBOW, WRIST, AND HAND CONDITIONS

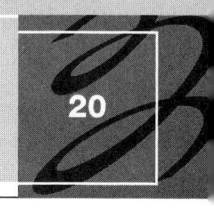

20

I. **BASIC EXAMINATION**
   A. **History.** As with any medical problem, the history of events leading up to the patient's visit to the physician with an upper extremity problem is critical. The history should contain family history, social history, personal medical history unrelated to the musculoskeletal system, infectious disease history, and risk behavior history. Some additional key facts to record include the following:
   1. **Handedness.** Is the patient right- or left-handed?
   2. **Work-relatedness.** If the patient believes a problem is related to work or a series of events, it is the physician's job to document the patient's beliefs. The physician can do this by "quoting" the patient exactly. It **is not** the physician's job or duty to question the veracity of a patient's complaint.
   3. **Mechanism of onset.** Record the details of the incident or accident as completely as possible. This is particularly relevant for motor vehicle accidents. Record details such as whether the patient was in the car, whether the air bags were deployed, whether the steering wheel was bent (particularly if the injured person was the driver), and the amount of damage done to the car.
   4. **Date of most recent tetanus booster.** This is important with any direct trauma. **Do not** assume that another first examiner has resolved this issue.

   B. **Physical examination**
   1. **General.** At first glance, the upper extremity is a mirror of the lower. But, several key differences are obvious:
      a. The **shoulder** has more freedom of motion and is consequently less stable than the hip.
      b. The "patella" of the elbow is fused to the ulna as the **olecranon**. However, it performs a similar function to the patella in that it increases the "lever arm" for the attached muscle (triceps in the arm, quadriceps in the leg).
      c. The **elbow and wrist** participate equally in guiding forearm rotation (supination and pronation). A similar motion is not available in the lower extremity.
      d. The **wrist** has more motion and less bony stability than the ankle.
      e. The **fingers** are longer in proportion to the palm than the toes in relationship to the midfoot.
      f. The **thumb** is longer and is opposable to the digits.
   2. **Region specifics**
      a. **Elbow**
         i. The elbow joint moves in a hinge manner at its articulation between the humerus and ulna. Thus, the ulnar-humeral articulation is uniaxial. In addition to its critical role in forearm rotation, the radius can transmit load to the humerus in "high-strength" situations. This issue is even more important if the elbow ligaments are injured. In general, the elbow gains minimal stability from muscle support and is reliant upon ligament support to guide joint motion.
         ii. Examination of this joint should document the active and passive arc of flexion and extension. Varus (lateral ligament loading) and valgus (medial ligament loading) should be assessed.
         iii. Standard radiographs include anteroposterior (AP) and lateral views.

b. Forearm
   i. Rotation of the forearm is guided by bone support at the proximal and distal radioulnar joints (PRUJ and DRUJ, respectively). Additional stability and guidance for this motion is provided by the interosseous membrane.
   ii. Examination should record the active and passive arc of supination and pronation. Crepitance or pain at the PRUJ or DRUJ should be noted. Pain or swelling in the mid-forearm should be assessed.
   iii. Standard radiographs include AP and lateral views.

c. Wrist
   i. The **wrist moves in a multiaxial manner.** The carpus is divided into a proximal (scaphoid, lunate, triquetrum) and distal (hamate, capitate, trapezoid, trapezium) row. Some of the key intercarpal articulations have more easily described relationships (the scaphoid moves relative to the lunate in flexion and extension). However, taken as a whole, the wrist is multiaxial and its motion is highly dependent on ligament function. There is no direct attachment of an extrinsic (forearm based) muscle or tendon to the bones of the proximal wrist. Thus, these bones (scaphoid, lunate, and triquetrum) are 100% dependent on ligament integrity for function.
   ii. **Examination** should record passive and active arcs of flexion, extension, radial deviation, and ulnar deviation. Obvious pain or crepitance should be recorded as specifically as possible.
   iii. **Standard radiographs** include posteroanterior (PA) or AP and lateral views. If the scaphoid is the focus of attention, AP and lateral views of the scaphoid should be specifically requested. These are oblique to the normal PA and lateral views of the wrist.

d. Hand
   i. The **hand** contains uniaxial (interphalangeal), multiaxial-stabilized (metacarpal phalangeal), and multiaxial-unstabilized (first and fifth carpometacarpal) articulations. Thus, these joints have varying degrees of ligamentous or muscle stability requirements. For example, the proximal interphalangeal joint of the index finger is dependent on ligament support. Whereas, the index finger's metacarpophalangeal joint can be partially stabilized by hand intrinsic muscle support.
   ii. **Examination** should record active and passive arcs of flexion and extension for all joints. Thumb examination should additionally include ability to abduct (palmar and radial), adduct, retropulse (extend), and oppose. Joint stability should be tested and any masses or tenderness noted.
   iii. **Standard radiographs** include PA and lateral views. Note: To obtain a lateral view of a finger, the adjacent digits need to be moved aside. Similar to the scaphoid, "normal" thumb views are oblique to the hand.
   iv. **Note:** Always examine the opposite or unaffected side. This is particularly important when assessing stability.

II. DEVELOPMENTAL DIFFERENCES
A. Developmental birth conditions
  1. **Radial agenesis.** Absence of the radius can be full or complete. Occasionally, this longitudinal deficiency is accompanied by thumb agenesis. An even more rare condition is presence of the radius and absence of the ulna. In either event, stability of the wrist is compromised. The deformity is often characterized with a "club hand." The absence of the radius would then be termed a radial club hand. Full assessment of this condition requires complete assessment of the child to include renal, cardiovascular, neural, and other musculoskeletal regions (shoulder, elbow, and hand). If the child has associated anomalies, correction of the deformity at the forearm carpal articulation may actually compromise function. Thus, any direct treatment must consider the whole forearm and carpal articulation.

2. **Syndactyly**
   a. This is the most common congenital hand condition (1 in 2,000 live births). The cause is not known. It is divided into **simple** (soft-tissue joining of two or more digits with no associated bone or joint anomaly) and **complex** (joining of two or more digits to include soft tissue and bones or joints) categories. Further subdivision is possible based on the length of the syndactyly. **Complete** syndactyly involves the whole length of the finger, whereas **incomplete** syndactyly does not. Simple syndactyly differences are often completely correctable. The complex differences, however, can occur in combination with other congenital differences (Apert syndrome).
   b. In general, surgical correction of this difference should be performed as soon as is anesthetically feasible. Correction of a multiple finger difference is done in stages. Limitations of correction are often related to digital blood supply; usually, full-thickness skin grafts are required at surgery.
3. **Polydactyly**
   a. This difference is classified into **preaxial duplication** (involvement of the thumb), central duplication (index, middle, or ring involvement), and postaxial duplication (small finger involvement). **Postaxial duplication** has a clear genetic component and is seen in as many as 1 in 300 live births. Correction of this difference usually involves excision. The degree of duplication and joint involvement determines the complexity of the procedure.
   b. **Treatment methods** for thumb duplication generally focus on excision of an unstable duplicate thumb. Duplication of the thumb has been characterized to occur in at least seven different patterns. The outcome of thumb reconstruction depends on the ability to create a thumb of appropriate length, rotation, stability, and mobility and to integrate the thumb into the child's daily routine. It is on this basis that earlier correction is generally recommended.
4. **Madelung's deformity.** First described by Malgaigne in 1855 and later by Madelung in 1878, this difference of growth related to the distal epiphysis of the radius is believed to be congenital in nature, although it is usually not noted before adolescence. It is a rare, genetic condition transmitted in an autosomal dominant pattern. Because of incomplete growth of the radius, the clinical presentation may be prominence of the ulnar head (distal ulna). Alternatively, abnormal forearm rotation may be the presenting complaint. At present, pain may not be a component. The method of surgical correction (shortening of the ulna versus lengthening of the radius) is less important than the goal of obtaining and preserving stable, painless forearm rotation with full and unrestricted use of the wrist.
5. **Brachial plexus**
   a. The brachial plexus comprises a coalescence of cervical and upper thoracic spine nerve roots. It traverses the space between neural foramina and the infraclavicular region where it again separates into individual nerves. Birth injuries relating to the brachial plexus are thought to represent an avulsion or stretch of the upper (**Erb's**), lower (**Klumpke's**), or both aspects (combined) of the brachial plexus. These injuries occur generally in the process of vaginal delivery of the child.
   b. Critical to the **examination** of any child with a presumed brachial plexus lesion is verification of normal shoulder bony anatomy. The physician should document this by way of physical examination and shoulder radiographs confirming the shoulder (glenohumeral joint) is located.
   c. Occasionally a child with nothing more than **a fractured clavicle (birth related)** will be mistaken to have a brachial plexus injury. Thus, it is important to include the clavicle in the physical examination of the infant. Generally speaking, a single AP chest radiograph suffices to detect such a fracture in the neonate.

d. **Management** of brachial plexus injuries at birth should include the following:
      i. Documentation of glenohumeral joint status (located)
      ii. Documentation of passive mobility of all upper extremity joints, including cervical spine mobility
      iii. Documentation of observed active motion in shoulder, upper arm, elbow, forearm, wrist, and hand
      iv. Initiation of twice-daily active-assisted "whole-arm" mobilization program to be completed by the **care team** or parents
      v. Plan for follow-up examination on a frequent interval to verify understanding and completion of passive and active-assisted exercises and available joint motion (both passive and active—looking for change or improvement)
   e. The **prognosis** for many brachial plexus injuries is for complete or near complete recovery. Children whose function remains compromised are evaluated and occasionally operated upon within the first 6 to 18 months of age. The treating physician who cannot document substantial improvement early (less than 6 months of age) should arrange further evaluation by an upper extremity specialist.

B. **Delayed presentation of developmental differences**
   1. **Cerebral palsy**
      a. Patients with cerebral palsy constitute the largest group of pediatric patients with neuromuscular disorders. The frequency varies from 0.6 to 5.9 patients per 1,000 live births. Difficulties related to this problem persist into adulthood. However, unlike many neuromuscular disorders, this condition does not progress. Relative progression of the disorder may occur in relation to growth, weight gain, or onset of degenerative change. However, any real progression should cause review of the original diagnosis. Generally, the problem relates to prenatal, natal, or early postnatal brain injury. The injury can express itself in a wide pattern, ranging from single limb to whole body involvement. Two clinical types of injury are seen:
         i. **Spastic type**—represents an injury to pyramidal tracts in the brain. Exaggerated muscle stretch reflex and increased tone are seen.
         ii. **Athetoid type**—probably a lesion in the basal ganglia. Continuous motion of the affected part is present; this type is more rare.
      b. **Diagnosis** is the first component of treatment. In cases with lesser involvement, diagnosis may not be obvious until the child fails to reach normal motor milestones or has difficulty with coordinated tasks. In some cases, the diagnosis is suspected because of early "under-use" of a part. For example, a child does not have a strong hand preference before 18 months of age.
      c. **Treatment** of cerebral palsy should always focus on functional improvement. Surgery generally has a cosmetic benefit, but the initial goal should be to improve a specific function. Intelligence and sensory awareness of the child are the two biggest determinants for functional improvement after surgery. Improvements of arm function are possible by improvement in the position of the shoulder, elbow, forearm, wrist, hand, and thumb. Three of the more successful surgeries are release of an internal rotation/adduction spastic contracture involving the shoulder, release/rebalancing of a flexed and pronated spastic wrist/forearm, and release/rebalancing of a thumb into palm deformity.

III. **ACQUIRED NONACUTE DYSFUNCTION OF THE ELBOW, WRIST, AND HAND**
   A. **Nerve.** Nerve tissue is responsible for communication in two directions between the brain and the external environment (peripheral). Like the brain, nerve function is highly dependent on oxygen. Although depolarization of a single axon is energy independent, repolarization of the axon is dependent on adenosine triphosphate to run the Na^+/K^+ pump to "recharge" the axon potential. Thus, although local loss of O_2 will not cause death of the peripheral axon cell body, local loss of O_2 will affect the ability of the axon to conduct **information.** This change in conduction is generally transient, depending on O_2 availability. However, frequent episodes of

reduced O_2 can produce permanent change in function. Common sites for nerve dysfunction to occur in the arm are the carpal canal (median nerve), the cubital tunnel (ulnar nerve), and the arcade of Froshe (posterior interosseous branch of the radial nerve).

1. **Carpal tunnel syndrome (CTS)**
   a. **Fig. 20-1** depicts the carpal tunnel as seen from end on. The carpal tunnel is seen to be formed by the three bony borders of the carpus (trapezium, lunate, hook of hamate) and the transverse carpal ligament. As such, it is a defined space with a fixed volume. Changes in the fixed volume can occur as a result of actual changes in the bony outline resulting from late effects of trauma or arthritis. Also, relative change in volume available can be the result of mass effect occurring from tendon or muscle swelling or synovitis, presence of an anomalous muscle, or presence of an actual mass (e.g., lipoma). The patient with reduction in available volume is less able to tolerate or accommodate increases in pressure within the carpal canal. Thus, in patients with reduced carpal canal volume, provocative maneuvers such as Tinel's (tapping or percussion of a nerve in a specific location), Phalen's (flexion of the wrist causing indirect nerve pressurization), or Durkin's compression test (manual pressure by examiner upon the median nerve) are more likely to be positive.
   b. **Presenting complaint** is most commonly pain in the median nerve distribution. Pain is often exacerbated at night or by specific activities (1). As the syndrome advances, numbness occurs in the distribution of the median nerve. Weakness of the thenar muscles with associated wasting is a late stage event.
   c. **Laboratory testing.** Radiographs to check for degenerative joint disease (DJD) or old fractures are occasionally of benefit. The most widely accepted diagnostic method is electrodiagnostic testing [electromyogram/nerve conduction velocity (EMG/NCV)]. This test can document slowing of nerve

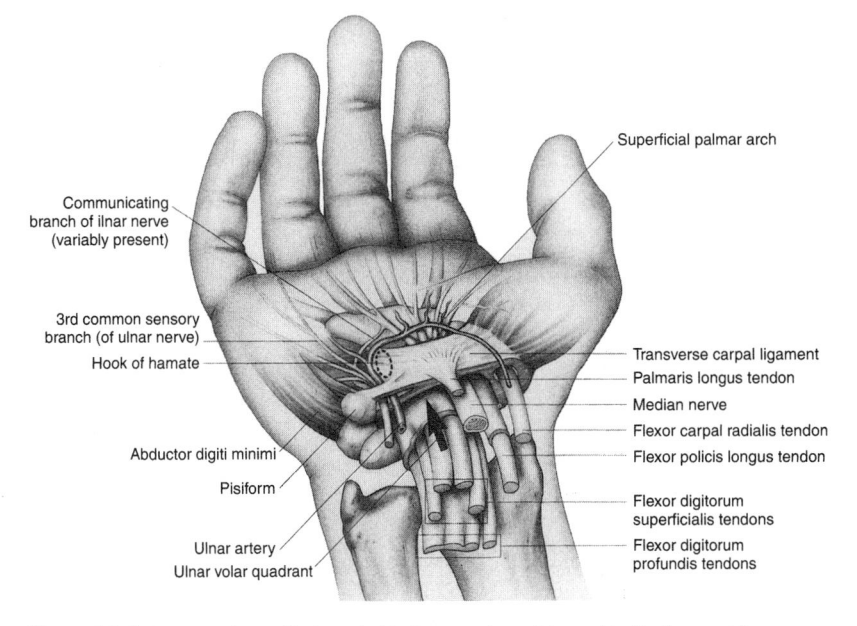

Figure 20-1. The carpal tunnel is bounded by bone on three sides and by the ligament (transverse carpal) on one side. Guyon's canal overlies the ulnar side of the carpal tunnel. The median nerve lies in the radial volar quadrant of the carpal canal. Generally, it is immediately below or slightly radial to the palmaris longus.

conduction and early muscle denervation. The EMG is most specific if the symptoms have been present for at least 1 month. Given the association of hypothyroidism and rheumatologic discorders, testing of the thyroid stimulating hormone (TSH) and rheumatoid factor (RF) should be strongly considered. Finally, carpal tunnel syndrome is very common in pregnancy, and symptoms frequently resolve after delivery.

    d. **Treatment** of CTS focuses on relief of pain. Initial therapy can include medication to relieve pain and swelling [nonsteroidal anti-inflammatory drugs (NSAIDs)], splint support, and exercises to increase mobility. No test or study has shown definite value for NSAIDs in management of CTS, except as they are related to relief of pain. An injection of corticosteroid into the carpal tunnel may be effective. There is some benefit from vitamin B_6 and C oral therapy.

    e. **Surgery** for relief of CTS symptoms is generally successful, with patient satisfaction exceeding 95% and complications less than 1%. The surgery can be completed by a variety of methods (open surgery versus percutaneous or arthroscopic-assisted release) without a clear benefit to one method versus another, as long as complete longitudinal division of the transverse carpal ligament is achieved along the ulnar half (1–4). Return to unrestricted activity after CTS surgery requires 4 to 8 weeks.

2. **Cubital tunnel syndrome**

    a. The **cubital tunnel** is formed by the bony borders of the medial epicondyle and medial ulna and overlying soft-tissue constraints including the entrance between the ulnar and humeral head of the bipennate flexor carpi ulnaris. It is a defined space with a fixed volume. Changes in the fixed volume can occur as a result of actual changes in the bony outline as a result of late effects of trauma or arthritis (osteoarthritis or rheumatoid arthritis). Relative change in volume available can be the result of mass effect occurring from tendon and muscle swelling or synovitis. Laxity of the soft-tissue–supporting structures can allow the ulnar nerve to migrate out of the cubital tunnel and over the medial epicondyle during flexion. This motion is often referred to as subluxation of the ulnar nerve and produces a "Tinel-like" distal sensory disturbance.

    b. **Presenting complaint** is most commonly pain in the distribution of the ulnar nerve distribution (5). Pain is often exacerbated at night or by specific activities. As the syndrome advances, numbness occurs in the distribution nerve. Weakness or atrophy of the hypothenar muscles is a late stage event.

    c. **Laboratory testing** (thyroid function tests and rheumatoid factor) and radiographs (DJD, old fractures) are occasionally of benefit. The most widely accepted diagnostic test method is electrodiagnostic testing (EMG/NCV). This test can document slowing of nerve conduction and early muscle denervation. Again, the EMG is most sensitive if symptoms have been present for at least 1 month.

    d. **Treatment** of cubital tunnel syndrome focuses on relief of pain (6). Initial therapy can include medication (NSAIDs) to relieve pain and swelling, provision of antielbow flexion splint support or pad, and exercises to increase mobility. No test or study has shown definite value for NSAIDs in management of cubital tunnel syndrome, except as related to relief of pain.

    e. **Surgery** for relief of cubital tunnel symptoms is substantially less successful than surgery for relief of CTS. The surgery can be completed by a variety of methods (small versus large surgical exposure) without a clear benefit to one method versus another as long as the point of observed nerve compression is released (7). The patient returns to unrestricted activity 12 to 24 weeks after surgery.

3. **PIN compression/other**

    a. The **PIN (posterior interosseous)** branch of the radial nerve travels through a defined space with a fixed volume. The tightest region of this space is formed by a fascial connection at the proximal margin of the two heads of the supinator muscle in the proximal forearm (arcade of Froshe). Changes in the fixed volume can occur as a result of actual changes in the bony outline that result from late effects of trauma or arthritis. Relative change in volume available can be the result of mass effect occurring from tendon and muscle swelling or synovitis, presence of an anomalous muscle, or presence of an actual mass (e.g., lipoma). The most common cause of nerve irritation in this region is believed to be the result of thickening of the facial margin in response to time (age) and stress.

   b. **Presenting complaint** is most commonly pain in the general region of the supinator muscle. Pain is often exacerbated at night or by specific activities. As the syndrome advances, numbness does not occur. Weakness of the PIN innervated muscles with associated wasting is a late stage event.
   c. The most widely accepted **diagnostic test** method is electrodiagnostic testing (EMG/NCV). PIN compression with this test is of substantially less benefit when compared with other nerve compression syndromes. Nonetheless, it shows muscle denervation in some cases.
   d. **Treatment** of PIN syndrome focuses on relief of pain. Initial therapy can include medication to relieve pain or swelling (NSAIDs) and exercises to increase mobility. Splints may exacerbate the problem if placed over the nerve. Wrist splints to reduce load on wrist extensors (the wrist extensors cross over the supinator) are occasionally helpful. As with the other nerve compression syndromes, no test or study has shown definite value for NSAIDs in management of PIN syndrome.
   e. **Surgery** for relief of PIN symptoms is substantially less successful than surgery for relief of CTS. A variety of surgical approaches have been described. The arcade of Froshe is identified and released. Return to unrestricted activity after surgery requires 12 to 24 weeks.
4. **Other.** Nerve compression can essentially occur wherever a nerve exits or enters a fascial plane/transition zone. The foregoing are the most common sites. Knowledge of extremity anatomy will aid the student in assessing other sites of suspected nerve entrapment.

B. **Muscle and tendon.** Muscles and tendons work together to generate and transmit force. The effect of load transfer depends on stable points of origin and insertion. Thus, at least **three locations of function failure** are apparent: (1) bone–muscle origin, (8) muscle–tendon junction, and (9) tendon–bone insertion. An example of each is provided.
   1. **Bone–muscle origin interface failure:** lateral epicondylitis (**Fig. 20-2**)
      a. **Failure of the muscle origin** of forearm extensors (lateral) or flexors (medial) is a common condition. The condition is uncommon in youths or persons of advanced age. It is occasionally seen in conjunction with working activities. Most often, the condition begins after a period of repetitive stress.
      b. **Presenting complaint** is usually pain focused at the muscle origin. Resisted use of the muscle aggravates the condition. The pain usually subsides with rest. Swelling is rarely present; no mass is seen with this condition. Range of motion may be uncomfortable; but a full active or active-assisted range of motion should be possible.
      c. **Laboratory testing** is of no particular value. Screening roentgenograms may be obtained but are generally normal for age. An injection test may be of confirmatory benefit (9). This is performed as outlined in **Fig. 20-2**. In this situation, the hope is that a precise injection of lidocaine with steroid into the area of extensor origin will eliminate or significantly alleviate the pain.
      d. **Treatment** of epicondylitis focuses on reducing the stress at the "inflamed" interface. Theoretically, if the stress is low enough, the healing process can succeed in healing the injured interface. Thus, use of splints (Froimson barrel or forearm band) to reduce the load on the injured muscle origin, massage to increase the blood supply for healing, and stretching exercises to increase muscle excursion are all measures that are likely to

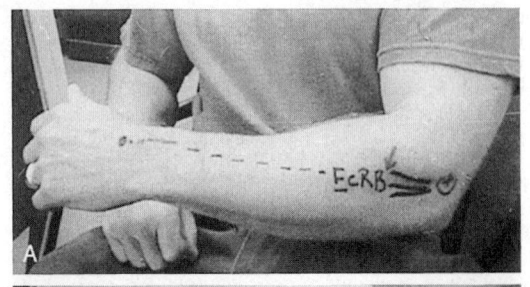

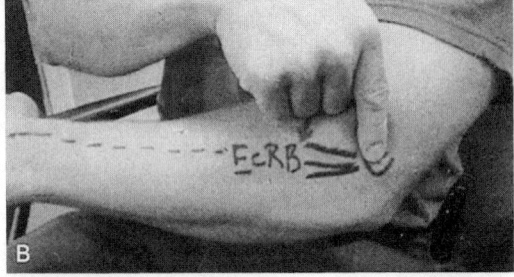

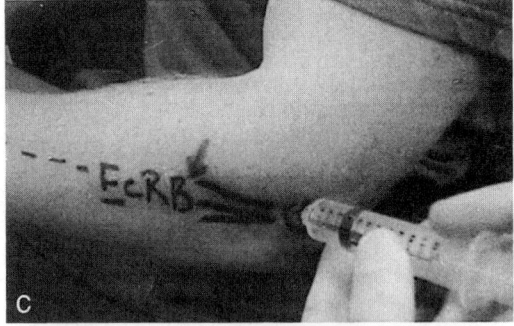

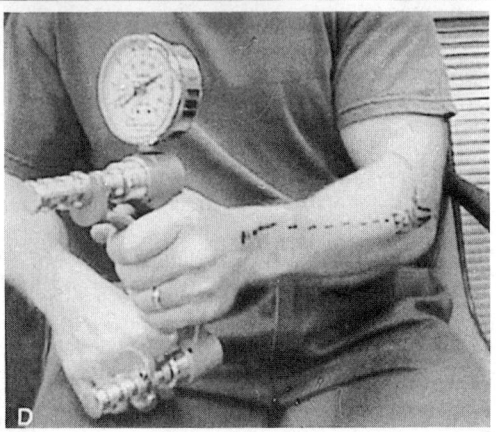

Figure 20-2. A: The path of the extensor carpi radialis brevis (ECRB) from lateral epicondyle to the base of the third metacarpal. **B:** The center of the epicondyle is the usual pain foci. **C:** Injection of lidocaine at the painful site. This should eliminate the pain. The injection is into the muscle origin, below the fascia. **D:** Postinjection strength testing usually reveals greater strength after pain is eliminated (successful injection). (From Putnam MD, Cohen M. Painful conditions around the elbow. *Orthop Clin North Am* 1999;30(1):109–118.)

provide success. The value of injections versus oral NSAIDs, rest, and splint support has not been clarified.
2. **Muscle–tendon pathway failure** results in trigger finger, trigger thumb, and de Quervain's tenosynovity.
   a. The **junction** between a specific muscle and its tendon is a potential site of failure. However, failure or pain at this location is uncommon in the upper extremity. Achilles tendinitis represents a condition occurring in the lower extremity. A similar condition does not occur in the upper extremity with any frequency. Problems along the tendon pathway, however, do occur.
   b. Commonly referred to as **trigger digits**, snapping of flexor tendon function caused by bunching of the flexor synovium at the annular one (A1) pulley does occur. This condition is seen more often in older patients, although a congenital version is also common. The condition occurs more often in patients with diabetes. Patients with active tenosynovitis (rheumatoid arthritis) may have a condition that is often confused for tendon triggering. But, rheumatoid arthritis and synovitis in other patients can be distinguished from true trigger digit by the inability to obtain complete active flexion. This is the result of too much synovium "blocking" the active flexion of the digit (the excursion of the flexor tendon is blocked). In the case of de Quervain's tenosynovitis, the problem is focused within the first dorsal extensor compartment of the wrist. The pathophysiology is the same, but this condition results in pain and crepitus along the tendon rather than triggering. The problem and degree of discomfort varies with time of day and activity.
   c. **Clinical diagnosis** of trigger dysfunction is made based on pain or tenderness, crepitance, and locking focused at the A1 pulley of a specific digit.
   d. **Laboratory studies** are essentially within normal limits. Radiographic studies are not generally useful. In the case of de Quervain's tenosynovitis, a special clinical test (Finkelstein's) is routinely performed. Finkelstein's test is positive if ulnar wrist deviation combined with thumb adduction and flexion of the metacarpal phalangeal joint reproduces the patient's complaint of pain.
   e. **Treatment** of trigger digit and de Quervain's synovitis includes rest, stretching exercises, steroid injection into the tendon sheath, and surgical release of the tendon sheath (3–8,11). If conservative care fails, response to supportive modalities is variable. In up to 60% of patients, the condition resolves after steroid injection (12). Surgical release of the sheath is thought to be 95% effective in those who fail to respond to lesser treatments (13).
3. **Tendon–bone insertion failure** results in mallet finger and biceps rupture.
   a. **Failure** at the distal point of muscle action can occur as a result of attrition or age-related change, or excessive load. Occasionally, both methods are involved. Patients are usually seen for diagnosis soon after the failure occurs. Pain is usually less an issue than is weakness or dysfunction.
   b. These conditions are **diagnosed** based on findings observed on clinical examination. Laboratory studies and roentgenographic findings are generally normal, the exception being when the extensor tendon involved with a Mallet finger pulls off a piece of the proximal aspect of the distal phalanx (thus, a "bony Mallet"). Larger tendon ruptures can be further clarified using magnetic resonance imaging (MRI) if there are unclear physical findings.
   c. **Treatment** is based on the ability to reposition the specific insertion and maintain this in a resting position. For the terminal extensor–mallet finger, 6 weeks of a conservative extension splint treatment is generally successful (8,10). Conversely, distal biceps ruptures will not heal without surgery because the tendon cannot be reliably positioned. However, because the muscle is a supporting elbow flexor (not the only elbow flexor), patients who do not require forceful supination (the biceps is the prime supinator) may choose to forego repair (and tolerate the functional limitations).

C. **Joint.** Painless, stable joint function is maintained by a combination of healthy cartilage, retained shape of the joint surface, ligamentous integrity, and muscle/tendon strength. Change in any of these four factors begins a process of increasing joint wear and dysfunction. Aging alone causes changes in the surface of the joint that accelerate wear. Most **arthritic conditions** of the arm are a combination of load, genetics, and history. However, it is occasionally possible to point to a single event many years earlier that has gradually led to joint dysfunction. Processes such as rheumatoid arthritis are usually the sole cause of dysfunction. Even in these diseases, isolated or cumulative trauma can play a role.
  1. **Thumb carpometacarpal (CMC)** (**Fig. 20-3**), wrist, and elbow DJD occur with decreasing frequency. Thumb CMC DJD may be the most common site of arthritic presentation. In any of the upper extremity sites, the most common presenting complaint is pain. To the degree that a specific joint is unstable, incongruous, or both, motion and stress aggravate symptoms. Certain activities and prior injury may predispose to arthritis, but underlying genetics is likely the most predominant cause.
  2. **Diagnosis** is a combination of history, examination, laboratory study, and plain radiographs. MRI or computed tomography (CT) methodology is rarely useful. Most patients complain of pain after activity that is relieved by rest. Oral NSAIDs are of some benefit. However, care must always be taken with long-term administration of these medications, particularly in elderly patients.
  3. **Treatment** begins with supportive splints and hot/cold modalities. Hand-based flexible splints are particularly helpful for thumb CMC.
  4. At some point, many patients can no longer "tolerate" the pain. This is the time to consider **surgery**. Unlike the lower extremity, upper extremity arthritic surgery can offer patients reliable joint rebuilding procedures without resorting to joint replacements. An example of such an excisional arthroplasty is shown in **Fig. 20-4**. Such procedures report greater than 90% success rate relative to pain relief.
  5. In the event that first-stage arthritic procedures do not work, newer and increasingly durable total **joint replacement** options are becoming available for the elbow, wrist, and the proximal interphalangeal joints.
D. **Bone.** Skeletal support is essential for function of the legs and arms. As such, immediate change (fracture) or gradual change (e.g., avascular necrosis, tumor) will alter the function of the arm or leg. Gradual change is rarely as painful as acute or fracture change in bone support. This may explain the late presentation for treatment of patients whose slow change process has progressed to the point at which curative or reconstructive treatment is no longer an option. Avascular necrosis of bone is a condition in which presentation and diagnosis are often delayed. As such, it is a good model to discuss the workup of bone pain.
  1. **Avascular necrosis, Kienböck's (lunate)** (**Fig. 20-4**), **Presiser's (scaphoid), and Panner's (humeral capitellum)** are focal avascular lesions of bone seen in the upper extremity. Genetics, overload, endocrine and systemic illness, and steroid use may play contributory roles. Patients usually have pain in the focal area and, on testing, it is usually possible to document a reduction in motion. Age of presentation varies from adolescence to late adulthood. Plain radiographs may reveal a change in bone density. In more advanced cases, the shape of the bone is altered. Change in shape is a precursor to diffuse arthritis.
     a. **Conservative treatment** starts with making a definite diagnosis. This is true for any unexplained pain in bone. If the diagnosis confirms a focal change in bone vascularity without change in bone shape, initial treatment may focus on joint support. However, many patients, particularly those with Kienböck disease, do not gain sufficient pain relief from splints, and other joint "unloading" treatments are sought.
     b. **Surgical treatments** for these processes can be broken down into treatments that reduce load on the injured bone segment, debride the injured bone segment, or replace/excise the injured bone segment. These treatments are likely to relieve pain in more than 80% of patients; however, full functional recovery rarely occurs.

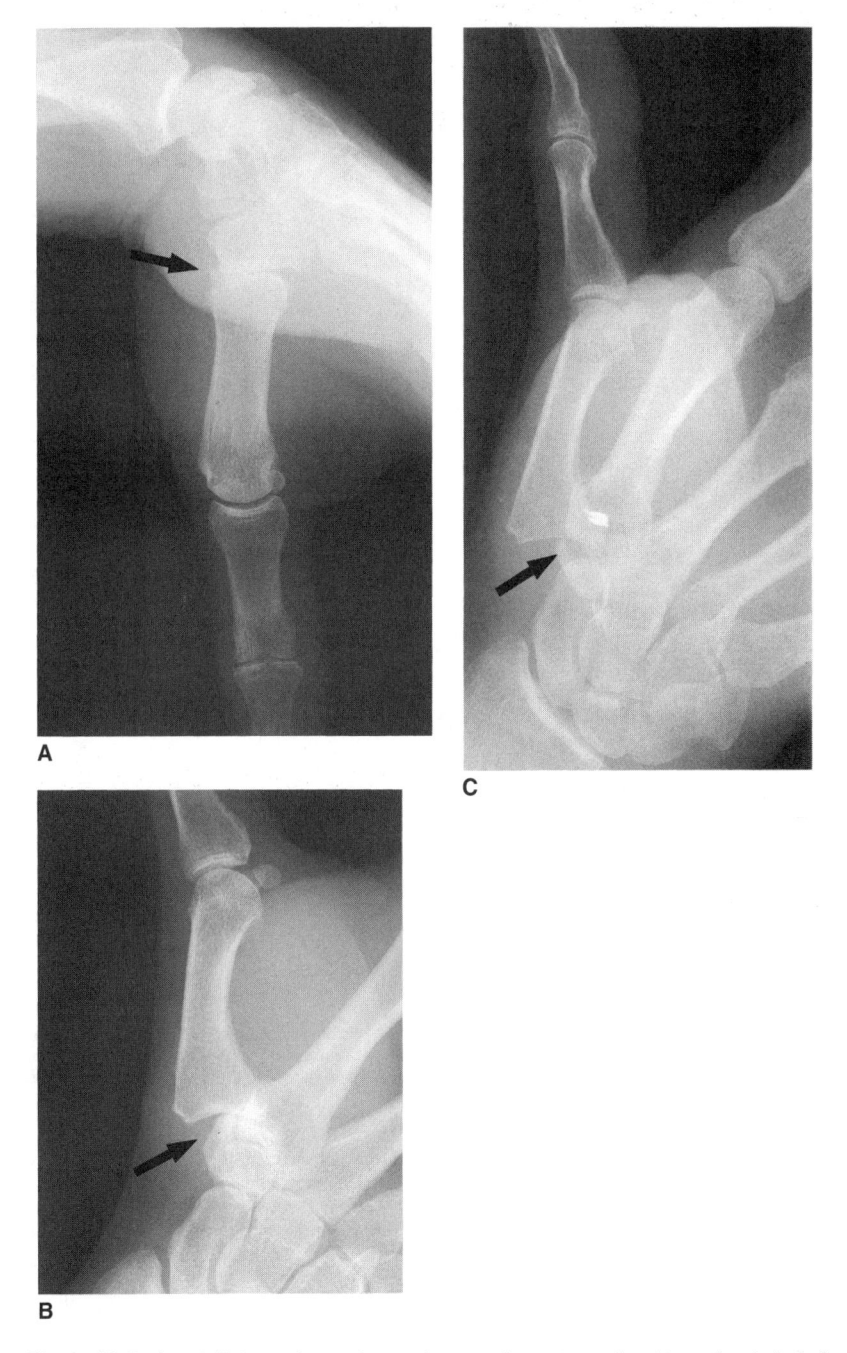

Figure 20-3. A and **B:** Loss of normal space between the metacarpal and trapezium typical of basilar joint thumb arthritis. **C:** After trapezial resection and stabilization of the first to second metacarpal, a new space for thumb carpometacarpal motion has been "created."

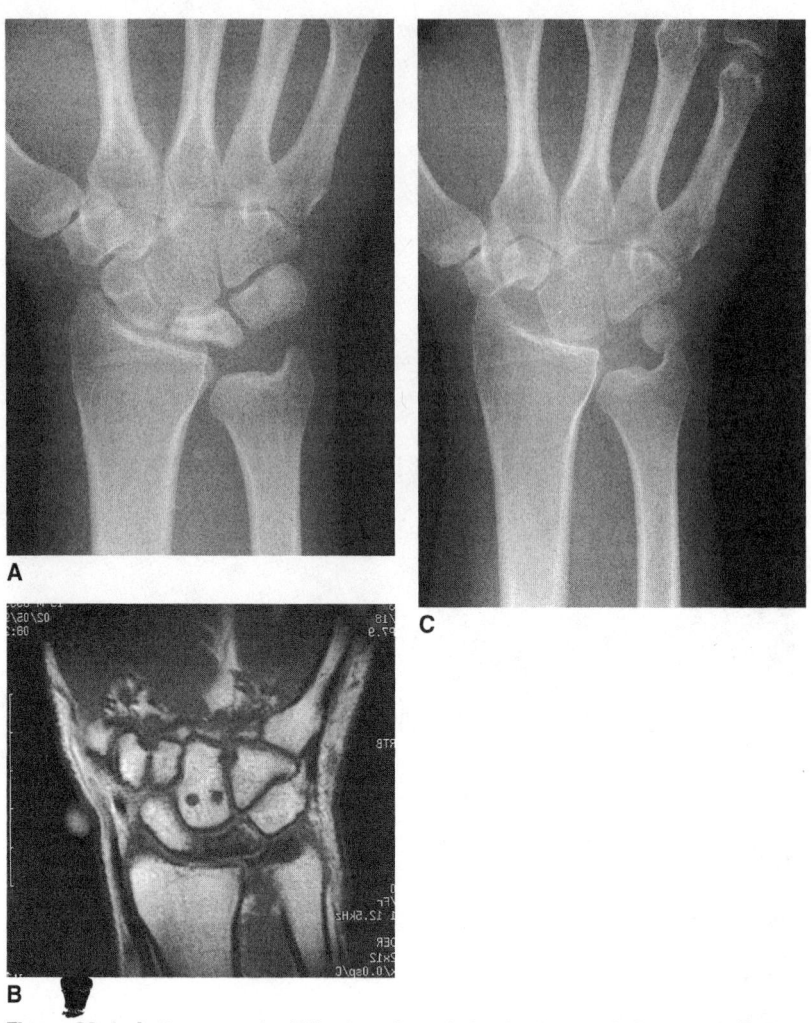

294 Chapter 20: Nonacute Elbow, Wrist, and Hand Conditions

Figure 20-4. A: Posteroanterior (PA) wrist radiograph showing "collapse" of the lunate. **B:** Magnetic resonance imaging study of the same wrist from the same point in time showing essentially no vascular signal within the lunate marrow. **C:** PA wrist radiograph showing the capitate "seated" in the lunate fossae after excision of the lunate.

- **E. Tumors.** The upper extremity is the site of a variety of tumors, many of which are rare, some appearing almost exclusively on the hand and the arm, and still others are common to all regions of the body. Although most tumors of the upper extremity are benign, few present simple therapeutic problems. The close anatomic relation of the tumor to the nerves, vessels, and muscles in the upper extremity presents a great challenge to the treating surgeon.
    1. Surgeons who treat hand and upper extremity tumors must be familiar with the wide range of **possible diagnoses**. Tumors that look innocent may not be; every mass should be considered potentially dangerous. This section focuses on primary malignant bony tumors of the upper extremity: diagnosis, evaluation, pathology, and treatment recommendations.

2. **Symptomatic tumors**, especially those that have increased in size, must be diagnosed and then classified as to stage. The patient's clinical and family history, the physical characteristics of the lesion, and diagnostic images provide information to determine whether the growth is aggressive and should be "staged."
3. **Diagnostic strategies** to accurately stage the lesion should be pursued before obtaining a biopsy. Appropriate evaluation includes a detailed history and proficient physical examination, imaging, and laboratory studies. The history should determine the length of time a lesion has been present, associated symptoms, and any incidence of family history. Physical examination requires detailed evaluation of the entire limb and testing, especially for sensibility, erythema, fluctuance, range of motion, tenderness, and adenopathy.
4. There are a few lesions that have significant associated **blood chemistry changes**. These include the elevated sedimentation rate of Ewing's sarcoma and the serum protein changes in multiple myeloma. Serum alkaline phosphatase is elevated in metabolic bone disease and in some malignancies. A serum immunoelectrophoresis determines whether multiple myeloma is present.
5. **Imaging** further aids in determining the location of the tumor and the presence or absence of tumor metastasis. There are a variety of imaging techniques that are useful tools.
    a. **Plain films and tomography.** Radiographs are of great importance in the diagnosis of bone tumors. Excellent technique is required to ensure good resolution of bone and adequate soft tissue surrounding the lesion. Plain films are the benchmark in predicting presence and location of bone involvement. Tomography or CT affords improved resolution.
    b. **MRI** has recently developed as one of the more important tools for diagnosing bone tumors. It offers excellent delineation of soft-tissue contrast as well as the ability to obtain images in axial, coronal, and sagittal planes. Additionally, MRI can visualize nerve, tendon, and vessels and, with advanced protocols, cartilage can also be evaluated.
6. **Classification of lesions.** Correct treatment must always take into consideration the location and size of the tumor, the histologic grade and clinical behavior, and the potential for metastasis. If a lesion increases in size or becomes symptomatic, or if the physical or radiographic appearance suggests an aggressive lesion, appropriate staging studies including a tissue diagnosis (biopsy) must be obtained.
7. **Specific tumors**
    a. **Benign**
        i. **Lipoma.** This common tumor occasionally presents in the hand or wrist as a firm mass within a nerve or vascular passageway. As such, it may be associated with carpal tunnel syndrome. Its nature may be suspected based on clinical examination alone (mass). To understand its dimensions and relationship to adjacent tissues, an MRI scan is usually obtained. Excision (marginal) is the treatment of choice.
        ii. **Enchondromas** (**Fig. 20-5**) of the hand are common; they are sometimes multiple and often present after a fracture. Initial treatment in this circumstance is aimed at satisfactory fracture healing. They can clinically be confused with osteochondromas. Radiographic examination easily differentiates the two processes. Most randomly identified lesions can be observed; any lesion associated with pain or increasing size in adulthood should be more carefully studied. Treatment is either observation or intralesional excision. Occasionally, previously benign lesions recur or undergo malignant transformation (**Fig. 20-5**). Any such lesion should be biopsied and carefully considered for wide excision.
    b. **Malignant**
        i. **Melanoma.** The hand, wrist, and forearm are common sites of melanoma. Any change in a pigmented lesion warrants biopsy.

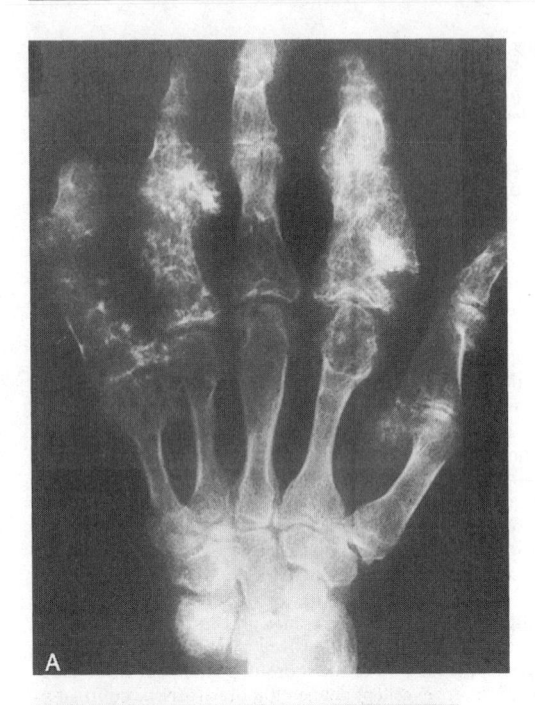

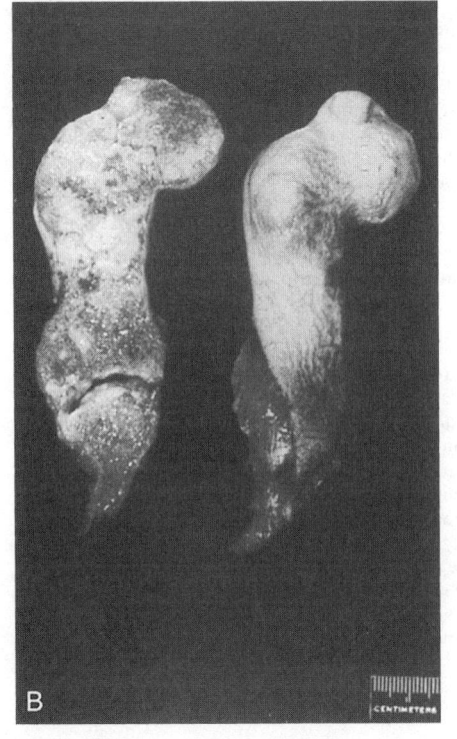

296 Chapter 20: Nonacute Elbow, Wrist, and Hand Conditions

Figure 20-5. A: Posteroanterior radiograph showing bone changes consistent with multiple enchondromas. **B:** Longitudinal section of the small finger. Pathology seen was consistent with low-grade chonorosarcoma. **C:** Preoperative clinical photo showing multiple digit enlargements. In this case, the patient noted rapid enlargement of the small finger during several months before surgery. (From Putnam MD, Cohen M. Malignant bony tumors of the upper extremity. *Hand Clin* 1995;11(2):265–286.) *(continued)*

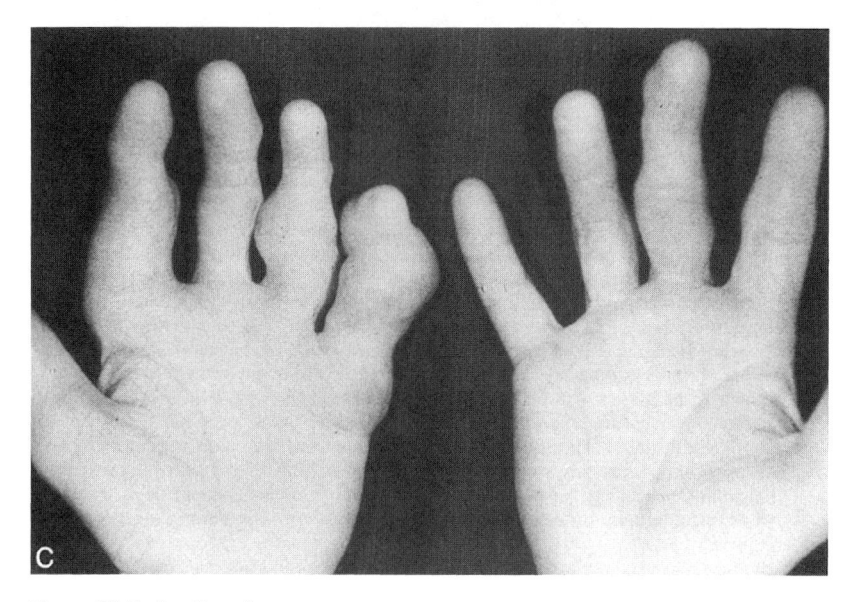

Figure 20-5. *(continued).*

- ii. **Osteosarcoma and chondrosarcoma.** Malignant bone lesions do occur in the arm. Most distal lesions are likely to represent degenerative change of benign processes (**Fig. 20-5**). Any bone or enlarging soft-tissue mass must always receive a complete evaluation (staging and biopsy) leading to a definitive diagnosis.
  8. **Metastasis.** Lesions from elsewhere appearing as metastasis are the most common form of malignancy in the hand. This should be kept in mind, particularly for the patient who is not known to have a malignancy and whose lesion is not in keeping with local origin. A search for the primary tumor is appropriate.
- F. **Other factors: Workmen's compensation.** The hand is often the first tool in and last tool out of a dangerous situation. As such, it is the frequent site of workplace injuries (14). Not all injuries are clearly documented. It is the physician's responsibility to remain the patient's advocate while at the same time remaining an objective observer. Occasionally, these tasks are in conflict. Three simple rules apply in these situations:
  1. Remain a dispassionate recorder of medical facts.
  2. Search for an accurate diagnosis.
  3. Offer no treatment without a specific diagnosis.

References

1. D'Arcy CA, McGee S. Does this patient have carpal tunnel syndrome? *JAMA* 2000;283:3110–3117.
2. Katz JN, Keller RB, Simmons BP, et al. Maine carpal tunnel study: outcomes of operative and nonoperative therapy for carpal tunnel syndrome in a community-based cohort. *J Hand Surg (Am)* 1998;23:697–710.
3. Kay NR. De Quervain's disease. Changing pathology or changing perception. *J Hand Surg (Br)* 2000;25:65–69.
4. Keller RB, Largay AM, Soule DN, et al. Maine carpal tunnel study: small area variations. *J Hand Surg (Am)* 1998;23:692–699.

5. Posner MA. Compressive neuropathies of the ulnar nerve at the elbow and wrist. *Instr Course Lect* 2000;49:305–317.
6. Mowlavi A, Andrews K, Lille S, et al. The management of cubital tunnel syndrome: a meta-analysis of clinical studies. *Plast Reconstr Surg* 2000;106:327–334.
7. Kleinman WB. Cubital tunnel syndrome: anterior transposition as a logical approach to complete nerve decompression. *J Hand Surg (Am)* 1999;24:886–897.
8. Foucher G, Binhamer P, Cange S, et al. Long-term results of splintage for mallet finger. *Int Orthop* 1996;20:129–131.
9. Smidt N, Assendelft WJ, van der Windt DA, et al. Corticosteroid injections for lateral epicondylitis: a systematic review. *Pain.* 2002;96(1–2):23–40.
10. Geyman JP, Fink K, Sullivan SD. Conservative versus surgical treatment of mallet finger: a pooled quantitative literature evaluation. *J Am Board Fam Pract* 1998;11:382–390.
11. Rankin ME, Rankin EA. Injection therapy for management of stenosing tenosynovitis (de Quervain's disease) of the wrist. *J Natl Med Assoc* 1998;90:474–476.
12. Zingas C, Failla JM, Van Holsbeeck M. Injection accuracy and clinical relief of de Quervain's tendinitis. *J Hand Surg (Am)* 1998;23:89–96.
13. Ta KT, Eidelman D, Thomson JG. Patient satisfaction and outcomes of surgery for de Quervain's tenosynovitis. *J Hand Surg (Am)* 1999;24:1071–1077.
14. Piligian G, Herbert R, Hearns M, et al. Evaluation and management of chronic work-related musculoskeletal disorders of the distal upper extremity. *Am J Ind Med* 2000;37:75–93.

Selected Historical Readings

de Quervain F. On a form of chronic tendovaginitis by Dr. Fritz de Quervain in la Chaux-de-Fonds. 1895. Illgen R, Shortkroffs, trans. *Am J Orthop* 1997;26:641–44.

FRACTURES OF THE PELVIS   21

I. **INCIDENCE AND MECHANISM OF INJURY.** Pelvic fractures are a common cause of death associated with trauma; head injuries are the most common cause (1–3). Approximately two thirds of pelvic fractures are complicated by other fractures and injuries to soft tissues. The fatality rate from pelvic hemorrhage with current management techniques ranges from 5% to 20% (4,5). Pelvic fractures generally are the result of direct trauma or of transmission of forces through the lower extremity. The importance of these fractures lies more in the associated soft-tissue injury and hemorrhage than in the fracture per se (1,5,6).

II. **CLASSIFICATION OF PELVIC FRACTURES.** Numerous systems have been proposed, but the **Tile system**, which expands on Pennel's work, is the most widely used (7). Burgess has expanded on this work by adding a combined mechanism notion (1).
   A. Types
      1. Type **A:** stable
      2. Type **B:** rotationally unstable, but **vertically** and **posteriorly** stable
      3. Type **C: rotationally** and **vertically unstable**
   B. **Subtypes**, which have important influences on treatment, are presented in **Table 21-1** and illustrated in **Figs. 21-1, 21-2,** and **21-3.**
   C. **Fractures of the acetabulum** are discussed in **Chap. 22.**
   D. Note for historical purposes that a **Malgaigne fracture** is a vertical fracture or dislocation of the posterior sacroiliac joint complex involving one side of the pelvis.

III. **EXAMINATION**
   A. Pelvic fractures are suspected because of pain, crepitus, or **tenderness over the symphysis pubis, anterior iliac spines, iliac crest, or sacrum,** but a good roentgenographic examination is essential for diagnosis. Patients with these injuries are often unconscious or intubated, so the examination for stability is helpful. The iliac wings are grasped and force-directed to the midline; instability can be detected with this maneuver. Gentle handling of the patient minimizes further bleeding and shock.
   B. **Specific studies.** Patients with all but minimal trauma should have an indwelling urinary catheter for the dual purposes of measuring urine output while the associated shock is being treated and investigating possible bladder trauma. If there is blood at the penile meatus, then a retrograde urethrogram should be performed before passage of the catheter (1,2,6). This prevents completion of a partial urethral tear. Intravenous pyelography (IVP) and cystography document renal function, bladder anatomy, and help delineate the size of any pelvic or retroperitoneal hematoma. When the initial urinalysis reveals less than 20 red blood cells per high powered field rbc/hpf, an IVP is generally not necessary (8). Despite the difficulties involved, a pelvic (in women) and rectal examination should be done to check for fresh blood and open wounds, perineal sensation in a conscious patient, a displaced unstable prostate, and sphincter tone. These fractures frequently are associated with neurologic damage, so a careful neurologic evaluation should be done in all patients.

IV. **PELVIC HEMORRHAGE** (1,5)
   A. **Symptoms and signs.** At presentation, approximately 20% of patients are in shock. Severe backache can help differentiate the pain of retroperitoneal bleeding from the pain of intraabdominal bleeding.
   B. **Treatment.** Pneumatic antishock garments (MAST trousers) help reduce the pelvic volume by compression of the iliac wings. MAST trousers are not useful as

TABLE 21-1	Substances of Pelvic Fractures

Type A: Stable
A1 Fractures not involving ring; avulsion injuries
    A1.1 Anterior superior spine
    A1.2 Anterior inferior spine
    A1.3 Ischial tuberosity
A2 Stable, minimal displacement
    A2.1 Iliac wing fractures
    A2.2 Isolated anterior ring injuries (four-pillar)
    A2.3 Stable, undisplaced, or minimally displaced fractures of the pelvic ring
A3 Transverse fractures of sacrum and coccyx
    A3.1 Undisplaced transverse sacral fractures
    A3.2 Displaced transverse sacral fractures
    A3.3 Coccygeal fracture

Type B: Rotationally unstable; vertically and posteriorly stable
B1 External rotation instability; open-book injury
    B1.1 Unilateral injury
    B1.2 Less than 2.5-cm displacement
B2 Internal rotation instability; lateral compression injury
    B2.1 Ipsilateral anterior and posterior injury
    B2.2 Contralateral anterior and posterior injury; bucket-handle fracture
B3 Bilateral rotationally unstable injury

Type C: Rotationally, posteriorly, and vertically unstable
C1 Unilateral injury
    C1.1 Fracture through ilium
    C1.2 Sacroiliac dislocation or fracture-dislocation
    C1.3 Sacral fracture
C2 Bilateral injury, with one side rotationally unstable and one side vertically unstable
C3 Bilateral injury, with both sides completely unstable

From Tile M. Pelvic ring fractures: should they be fixed? *J Bone Joint Surg* 1988;70B:I.

a routine transfer aid for patients with blunt trauma (9). These garments are useful in transport of patients where there is a high degree of suspicion of a pelvic fracture, but should be removed as soon as resuscitation is underway because they are associated with compartment syndrome in the legs (10). Most causes of hemorrhage are adequately handled by rapid replacement and maintenance of blood volume, followed by reduction (when appropriate) and stabilization of the fractures as described in **VI.** Adequate blood replacement is the first priority, and its effectiveness is monitored by the patient's pulse, blood pressure, central venous pressure, urine output, and so on, as described in **Chap. 1.** Blood loss of 2500 mL is common, and blood replacement is usually necessary even without evidence of an open hemorrhage. Diagnostic peritoneal lavage is a useful test to rule out intraabdominal injury at the site of hemorrhage (6). Abdominal computed tomography (CT) scan and abdominal ultrasound are effective (first) screening tests for this condition (2,5). The surgeon must follow the patient's platelet count and coagulation studies after 4 units of blood have been given because disseminated intravascular coagulation can result from dilution of these components. The use of angiography and embolization of distal arterial bleeding points with blood clot, Gelfoam, or coils has been proven to be useful (1,2). Because only 10% of patients have identifiable arterial bleeding, the authors prefer to stabilize the pelvis first with internal or external fixation (1,2,5,11–13). Anterior external fixation with one or two pins in each iliac wing is an effective means of stabilizing the pelvis

Chapter 21: Fractures of the Pelvis 301

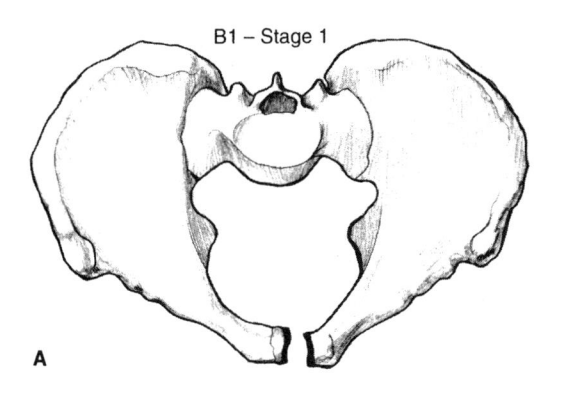

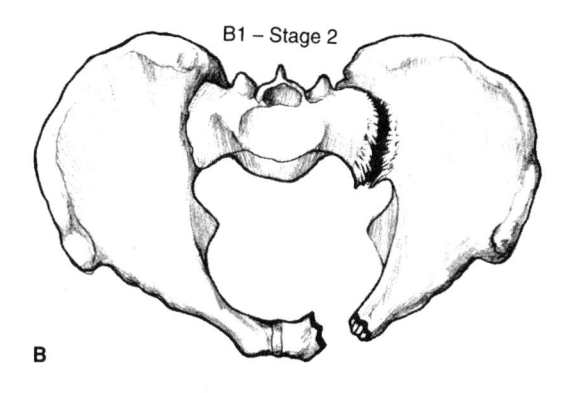

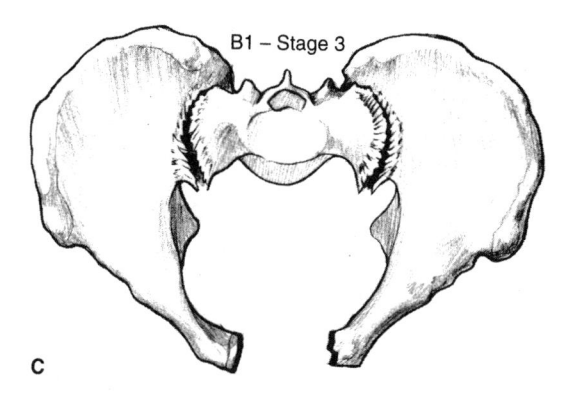

Figure 21-1. A: Type B1, stage 1 symphysis pubis disruption. **B:** Type B1, stage 2 symphysis pubis disruption. **C:** Type B1, stage 3 symphysis pubis disruption. (From Hansen ST, Swiontkowski MF. *Orthopaedic trauma protocols.* New York: Raven, 1993:228.)

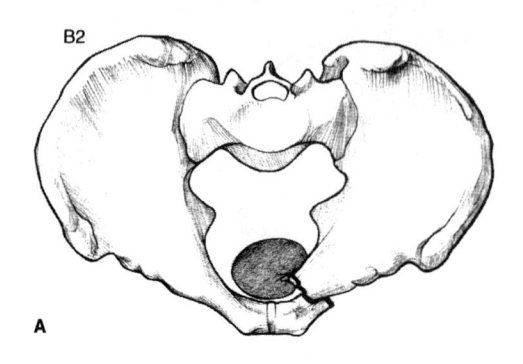

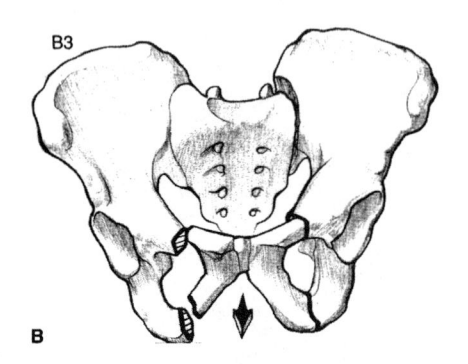

Figure 21-2. A: Type B2 lateral compression injury (ipsilateral). **B:** Type B3 lateral compression injury (contralateral). (From Hansen ST, Swiontkowski MF. *Orthopaedic trauma protocols.* New York: Raven, 1993:228.)

when the traumatic pattern allows its use (11,14,15). Alternatively, wrapping the patient in a hospital sheet at the level of the iliac rings or in a commercially available pelvic binder have been proven to be effective simple methods of decreasing the pelvic volume (4). If the pelvic injury involves the posterior wing with a sacral fracture or unstable sacroiliac joint injury, the antishock clamp can be lifesaving. It requires skill, familiarity with the device, and fluoroscopic control (16). Spica casting can also be used if the necessary expertise or equipment is not available (17). Distal femoral pins must be incorporated into the cast. If this does not control the bleeding, then arteriography and embolization are indicated (2).

V. ROENTGENOGRAMS

- **A. An anteroposterior view of the pelvis** is made routinely in all patients who have suffered severe trauma or who complain of pain in and around the pelvic region. After the patient's general condition has stabilized following a pelvic fracture, special films are indicated, including a 60-degree caudad-directed inlet view and a 40-degree cephalad-oriented tangential (or outlet) view (7,12). The former helps visualize the posterior pelvic ring, and the latter is for the anterior ring.
- **B. CT scans** can be most useful in defining posterior ring fractures (1,2,13). Fifty percent of sacral fractures are missed on plain roentgenograms, but they are well visualized on CT scans.

VI. TREATMENT

- **A. Stable A type fractures** are treated symptomatically. Turn the patient by logrolling or begin treatment on a Foster frame until the severe pain subsides. As soon as the patient can move comfortably in bed, he or she can ambulate in a walker and progress to walking with crutches. The fractures are through cancellous bone that has good blood supply, and stability of the fracture usually is present in 3 to 6 weeks, with excellent healing expected within 2 months. Because of the

Chapter 21: Fractures of the Pelvis **303**

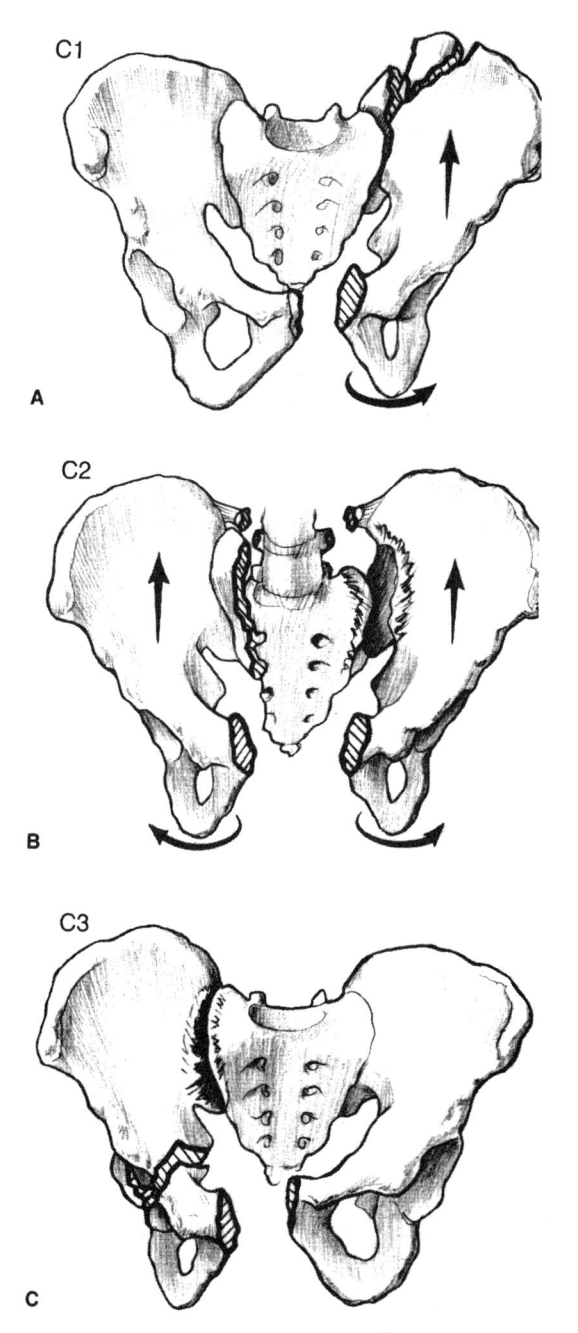

Figure 21-3. A: Type C1 pelvic injury. **B:** Type C2 pelvic injury. **C:** Type C3 pelvic injury. (From Hansen ST, Swiontkowski MF. *Orthopaedic trauma protocols.* New York: Raven, 1993:229.)

dense plexus of nerves about the sacrum and coccyx, injuries to this area may produce chronic pain, especially if the patient is not encouraged to accept some discomfort and start an early active exercise program.
- B. **Type B fractures** (rotationally unstable, but vertically and posteriorly stable) must be treated on an individual basis. Fracture displacements, associated injuries, age of the patient, and functional demands should be taken into account (1,5,13). In open-book fractures, disruption of the anterior sacroiliac joints and sacrospinous ligaments occurs if the displacement is more than 2.5 cm. These may be reduced and stabilized by external fixation or plate fixation across the symphysis (11,12). The authors generally prefer plate fixation because of the problems with patient comfort, pin tract infection, and loosening and loss of reduction with external fixation (5,14,18). Minimally displaced B1, B2, and B3 injuries may be treated conservatively with bed to wheelchair mobilization for 6 to 8 weeks, followed by crutch ambulation with weight bearing to tolerance on the side of the pelvis where the posterior ring is uninjured or more stable. Internal fixation is used for more widely displaced and unstable injuries (2,12,13). Traction is not recommended because of patient morbidity and the inability to improve fracture displacements.
- C. **Type C** minimally displaced isolated injuries, especially those involving the ilium, may be treated conservatively as in **B.** However, patients need to be followed up closely roentgenographically and, if fracture displacement is increasing, reduction and fixation is indicated. Some centers utilize simulated weight-bearing radiographs as a method for detecting fracture instability. Improved results with internal fixation over traction treatment have been documented (12). If seen early on, then fractures of the sacrum and sacroiliac joints can be managed with closed reduction and percutaneous lag screw fixation (2,13). Because of the complexity of reduction and fixation techniques as well as the potential for high morbidity resulting from adjacent neurovascular structures, patients with type C injuries should be referred to an experienced pelvic and acetabular surgeon.

VI. COMPLICATIONS
- A. Complications from **associated injuries** (e.g., of the bladder, cranium, chest)
- B. **Persistent symptoms from sacroiliac joint instability,** including pain and leg length inequality
- C. **Chronic pain patterns** from injuries around the coccyx and sacrum and sacroiliac joint (19,15), including dyspareunia
- D. **Persistent neurologic deficit** from nerve root injury with L5, S1, and distal sacral root injuries most common; erectile dysfunction is common in males
- E. Pulmonary and fat emboli
- F. Infection from bacterial seeding of the large hematomas or from open pelvic fractures (20). Injuries to the large bowel are not uncommon.

HCMC Treatment Recommendations

Pelvic Ring Fractures

  Diagnosis: Anteroposterior pelvic radiograph, inlet-outlet views, physical examination, CT scan

  Treatment: Management of hemorrhage, limited weight bearing (6–8 weeks) for lateral compression fractures that do not have significant deformity, non–weight bearing for other nondisplaced patterns for 8 to 12 weeks, follow-up radiographs to check for late instability

  Indications for surgery: Ongoing hemorrhage (external fixation or posterior pelvic clamp), displaced posterior pelvic injury, symphysis widening more than 2.5 cm, unacceptable pelvic deformity

  Recommended technique: Symphysis plating, posterior iliosacral screws. Open reduction and iliosacral screw placement is safest; consider percutaneous iliosacral screws in thin patient with minimal deformity. Occasionally, anterior sacroiliac joint fixation is performed if posterior skin is not safe or if the injury is associated with an ipsilateral acetabular fracture.

References
1. Burgess AR, Eastridge BJ, Young JWR, et al. Pelvic ring disruptions: effective classification system and treatment protocol. *J Trauma* 1990;30:848–856.
2. Gruen GS, Leit ME, Gruen RJ, et al. The acute management of neurodynamically unstable multiple trauma patients with pelvic ring fractures. *J Trauma* 1994;36:706–713.
3. Poole GV, Ward EF, Muakkassa FF, et al. Pelvic fractures from major blunt trauma; outcome is determined by associated injuries. *Ann Surg* 1991;213:532–539.
4. Bottlang M, Krieg JC, Mohr M, et al. Emergent management of pelvic ring fractures with use of circumferential compression. *J Bone Joint Surg (Am)* 2002;84:43–47.
5. Failinger MS, McGanity PL. Unstable fractures of the pelvic ring. *J Bone Joint Surg (Am)* 1992;74:781–791.
6. Mendez C, Grubler KD, Maier RV. Diagnostic accuracy of peritoneal lavage in patients with pelvic fractures. *Arch Surg* 1994;129:477–481.
7. Tile M. Pelvic ring fractures: should they be fixed? *J Bone Joint Surg (Br)* 1988;70:1.
8. Lieu TA, Fleisher GR, Mahboubi S, et al. Hematuria and clinical findings as indications for intravenous pyelography in pediatric blunt renal trauma. *Pediatrics* 1988;82:216–222.
9. Mattox KL, Bickell W, Pepe PE, et al. Prospective MAST study in 911 patients. *J Trauma* 1989;29:1104–1112.
10. Apprahamian C, Gessert G, Bandyk D, et al. MAST–associated compartment syndrome (MACS): a review. *J Trauma* 1989;29:549–555.
11. Kellam JF. The role of external fixation in pelvic disruptions. *Clin Orthop* 1989;241:66.
12. Matta JM, Saucedo T. Internal fixation of pelvic ring fractures. *Clin Orthop* 1989;242:83–97.
13. Routt ML Jr, Kreger PI, Simonian PT, et al. Early results of percutaneous iliosacral screws placed with the patient in the supine position. *J Orthop Trauma* 1995;9:207–214.
14. Hupel TM, McKee MD, Waddell JP, et al. Primary external fixation of rotationally unstable pelvic fractures in obese patients. *J Trauma* 1998;45:111–115.
15. Nepola JV, Trenhaile SW, Miranda M, et al. Vertical shear injuries: is there a relationship between residual displacement and functional outcome? *J Trauma* 1999;46:1024–1030.
16. Ganz R, Krushell RJ, Jakob RP, et al. The antishock pelvic clamp. *Clin Orthop* 1991;267:71–78.
17. Cotler HB, LaMont JB, Hansen ST. Immediate spica cast for pelvic fractures. *J Orthop Trauma* 1988;2:222–228.
18. Lindahl J, Hirvensalo E, Bostman O, et al. Failure of reduction with an external fixator in the management of injuries of the pelvic ring—long-term evaluation of 110 patients. *J Bone Joint Surg (Br)* 1999;81:955–962.
19. Copeland CE, Bosse MJ, McCarthy ML, et al. Effect of trauma and pelvis fracture on female genitourinary, sexual and reproductive function. *J Orthop Trauma* 1997;11:73–81.
20. Hak DJ, Olson SA, Matta JM. Diagnosis and management of closed internal degloving injuries associated with pelvic and acetabular fractures: the morel-lavallee lesion. *J Trauma* 1997;42:1048–1051.

Selected Historical Readings
Bucholz RW. The pathological anatomy of the Malgaigne fracture-dislocation of the pelvis. *J Bone Joint Surg* 1981;63A:400–404.
Peltier LF. Complications associated with fractures of the pelvis. *J Bone Joint Surg (Am)* 1965;47:1060–1069.
Rafii M, Firooznia H, Golimbu C, et al. The impact of CT in clinical management of pelvic and acetabular fractures. *Clin Orthop* 1983;178:228–235.
Saibil EA, Maggisano R, Witchell SJ. Angiography in the diagnosis and treatment of trauma. *J Can Assoc Radiol* 1983;34:218–227.

HIP DISLOCATIONS, FEMORAL HEAD FRACTURES, AND ACETABULAR FRACTURES

22

I. **INTRODUCTION.** A hip dislocation, with or without associated acetabular fracture, is a major injury. The forces needed to cause hip dislocation are considerable, and, in addition to the disruption noted on roentgenography, soft-tissue injury is significant. Occasionally, small osseous or cartilaginous fragments remain in the hip joint. The injury is most frequently caused by an automobile or automobile-pedestrian accident, so significant injury elsewhere in the body is likely. A fracture or fracture-dislocation at the hip can easily be missed when associated with an ipsilateral extremity injury. Such an injury emphasizes the rule: always visualize the joint above and the joint below the diaphyseal fracture. Because injuries about the pelvis can be missed in a seriously traumatized patient, most authorities advocate a routine pelvic roentgenogram for all patients involved in severe blunt trauma. The condition is viewed as an orthopaedic emergency. In general, the sooner the reduction is achieved, the better is the end result (1,2).

II. **CLASSIFICATION OF DISLOCATIONS**
   A. **Anterior dislocations**
      1. **Obturator**
      2. **Iliac**
      3. **Pubic**
      4. **Associated femoral head fractures** (see **V**)
   B. **Posterior dislocations**
      1. **Without fracture**
      2. **With posterior wall fracture** (see **IV**)
      3. **With femoral head fracture** (see **V**)

III. **ANTERIOR DISLOCATIONS**
   A. This injury usually occurs in an automobile accident, in a severe fall, or from a blow to the back while squatting. The **mechanism of injury** is forced abduction. The neck of the femur or trochanter impinges on the rim of the acetabulum and levers the femoral head out through a tear in the anterior capsule. If in relative extension, an iliac or pubic dislocation occurs; if the hip is in flexion, an obturator dislocation occurs. In many instances, there is an associated impaction or shear fracture of the femoral head as the head passes superiorly over the anteroinferior rim of the acetabulum. These injuries are associated with poor long-term results (3,4).
   B. On **examination** with an **obturator dislocation**, the hip is abducted, externally rotated, and flexed, but in the **iliac or pubic dislocation**, the hip may be extended. The femoral head can usually be palpated near the anterior iliac spine in an iliac dislocation or in the groin in a pubic dislocation. In all patients, carefully assess the circulatory and neurologic status before attempting a reduction. The diagnosis is readily apparent on roentgenogram, which shows the femoral head out of the acetabulum in an inferior and medial position.
   C. **Treatment** (2,3). Early closed reduction is the treatment of choice, but open reduction may be necessary. Reduction is optimally attempted under spinal or general anesthesia, which ensures complete muscle relaxation. In the multiply injured patient, reduction may be attempted in the emergency department with sedation or pharmacologic paralysis after the airway is controlled. Initiate strong but gentle traction along the axis of the femur while an assistant applies stabilization of the pelvis by pressure on the anterior iliac crests. For the **obturator dislocation**, the

traction is continued while the hip is gently flexed, and the reduction is accomplished usually by gentle internal rotation. A final maneuver of adduction completes the reduction but should not be attempted until the head has cleared the rim of the acetabulum with traction in the flexed position. For the **iliac or pubic dislocation**, the head should be pulled distal to the acetabulum. The hip is gently flexed and internally rotated. No adduction is necessary. If the hip does not reduce easily, forceful attempts are not indicated. Failure to obtain easy reduction with the above maneuvers usually indicates that traction is increasing the tension on the iliopsoas or closing a rent in the anterior capsule, producing a "buttonhole" effect. Forced maneuvers only increase the damage. Because the closed reduction may fail, the patient is initially prepared for an open procedure. The open reduction can be accomplished through a muscle-splitting incision, using the lower portion of the standard anterior Smith-Peterson approach. The structures preventing the reduction are released. The postreduction treatment is the same as for a posterior dislocation of the hip, except it is important to avoid excessive abduction and external rotation.

D. **Prognosis and complications.** Excellent reviews of hip dislocations have been published; anterior dislocations occur in approximately 13% of some 1,000 hip dislocations. Early reduction is necessary if a satisfactory result is to be obtained, and although the end result is frequently excellent in the child, traumatic arthrosis and, occasionally, avascular necrosis make the prognosis guarded in the adult. Recurrent dislocation is rare in an adult (1–3).

IV. **POSTERIOR DISLOCATIONS**
A. The **mechanism of injury** is usually a force applied against the flexed knee with the hip in flexion, as occurs most commonly when the knee strikes the dashboard of an automobile during a head-on impact. If the hip is in neutral or adduction at the time of impact, a simple dislocation is likely, but if the hip is in slight abduction, an associated fracture of the posterior or posterosuperior acetabulum can result. As the degree of hip flexion increases, it is more probable that a simple dislocation is produced.

B. **Physical examination** reveals that the leg is shortened, internally rotated, and adducted. A careful physical examination should be carried out before reduction including sensory exam and muscle group motor strength grading. Sciatic nerve injury is associated with 10% to 13% of these injuries (5). Associated bony or ligamentous injury to the ipsilateral knee, femoral head, or femoral shaft is not uncommon. When associated with a femoral shaft fracture, a dislocation may go unrecognized because the classic position of flexion, internal rotation, and adduction is not apparent. In this situation, the diagnosis is confirmed by a single anteroposterior roentgenogram of the pelvis as part of the initial trauma roentgenographic series. This single examination does not allow adequate assessment of any associated acetabular fracture (6–8), however, so more roentgenograms are needed for treatment planning before carrying out a reduction if an acetabular fracture is identified. The patient, not the x-ray beam, is moved to obtain the following films: the anteroposterior obturator oblique and the iliac oblique views (6,9). This is best accomplished by keeping the patient on a backboard and using foam blocks to support the oblique position of the board (**Fig. 22-1**). If necessary, computed tomography (CT) scanning can also be performed; optimally, this is done after the closed reduction of the hip joint to reestablish femoral head circulation. Although some authors question its routine use after uneventful closed reduction, others report a 50% incidence of bony fragments being identified with CT (9–12).

C. **Treatment**
1. **Posterior dislocation without fracture.** This dislocation is reduced as soon as possible and always within 8 to 12 hours when possible. Reduction is accomplished with the Allis maneuver under spinal or general anesthesia to overcome the significant muscle spasm. The essential step in a reduction is traction in the line of the deformity, followed by gentle flexion of the hip to 90 degrees while an assistant stabilizes the pelvis with pressure on the iliac spine. With continued traction, the hip then is gently rotated into internal

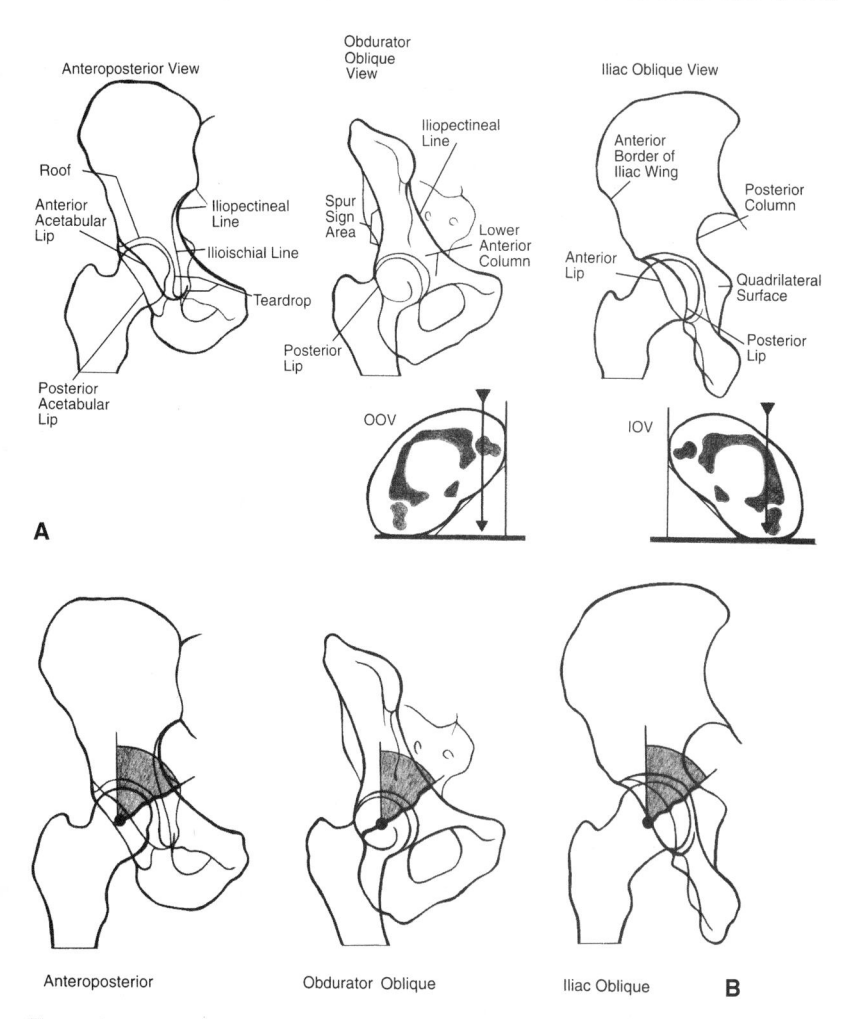

Figure 22-1. Radiographic assessment of acetabular fractures. **A:** The anteroposterior, obturator oblique, and iliac views are essential for the definition of the fracture. **B:** The "roof arc" measurement is made between a vertical line and the angle of the fracture. Angles greater than 40 degrees on all three views indicate a fracture which may be treated nonoperatively. (From Hansen ST, Swiontkowski MF. *Orthopaedic trauma protocols.* New York: Raven, 1993:249.)

and external rotation, which usually brings about a prompt restoration of position. Because considerable traction is required, even with good muscle relaxation, the alternative method of Stimson may be attempted. The patient is placed prone with the hip flexed over the end of the table, and an assistant fixes the pelvis by extending the opposite leg. The same traction maneuvers described earlier are completed, but the pull is toward the floor with pressure behind the flexed knee. Although considerable traction is necessary, under no circumstances should rough or sudden manipulative movement be attempted. Postreduction stability should be confirmed on physical examination and by a roentgenogram obtained in the operating room to be sure there are no fractures around the femoral head or neck.

a. **Postreduction treatment.** Isometric exercises for the hip musculature are instituted as soon as pain subsides sufficiently. Continuous passive motion (CPM) may be useful to maintain joint motion but is not essential. There is no consensus in the literature as to the length of time the patient should be restricted from weight bearing. The authors favor bed rest until the patient is pain free and has established near-normal abduction and extension muscle power. The patient then is allowed to move around, using crutches for protective weight bearing until it is determined that he or she can ambulate without pain or an antalgic limp; this generally takes 3 to 6 weeks. At that time, full weight bearing is permitted.
b. **Prognosis and complications**
   i. Sciatic nerve injuries are discussed in **IV.2.c** and **e**.
   ii. **Avascular necrosis of the femoral head** is the most feared delayed complication from a simple posterior dislocation of the hip. It occurs late, but various authors have noted an average time of 17 to 24 months from injury to time of diagnosis. Rates of approximately 6% to 27% are variously reported, and figures show an incidence of 15.5% for early closed reductions, increasing to 48% if reduction is delayed. There were no good results if reduction was delayed more than 48 hours. In Epstein's classic study of 426 cases, better results were obtained with open reduction and internal fixation in patients who had associated fractures (see Selected Historical Readings). The overall rate of avascular necrosis was 13.4% with a higher rate of 18% in patients with associated fractures. For fracture-dislocations treated by open means, the avascular necrosis rate was only 5.5%. Treatment of avascular necrosis is discussed in **Chap. 23, I.I.2**.
   iii. Epstein also reported an overall rate of **traumatic osteoarthritis** of 23% following posterior hip dislocations, with a rate of 35% in dislocations treated by closed means and a rate of 17% in those treated by open means. In another series, after 12 to 14 years of follow-up, 16% of patients had posttraumatic arthritis, and arthritis developed in an additional 8% as a result of avascular necrosis (2). Similar results have been reported from other centers (1,2).
2. **Posterior dislocation with associated acetabular fracture**
   a. As previously noted, the **dislocation is reduced as soon as possible considering the patient's other injuries**. If the patient needs to undergo a lengthy trauma evaluation, then an attempt can be made in the emergency department to reduce the hip with sedation. In the patient who has been intubated for airway control, chemical paralysis totally eliminates muscle spasm. If reduction attempts fail, then the urgency for hip reduction must be transmitted to the trauma team leader so the patient can be brought to the operating room earlier in the evaluation phase. An alternative to standard closed reduction maneuvers involves inserting a 5-mm Schanz pin into the ipsilateral proximal femur at the level of the lesser trochanter. This allows more focused lateral and distal traction by a second assistant to accompany the reduction maneuver. If this maneuver fails, then open reduction is preferred via a posterior approach. A posterior wall fracture is internally fixed with lag screws and a neutralization plate after joint lavage. If a more complex acetabular fracture is present, then an experienced acetabular and pelvic surgeon should be consulted (13). If the basic posterior acetabular anatomy appears intact and the joint debridement is complete, then a CT scan should be obtained to check on the adequacy of debridement and to evaluate for associated fractures (4,11).
   b. **Postoperative treatment.** Historically, traction has been used postoperatively, but this is no longer recommended. With stable internal fixation, early motion is advised starting with CPM. Flexion is generally limited to 60 degrees for the first 6 weeks postoperatively for large posterior wall fractures (13). Weight bearing is limited and crutches are used for 12 weeks (6–9).

c. **Sciatic nerve injury.** Direct contusion, partial laceration by bone fragments, a traction injury, or occasionally an iatrogenic injury resulting from malplacement of retractors during open reduction can cause this injury. Nerve injury should be evaluated early by a careful motor and sensory examination before reduction. If the nerve function is normal before reduction and is abnormal after reduction, then this may represent sciatic nerve entrapment in a fracture line. Emergent open reduction and nerve exploration are indicated (6–9). The peroneal portion of the sciatic nerve is most commonly injured because it lies against the bone in the sciatic notch. When the entire distal sciatic nerve function is abnormal, the tibial portion of function returns nearly 100% of the time. The peroneal portion of function is regained in 60% to 70% of cases: The more dense the motor injury, the less likely is the return of good function (5). The postinjury foot drop is generally easily managed by a plastic ankle-foot orthotic. Tendon transfers at a later date remain an option.
d. **Prognosis and complications.** Late traumatic arthritis and femoral head avascular necrosis can result in 20% to 30% of cases (6–9,13). Of all acetabular fractures, the posterior wall injury, despite its being the simplest pattern, has the worst prognosis with regard to these complications (14–16). Total hip arthroplasty is the most acceptable reconstruction option when these complications occur; long-term results in this situation are not as predictable as with total hip arthroplasty for arthritis (2,15). Rarely total hip arthroplasty is indicated as the initial surgical therapy in elderly patients with complex fracture patterns (17). Most patients who sustain these injuries are younger than 50 years of age, so loosening of the components over the patient's lifetime is a real concern (16).

V. **FRACTURES OF THE FEMORAL HEAD**
   A. **Diagnosis.** Fractures of the femoral head generally occur with an associated hip dislocation. They are seen as abrasion or indentation fractures of the superior aspect of the head in association with an anterior dislocation or as shear fractures of the inferior aspect of the head in association with a posterior dislocation. Comminuted head fractures occasionally occur with severe trauma. Femoral neck or acetabular fractures may be involved. The diagnosis is established by roentgenograms and CT scan.
   B. **Treatment**
      1. **Emergent.** Early treatment must focus on reducing the hip dislocation and diagnosing the fracture pattern. Diagnosis, made by clinical examination, is confirmed by the admission anteroposterior pelvic roentgenogram. Great care should be given in evaluating the roentgenograms before reducing the hip because nondisplaced associated femoral neck fractures may be displaced with the reduction maneuver. If these are noted, the reduction should be performed in the operating room under fluoroscopy so that, if the femoral neck fracture appears unstable with the reduction maneuver, the surgeon can proceed with an open reduction. If the closed reduction is successful, a repeat roentgenogram is obtained to confirm the reduction and a CT scan should be obtained for treatment planning.
      2. **Definitive.** If the femoral head fracture is an indentation fracture associated with an anterior dislocation, early CPM and mobilization with crutches (partial weight bearing) are indicated. The prognosis regarding degenerative joint disease is poor, however (3,4,18).
         a. If the femoral head fracture is a shear fracture associated with a posterior dislocation and is of small size (**Pipkin type I, infrafoveal**), the treatment can involve a brief period of traction for comfort followed by mobilization with a restriction of flexion to less than 60 degrees for 6 weeks. Indications for surgery include a restriction of hip motion resulting from an incarcerated fragment and multiple associated injuries. The fracture should be approached anteriorly for best visualization (18).
         b. If the fracture is of larger size (**Pipkin type II, suprafoveal**), the reduction should be anatomic or within 1 mm on the postreduction CT to proceed with conservative treatment as outlined earlier. If it is displaced,

open reduction and internal fixation with well-recessed (countersink) screws using an anterior approach is indicated (18).
- c. If the fracture is associated with a femoral neck fracture (**Pipkin type III**), both fractures should be internally fixed via an anterior approach, and early motion with CPM should be initiated. The prognosis for this combination injury is not as favorable as with isolated femoral head fractures because of the higher incidence of posttraumatic osteonecrosis associated with the neck fracture.
- d. Femoral head fractures associated with acetabular fractures (**Pipkin type IV**) should be managed in tandem with the acetabular fracture. Generally this is accomplished operatively by an experienced pelvic surgeon (6–8).

VI. ACETABULAR FRACTURES WITHOUT POSTERIOR DISLOCATION
- A. **Mechanism of injury.** These fractures result from a blow on the greater trochanter or with axial loading of the thigh with the limb in an abducted position.
- B. **Physical examination.** These patients often have multiple injuries, so the management of the patient is the same as outlined in **Chap. 1**. A careful examination of the sciatic nerve function must be conducted with detailed sensory exam to light touch and motor grading of all distal muscle groups. The muscles innervated by the femoral and obturator nerves must also be examined because they can occasionally be injured with complex anterior column fractures. The anteroposterior pelvis admission trauma film and the two 45-degree pelvic oblique views described by Judet (see Selected Historical Readings) (**Fig. 22-1**), as well as a CT scan of the pelvis (6–9), are used to evaluate the fracture pattern. The scan is helpful in determining the presence of intraarticular bone fragments, femoral head fractures, and displacement in the weight-bearing region of the acetabulum (12). Roof arc measurements are useful for treatment planning (**Fig. 22-1**).
- C. **Treatment**
    1. **Nonoperative.** Traction was once the recommended definitive treatment for all acetabular fractures (19). With modern techniques, nearly all significantly displaced acetabular fractures can be fixed safely and effectively, even in elderly individuals (20,13,6–9). As definitive therapy, traction is not currently generally recommended, with the exception of elderly patients with multiple medical comorbidities. It is generally reserved for temporary treatment of displaced transverse acetabular fractures in which the femoral head is articulating on the ridge of the fracture edge on the lateral portion of the joint. Traction prevents further cartilage injury and femoral head indentation; however, it must be heavy (35–50 lb) and with a distal femoral pin. Trochanteric pins to provide a lateral traction vector should never be used if open reduction is an option at any time in the patient's management. If nonoperative management is selected, then bed-to-chair mobilization for 6 to 8 weeks is the best option, followed by gradual return to weight bearing. Total hip arthroplasty is an effective salvage technique as long as the acetabular anatomy is not too distorted (15,16).
    2. **Operative.** In young patients, displacement of 2 to 3 mm in the major weight-bearing portions of the acetabulum is an indication for open reduction (6–9). Numerous surgical approaches to reduction are available, including the Kocher-Langenbach posterolateral approach, the ilioinguinal, the extended iliofemoral, and combined approaches. These procedures should be undertaken by experienced acetabular surgeons because the techniques for reduction and fixation are numerous and require much special equipment; inferior results are documented by surgeons who are inexperienced (13). Postoperatively, CPM is occasionally used; patients are mobilized with 12 weeks of "touch down" weight bearing with crutches. If posterior wall involvement is significant, then flexion is restricted to 60 degrees for the first 6 weeks. Complications include infection (1%–2%), heterotopic ossification (4%–6% functionally limiting), avascular necrosis (5%), deep venous thrombosis (10%–20%), pulmonary embolus (1% fatal), degenerative arthritis (20%–30%, generally associated with posterior wall fractures), and sciatic nerve injury (2%–5%) (13,14,20,21,22,23). Occasionally, acute hip replacement is indicated in older patients with complex fractures.

Heterotopic ossification is most commonly associated with extended posterior (the extended iliofemoral) and combined approaches (21). All of these complications occur more often when surgeons are inexperienced. Effective prophylaxis includes indomethacin, 25 mg t.i.d for 6 weeks, and low-dose irradiation (800–1,000 R) in the first week postoperatively (13,22). The use and relative benefits of radiation therapy and indomethacin remain controversial.

VI. **ACETABULAR FRACTURES IN ASSOCIATION WITH FRACTURES OF THE FEMORAL HEAD, NECK, OR SHAFT.** Associated injuries of the femur are not uncommon. They should be dealt with by internal fixation; then the acetabular injury should be treated as outlined previously (6–9). Attempts at treating both injuries by traction have not been satisfactory.

VII. **TRACTION.** The use of traction in the lower extremity is discussed in **Chap. 9, VII.** Classic balanced traction with a half or a full ring Thomas splint is not only cumbersome but also restricts the use of the hip in the muscle rehabilitation program. A hip exerciser such as that described by Fry should be considered. These techniques must be learned because they are occasionally needed in treating problems associated with severe preexisting systemic disease or local skin problems.

VIII. **TRAUMATIC DISLOCATION OF THE HIP JOINT IN CHILDREN.** This condition is fairly uncommon.
   A. **Immediate reduction is essential.** Delaying reduction for more than 24 hours increases the incidence of avascular necrosis.
   B. **Weight bearing should be prohibited for 3 months** (a spica cast is recommended for children younger than 8 years of age), at which time it usually is possible to determine the degree of avascular necrosis, although a 3-year follow-up period is necessary to assess this complication fully. Institution of prompt treatment and protected weight bearing as for Legg-Calvé-Perthes disease probably is indicated. Recurrent dislocation can occur in children who are not immobilized.
   C. When reduction is achieved rapidly with no gross associated trauma, the **results are usually satisfactory**, especially in patients younger than 6 years old. The incidence of avascular necrosis, however, has been reported to be approximately 5% to 10%.

HCMC Treatment Recommendations

Hip Dislocations

Diagnosis: Anteroposterior pelvic radiograph and physical examination. Leg is shortened and internally rotated for posterior dislocation and flexed and externally rotated for anterior dislocation. Judet views and CT scan are obtained after redcuction.

Treatment: Reduction in emergency department with sedation and analgesia; reduction in operating room if other injuries so require

Indications for surgery: Irreducible dislocation, intraarticular loose bodies diagnosed on postreduction radiographs or CT scan

Recommended technique: Hip arthroscopy for small loose bodies, arthrotomy with posterior approach for irreducible dislocation

---

HCMC Treatment Recommendations

Femoral Head Fractures

Diagnosis: Anteroposterior pelvis radiograph and physical examination—these nearly always accompany a hip dislocation, 90% of which are posterior dislocations

Treatment: Closed reduction of hip (see previous discussion) followed by CT scan to assess size and reduction of fragment. If reduction is anatomic, limited weight bearing with crutches for 6 weeks

Indications for surgery: Displaced large head fragment (Pipkin II, >2 mm displaced) or displaced type III or IV fracture

Recommended technique: Open reduction with internal fixation (ORIF) via anterior approach, fixation with counter sunk lag screws

HCMC Treatment Recommendations
Acetabular Fractures
   Diagnosis: Anteroposterior pelvic and Judet views, CT scan, physical examination
   Treatment: ORIF of displaced (>2 mm) intraarticular components, 6–8 weeks of partial weight bearing for nondisplaced fractures
   Indications for surgery: Displaced articular component
   Recommended technique: Surgical approach of ilioinguinal, Kocher-Langenbach or extended approach based on fracture pattern and experience of surgeon; fixation with lag screws and reconstruction plates; limited weight bearing for 12 weeks

References

1. Dreinhofer KE, Schwarzkupf SR, Haas NP, et al. Isolated traumatic dislocation of the hip; long-term results in 50 patients. *J Bone Joint Surg (Br)* 1994;76:6–12.
2. Upadhyay SS, Moulton A, Srikrishnamurthy K. An analysis of the late effects of traumatic posterior dislocation of the hip without fractures. *J Bone Joint Surg (Br)* 1983;65:150–152.
3. DeLee JC, Evans JA, Thomas J. Anterior dislocation of the hip and associated femoral head fractures. *J Bone Joint Surg (Am)* 1980;62:960–964.
4. Konrath GA, Hamel AI, Guemin J, et al. Biomechanical evaluation of impaction fractures of the femoral head. *J Orthop Trauma* 1999;13:407–413.
5. Seddon HJ. *Surgical disorders of the peripheral nerves*, 2nd ed. New York: Churchill Livingstone, 1975.
6. Matta JM, Anderson LM, Epstein HC, et al. Fractures of the acetabulum: a retrospective analysis. *Clin Orthop* 1986;205:230–240.
7. Matta JM. Fractures of the acetabulum: accuracy of reduction and clinical results in patients managed operatively within three weeks after the injury. *J Bone Joint Surg (Am)* 1996;78:1632–1645.
8. Matta JR, Mehne DK, Roffi R. Fractures of the acetabulum: early results of a prospective study. *Clin Orthop* 1986;205:241–250.
9. Mayo KA. Fractures of the acetabulum. *Orthop Clin North Am* 1987;18:43–57.
10. Frick SL, Sims SH. Is computed tomography useful after simple posterior hip dislocation? *J Orthop Trauma* 1995;9:388–391.
11. Hougaard K, Jaersgaard-Anderson P, Kuut E. CT scanning following traumatic dislocation of the hip. *Int J Orthop Trauma* 1994;4:68–69.
12. St. Pierre RK, Oliver T, Somoygi J, et al. Computerized tomography in the evaluation and classification of fractures of the acetabulum. *Clin Orthop* 1984;188:234–237.
13. Kaempfte FA, Bone LB, Border JR. Open reduction and internal fixation of acetabular fractures: heterotopic ossification and other complications of treatment. *J Orthop Trauma* 1991;5:439–445.
14. Moed BR, Willson Carr SE, Gruson KI, et al. Computed tomographic assessment of fractures of the posterior wall of the acetabulum after operative treatment. *J Bone Joint Surg (Am)* 2003;85:512–522.
15. Rumness DW, Lewallen D. Total hip arthroplasty after fracture of the acetabulum. *J Bone Joint Surg (Br)* 1990;72:761–764.
16. Weber M, Berry DJ, Harmsen WS. Total hip arthroplasty after operative treatment of an acetabular fracture. *J Bone Joint Surg (Am)* 1998;80:1295–1305.
17. Mears DC, Velyvis JH. Acute total hip arthroplasty for selected displaced acetabular fractures: two to twelve year results. *J Bone Joint Surg (Am)* 2002;84:1–9.
18. Swiontkowski MF, Thorpe M, Seiler JG, et al. Operative management of displaced femoral head fractures: case matched comparison of anterior versus posterior approaches for Pipkin I and Pipkin II fractures. *J Orthop Trauma* 1992;6:437–442.
19. Hesp W, Goris R. Conservative treatment of fractures of the acetabulum: results after long-term follow-up. *Acta Chir Belg* 1988;88:27–32.
20. Helfet DL, Borrelli J, DiPasquale T, et al. Stabilization of acetabular fractures in elderly patients. *J Bone Joint Surg (Am)* 1992;74:753–764.

21. Ghalambour N, Matta JM, Bernstein L. Heterotopic ossification following operative treatment of acetabular fracture. An analysis of risk factors. *Clin Orthop* 1994;305:96–105.
22. McLaren AC. Prophylaxis with indomethacin for heterotopic bone after open reduction of fractures of the acetabulum. *J Bone Joint Surg (Am)* 1990;72:245–247.
23. Webb LX, Rush PT, Fuller SB, et al. Greenfield filter prophylaxis of pulmonary embolism in patients undergoing surgery for acetabular fracture. *J Orthop Trauma* 1992;6:139–145.

Selected Historical Readings

Epstein HC. *Traumatic dislocations of the hip*. Baltimore, MD: JB Lippincott Williams & Wilkins, 1980.

Epstein HC. Posterior fracture-dislocations of the hip. *J Bone Joint Surg (Am)* 1974;56:1103–1127.

Epstein HC, Harvey JP. Traumatic anterior dislocations of the hip. *Orthop Rev* 1972;1:33.

Funk FJ Jr. Traumatic dislocations of the hip in children. *J Bone Joint Surg (Am)* 1962;44:1135–1145.

Judet R, Judet J, Letournel E. Fractures of the acetabulum: classification and surgical approaches for open reduction. *J Bone Joint Surg (Am)* 1964;46:1615–1646.

Letournel E. *Fractures of the acetabulum*. New York: Springer-Verlag, 1981.

Moore TM. Central acetabular fracture secondary to epileptic seizure. *J Bone Joint Surg (Am)* 1970;52:1459–1462.

Pearson DE, Mann RJ. Traumatic hip dislocation in children. *Clin Orthop* 1973;92:189–194.

Pipkin G. Treatment of grade IV fracture-dislocation of the hip. *J Bone Joint Surg (Am)* 1957;39:1027–1042.

Stewart MJ, Milford LW. Fracture-dislocation of the hip. *J Bone Joint Surg (Am)* 1954;36:315–342.

FRACTURES OF THE FEMUR   23

I. **FRACTURES OF THE FEMORAL NECK**
   A. **Mechanism of injury.** Femoral neck fractures account for just over half of all proximal femoral fractures and are most common in patients older than the age of 50 years; elderly patients account for approximately 95% of the total number of cases (1,2). These fractures become more common with increasing age because of the unhappy combination of osteoporosis and an increasing propensity for falls. Besides osteoporosis, other factors associated with an increased risk of femoral neck fracture are early menopause (or low estrogen state), alcoholism, smoking, low body weight, steroid therapy, history of stroke, phenytoin treatment, and lack of exercise. Excessive use of sedative drugs has also been implicated (3). Typical patients are female, fair, and thin. Eating a high fat diet is "poor dietary habit," but does not put one at risk. Efforts at preventing falls in elderly persons seem to have the most potential for controlling this phenomenon. Trochanteric pads may lessen the risk of fracture with falls (4), but compliance is poor and their usefulness has been questioned (5). In the elderly, hip fractures result in an increased 1-year mortality rate of 12% to 18%.

   Femoral neck fractures in younger patients usually result from high-energy trauma. In addition to traumatic injuries, stress fractures of the femoral neck may occur in active patients. Stress fractures that occur along the superior aspect of the femoral neck are called **tension fractures** and have a high propensity to progress to complete fractures. The **compression** stress fracture, which occurs at the base of the femoral neck, is less likely to displace.

   B. **Classification of fractures.** From the clinical standpoint, femoral neck fractures are of **four basic types**: displaced, nondisplaced, impacted, and the stress fracture. Radiographs can distinguish these, although some nondisplaced fractures may be radiographically occult and are only diagnosed after magnetic resonance imaging (MRI). Approximately two thirds of femoral neck fractures are displaced (2).

   C. **Symptoms and signs of injury.** Patients with stress fractures, nondisplaced fractures, or impacted fractures may complain only of **pain in the groin** or sometimes pain in the ipsilateral knee. The patients with stress fractures have a history of a recent increase in activity and may believe themselves to have a muscle strain. In contrast, patients with nondisplaced or impacted fractures have some history of trauma. They generally have a higher intensity of pain, can associate the onset with a traumatic event, and are seen early for medical treatment. In all three groups of patients, there is no obvious deformity on physical examination, but there is generally pain with internal rotation. A high index of suspicion must be maintained to avoid delay in diagnosis. Patients with displaced femoral neck fractures complain of pain in the entire hip region and lie with the affected limb shortened and externally rotated. Anteroposterior and high-quality cross-table lateral (obtained by flexing the uninjured, not the injured, hip) radiographs of the hip are necessary and sufficient to diagnose displaced, nondisplaced, and impacted fractures and for planning treatment. MRI (with Short TI Inversion Recovery STIR images) has been shown to be the quickest, most cost-effective way of correctly identifying radiographically occult fractures. Pending treatment, patients should be non–weight bearing and allowed to rest with the limbs in the most comfortable position, which is generally in slight flexion on a pillow. Traction is not necessary and may increase pain.

D. Treatment

1. **Stress fractures.** These fractures commonly occur in young, vigorous individuals and require careful evaluation. A high index of suspicion for this injury should be kept for active patients presenting with groin pain (6). Patients with femoral neck stress fractures often have decreased bone density compared to age-matched controls (7). Femoral neck stress fractures often heal uneventfully but have the potential to displace, especially if on the superior/lateral side. Upon diagnosis, patients should be treated by restricted weight bearing. Use of crutches or a walker is mandatory, but patients should also be cautioned not to attempt straight-leg raising exercises and not to use the leg for leverage in rising or in changing positions, particularly getting up out of a chair. Partial weight bearing is safe within 6 weeks, with full weight bearing in 12 weeks, as long as the fracture shows roentgenographic evidence of healing, which is evidenced by sclerosis at the superior femoral neck. Because of the potentially severe complications of displacement (nonunion, osteonecrosis, need for surgery), in-situ pinning should be considered in active or unreliable patients or any patient with a tension (superior) fracture. Compression types of fractures in elderly individuals generally do well with limiting activity as outlined above. Functional complaints may persist for years in patients with femoral neck stress fractures (8).

2. **Impacted fractures**
   a. These can be treated either **nonoperatively** or **operatively** (1,9). With the nonoperative method, the patient usually is kept in bed for a few days with the leg protected from rotational stresses until the muscle spasms subside. A program of protected ambulation, as outlined for stress fractures, is then initiated. In a series of over 300 patients with impacted femoral neck fractures treated nonoperatively, displacement only occurred in 5% of younger, healthy patients (9). When displacement occurred in these patients, operative treatment led to a successful outcome in all cases (9). Although the authors of this study suggest that surgery is only necessary in patients over age 70 with multiple medical problems, others would argue that even a 5% risk of late displacement is unacceptable.
   b. **Internal fixation** of impacted fractures has many advantages over nonoperative methods, especially using percutaneous technique. Although the rate of avascular necrosis may not be different, a union rate of 100% in operative cases has been reported, compared to 88% with closed management. The authors recommend multiple screw fixation, either percutaneous or by open technique, because it allows immediate weight bearing and avoids the risk of late displacement (10) (see **I.F**).

3. **Displaced fractures.** The management of displaced femoral neck fractures continues to be an area of controversy. The treatment decision is best based on the activity level of the patient before the fracture because this is a direct measure of the functional demands of the patient that should be restored and because activity level correlates with bone density (1). Patient's must be treated with understanding of their physical and mental abilities. Those that are most debilitated often need the surgery most. For example, the patient with poor cardiac function, while not an ideal surgical candidate, also needs to be as active as possible. The patient with dementia may need surgery as many do not understand recommendation for non–weight bearing. It is important to rapidly arrange family discussions and indepthly explain the risks and benefits of surgical intervention.
   a. Currently, there is disagreement about how to best manage displaced fractures in active patients. Certainly, fractures in healthy patients less than age 60, with or without slight comminution, should be **reduced, impacted,** and **internally fixed.** Such surgery should be done as quickly as possible. When surgical repair was carried out within the first 12 hours, a 25% rate of avascular necrosis was reported, increasing to 30% with surgery between 13 and 24 hours, 40% between 24 and 48 hours, and 100% after 1 week.

Intracapsular tamponade from fracture hematoma has an unfavorable effect on femoral head blood flow, as does nonanatomic position, so there is a rationale for proceeding with some urgency (1,11–16). However, patients with dehydration or unstable cardiac conditions should be medically stabilized before surgery to minimize the risk of fatality (17). There is consensus that accurate reduction and impaction at the fracture site are essential to a good end result.
- i. Authorities who stress an **anatomic reduction with impaction** believe that this allows the maximum opportunity for reestablishment of the vascular supply. Any stretch or kinking of the vessels of the ligamentum teres or retinaculum is avoided while stability of the fracture is optimized (13). Internal fixation with three pins or screws secures fracture stability; there is no value in using more than three implants (10). An exception to this generalization is the fracture comminuted with posterior comminution; in this instance the addition of a fourth screw may confer a little more stability (18).
- ii. Authorities who stress a **valgus reduction** believe that this position allows for maximum bone-on-bone stability and a reduced varus moment arm on the repaired fracture. In a valgus nailing, the nail or screw is near the center of the head, but the nail is rested along the calcar of the femoral neck to reduce the distance between the fulcrum of the nail or screw and the head. This positioning produces a shorter biomechanical moment and less stress on the device. Concern that the fixation cuts out superiorly or anteriorly can be eliminated by proper impaction of the fracture and the use of multiple pins or a sliding fixation apparatus (10,13). When valgus nailing is performed, it is more likely that screws will exit the femoral shaft at or distal to the lesser trochanter, which increases the risk of late subtrochanteric fracture.

  b. **The authors believe that an anatomic reduction is preferable to the valgus reduction, but when faced with a choice between slight valgus and any varus, then slight valgus is chosen.**

E. **Reduction techniques**
  1. The authors favor a **closed reduction** on a fracture table that then allows for the insertion of internal fixation under two-plane image-intensifier control. Manipulative reduction should be gentle, and the authors have found the techniques of McElvenny and Deyerle to be the most satisfactory. Frequently, however, the fracture is reduced by the maneuver of applying traction on the limb with neutral adduction-abduction with internal rotation to bring the femoral neck parallel to the floor. Nonanatomic reduction should not be accepted; if acceptable reduction is not obtainable by closed means then open reduction should be considered.
      a. In **McElvenny's technique**, both extremities are placed in traction with the hips in extension. The affected leg is lined up with the long axis of the body and is then maximally internally rotated by rotating the knee rather than the foot to reduce stress on the knee ligaments. Traction then is released on the contralateral side. After viewing follow-up radiographs, if more valgus is required, the traction may be reapplied to the affected leg. Just before releasing the traction on the opposite leg, an abduction force at the knee is applied along with a simultaneous pushing inward over the trochanter.
      b. The **Deyerle technique** achieves final alignment of the femoral neck and head in the lateral plane by a direct push posteriorly by two hands placed anteriorly over the greater trochanter while the pelvis on the contralateral side is supported to prevent ligament stress. This procedure is carried out after traction and internal rotation have reduced the fracture in the anteroposterior plane and before placement in slight valgus as described in **a.**
  2. **Open methods.** Open reduction is performed through either a **Smith-Petersen anterior approach** or a **Watson-Jones anterolateral approach**

when a satisfactory closed reduction cannot be obtained in a patient in whom prosthetic replacement is contraindicated (1). Although fracture site visualization may be best with the anterior approach, the screws have to be inserted through a separate lateral incision. The Watson-Jones interval is a more familiar approach for many surgeons, but fracture visualization may be a little more difficult.

F. **Operative techniques**
   1. **Multiple screws.** The multiple screw method, using three implants, is the simplest method of obtaining internal fixation. This method can be a percutaneous procedure, thus reducing the risk of infection and the operative morbidity in elderly patients, extremely poor-risk patients, and bedridden patients. The alternative of prosthetic replacement in the low functional demand patient is chosen except when these criteria apply (19). When an adequate (anatomic) closed reduction is obtained, the screws can be placed through a small lateral incision, but a capsulotomy is recommended by extending the deep dissection anteriorly. When the reduction is nonanatomic, open reduction is advised (1,16).
   2. **Sliding hip screw fixation** is an alternative to multiple screw fixation. With anatomic reduction, no mechanical advantage is obtained with the hip screw because fracture stability is most dependent on the quality of the reduction and the density of the bone in the femoral head. However, with a nonanatomic reduction, there is an advantage to the use of a hip screw because the fixation relies on the lateral cortex rather than opposition of the fracture surface (10,13). A sliding screw plate appears to have the advantage of firm fixation of the head, as well as allowing for impaction through sliding in a fitted barrel. An additional threaded pin or cancellous screw should be placed superiorly in the neck and head for improved torsional control (13). Regardless of the particular type of mechanism used, it is essential to obtain maximum holding capacity in the head, which necessitates the use of a 135-degree angle device in most individuals when anatomic reduction is obtained. When a valgus reduction is chosen, it is important to use a 150-degree nail plate device and to position the nail or screw in the deepest portion of the head.
   3. **Prosthetic replacement.** Many studies have demonstrated improved functional outcomes and dramatically lower reoperation rates with hemiarthroplasty and total hip replacement when compared with internal fixation of displaced femoral neck fractures. However, arthroplasty procedures carry a higher risk of deep infection, dislocation, and potential need for revision (20). Use of an anterior or lateral approach significantly decreases the risk of dislocation (20). Hemiarthroplasty of the hip may be performed with unipolar or bipolar components. Traditionally, a unipolar prosthesis is used for patients with very low functional demand, while bipolar devices are used in patients with higher functional demands. However, recent studies have failed to demonstrate any significant difference in outcomes with either type of device (21), while bipolar components may contribute polyethylene wear particles with time (22). Total hip arthroplasty provides the best functional results but is considered to be associated with a higher risk (10%) of dislocation (23). Fortunately, the risk of recurrent dislocation and reoperation are not different than those after primary total hip arthroplasty (24). The use of larger femoral heads with cross-linked polyethylene and avoidance of posterior approaches should reduce the risk of dislocation, although this has not yet been demonstrated in the literature. Total hip replacement is the procedure of choice when femoral neck fractures occur in patients with rheumatoid arthritis. Such fractures are exceedingly rare in patients with degenerative arthritis of the hip, but total hip arthroplasty would also be appropriate in these cases.
   4. The **authors' preference.** Multiple screw fixation or a sliding hip screw with an additional pin or screw appears to offer optimum fixation (1,16).

The techniques are not easily learned or applied and are only effective with anatomic reduction and maximum fracture impaction at the time of surgery. Given the difficulties inherent with either technique, the uncertain end-results if anatomic reduction is not obtained, and **the minimum of a 12% avascular necrosis rate**, the surgeon should consider femoral prosthetic replacement as an alternative in the older patient with low functional demands and poor bone quality or the very active older patient who will have the best function after total hip replacement (20).

G. **Failed primary fixation.** The most frequent complications following internal fixation of displaced femoral neck fracture are loss of reduction, protrusion of the screw or pins into the acetabulum, and collapse with symptomatic avascular necrosis. All of these complications are reliably salvaged by total hip arthroplasty.

H. **Postoperative care and rehabilitation.** The aim of treatment is to return the patient to preoperative status by the quickest, safest method. Therefore, rehabilitation planning should begin at the time of admission because most patients are elderly and do not tolerate prolonged periods away from familiar environments (17). Surgery is carried out as soon as possible, and the procedure should be one that allows immediate partial or full weight bearing, the first step in rehabilitation. Attempting to maintain a patient in non–weight-bearing status is frustrating for the surgeon, therapist, and family. The use of bedpans and the practice of straight-leg raising of the intact leg while in bed have been shown to produce considerable stress across the femoral neck. It is fallacious to attempt to protect the hip by non–weight-bearing with crutches, because approximately half the body weight is transmitted across the so-called non–weight-bearing hip. If the knee and hip are fully flexed, the forces at the hip approximate total body weight. The dependent position without the normal pumping action of muscles also predisposes to edema, venous stasis, and thrombophlebitis. The authors' experience indicates that, as long as stable internal fixation is achieved, gains from early weight bearing far outweigh the risks. Patients are encouraged to ambulate and to apply as much weight as is comfortable. Initially, a walker is used, and then gradual progress is made to crutches, if practical, and eventually a cane. In the case of the patient with balance problems, the walker or cane may be used indefinitely to help prevent more falls.

I. **Nonunion and avascular necrosis**
1. In the past, **nonunion** has been an important complication, but with proper reduction, impaction, and internal fixation, its incidence should be reduced to less than 10% (1,20). Most fractures heal promptly and the union is well established within 4 months. Occasionally, there is some resorption at the fracture site, probably a result of insufficient impaction at surgery and therefore some fracture instability. Further impaction and eventual healing usually occur, but the incidence of avascular necrosis is significantly higher than in patients who obtain primary union.
2. **Avascular necrosis**
   a. The **roentgenographic signs** of avascular necrosis, with associated collapse, can occur at any time postoperatively. For practical purposes, however, changes with collapse are usually seen within 3 years. The incidence of avascular necrosis is variously reported to be within 12% to 35%, and it must be appreciated that for displaced femoral neck fractures, the head, or at least a major portion of it, is rendered avascular at the time of injury (1,20). The lower figure of 12% is identical to that reported by most authors for impacted valgus fractures and probably represents the lowest possible incidence. When avascular changes are identified, the patient should be managed according to symptoms. In many older patients, the condition may not be severe enough to warrant any further surgery, but in patients with complete collapse of the femoral head and increasing pain, early total hip replacement is the treatment of choice.
   b. **The role of bone grafting for either prevention or treatment of avascular necrosis remains uncertain.** Currently, evidence for use of bone grafting for either of these conditions on a routine basis is lacking.

J. **Prognosis.** Anticipated complications and end results have been discussed for each fracture. Because of the advanced age of the typical patient, development of degenerative articular changes over a long period is difficult to assess, but it does not appear to be a frequent complication. The **morbidity and mortality rates (12% for the 12 months following fracture) are high, but they can be notably decreased by treating this fracture with early reduction and early ambulation.** The mortality rates return to those of age-matched control subjects after 1 year.
K. **Fractures of the neck of the femur in children** (25–27)
  1. **Treatment**
    a. **Transepiphyseal fractures** are uncommon, and there is no series of sufficient size to make any conclusions about the treatment of choice. The authors recommend reduction with capsulotomy and fixation with smooth pins (27).
    b. **Undisplaced and minimally displaced cervicotrochanteric fractures** carry a risk of avascular necrosis. The pathophysiology may involve intracapsular tamponade of the vessels supplying the femoral head (27). The authors recommend capsulotomy, reduction if necessary, and fixation with lag screws short of the femoral head epiphysis. The screws are generally sufficient because of the density of the bone. In children 8 years old and younger, postoperative spica cast immobilization is also used for 6 to 12 weeks. Displaced fractures are treated in the same way. These fractures must be treated emergently to minimize the complication of avascular necrosis.
  2. **Prognosis.** These fractures have nearly a 100% rate of union with optimum management.
  3. **Complications**
    a. **Coxa vara.** Although this complication is commonly reported, it is generally associated with nonoperative management.
    b. **Avascular necrosis.** This complication affects 0% to 17% of patients who undergo emergent treatment. The long-term consequence is generally degenerative arthritis, which requires total hip arthroplasty in patients in their 40s to 60s.
    c. **Premature closure of the epiphysis** occurred in 7% of the patients in Lam's series (26). This complication is not a significant long-term problem except when it occurs in children younger than 8 years.
II. **Intertrochanteric fractures** (28)
  A. **Surgical anatomy**
    1. **The classic intertrochanteric fracture occurs in a line between the greater and lesser trochanters.** Although in theory such a fracture is totally extracapsular, the distinction between an intertrochanteric fracture and a basilar femoral neck fracture is not always clear. In peritrochanteric fractures, the internal rotators of the hip remain with the distal fragment, whereas usually at least some of the short, external rotators are still attached to the proximal head and neck fragment. This factor becomes important in reducing the fracture because, in order to align the distal fragment to the proximal one, the leg must be in some degree of external rotation. This is in contrast to the internal rotation often needed to reduce transcervical femoral neck fractures and requires a distinctly different maneuver in the operating room with the patient on the fracture table to reduce the fracture.
    2. When the forces producing the fracture are increased, the greater trochanter and lesser trochanter can be separately fractured and appear as separated fragments **(three- and four-part fractures).** Secondary comminution is not infrequent and usually involves one of the four major fragments. Anatomic restoration becomes a major undertaking but is not necessary to obtain a satisfactory result from a functional point of view. Occasionally, a subtrochanteric extension of the fracture is encountered.
  B. **Mechanism of injury.** The intertrochanteric fracture almost invariably occurs as a result of a fall in which both direct and indirect forces are acting. Direct forces act

along the long axis of the femur or directly over the trochanter. Indirect forces include the pull of the iliopsoas muscle on the lesser trochanter and that of the abductors on the greater trochanter.
C. **Classification.** A number of classifications and subclassifications have been proposed (29,30). From the standpoint of treatment and prognosis, a simple classification into stable or unstable fractures is most satisfactory.
  1. A **stable intertrochanteric fracture** is one in which it is possible for the medial cortex of the femur to butt against the medial cortex of the calcar of the femoral neck fragment. Not uncommonly, the lesser trochanter is fractured off as a small secondary fragment, but this does not interfere with the basic stability of the fracture.
  2. The **unstable intertrochanteric fracture** is one in which there is comminution of the posteromedial-medial cortex (along the calcar femorale). In the most common unstable pattern, a large posteromedial fragment encompasses the lesser trochanter, with or without a fracture through the greater trochanter (four-part fracture). A fracture with high obliquity may be considered unstable because of the high shearing force at the fracture site despite anatomic reduction and internal fixation.
D. **Physical examination.** The fracture occurs primarily in the elderly, the average age reported being 66 to 76 years, which is slightly older than for femoral neck fractures. There is a predominance in women, with a ratio of occurrence in women to men of 2:1 to 8:1. The leg is shortened and lies in marked external rotation. Any movement of the extremity is painful and should not be attempted. If traction is applied with a Thomas splint for patient transport, it should be removed before radiographs are obtained because the ring interferes with proper assessment of the fracture. Both anteroposterior and lateral radiographs should be made to confirm the diagnosis and to delineate the fracture pattern. The lateral film is obtained as a cross-table view, which can be obtained by flexing the uninjured hip.
E. **Treatment.** Operative treatment is the procedure of choice if a skilled anesthesiologist and surgeon are available. The more debilitated the patient, the more urgent the indications. The goal of treatment must be to restore the patient to preoperative status as early as possible, which can be achieved best through reduction and internal fixation in a stable fashion so as to allow early ambulation. As with intracapsular fractures, if the patient is first seen with unstable medical conditions, these should be stabilized before surgery to minimize the risk of perioperative morbidity and mortality (17). If there are complicating injuries or illnesses that make it impossible to carry out operative reduction and fixation, well-leg traction is remarkably well suited to this situation. The leg must be held in some external rotation to maintain reduction of the fracture. This treatment allows movement from bed to chair and eliminates cumbersome traction apparatus for transport. Because treatment necessitates the use of crutches following the period of bed rest, weights should be used for strengthening the upper extremities. Great care must be taken to avoid secondary complications such as pressure areas over the sacrum and the heels, equinus contractures of the foot, and thromboembolic disease. Traction must be maintained until there is callus seen on radiographs—usually approximately 8 weeks. Following this period, mobilization may begin using non–weight bearing and parallel bars, a walker, or crutches. The hip must be protected until there is mature callus and bridging bone—an additional 4 to 6 weeks. The use of a cane in the opposite hand should be encouraged indefinitely to help prevent subsequent falls and injury.
  1. **Operative treatment of intertrochanteric fractures.** Currently, the sliding hip screw is the "gold standard" for the fixation of stable and unstable trochanteric fractures of the femur (31). "Fixed angle" devices that do not allow collapse of the fracture produce inferior results (29). There has been renewed interest in the use of intramedullary devices whose use is perceived as less invasive and associated with less perioperative morbidity. However, structured literature reviews show no difference in outcomes between intramedullary devices and sliding hip screws, except for a greater incidence of

both intraoperative and late femur fracture associated with intramedullary fixation (32,33). Most of the current available internal fixation devices for treatment of intertrochanteric fractures can be expected to yield satisfactory results.

    a. When using a **sliding hip screw**, the fracture must be reduced to a stable position; that is, the medial cortices must abut each other anatomically. What is potentially a stable fracture can be converted into an unstable situation by inadequate reduction of the medial cortices. The reduction is accomplished on a fracture table by direct traction, slight abduction, and external rotation. If these maneuvers do not produce an anatomic reduction, the fracture site should be opened to ensure stability of the reduction. Not infrequently, there is some posterior displacement at the fracture site that requires the femur shaft to be lifted anteriorly to secure an anatomic reduction at the time of fixation. Regardless of the internal fixation used, in the elderly osteoporotic patient, the neck itself might be little more than a hollow tube; to gain purchase, it is essential to insert the nail or screw well into the head. The authors recommend insertion to within 0.5 inch of the subchondral bone. The position should be in the center of the femoral head on both views (34,35). Baumgaertner has popularized the "tip-apex distance" as a way to emphasize the center/center position within the femoral head. The plate should be securely fixed across both femoral cortices by four screws. **The authors believe that a properly inserted sliding screw plate with the wide, threaded, blunt-nosed screw offers the best mechanical fixation for intertrochanteric fractures (Fig. 23-1).** With unstable fracture patterns, a trochanteric plate may be used to prevent excessive collapse (31).

    b. When **intramedullary devices** such as the Gamma nail are used, one must be careful to ream adequately and always insert the nail by hand to avoid intraoperative fracture. Long devices should be used to prevent later fracture at the tip of the stem; however, long intramedullary implants risk perforation of the distal anterior femoral cortex (33,36,37).

    c. In **osteoporotic patients** with highly comminuted fractures, hemiarthroplasty in total hip replacement may rarely be indicated (38). Comparative data are lacking to know whether outcomes are any different with arthroplasty compared to internal fixation.

    d. A special fracture that deserves mention is the **reverse obliquity fracture** (**Fig. 23-2**). With this pattern, the primary fracture line is parallel to the axis of the femoral neck and the sliding vector of the hip screw. This results in tremendous instability and very high failure rates when sliding hip screws are used (39). Fractures with this pattern are better stabilized with intramedullary implants or fixed-angle 95-degree devices.

F. Postoperative treatment. There is little agreement in the literature as to what constitutes the best postoperative management of intertrochanteric fractures. Our recommendation for rehabilitation is that patients be moved to at least a sitting position on the first postoperative day. In 2 to 3 days, they should be taken to the physical therapy department where ambulation can be started using the parallel bars. Patients may be allowed to place as much weight on the fractured extremity as they wish. They are not forced to go beyond what is comfortable for them but are reassured that some weight bearing is desirable and not to be feared. As soon as they feel secure using the parallel bars, patients should be transferred to a walker or crutches, depending on their abilities based on their prefracture status. With this program, it is rare that individuals who were able to walk without support before fracture cannot be returned to a self-sufficient state within 10 to 14 days using either a walker or crutches. Patients may disregard the walker or crutches at any time they feel secure. The long-term use of a cane is encouraged as a preventive measure in elderly patients to avoid falls and injury.

G. Prognosis and complications. Because of the age of patients (many suffer from other debilitating conditions at the time of injury), **mortality and morbidity rates**

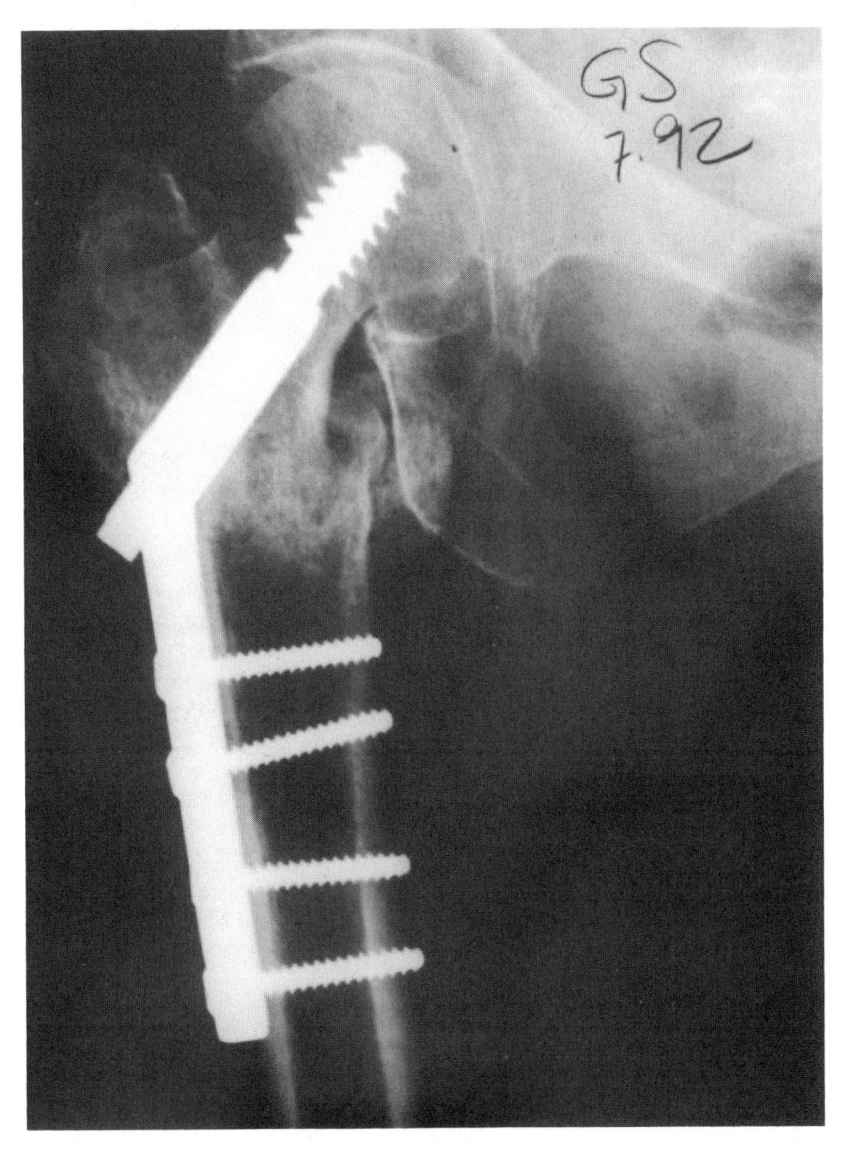

Figure 23-1. A sliding screw plate. Note the proper positioning for maximum fixation with the screw centrally seated in the head within 1 cm of the subchondral bone. Four screws are used to insert the slide plate onto the femur.

will always be significant. With an aggressive treatment program, mortality rate should be 10% to 15% for the first year after the fracture; subsequently, the mortality rate returns to that of age-matched controls. Mechanical failure and nonunion can be reduced to 1% or less. Avascular necrosis is rare but has been reported (40). Infection is still a problem, with most series reporting an incidence of deep infections of 1% to 5%. This rate can be significantly decreased by careful soft tissue technique (11,41) and the use of prophylactic antibiotics for 24 hours.

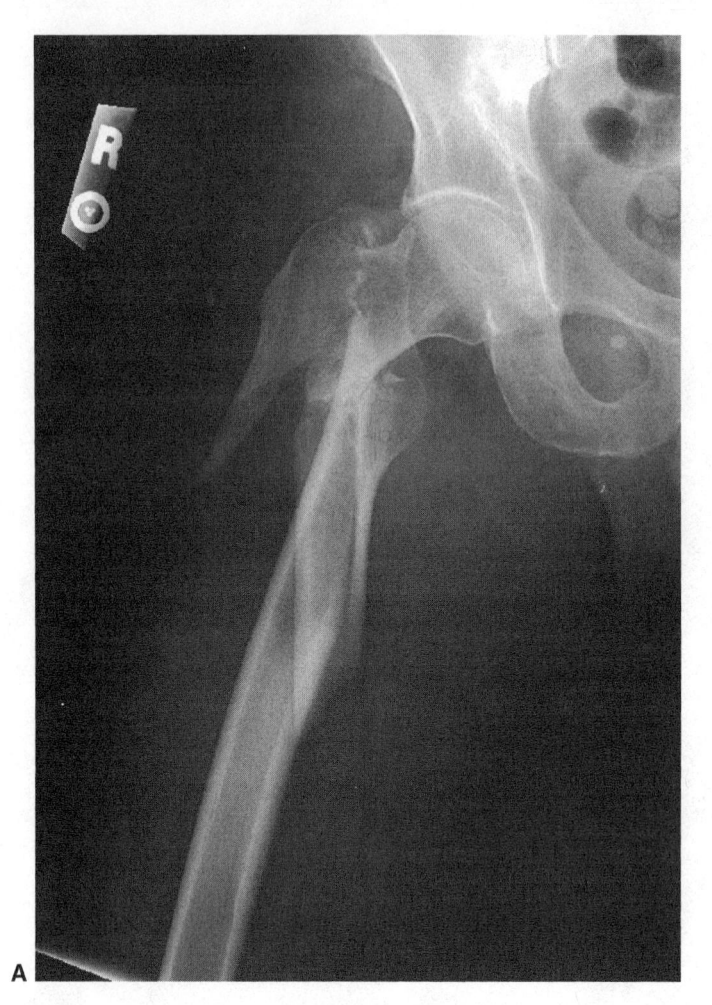

Figure 23-2. Reverse obliquity fracture *(continued)*.

With prompt internal fixation and an aggressive postoperative rehabilitation program stressing early weight bearing, complications from thromboembolic disease can be sharply reduced. The authors recommend the use of sequential compression devices and aspirin for all patients with the use of a low-dose warfarin of enoxaparin regimen. **Even with optimum treatment, it is scarcely possible to return more than 40% of the patients to their true prefracture status, but one can obtain satisfactory results from treatment in approximately 80% of patients.** Prophylactic antibiotics are recommended as discussed in **Chap. 8, IV.E,** and **Chap. 10, I.B.2.**

III. GREATER TROCHANTERIC FRACTURES
A. Isolated avulsion or comminuted fractures of the greater trochanter occasionally are seen. **Unless displacement of the fragment is greater than 1 cm,** the fracture is treated as a soft-tissue injury with protected weight bearing until the patient is asymptomatic. Several days of bed rest are usually required, followed by walker

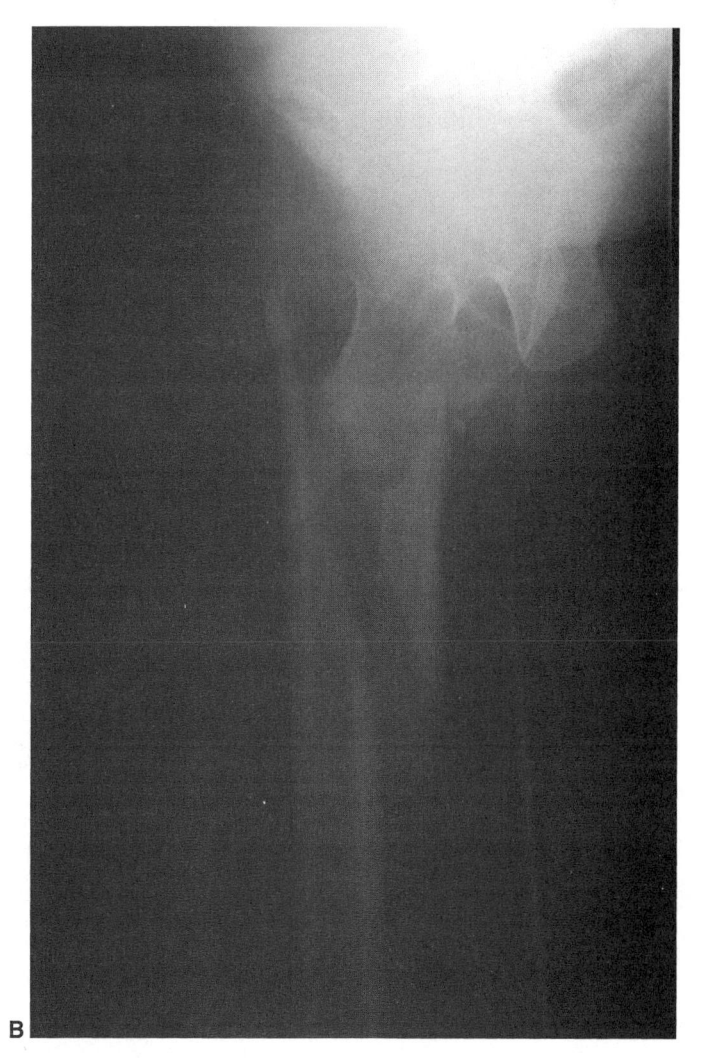

Figure 23-2. *(continued).*

or crutch ambulation for 3 to 4 weeks. **In elderly patients, even with separation greater than 1 cm, operative treatment with internal fixation rarely is indicated.**

B. In the younger patient, **when displacement is greater than 1 cm**, it is advisable to fix the fracture fragment internally with either two cancellous screws or a wire loop to secure fragments. This maneuver reconstitutes the functional integrity of the abductor mechanism. Postoperatively, the extremity is protected until soft-tissue healing is secured. Then the patient is allowed to ambulate without weight bearing for 3 to 4 weeks, followed by partial weight bearing for another 3 to 4 weeks until limp-free walking can be achieved.

IV. ISOLATED AVULSION FRACTURES OF THE LESSER TROCHANTER
   A. These fractures are seen mainly in children and athletic young adults. If they occur in an older patient, one must consider the possibility of metastatic disease. **Unless**

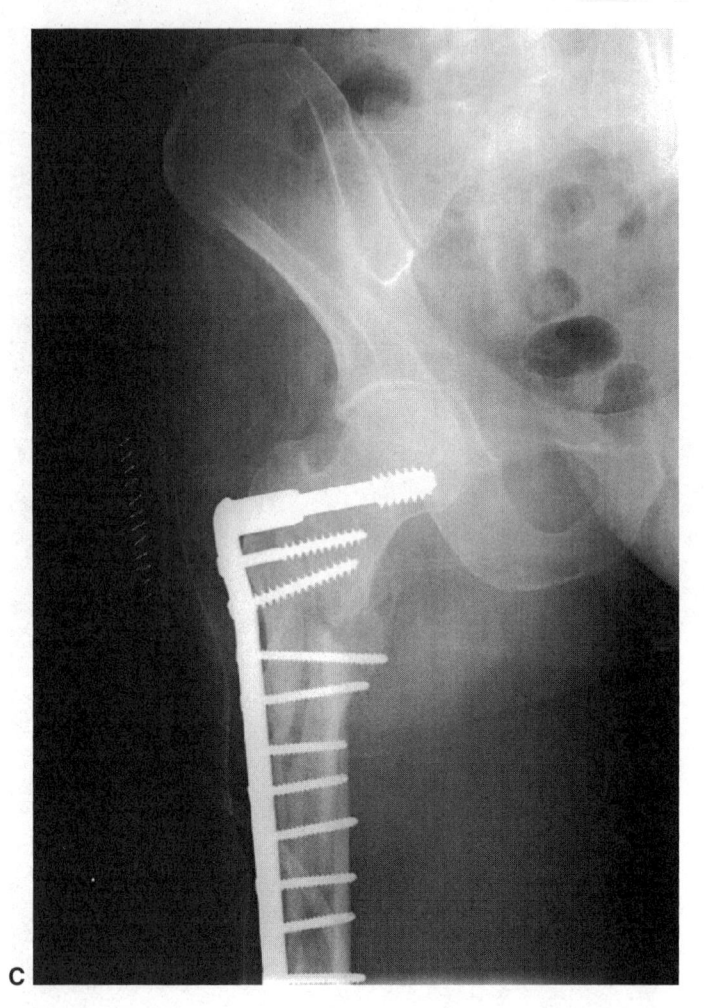

Figure 23-2. *(continued).*

       displacement is greater than 2 cm, operative fixation is not indicated and the end result is excellent.
    B. With displacement greater than 2 cm, it is advisable to stabilize the avulsed fragment with a cancellous screw or a cortical screw, securing it to the opposite cortex. This procedure is most readily accomplished through a medial approach to the hip. Complications are minimal, and the end result is most satisfactory.
V. SUBTROCHANTERIC FRACTURES
    A. Subtrochanteric fractures occur as extensions of intertrochanteric fractures or as independent entities (11). The mechanism is direct trauma, and significant forces usually are required. This type of fracture is ordinarily seen in younger individuals as compared with the intertrochanteric or femoral neck fracture. Subtrochanteric fractures, which are extensions of intertrochanteric fractures, are also seen in elderly patients. Thus, these fractures have a bimodal distribution.

B. **Classification.** Fielding (see Selected Historical Readings) classified subtrochanteric fractures as occurring in three zones: zone I, those at the level of the lesser trochanter; zone II, those 1 to 2 in below the upper border of the lesser trochanter; zone III, those 2 to 3 in below the upper border of the lesser trochanter. Seinsheimer's classification and results have emphasized the importance of the posteromedial fragment. Internal fixation then acts as a tension band on the outer (distracting) cortex and allows for impaction and weight bearing directly through the medial cortex. If this internal fixation is not possible, the fracture pattern is unstable. The most practical classification of subtrochanteric fractures is the system of Russell (75) et al., which divides such injuries into high and low fractures and has direct implications for the most appropriate type of internal fixation (39). High fractures occur above the lesser trochanter and may or may not involve the greater trochanter and piriformis fossa of the proximal femur. Fractures that involve the piriformis fossa require plate fixation or trochanteric nailing. High fractures not involving the piriformis fossa may be treated by reconstruction nailing. Low fractures occur below the lesser trochanter, may or not be comminuted, and have varying degrees of extension down the femoral shaft. These fractures, regardless of pattern, are readily treated with standard intramedullary nails.

C. **Physical examination.** Because the forces required to produce the fracture are substantial, other injuries in the same extremity and elsewhere in the body often occur. Emergency splinting in a Thomas splint generally is required. Hemorrhage in the thigh may be significant, so the patient should be monitored for hypovolemic shock, and blood replacement may be necessary. Good anteroposterior and lateral radiographs are necessary to clearly assess the extent of the fracture.

D. **Treatment.** Operative stabilization to allow early rehabilitation is the treatment of choice. Traction may rarely be necessary for the severely comminuted fracture, but the healing time is longer than for an intertrochanteric fracture, and delayed unions and malunions frequently are encountered. Skeletal traction should be used and applied in such a way as to align the distal fragment to the proximal fragment. If the lesser trochanteric fragment with its attached iliopsoas muscle remains intact on the head and neck fragment, it is necessary to flex and externally rotate the distal fragment to obtain reduction. The strong adductors attached to the femoral shaft tend to cause varus angulation, and attempts to correct this by abduction of the hip often exert pull on the adductors and cause bowing at the fracture site or medial displacement of the shaft fragment. In this event, it is best for the patient to undergo treatment in a neutral position with reference to abduction-adduction and to increase the traction. When the fracture is comminuted and the lesser trochanter is off as a separate piece, treatment is the same as for intertrochanteric fractures. If traction treatment is used, it should be maintained until there is roentgenographic evidence of union. The patient is then placed in a single spica cast or hip abduction brace for protected weight bearing until the callus matures.

E. **Operative treatment**
  1. **Fractures involving the lesser trochanter** (Fielding zone I). Fractures in this region not involving the piriformis fossa may be treated with intramedullary nailing using a second-generation (reconstruction) nail with fixation into the femoral neck and head. When there is **comminution involving the piriformis**, there are two potential options. The first is to proceed with intramedullary nailing using a trochanteric nail, again with proximal fixation in the femoral neck and head. This may be difficult because the nail may still need to be inserted directly through the fracture site. In the author's opinion, use of a **95-degree fixed-angle device** such as a blade plate or dynamic condylar screw is the ideal method for these fractures. With either method, the procedure is facilitated by use of a fracture table and with the patient in the lateral position. **Indirect reduction techniques** should be used to restore length, rotation, and alignment; it is not necessary to expose, manipulate, or bone-graft the comminuted region of the lesser trochanter.
  2. **Fractures below the lesser trochanter** (Fielding zones II and III). These fractures represent proximal femoral shaft fractures and are usually amenable to

the same techniques of fixation (i.e., intramedullary nailing) (42). Compression plating is equally satisfactory in the hands of persons familiar with its application, but it is not used routinely because of the large surgical dissection required.
- **F. Postoperative management.** Stable subtrochanteric fractures or those that can be rendered stable by operative treatment can be managed much as intertrochanteric fractures. The unstable subtrochanteric fracture must be supported and protected from weight bearing until the union is secure.
- **G. Complications.** In the event of a frank nonunion or a delay in union of an intertrochanteric or subtrochanteric fracture, a careful assessment of the cause of this failure should be made. Too often it is caused by less-than-strict adherence to the treatment principles outlined. If the fixation is secure and the reduction adequate, bone grafting may suffice. As soon as problems with union are recognized, optimal position of the fracture should be obtained and standard internal fixation combined with fresh autogenous cancellous grafting carried out. Osteotomy may be required, especially if there is varus malposition of the proximal femur. Once this process is completed, the management is the same as for a fresh fracture, except that it may be necessary to delay patient activity until discomfort from the graft donor site has subsided.

VI. INTERTROCHANTERIC AND SUBTROCHANTERIC FRACTURES IN CHILDREN.
These fractures may be treated in **balanced skeletal traction**, aligning the distal fragment to the proximal one. Often, this requires that traction be applied with the hip and knee flexed (90-90 traction). Traction is maintained until the fracture is stable (4–6 weeks), at which time the extremity is placed in a single spica cast for immobilization until union is solid (approximately 12 weeks). Increasingly, percutaneous pin or screw fixation with supplemental spica casting is used. The authors favor reduction and percutaneous Steinmann pin fixation followed by supplemental spica casting.

VII. FEMORAL DIAPHYSEAL FRACTURES IN ADULTS (43–45)
- **A.** Diaphyseal fractures of the femur are the result of significant trauma and usually are associated with considerable **soft-tissue damage**. Blood loss of 2 to 3 units is common. In addition, these fractures have a high incidence of associated injury in the same extremity (46,47), including fractures of the femoral neck (48), posterior fracture-dislocations of the hip, tears of the collateral ligaments of the knee (47), and osteochondral fractures involving the distal femur or patella and fractures of the tibia (46).
- **B. Examination.** Diagnosis usually does not present any clinical problem if care is taken to rule out the other associated injuries by physical examination and radiographs.
- **C. Radiographs.** Films are obtained primarily to confirm the diagnosis and for preoperative planning. It is **essential** to view the joint above and the joint below the fracture. Films of the uninjured femur are helpful for selecting the appropriate internal fixation device. An anteroposterior and lateral roentgenogram of the injured femur should be supplemented by the anteroposterior pelvis to obtain optimum views of the femoral neck (49). Unpublished data indicate that routine computed tomographic (CT) imaging of the femoral neck reduces the rate of missed ipsilateral femoral neck fracture.
- **D. Treatment**
    1. Emergency treatment consists of the immediate application of a Thomas or Hare splint before radiographs are obtained. Unless there is gross comminution or the patient is not a surgical candidate, fractures of the shaft of the femur from the lesser trochanter to approximately 10 cm above the knee joint should be treated by **closed antegrade interlocking nailing** (see **Fig. 25-3**), with reaming of the canal using flexible reamers and prebent nails (44,45). Current areas of controversy include the role of retrograde nailing and the timing of surgery. In general, once associated body cavity and other extremity injuries are ruled out, the patient should receive urgent operative stabilization. The more severely injured the patient, the more critical stable fixation of the femur fracture becomes. Early fixation has been shown to be

associated with decreased narcotic use, reduced pulmonary complications (e.g., adult respiratory distress syndrome), and decreased mortality rate (43). Even patients with isolated femoral shaft fractures, including elderly patients, benefit from urgent (within 24 hours of admission) stabilization of the femur with an interlocking nail (43,50,51). These procedures are carried out on a fracture table in the operating room under fluoroscopic control, although some authors report good results with nailing on a standard radiolucent table (52). Although many authors recommend routine supine positioning because of the ease of placement of locking bolts, we favor the lateral position on the fracture table when the patient does not have chest, abdominal, or pelvic injuries. This allows greater ease of access to the greater trochanter and use of smaller incisions in large patients. When the patient is severely traumatized, especially those with traumatic brain injuries at risk for secondary brain insults, fracture stability can be achieved with external fixation or plates much more rapidly on a standard table. The fixator is generally exchanged for an interlocking nail within the first 5 to 7 days when the patient's condition has stabilized. Primary interlocking nailing immediately following debridement is the procedure of choice for most open femoral shaft fractures (53). Some advocate the use of small diameter locked nails without reaming, especially in patients with severe cardiopulmonary trauma; this has been associated with longer healing time and implant failure (54–56).
   2. Recently, implants for retrograde locked nailing have been developed (57,58). Indications for retrograde nailing include severe obesity, pregnancy, bilateral fractures, and ipsilateral tibia, patella, or acetabular fractures (that require repair via a posterior hip approach) (59).
   3. Balanced suspension skeletal traction may be used until a cast-brace can be applied only when the equipment or expertise necessary for locked nailing is unavailable and when the patient cannot be transported (60).
  E. Complications
   1. **Associated vascular and nerve damage**, especially a transient peroneal or pudendal nerve palsy, is not uncommon. These problems are generally associated with excessive or prolonged traction.
   2. **Shortening and malrotation** of the extremity frequently occur (61), even with intramedullary nailing. Slight shortening is associated with earlier fracture union, and shortening up to 0.5 inch should be accepted without hesitation.
   3. **Skin breakdown** over bony prominences and pin track infections are complications of traction.
   4. **Infection is extremely rare with the closed nailing technique** (62).
   5. **Nonunion** occurs in approximately 1% of fractures treated with nailing. This problem is easily managed with nail removal, reaming, and repeat nailing. Healing complications are more common when small-diameter nails are used.
   6. Rotational malunion occurs in 10% to 20% of patients; the deformity is generally external rotation (63).
   7. Weakness of the abductor muscles and hip pain can occur in one third of patients (64,65).
   8. Knee injuries are common after femoral shaft fractures (66).
VIII. **DIAPHYSEAL FEMUR FRACTURES IN CHILDREN**
  A. **For children younger than 6 to 8 years** with an uncomplicated, isolated femoral shaft fracture, a spica cast can be used for primary treatment. The technique is as follows (67):
   1. When the patient's general condition has stabilized, usually after at least 24 hours of observation in 2 to 3 lb of Buck's traction, the patient is placed under general anesthesia on a fracture table. The feet are placed in stirrups, and traction is applied. If necessary, a sling attached to an overhead bar may support the fractured thigh to restore the normal anterior bow of the femur. For a

child younger than 2 years, it may be desirable to flex the hip and knee to 90 degrees. For the older child, the hip is flexed approximately 20 to 30 degrees, abducted 20 degrees, and externally rotated to best align the distal fragment to the proximal fragment. The knees are kept extended. Radiographs are made to verify the reduction. The object of manipulation is to provide approximately 1 cm of overriding of the fragments (bayonet apposition in good alignment in both planes). When this position has been achieved, the skin between the knees and ankles is then sprayed with medical adhesive. A single layer of bias-cut stockinet is wrapped over the entire area as described for extremity casting (see **Chap. 7**). Quarter-inch felt, sponge rubber, or several additional turns of Webril may be used over bony prominences except between the knee and ankle. A **double hip spica cast** is then applied, molded carefully around the pelvis, and extended to embrace the rib margin. When the cast has hardened, the foot pieces of the fracture table are removed, and if radiographs confirm the proper position, the cast is extended to include both feet and ankles, which are well padded, in a neutral position. A crossbar is added to the cast.

   2. **Postcasting treatment.** Follow-up radiographs are made at 1, 2, and 3 weeks to be certain of the maintenance of position. The cast is worn for 6 to 12 weeks, depending on the age of the patient and the type of fracture. The family must be instructed in cast care and told to alert the physician if there is any evidence of pain, fever, or loss of extension of the great toe.
- B. **Children older than 8 years** are not ideally managed with spica casts and usually receive some sort of operative fixation. Antegrade interlocking nails, as used in adults, are not appropriate in skeletally immature patients because of the risk of osteonecrosis of the hip. For transverse, length stable fractures, retrograde flexible nailing has gained increased acceptance (68). Trochanteric nails may be considered for the teenage child with fractures of the diaphysis of the femur. The starting point for the nail should be moved slightly lateral to decrease the risk of avascular necrosis. Compression plating remains a very good option (69); percutaneous submuscular plating is another recent option.
- C. **Children with head injuries** or multiple trauma should be managed with operative stabilization. In patients younger than 12 years, this should involve plates, retrograde flexible nails, or external fixators. Children older than 12 years may undergo treatment with intramedullary nails.

IX. **UNICONDYLAR, SUPRACONDYLAR, AND INTRACONDYLAR FRACTURES** (62)
- A. **Mechanism of injury.** In older individuals, these fractures are sustained with minimal trauma. In young people, these fractures generally are caused by massive trauma and often are associated with vascular and other soft-tissue injuries. This fracture has a bimodal age distribution as well.
- B. **Examination.** A careful assessment of nerve and vascular status distal to the fracture is critical here as with any fracture. Care must be taken to ascertain any injuries to the soft tissues about the knee and whether the fracture extends into the joint.
- C. **Radiographs.** Anteroposterior, lateral, and, occasionally, oblique views are necessary.
- D. **Treatment**
   1. **Displaced unicondylar fractures** should be treated by open reduction and internal fixation. Although good results can be anticipated with use of traditional devices such as the dynamic condylar screw or blade plate (35), newer periarticular plates may be an advantage. Retrograde nailing is advocated by many; its advantages include a less invasive approach and better stabilization in severely osteoporotic patients.
   2. **Undisplaced supracondylar fractures** or fractures displaced less than 1 mm involving the joint surface may be treated by percutaneous screw fixation, generally with cannulated screw systems. Alternatively, a hinged knee brace or cast-brace may be used, but frequent radiographs must be obtained. In either case, early motion must be initiated to optimize results.

Inferior results with nonoperative management for these fractures has been documented (70).
3. **Extra-articular distal femur fractures** or those occurring above total knee replacements can be nicely managed with retrograde supracondylar nails (71,72) or standard antegrade nails (73).
4. **Displaced intra-articular or supracondylar fractures** are managed by internal fixation (41,58,74,75). The fracture requires open reduction of the joint surface via a lateral or anterolateral approach to ensure that it is anatomically reduced. Minimal stripping of the soft-tissue attachments to the extra-articular fragments must be completed. This speeds union and decreases the need for bone grafting while minimizing infection (76). A 95-degree condylar blade plate or dynamic condylar screw is the optimum device for fixing these fractures, but they require 1.5 to 2.0 cm of intact bone proximal to the compression screw or blade (75). With extremely comminuted fractures, a condylar buttress plate is required, which allows for more screws into the distal fragment. Fixed-angle locking plates have revolutionized the care of these fractures (74). Medial or varus collapse is prevented, and fixation in osteoporotic bone is improved. Minor malunion is common with the use of fixed angle devices (77). If the expertise or equipment to perform these procedures does not exist and the patient cannot be transported to a facility where they are available, skeletal traction can be used. A tibial pin is inserted with the knee flexed 20 degrees, and balanced suspension is used. Early active quadriceps exercises are necessary to prevent joint fibrosis. Because of the pull of the gastrocnemius, which extends the fracture, the flexed position should be maintained for the first several weeks. The distal fragment must be aligned to the proximal fragment, which is usually in external rotation.

E. **Postoperative care.** Continuous passive motion is used while the patient is in the hospital and may be extended to the early posthospitalization period (first 3 weeks) in most cases in which stable internal fixation has been achieved. A hinged-knee brace is generally used for 6 weeks. The goal of full extension and 120 degrees of flexion by 6 weeks postoperatively is standard. Full weight bearing is delayed for 10 to 12 weeks. Strengthening exercises can then be initiated. Patients in traction require aggressive physical therapy to regain full extension and 90 degrees of flexion. Active and gentle passive motion protocols are initiated once the fracture is clinically and radiographically healed at about 8 weeks after injury. Some permanent loss of motion is expected for fractures treated this way as well as for severe intra-articular fractures managed operatively (74).

HCMC Treatment Recommendations
Femoral Neck Fractures
  Diagnosis: Anteroposterior pelvis and lateral radiographs, physical examination. Patient's leg will be shortened and internally rotated.
  Treatment: Open reduction internal fixation (ORIF) of fracture with multiple pins/screws for all impacted and nondisplaced fractures and for displaced fractures in active patients with good bone density. Patients with pre-existing arthritis or significant osteoporosis should receive a prosthetic replacement (hemiarthroplasty or total hip replacement).
  Indications for surgery: Femoral neck fracture
  Recommended technique: Hemiarthroplasty done through an anterior or posterior approach to the hip—rehabilitation is easier with the anterior approach but access to the proximal femur is slightly more difficult. In active elderly patients, total hip replacement is considered, and when done, a large (36–40 mm) head is used with highly cross-linked polyethylene.

HCMC Treatment Recommendations
Intertrochanteric Hip Fractures
   Diagnosis: Anteroposterior pelvis and lateral hip radiographs, clinical examination. Patient's leg will be shortened and externally rotated.
   Treatment: ORIF of fracture with sliding hip screw or trochanteric nail. The latter is used for reverse oblique fractures and at surgeon discretion. Rarely, extremely comminuted fractures in extremely osteoporotic individuals are treated with prosthetic replacement.
   Indications for surgery: Any intertrochanteric fracture, displaced or nondisplaced
   Recommended technique: Sliding hip screw applied with patient on the fracture table with C-arm control.

HCMC Treatment Recommendations
Subtrochanteric Femur Fractures
   Diagnosis: Anteroposterior pelvis and lateral proximal femur radiographs, clinical examination. Again, patient's leg will be shortened and externally rotated.
   Treatment: Depends on involvement of the piriformis fossa. Fractures below the piriformis fossa are treated by closed reduction and interlocking nail placement. Open reduction may be required in certain fracture patterns to ensure proper placement of the implant. If the lesser trochanter is not attached to the proximal fragment, a "second-generation" interlocking nail where the proximal interlocking screws are directed into the femoral head and neck are required. Fractures above the piriformis fossa may be treated by a sliding hip screw, 95-degree condylar screw, blade plate, or proximal femoral nail.
   Indications for surgery: All subtrochanteric femur fractures
   Recommended technique: For isolated fractures, the implant is inserted with the patient on the fracture table in the lateral decubitus position. Nailing of fractures as described is preferred; rarely a 95-degrees device such as a condylar screw or blade plate is preferred based on fracture pattern considerations.

HCMC Treatment Recommendations
Femoral Shaft Fractures
   Diagnosis: Anteroposterior and lateral radiographs of the femur, clinical examination. CT imaging of the hip is routinely reviewed for occult femoral neck fracture.
   Treatment: Closed reduction and insertion of reamed interlocking nail
   Indications for surgery: All femoral shaft fractures in adult patients
   Recommended technique: For isolated fractures, closed interlocking nail placement on the fracture table with the patient in the lateral decubitus position. For patients with multisystem trauma, the nailing can be done with the patient supine on a radiolucent table with a C-arm. Rarely, a plate or the temporary use of an external fixator followed by conversion to an interlocking nail is indicated within the first 2 weeks after injury. Retrograde nails are used for specific indications, including the morbidly obese and ipsilateral tibial or patellar fractures.

HCMC Treatment Recommendations
Distal Femur Fractures
   Diagnosis: Anteroposterior and lateral radiographs of the distal femur, including the knee joint, clinical examination
   Treatment: Internal fixation to allow range of motion of the knee joint
   Indications for surgery: All displaced supracondylar fractures of the femur with or without joint extension
   Recommended technique: ORIF with plate and screws for most younger patients with articular extension. Retrograde nailing with or without lag screws for patients who are obese, osteoporotic, have a fracture above a knee prosthesis. Active range-of-motion (AROM) and limited weight bearing for 12 weeks.

References

1. Swiontkowski MF. Femoral neck fractures: current concept review. *J Bone Joint Surg (Am)* 1994;76:129–138.
2. Thorngren KG, Hommel A, Norrman PO, et al. Epidemiology of femoral neck fractures. *Injury* 2002;33(Suppl 3):C1–C7.
3. Ray WA, Griffin MR, Downey W. Benzodiazepines of long and short elimination half-life and the risk of hip fracture. *JAMA* 1989;262:3303–3307.
4. Kannus P, Parkkari J, Niemi S, et al. Prevention of hip fracture in elderly people with use of a hip protector. *N Engl J Med* 2000;343:1506–1513.
5. Patel S, Ogunremi L, Chinappen U. Acceptability and compliance with hip protectors in community-dwelling women at high risk of hip fracture. *Rheumatology* 2003;42:769–772.
6. Clough TM. Femoral neck stress fracture: the importance of clinical suspicion and early review. *Br J Sports Med* 2002;36:308–309.
7. Muldoon MP, Padgett DE, Sweet DE, et al. Femoral neck stress fractures and metabolic bone disease. *J Orthop Trauma* 2001;15:181–185.
8. Weistroffer JK, Muldoon MP, Duncan DD, et al. Femoral neck stress fractures: outcome analysis at minimum five-year follow-up. *J Orthop Trauma* 2003;17: 334–337.
9. Raaymakers EL. The non-operative treatment of impacted femoral neck fractures. *Injury* 2002;33(Suppl 3):C8–14.
10. Swiontkowski MF, Harrington RM, Keller TS, et al. Torsion and bending analyses of internal fixation techniques for femoral neck fractures: the role of implant design and bone density. *J Orthop Res* 1987;5:433–444.
11. Mast J, Jakob R, Ganz R. *Planning and reduction techniques in fracture surgery*. New York: Springer-Verlag, 1989:1–254.
12. Melberg PE, Korner L, Lansinger O. Hip joint pressure after femoral neck fracture. *Acta Orthop Scand* 1986;57:501–504.
13. Ort PJ, Lamont T. Treatment of femoral neck fractures with a sliding hip screw and the knowles pins. *Clin Orthop* 1984;190:158–162.
14. Sevitt S, Thompson RG. The distribution and anastomosis of arteries supplying the head and neck of the femur. *J Bone Joint Surg (Br)* 1965;47:560–573.
15. Stromqvist B. Femoral head vitality after intracapsular hip fracture: 490 cases studied by intravital tetracycline labeling and TC-MDP radionuclide imagery. *Acta Orthop Scand* 1983;54(S200):1–71.
16. Swiontkowski MF, Winquist RA. Displaced hip fractures in children and adolescents. *J Trauma* 1986;26:384–388.
17. Kenzora JE, McCarthy RE, Lowell JD, et al. Hip fracture mortality: relation to age, treatment, preoperative illness, time of surgery, and complications. *Clin Orthop* 1984;186:45–56.
18. Kauffman JI, Simon JA, Kummer FJ, et al. Internal fixation of femoral neck fractures with posterior comminution: a biomechanical study. *J Orthop Trauma* 1999;13:155–159.
19. Sikorski JM, Barrington R. Internal fixation vs. hemiarthroplasty for the displaced subcapital fracture of the femur: a prospective randomized study. *J Bone Joint Surg (Br)* 1981;63:357–361.
20. Lu-Yao GL, Keller RB, Littenberg B, et al. Outcomes after displaced fractures of the femoral neck: a meta-analysis of one hundred and six published reports. *J Bone Joint Surg (Am)* 1994;76:15–25.
21. Raia FJ, Chapman CB, Herrera MF, et al. Unipolar or bipolar hemiarthroplasty for femoral neck fractures in the elderly? *Clin Orthop* 2003;414:259–265.
22. Coleman SH, Bansal M, Cornell CN, et al. Failure of bipolar hemiarthroplasty: a retrospective review of 31 consecutive bipolar prostheses converted to total hip arthroplasty. *Am J Orthop* 2001;30:313–319.
23. Delamarter R, Moreland JR. Treatment of acute femoral neck fractures with total hip arthroplasty. *Clin Orthop* 1987;218:68–74.
24. Abboud JA, Patel RV, Booth RE, et al. Outcomes of total hip arthroplasty are similar for patients with displaced femoral neck fractures and osteoarthritis. *Clin Orthop* 2004;421:151–154.

25. Cheng JC, Tang N. Decompression and stable internal fixation of femoral neck fractures in children can affect the outcome. *J Pediatr Orthop* 1999;19:338–343.
26. Lam SF. Fractures of the neck of the femur in children. *J Bone Joint Surg (Am)* 1971;53:1165–1179.
27. Swiontkowski MF, Winquist RA, Hansen ST. Fractures of the femoral neck in patients between the ages of twelve and forty-nine years. *J Bone Joint Surg (Am)* 1984b;66:837–846.
28. Lorich DG, Geller DS, Nielson JH. Osteoporotic pertrochanteric hip fractures: management and current controversies. *Instr Course Lect* 2004;53:441–454.
29. Bannister GC, Gibson GF, Ackrund CE, et al. The fixation and prognosis of trochanteric fractures. A randomized, prospective controlled trial. *Clin Orthop* 1990;254:242–246.
30. Larsson S, Friberg S, Hansson LI. Trochanteric fractures; influence of reduction and implant position in impaction and complications. *Clin Orthop* 1990;259:130–138.
31. Lindskog DM, Baumgaertner MR. Unstable intertrochanteric hip fractures in the elderly. *J Am Acad Orthop Surg* 2004;12:179–190.
32. Parker MJ, Handoll HH. Gamma and other cephalocondylic intramedullary nails versus extramedullary implants for extracapsular hip fractures. *Cochrane Database Syst Rev* 2002;1:pCD000093.
33. Parker MJ, Pryor GA. Gamma versus DHS nailing for extracapsular femoral fractures; metanalysis of 10 randomized trials. *Int Orthop* 1996;20:163–168.
34. Baumgaertner MR, Curtin SL, Lindskog DM, et al. The value of the tip-apex distance in predicting failure of fixation of peritrochanteric fractures of the hip. *J Bone Joint Surg (Am)* 1995;77:1058–1064.
35. Baumgaertner MR, Solberg BD. Awareness of tip-apex distance reduces failure of fixation of trochanteric fractures of the hip. *J Bone Joint Surg (Br)* 1992;79:969–971.
36. Handy DCR, Descamps PY, Krallis P, et al. Use of an intramedullary hip-screw compared with a compression hip-screw with a plate for intertrochanteric femoral fractures: a prospective, randomized study of one hundred patients. *J Bone Joint Surgery (Am)* 1998;80:618–630.
37. Herscovici D, Ricci WM, McAndrews P, et al. Treatment of femoral shaft trauma. *J Orthop Trauma* 2000;14:10–14.
38. Green S, Moore T, Proano F. Bipolar prosthetic replacement for the management of unstable intertrochanteric hip fractures in the elderly. *Clin Orthop* 1987;224:169–177.
39. Haidukewych GJ, Israel TA, Berry DJ. Reverse obliquity fractures of the intertrochanteric region of the femur. *J Bone Joint Surg (Am)* 2001;83A:643–650.
40. Mann RJ. Avascular necrosis of the femoral head following intertrochanteric fractures. *Clin Orthop* 1973;92:108–115.
41. Bolhofner BR, Carmen B, Clifford P. The results of open reduction and internal fixation of distal femur fractures using a biologic (indirect) reduction technique. *J Orthop Trauma* 1996;6:372–377.
42. Wiss D, Fleming CH, Matta JM, et al. Comminuted and rotationally unstable fractures of the femur treated with an interlocking nail. *Clin Orthop* 1986;212:35–47.
43. Bone LB, Johnson KD, Weigelt J, et al. Early versus delayed stabilization of femoral fractures: a prospective randomized study. *J Bone Joint Surg (Am)* 1989;71:336–340.
44. Winquist RA, Hansen ST, Clawson DK. Closed intramedullary nailing of femoral fractures. *J Bone Joint Surg (Am)* 1984;66:529–539.
45. Wolinsky PR, McCarty E, Shyr Y, et al. Reamed intramedullary nailing of the femur: 551 cases. *J Trauma* 1999;46:392–399.
46. Veith RG, Winquist RA, Hansen ST. Ipsilateral fractures of the femur and tibia. *J Bone Joint Surg (Am)* 1984;66:991–1002.
47. Walling AK, Seradge H, Spiegel PG. Injuries to the knee ligaments with fractures of the femur. *J Bone Joint Surg (Am)* 1982;64:1324–1327.
48. Ostermann PAW, Neumann K, Ekkernkamp A, et al. Long-term results of unicondylar fractures of the femur. *J Orthop Trauma* 1994;8:142–146.

49. Swiontkowski MF, Hansen ST, Kellam J. Ipsilateral fractures of the femoral neck and shaft. *J Bone Joint Surg (Am)* 1984a;66:260–268.
50. Cameron CD, Meek RN, Blachut PA, et al. Intramedullary nailing of the femoral shaft: a prospective, randomized study. *J Orthop Trauma* 1992;6:448–451.
51. Morgan CG, Gibson MJ, Cross AE. Intramedullary locking nails for femoral shaft fractures in elderly patients. *J Bone Joint Surg (Br)* 1989;72:19–22.
52. Stephen DJ, Kreder HJ, Schemitsch EH, et al. Femoral intramedullary nailing: comparison of fracture-table and manual traction. A prospective, randomized study. *J Bone Joint Surg (Am)* 2002;84:1514–1521.
53. O'Brien PJ, Meek RN, Powell JN, et al. Primary intramedullary nailing of open femoral shaft fractures. *J Trauma* 1991;31:113–116.
54. Bhandari M, Guyatt GH, Tong D, et al. Reamed versus nonreamed intramedullary nailing of lower extremity long bone fracture: a systematic overview and meta-analysis. *J Orthop Trauma* 2000;14:2–9.
55. Moed BR, Watson JT, Cramer KE, et al. Unreamed retrograde intramedullary nailing of fractures of the femoral shaft. *J Orthop Trauma* 1998;12:334–342.
56. Tornetta P, Tiburzzi D. Reamed versus nonreamed antegrade femoral nailing. *J Orthop Trauma* 2000;14:15–19.
57. Cole JD, Huff WA, Blum DA. Retrograde femoral nailing of supracondylar, intracondylar and distal fractures of the femur. *Orthopedics* 1996;19(Suppl 1):22–30.
58. Ostrum RF, DiCiccio J, Lakatis R, et al. Retrograde intramedullary nailing of femoral diaphyseal fractures. *J Orthop Trauma* 1998;12:464–468.
59. Patterson BM, Routt ML Jr, Benirschke SK, et al. Retrograde nailing of femoral shaft fractures. *J Trauma* 1995;38:38–43.
60. Johnson KD, Johnston DWC, Parker B. Comminuted femoral-shaft fractures: treatment by roller traction, cerclage wires, and an intramedullary nail, or an interlocking intramedullary nail. *J Bone Joint Surg (Am)* 1984;66:1222–1235.
61. Tornetta P, Ritz G, Kanton A. Femoral torsion after interlocking nailing of unstable femoral fractures. *J Trauma* 1995;38:213–219.
62. Schatzker J, Lambert DC. Supracondylar fractures of the femur. *Clin Orthop* 1979;138:77–83.
63. Braten M, Terjesen T, Rossvoll I. Torsional deformity after intramedullary nailing of femoral shaft fractures. *J Bone Joint Surg (Br)* 1993;75:799–803.
64. Bain GI, Zacest AC, Paterson DC, et al. Abduction strength following intramedullary nailing. *J Orthop Trauma* 1997;11:93–97.
65. Benirschke SK, Melder I, Henley MB, et al. Closed interlocking nailing of femoral shaft fractures: assessment of technical complications and functional outcomes by comparison of a prospective database with retrospective review. *J Orthop Trauma* 1993;7:118–122.
66. Moore TJ, Campbell J, Wheeter K, et al. Knee function after complex femoral fractures treated with interlocking nails. *Clin Orthop* 1990;261:238–241.
67. Staheli LT, Sheridan GW. Early spica cast management of femoral shaft fractures in young children. *Clin Orthop* 1977;126:162–166.
68. Greisberg J, Bliss MJ, Eberson CP, et al. Social and economic benefits of flexible intramedullary nails in the treatment of pediatric femoral shaft fractures. *Orthopedics* 2002;25:1067–1070.
69. Caird MS, Mueller KA, Puryear A, et al. Compression plating of pediatric femoral shaft fractures. *J Pediatr Orthop* 2003;23:448–452.
70. Butt MS, Krikler SJ, Ali MS. Displaced fractures of the distal femur in elderly patients; operative vs. non-operative treatment. *J Bone Joint Surg (Br)* 1995;77:110–114.
71. Brumback RJ, Toal TR, Murphy-Zane MS, et al. Immediate weight-bearing after treatment of a comminuted fracture of the femoral shaft with a statically locked intramedullary nail. *J Bone Joint Surg (Am)* 1999;81:1538–1544.
72. Henry SL. Management of supracondylar fractures proximal to total knee arthroplasty with the GSH supracondylar nail. *Contemp Orthop* 1995;31:231–238.

73. Leung KS, Shen WY, So WS, et al. Interlocking intramedullary nailing for supracondylar and intracondylar fractures of the distal part of the femur. *J Bone Joint Surg (Am)* 1991;73:333–340.
74. Kregor PJ. Distal femur fractures with complex articular involvement: management by articular exposure and submuscular fixation. *Orthop Clin North Am* 2002;33:153–175.
75. Russell TA, Taylor JC. Subtrochanteric fractures of the femur. In: Browner BD, Jupiter JB, Levine AM, et al. eds. *Skeletal Trauma*, 2nd ed. Philadelphia, PA: Saunders, 1992.
76. Ostrum RF, Geel C. Indirect reduction and internal fixation of supracondylar femur fractures without bone graft. *J Orthop Trauma* 1995;9:278–284.
77. Zehntner MK, Marohesi DG, Burch H, et al. Alignment of supracondylar/intracondylar fractures of the femur after internal fixation by AO/ASIF technique. *J Orthop Trauma* 1992;6:318–326.

Selected Historical Readings

Clawson DK. Trochanteric fractures treated by the sliding screw plate fixation method. *J Trauma* 1964;4:737–752.

Clawson DK, Smith RF, Hansen ST Jr. Closed intramedullary nailing of the femur. *J Bone Joint Surg (Am)* 1971;53:681–692.

Dimon JH, Hughston JC. Unstable intertrochanteric fractures of the hip. *J Bone Joint Surg (Am)* 1967;49:440–450.

Fielding JW. Subtrochanteric fractures. *Clin Orthop* 1973;92:86–99.

Garden RS. Malreduction and avascular necrosis in subcapital fractures of the femur. *J Bone Joint Surg (Br)* 1971;53:183–197.

Kempf I, Grosse A, Beck G. Closed locked intramedullary nailing: its application to comminuted fractures of the femur. *J Bone Joint Surg (Am)* 1985;67:709–720.

Kyle RF, Gustilo RB, Premer RF. Analysis of 622 intertrochanteric hip fractures. *J Bone Joint Surg (Am)* 1979;61:216–221.

Lesin BE, Mooney V, Ashby ME. Cast-bracing for fractures of the femur. *J Bone Joint Surg (Am)* 1977;59:917–923.

McElvenny RT. The importance of the lateral x-ray film in treating intracapsular fractures of the neck of the femur. *Am J Orthop* 1962;4:212.

Neer CS, Grantham SA, Shelton ML. Supracondylar fractures of the adult femur. *J Bone Joint Surg (Am)* 1967;49:591–613.

Olerud S. Operative treatment of supracondylar-condylar fractures of the femur. *J Bone Joint Surg (Am)* 1972;54:1015–1032.

Seinsheimer F. Subtrochanteric fractures of the femur. *J Bone Joint Surg (Am)* 1978;60:300–306.

Singh M, Nagrath AR, Main PS. Changes in trabecular patterns of the upper end of the femur as an index of osteoporosis. *J Bone Joint Surg (Am)* 1970;52:457–467.

Zickel RE. A new fixation device for subtrochanteric fractures of the femur. A preliminary report. *Clin Orthop* 1967;54:115–123.

KNEE INJURIES: ACUTE AND OVERUSE   24

I. **FOUNDATION OF INJURY DIAGNOSIS.** Knee injuries are common in active individuals. Both acute and overuse injuries occur, and they require different investigative processes to diagnose and treat them properly.
   A. Subdivision of clinical categories
      1. Acute injury is an injury that happens where a single application of force creates the musculoskeletal damage. This is common in athletics, motor vehicle trauma, etc.
      2. Acute or chronic injury is an injury that results in a disabled state that can be quiescent over time and result in a new injury episode at a later time. This new injury would represent an acute injury. However, this new injury did not depend on abnormal forces creating the injury but rather the fact that there was pre-existing damage to the musculoskeletal tissue. Common examples might be recurrent patella instability or recurrent shoulder subluxation.
      3. Overuse injury is an injury that is characterized by the absence of an injury or at least no injury significant enough to explain the current clinical situation. This kind of injury results from repetitive submaximal or subclinical trauma that results in macro- or microscopic damage to a structural unit and/or its blood supply. This overuse pattern can be seen in all musculoskeletal tissue but is most common in bone (overuse pattern resulting in stress fracture), bursal tissues (overuse pattern resulting in bursitis), and tendon (overuse pattern resulting in tendonosis).
   B. **Clinical correlation.** The clinical approach to a knee injury (acute/chronic/overuse) depends on four cornerstones:
      1. History
      2. Physical examination
      3. Tests and their interpretations
      4. Treatment

II. **APPROACH TO THE ACUTELY INJURED KNEE**
   A. History
      1. **Mechanism of injury.** This helps to identify potential structures that may have been damaged by the application of force, either direct (contact) or indirect (twisting mechanism). If the injury was a contact injury, one should look for external signs at the point of force application and what structures might have been injured as that force continues. For instance, a blow to the anterior tibia might create upper tibial bruising. This force creates a posterior displacement of the tibia on the femur, potentially injuring the posterior cruciate ligament. Non-contact injuries frequently involve rotatory twisting; the lower limb remains fixed as the upper body twists around the knee.
      2. **Was a pop heard or felt?** A pop is frequently associated with tearing of a ligament, most commonly the anterior cruciate ligament, or a bone bruise.
      3. **Return to play.** The degree of pain and/or disability cannot be used as a reliable indicator of the seriousness of an injury. However, continued play with little or no impairment in performance diminishes the likelihood of a serious knee injury.
      4. **Has the joint been previously injured?** Frequently this question uncovers an acute on chronic injury. Two common examples are recurrent kneecap dislocation and recurrent subluxation after initial anterior cruciate ligament injury.

5. **Joint swelling.** Knee joint swelling within 12 hours after an injury is, by definition, hemorrhage into the joint. An effusion that occurs after 12 hours suggests synovial fluid accumulation due to reactive synovitis, often due to cartilage or meniscus damage. (see **6.b** below).
6. The **differential diagnosis** of an acute knee hemarthrosis (1) (what inside the knee can bleed?) is:
   a. **Ligament injury.** The anterior cruciate ligament (ACL) and posterior cruciate ligament (PCL) are intraarticular/extra-synovial structures. The superficial medial collateral ligament (MCL) is an extraarticular structure. However, the deep MCL is a thickening of the joint capsule and is intraarticular. In a complete tearing of the MCL, both structures are torn. The lateral collateral ligament (LCL) is an extraarticular structure. It is rare that this ligament is torn in isolation. The most common ligament torn in acute hemarthrosis is the ACL (approximately 70%) (2).
   b. **Peripheral meniscus tear.** The outer, or peripheral, one third of the meniscus is vascular, and a tear in this region results in a hemarthrosis. Meniscus tears in this zone have the potential for healing and are repairable. Tears in the inner two thirds of the meniscus are more often associated with synovial irritation leading to a serous effusion that arises later (e.g., 24–48 hours) after the initial injury.
   c. **Fractures.** Any fracture that involves the joint surface results in a joint hemarthrosis. In addition to obvious condylar/patellar fractures, occult osteochondral fractures can be a source of hemarthrosis. These can include avulsion fractures of the PCL and ACL (more common in developing adolescents) and fractures secondary to patella dislocation.
   d. **Synovial/capsular tears.** Patella dislocations, even in the absence of fractures, are a source of hemarthrosis as the medial patellofemoral ligament and medial retinacular restraints are torn. Also, a significant contusion without a frank fracture or ligament/meniscus injury can create synovial bleeding. This is often considered a diagnosis of exclusion.

B. Physical Examination
1. **Inspection**
   a. **Swelling.** The absence of notable intraarticular swelling does not signify a less severe injury. Severe ligament disruptions are associated with large capsular disruptions, and fluid typically escapes into the surrounding tissue. The absence of knee swelling may indicate an extraarticular source of pain.
   b. **Localized bruises and abrasions.** These can be useful to identify the point of application of force in a contact injury. These can indicate the direction of the force, which helps to indicate what structures may be injured.
2. **Palpation**
   a. **Direct palpation** of the injured area corresponds to the anatomic structure underneath that area. This is most useful for diagnosis when surface anatomy is directly correlated such as iliotibial band tendonosis and patella tendonosis. Direct palpation of meniscal, patellofemoral, and MCL structures can be useful in distinguishing a differential diagnosis. The cruciate ligaments do not have a palpable attachment to the capsule, and, therefore, direct palpation of these structures is not possible. However, injury to the ACL is associated with anterolateral subluxation of the tibia on the femur and, therefore, anterolateral joint line tenderness is common.
   b. **Patella subluxation/dislocation.** This is associated with tenderness along the patella retinaculum, especially at the medial epicondyle where the medial patellofemoral ligament (MPFL) inserts and/or along the superior medial portion of the patella. Note that although the patella dislocates laterally, it is the medial based structures that are injured and thus are painful when palpated.
3. **Range of motion.** This is best assessed with the patient in the supine position. When the knee has an effusion, the knee's resting position prefers approximately 30 degrees of flexion (where potential capsular distention is largest). Full extension and full flexion should be compared to the opposite side, presuming

that side is normal. If the opposite side knee hyperextends, then an injured knee that goes just to zero would be considered lacking full extension.
- a. A **locked knee** is defined as the inability to obtain full passive motion of the joint secondary to a mechanical block. This does not mean that the knee is in one position, but rather that there is an inability to obtain full motion. Common causes are a displaced meniscus tear or loose body.
- b. A **pseudo locked knee** is defined as the inability to obtain full range of motion secondary to pain or intraarticular knee swelling. A torn meniscus without displacement can result in pain at the limits of flexion and/or extension. If the patient's knee "locks" in full extension and doesn't want to bend, the most common reason is an injury to the extensor mechanism, resulting in pain when the patient attempts to engage the kneecap in the trochlear groove.
- c. **Active range of motion** assesses the integrity of the motor units surrounding a joint. Even in a severely injured knee, the patient typically retains the ability to lift his or her leg. Therefore, active straight leg raising and range of motion should be assessed. Frequently missed acute knee injuries are disruptions of the extensor mechanism, which include quadriceps tendon and patella tendon injuries. In this instance, the patient will generally be incapable of a straight leg raise.
4. **Stability testing.** The *sine qua non* of a ligament disruption is the presence of pathologic joint motion.
   - a. **Straight plain instabilities** are the easiest instabilities to test on a knee. This represents the ability to move the tibia away from the femur in four known planes.
     - i. **Medial instability** is associated with injury to medial or tibial collateral ligament
     - ii. **Lateral instability** is associated with injury to lateral or fibular collateral ligament
     - iii. **Anterior instability** is associated with injury to ACL
     - iv. **Posterior instability** is associated with injury to PCL
   - b. **Rotary instabilities.** This refers to the rotation of the tibia around its vertical or longitudinal axis (**Fig. 24-1**).
     - i. **Anterolateral instability** is associated with ACL injury
     - ii. **Posterolateral instability** is associated with structures of the posterolateral corner of the knee (LCL, popliteal fibular ligament, popliteus tendon). These are frequently associated with PCL and/or ACL injuries.
     - iii. **Posteromedial injuries.** These injuries are rare and are commonly associated with PCL injury with or without MCL injury.
     - iv. **Anteromedial injuries** are associated with ACL/MCL injuries
   - c. **Extensor mechanism instability**
     - i. **Apprehension sign.** Passive lateral movement of the patella causing pain and/or quadriceps contraction is suggestive of patellofemoral subluxation/dislocation. This maneuver is typically done with the leg in full extension, quadriceps muscles relaxed.
     - ii. **Straight leg-raising against gravity** confirms integrity of the extensor mechanism, including quadriceps tendon, patella, and patella tendon. A "lag" sign represents the difference between passive and active extension of the knee. A lag signifies disruption and/or weakness of the extensor mechanism.
     - iii. **Medial/lateral patella restraints.** Stability testing of the patellofemoral joint involves assessing the degree of passive patella motion in a medial and lateral direction of the patella. This is typically measured against an imaginary midline of the patella in the resting position (**Fig. 24-2**). This maneuver tests the static restraints of the medial and lateral extensor retinaculum complex. Any change from the patient's "normal" measured

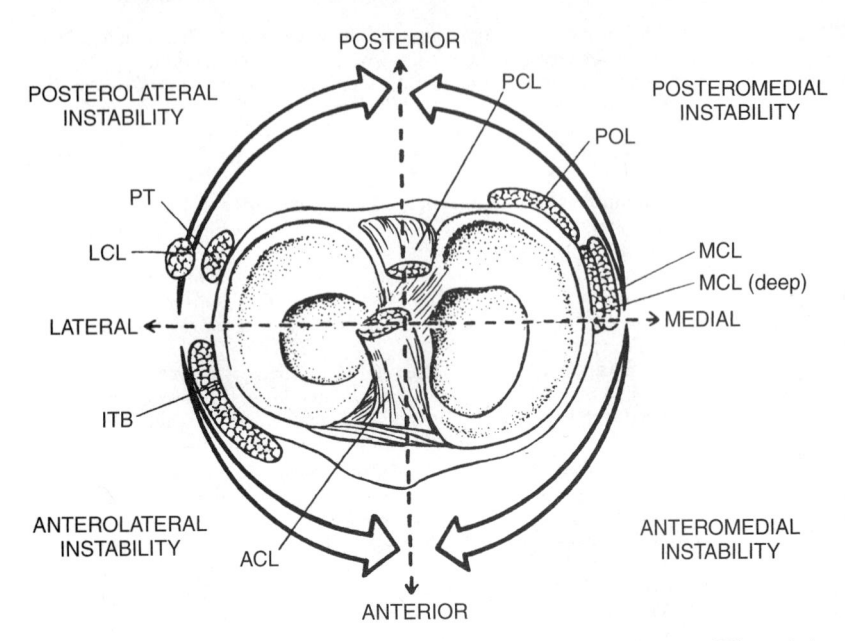

Figure 24-1. Rotatory instability of the knee. PCL, posterior cruciate ligament; POL, posterior oblique ligament; MCL, medial collateral ligament; ACL, anterior cruciate ligament; ITB, iliotibial band; LCL, lateral collateral ligament; PT, popliteal tendon. (From Arendt, EA. Assessment of the athlete with a painful knee. In: Griffin, LY, ed. *Rehabilitation of the injured knee*, 2nd ed. St. Louis, MO: Mosby, 1990, with permission.)

against their normal contralateral knee is suggestive of extensor mechanism disruption. Most particularly, an increase in lateral patella motion represents laxity or incompetence of the medial patella femoral ligament and medial retinacular structures associated with past or present patella dislocation.

C. Tests and their interpretation
1. **Plain radiographs**
    a. **Anterior/posterior view.** The primary utility of this view is to rule out diagnoses and assess overall tibiofemoral alignment. Standing views are preferred as they best assess tibial-femoral joint space. If pain/swelling limits full extension and/or full weight bearing, supine views are performed but provide less information.
    b. **Lateral view** evaluates the caudad/cephalad position of the kneecap. Patella alta, or increase in the cephalad position of the kneecap, suggests a patella tendon injury, especially when the injured side's kneecap is higher than the opposite side. Avulsion fractures, especially those of the PCL, are typically visualized along the posterior aspect of the tibia in this view.
    c. **Axial view** evaluates the position of the patella in its relationship to the femoral trochlear groove. Oftentimes, osteochondral fragmentation following a patella dislocation can be visualized on this view. Typically, one would see fragmentation of the medial patella facet and/or lateral femoral condyle in an acute patella dislocation (**Fig.24-3**). Different axial views have been established (Laurin's, Merchant's) (3). The clinician should become familiar with one technique. Axial views are a must for complete evaluation of all acute knee injuries.

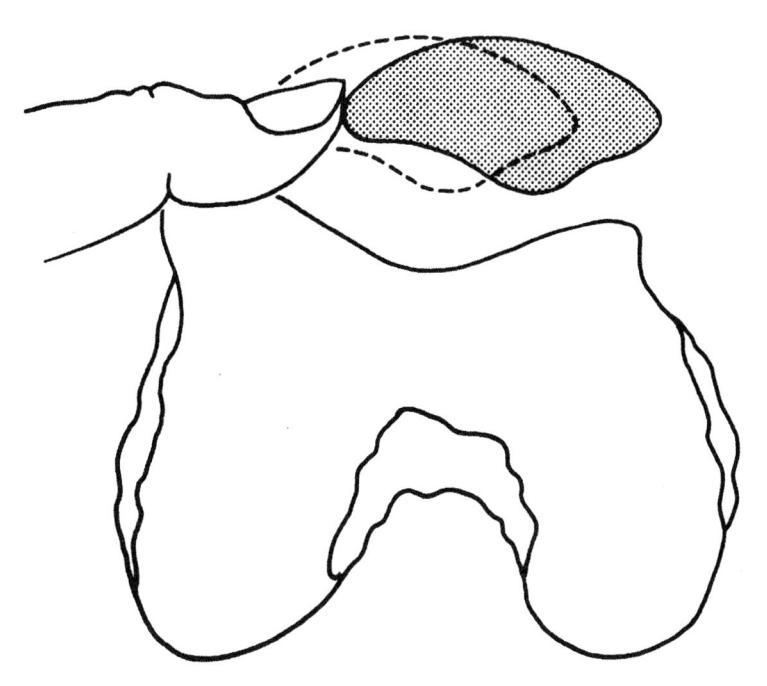

Figure 24-2. Demonstrates one quadrant medial "glide." The patella is divided visually into four quadrants. Holding the patella between the examiner's thumb and index finger, the limits of medial and lateral motion are assessed and recorded as "quadrants" of motion. (From Halbrecht JL, Jackson DW. Acute dislocation of the patella. In: Fox JM, Pizzo WD, eds. *The patellofemoral joint*. New York: McGraw-Hill, 1993, with permission.)

   d. **Notch or tunnel view** is most useful for evaluation of avulsion fractures of the tibia, osteochondritis dissecans, and loose bodies. This view is not standard for an acute knee injury.
2. **Magnetic resonance imaging (MRI)** for the knee. MRI has its largest application in evaluating meniscus and cruciate ligament injury. The overall accuracy is greater than 90% (4). An MRI is typically an adjunct test in the evaluation of an acutely injured knee. It should be performed only if it will alter the treatment protocol and is typically ordered by the physician who will be giving definitive treatment. It should never be used in the absence of a thorough and knowledgeable history and physical examination.

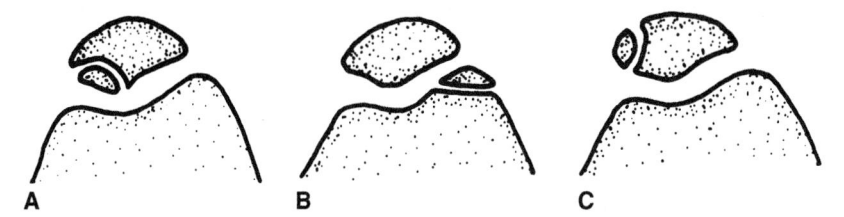

Figure 24-3. Three types of fractures associated with patella dislocation. **A:** osteochondral fracture of the medial patella facet. **B:** osteochondral fracture of the lateral femoral condylar. **C:** Avulsion fragment of medial patella femoral ligament off medial epicondyle (osseous-nonarticular). (From Halbrecht JL, Jackson DW. Acute dislocation of the patella. In: Fox JM, Pizzo WD, eds. *The patellofemoral joint*. New York: McGraw-Hill, 1993, with permission.)

Posterolateral knee structures are not well visualized in the standard knee MRI views.
3. **TcMDP** bone scans are most useful in occult infections and to rule out stress fractures. Their usefulness in diagnosing reflex sympathetic dystrophy is variable. This is not a common diagnostic test ordered for acute knee injuries.
4. **Computerized tomography (CT)** has few specific applications for routine imaging of acute knee injuries. It continues to have utility for evaluating complex fractures around the knee, especially those involving articular surfaces. When used with contrast, it can be useful to evaluate the cartilage integrity of osteochondral defects such as osteochondritis dissecans.
5. **Stress radiographs** can be utilized to document ligamentous disruption of the knee but are infrequently performed. Stress radiographs can be useful to help evaluate the stability of a fracture through the growth plate, typically used within a surgical setting. Stress views of the knee are recommended to evaluate the degree of PCL laxity, most often used in the subacute or chronic setting.

D. General treatment
1. **Joint aspiration** is rarely used to help with evaluation of an acute knee injury. It is classically taught that fat dropules in a bloody aspirate helps to diagnose a fracture through bone. When a tense effusion is present, an aspiration can be therapeutic. Aspiration continues to be used when a non-traumatic effusion is present and to rule out infection, rheumatological diseases, especially crystalline deposit diseases such as gout and pseudogout, and rarely synovial based tumors such as pigmented villonodular synovitis. Aspirations for non-traumatic effusions are usually complex with blood workup including complete blood count (CBC) with differential, erythrocyte sedimentation rate (ESR), C-reactive protein (CRP), rheumatoid factor (RF), flourescent antinucclear antibody test (FANA), and Lyme's titer.
2. **Immobilization/crutches.** This is the safest way to protect an injured knee until a repeat examination or a definitive diagnosis and/or treatment can be initiated by the same or a referral physician. However, if no significant/unstable fracture is present, removal of the brace to perform gentle range-of-motion exercise is useful to help resolve an effusion. Partial weight bearing, depending on the patient's comfort level and the working diagnosis can also be therapeutic and is encouraged. A knee immobilizer may be indicated for the acute knee injury when the patient's knee is unstable or the pain is severe with passive flexion. It is crucial to advise re-evaluation within a few days as prolonged immobilization can precipitate atrophy and may turn a small, self-limiting injury into a chronic problem.
3. **Reduction of swelling.** Strategies to reduce swelling should be included in the initial treatment recommendation. These include ice, gentle passive or active assisted range of motion, elevation, and compression.
4. **Repeat examination** is helpful in establishing a more firm diagnosis, especially when pain, swelling, and/or apprehension limit the initial examination.
5. **Antiinflammatory medication** is commonly used to control pain. The efficacy in the reduction of an acute effusion or inflammation of injured tissues is debated. Antiinflammatory medications also change the role of platelet function and can theoretically increase bleeding of an injured site. It is recommended that this class of medications be used only for analgesic reasons and should be taken as a *prn* drug.

III. SPECIFIC ACUTE KNEE INJURIES
A. Fractures of the patella
1. **Anatomic considerations.** The patella is a sesamoid bone that is contained within the extensor mechanism. Its main function is to provide a lever arm for superior mechanical functioning of the extensor mechanism and to help stabilize the limb in deceleration. The strong quadriceps muscle complex is attached to its superior pole.
2. Common types of **fractures**
   a. **Transverse fractures**, with or without comminution. These can be caused by direct or indirect trauma. They frequently are associated with disruption

of the extensor mechanism and need to be surgically stabilized in order to regain the mechanical function of the extensor mechanism.
- b. **Vertical fractures** of the patella frequently are due to a direct injury; infrequently they represent an overuse injury of the patella. When they are associated with no or minimal displacement, they do not constitute a disruption of the extensor mechanism and can be treated conservatively.
- c. **Chip fractures** of the medial border are commonly seen with a patella dislocation; infrequently, they can be associated with direct trauma. This variety will be more thoroughly discussed under patella dislocation.

3. **Treatment**
   - a. **Undisplaced or minimally displaced fractures** may be treated symptomatically without surgery. However, they must be protected from further damage. Immobilization in a knee immobilizer for 2 to 4 weeks is sufficient, with weight bearing as tolerated. Quadriceps isometric exercises can be performed during this time. Gentle, passive range of motion as per the patient's comfort level is recommended.
   - b. For **displaced fractures** involving the articular surface, an anatomic reduction is essential. Open reduction and internal fixation of the fragments with a tension band wire or lag screw is the treatment of choice (5).
   - c. **Comminuted fractures** require surgical treatment. A patellectomy is necessary if the entire patella cannot be internally fixed to gain stability. If more than half of the patella remains intact, then the comminuted pieces may be excised and the tendon sutured just above the subchondral bone into the remaining pole of the patella. Occasionally, fragments are large enough to fix with tension band wiring or 2.7-mm cortical lag screws (5).
   - d. If an **osteochondral fracture** is suspected, an arthroscopy to inspect the joint and remove small fragments of bone and cartilage may be of benefit. This is often the result of a patella dislocation and will be more thoroughly discussed below. At times, typically due to direct trauma, a large osteochondral fragment can be present. If the chondral fragment has an osseous layer, open or arthroscopic fixation should be attempted. This might be most readily accomplished by using bioabsorbable implants. Cartilage injuries are ominous for the future health of the joint; their treatment is beyond the scope of this text (6,7).
   - e. **Postoperative treatment** must be individualized according to the type of fracture and the security of the repair. Most knees are initially placed in a compressive dressing with a posterior splint or knee immobilizer. If rigid internal fixation is achieved and the patient is trustworthy, early protective passive range of motion is initiated, progressing to active motion. Typically, 6 weeks of some form of immobilization is necessary for healing of the fracture(s). Quadricep muscle strength within the limits of the allowed knee motion should be encouraged throughout this time.
   - f. The **prognosis** of patella fractures depends on the degree of articular damage and the ability to re-establish quadricep strength. Both are necessary for full recovery of the extensor mechanism complex. If articular damage is minimal, and good extensor mechanism strength can be restored, the prognosis of patella fractures is excellent.

B. **Patella dislocations**
   1. **Mechanism of injury.** This injury can result from a direct blow but is more commonly associated with a non-contact twisting injury involving an externally rotated tibia combined with a forceful quadriceps contraction. The patella is dislocated laterally which disrupts the medial retinaculum. Spontaneous reduction frequently occurs when the patient instinctively tries to straighten his or her leg. When the patella relocates, osteochondral fragments can occur as the medial patella facet abuts the lateral femoral condyle. These two areas, in particular, should be scrutinized for osteochondral damage (see **Fig. 24-3**).

Medial patellar dislocations are rare in knees which have not had previous surgery. It is most often associated with iatrogenic causes, in particular a lateral retinacular release (8).

2. **Physical examination.** The patient will invariably have medial retinacular tenderness, especially at the medial femoral condylar region. If an attempt is made to displace the patella laterally, the patient resists this (patella apprehension test). A straight leg raising effort should be requested. The patient should be able to lift the leg, although he or she will report pain with this maneuver. This is frequently associated with minimal extension lag (the difference between passive and active extension).

3. **Radiographs.** An axial view is necessary for a complete evaluation of patellofemoral or extensor mechanism injury. If the patient is seen prior to spontaneous reduction of the patella, axial views will reveal the dislocated patella. Once reduced, the axial view may reveal any residual tilt and/or subluxation as well as the presence of osteochondral fragmentation. Axial views taken in lower degrees of flexion (Laurin's 20-degree views or Merchant's 30-degree views) will be more likely to show minor degrees of continued subluxation (9–14).

   a. If the patella **remains dislocated**, then a reduction should be performed without delay to relieve pain. Achieve intravenous analgesia with morphine sulfate and a hypnotic before reduction is attempted. Once the patient's muscles are relaxed, the knee is placed in full extension and the patella is reduced into place by a gentle, medially directed pressure. Slight elevation of the medial border of the patella during this maneuver is ideal. On occasion the kneecap can be "trapped" by the condyle, and reduction can be difficult. After appropriate prep of the skin, grabbing the kneecap with a large towel clip and using it to gently unlever the kneecap can be a useful maneuver for difficult reductions. Due to large hematomas frequently associated with patella dislocations, and the fact that there is a large retinacular tear medially, the use of local intraarticular injections is not favored. General or regional block anesthetic is rarely required.

   b. If a large associated **hemathrosis** is present, aspiration is suggested as this can be therapeutic in relieving pain.

   c. There is no consensus in **surgical treatment** for patella dislocations. There is universal agreement that, if it is associated with radiographic osteochondral fragmentation, an arthroscopy with irrigation and debridement or fracture repair is advisable. Whether surgical repair of the injured retinacular structures is necessary and/or whether it produces superior functional outcome is unclear (12).

   d. When **acute surgical repair** is performed, it is directed at the medial retinacular structures, in particular the MPFL (12). Classically, this may also involve a lateral retinacular release and/or a medial transfer of the tibial tubercle (13), though these additional surgical procedures continue to be debated (13).

   e. If there is no evidence of a fracture or continued radiographic subluxation/tilt, **non-operative treatment** can be elected. Non-surgical treatment is directed at providing an environment where the patella does not dislocate. Typically, the patient should be treated initially with crutches and a knee sleeve, encouraging gentle motion. In the presence of a significant hemarthrosis, a compression dressing and immobilization in extension is appropriate until early motion is comfortable. The knee sleeve is used for 4 to 6 weeks while an aggressive quadriceps rehabilitation program is pursued. Typically 6 weeks of monitored activities, keeping the knee out of pivoting and twisting activities, is recommended. The most important thing to accomplish in the first 6 weeks post-injury is return of normal quadriceps strength. Return to full functional activities should be based on functional strength rather than a specific time period from the original injury (13).

4. **Complications**
    a. **Recurrent dislocation.** The main physical examination feature associated with recurrent dislocation is continued quadriceps weakness. Recurrent dislocators that have successfully accomplished strength comparable to their other side will likely need surgical reconstruction to stabilize their patella. Recurrent patella dislocations are frequently associated with recurrent effusions at the time that the patient dislocates; a history that "my knee gives out" following an initial patella dislocation may represent quad weakness and not necessarily a re-dislocation.
    b. **Degenerative joint changes** of the patellofemoral joint may occur when significant cartilage trauma is present from the initial/recurrent patella subluxations.

C. **Meniscus injuries** about the knee
   1. **Anatomic concerns.** Menisci are C-shaped structures that rest on the medial and lateral sides of the tibial plateau, whose main function is shock absorbency of the tibial–femoral knee articulation. Because their outer perimeter is thicker than their inner rim, some stability is afforded by their anatomic construct as well. This added stability is most important when cruciate ligament laxity is present.
   2. **Mechanism of injury.** Most isolated injuries of the meniscus (not associated with ligamentous injuries) occur with a rotatory stress on a weight-bearing knee. Isolated meniscal injuries occur from trapping of the meniscus between the femoral condyle and the tibia while the knee is weight bearing, typically in flexion. A history of locking or clicking is helpful, but it is frequently misleading.

      In a young patient (typically under age 30), significant trauma is necessary to injure a meniscus. However, in the older knee, a degenerative tear can occur from repetitive day-to-day activities.
   3. **Physical examination**
      a. Joint line tenderness is typically present along the medial (medial meniscus tear) or lateral (lateral meniscus tear) joint lines. This joint line pain increases with attempts at full extension or full flexion.
      b. The **McMurray test**. An audible, palpable, and often painful clunk is produced when the knee is extended from the full flexed position while the tibia is forcefully externally rotated (medial meniscus) or internally rotated (lateral meniscus). This sign is associated with a torn meniscus. Crepitus or pain along the joint line and when this maneuver is performed, even in the absence of an audible clunk, are also suggestive of a medial/lateral meniscus tear. The reliability of this test is low, though it is classically discussed in most textbooks (14).
      c. The presence of an **effusion** is frequent in a meniscus tear. Typically the normal knee has less than 15 mL of fluid and is not detectable on physical examination. Small amounts of fluid can be detected by "milking" the suprapatellar pouch, looking for a fluid wave as one tries to push the fluid from the lateral side of the knee to the medial side of the knee. This maneuver is the best way to detect small amounts of swelling.

         The presence of an effusion limits complete extension of the joint and may be a cause of a lack of full extension and/or flexion.
   4. **Radiographs**
      a. A meniscus tear is not seen on **plain x-ray**. However, in an older patient, medial or lateral joint space narrowing, best seen on standing films, may give some indication as to the likelihood of a degenerative meniscus tear.
      b. An **MRI** is frequently requested to confirm the presence of a meniscus tear. The MRI has high accuracy in diagnosing a meniscus tear (greater than 93%) (15,16).
   5. **Treatment**
      a. An **isolated meniscus tear** in the repairable zone in a young person should generally be repaired. The re-tear rate of a meniscus repair in a stable knee (not associated with a ligamentous tear) has a higher re-tear rate

than those meniscus tears associated with ligamentous instability when both meniscus and ligament injuries are surgically treated (17).
- b. A **symptomatic meniscus tear in the non-repairable zone** and/or a complex meniscus tear that persists despite conservative management should be arthroscopically debrided. However, in the older age group, consideration must be given to the fact that the symptoms may be the result of osteoarthritis and cartilage wear and not from the meniscal tear.
- c. In the **older age group**, where one suspects a degenerative meniscus tear, the meniscus tear is a reflection of generalized early arthritis of the knee joint. This "tear" should be treated symptomatically according to the patient and physician's discussion. The presence of a degenerative meniscus tear on MRI is not an indication to treat. If the symptoms associated with a degenerative meniscus tear can be quieted down with rest, relative rest, and/or medication, surgical treatment may not be necessary (18).

D. **Ligamentous injuries** of the knee
1. **Anatomic considerations.** The cruciate ligaments are intraarticular/extrasynovial structures. When the cruciate ligaments are torn they can create a hemarthrosis or bleed into the joint. The LCL and superficial MCL are extraarticular structures. The deep MCL is a thickening of the joint capsule and thus is intraarticular.
2. **Mechanism of injury**
   - a. **Ligamentous injuries** can be the result of a direct or indirect trauma. Indirect trauma frequently occurs when the body rotates around a relatively fixed foot/leg. Direct injuries are a consequence of force directed to the knee or limb. Typically, the ligament opposite the area of contact is the ligament which is the most vulnerable. For instance, a blow to the lateral side of the knee places the MCL most under stress for injury. Straight plain instabilities (anterior, posterior, medial, lateral) are most readily assessable by direct physical exam. Rotatory instability of the knee (anterior lateral and posterior lateral) requires more sophisticated physical exam skills.
   - b. In an **isolated tear of the MCL**, palpable discomfort can be detected anywhere along the ligament from its origin on the medial femoral condyle to its insertion on the tibia (approximately three finger breadths below the joint line). The deep capsular ligament is a thickening at the joint line. Medial joint line tenderness is also associated with MCL injuries. However, different from a meniscal injury, an MCL injury would create pain to stressing the knee in a valgus direction, as well as externally rotating the leg with the knee flexed. Although attached to the medial meniscus, the incidence of an in-substance medical meniscus tears in an isolated tear of the MCL is low (19).
   - c. **Isolated injuries of the LCL** are rare. Frequently accompanying complete tears of the LCL are tears of the posterolateral complex with or without cruciate involvement. If one suspects a lateral/posterior lateral injury, physical examination must include close inspection of peroneal nerve function distally in the leg and foot region. Complete (grade 3) injuries to the posterolateral region of the knee do not heal, and superior results are present if the injury is addressed in the acute phase (with repair of structures) rather than the chronic phase of this injury. Any increase in external rotation of the tibia with the femur fixed that is increased over the patient's opposite uninjured knee should be suspect for a posterolateral knee injury. This needs to be evaluated within days of the injury by a surgeon competent in treatment of multi-ligamentous injuries of the knee.
   - d. **Isolated tears of the PCL** are frequently associated with a hyperextension injury (indirect injury) or a blunt contusion to the front of the tibia (direct injury).
   - e. **Isolated ACL injuries** can be sustained through a number of mechanisms, most commonly a non-contact deceleration injury or landing from a jump. The potential causal mechanisms in non-contact ACL injuries have been

the subject of intense research in the last decade (20). Recent interventional studies suggest that neuromuscular training in improving bent knee landing and pivoting can be helpful in injury reduction (21).
3. **Physical examination.** The amount of joint line opening or motion between the tibia and femur that occurs with manual testing is graded according to American Medical Association (AMA) guidelines (4): grade 1 injuries would be less than 5 mm of joint line opening; grade 2 are 5 to 10 mm; and grade 3 injuries (complete tear) are more than 10 mm of opening (13).
   a. The main **clinical motion test** for providing an analysis of the severity of MCL complex injuries is a valgus stress test with the knee flexed at 30 degrees. The leg is put over the side of the examining table, the fingers are placed on the medial joint line to assess the amount of joint line opening and rotation, and a valgus stress is applied to the knee. The reverse of this, placing a varus stress on the knee, is the main clinical motion test to analyze LCL instability.
   b. Typically injuries to the LCL also involve injury to the **posterolateral complex**. Motion tests to determine the amount of injury to the posterior lateral complex of the knee are the most complex of all knee exams. It is beyond the scope of this text (22).
   c. The main clinical motion test for an analysis of ACL injuries is the **Lachman's test** (23) (**Fig. 24-4**). This is performed with the knee in approximately 20 degrees of flexion, with the leg in neutral rotation. The examiner holds firmly the distal femur in one hand and the proximal tibia in the other hand, then one places an anterior-directed force on the proximal tibia. Grading of displacement of the tibia on the femur is along the AMA guidelines. In addition to the Lachman's exam, ACL injuries are associated with anterior lateral rotatory tibial subluxation that is best evaluated through the pivot shift maneuver or Losee maneuver (24). The anterior drawer test (done at 90 degrees of knee flexion), though historically cited, is not as reliable as the manual test for laxity of the ACL (14).
   d. The main clinical motion test to detect injuries of the PCL is the **posterior drawer test.** This is performed by placing the knee at 70 to 90 degrees of flexion. A posterior force is applied to the tibia and the extent of translation and the quality of the endpoint is recorded. Again, AMA guidelines are used to assess the degree of translation. The key to this test is accurately assessing the starting point of the tibia (25).

   Another useful test in assessing PCL laxity in an awake patient is the "quads active" test: With the knee at 70 to 90 degrees of flexion, the patient is asked to activate his or her quads with the examiner holding the tibia in the position in which the tibia comes to rest. Posterior motion from this starting point is then assessed.
   e. An acute knee examination should include **all major ligamentous structures** within the knee. Significant anterior-posterior translation (>10 mm) with the drawer or Lachman's test may suggest an injury to both the ACL and the PCL. Varus and valgus stress testing should be performed both at 0 and 30 degrees of knee flexion. Asymmetry in varus or valgus laxity that exists at 0 degrees of knee extension suggests a posterior cruciate/posterior capsular injury as well as collateral ligament injury. Varus or valgus asymmetry laxity existing at 30 degrees of flexion but not at 0 degrees is indicative of at least an injury to a collateral ligament.
4. **Treatment**
   a. **Isolated tears** of ligamentous injuries
      i. **MCL.** Isolated tears of the MCL can be treated conservatively (19,26). For complete tears, progressive weight bearing on crutches, in a brace limiting valgus stress for 4 to 6 weeks is recommended. In the absence of a complete tear of the MCL, one can bear weight as pain and motion permits. Complete recovery after isolated MCL injuries is the norm, though distal MCL tears typically have more disability and take longer to heal (26).

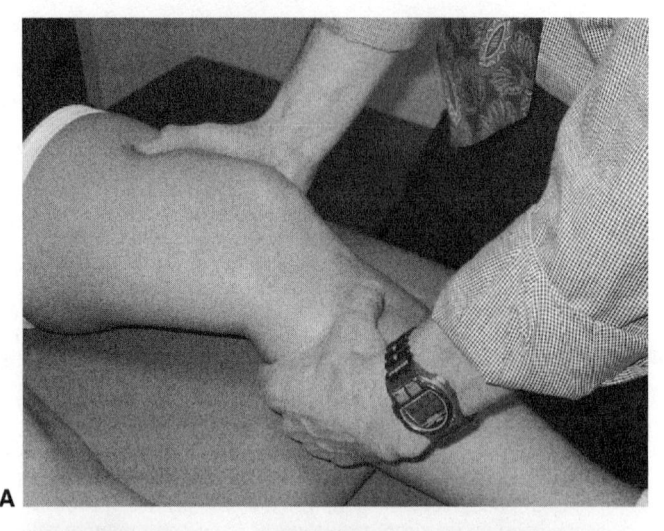

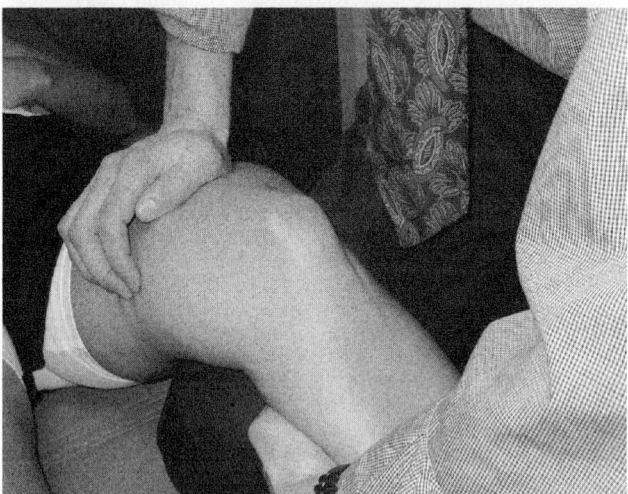

Figure 24-4. Lachman's exam of the knee: This is a test for deciding the degree of anterior translation of the tibia under the femur. The knee is held firmly in place at 20 to 30 degrees of flexion by the examiner's hand **(A)** or by resting the patient's leg over the examiner's knee **(B)**. With a firm hold of the proximal tibia, the examiner places an upward or anteriorly directed force on the tibia, judging both the distance of translation and the firmness of the endpoint.

    ii. **Isolated tears of the PCL** are frequently treated non-operatively. In the rehabilitation process, special emphasis on quad strength is important to maintain a muscular support to limit posterior displacement of the tibia.

    iii. **Isolated tears of the ACL** are prone to subluxation events when jumping and pivoting activities are performed. In young active patients, or middle-aged patients that have a high demand job or recreational aspirations, ACL reconstruction is typically advised. The goal of ACL reconstruction is to prevent future subluxation events which can be associated with meniscus and/or cartilage damage.

iv. **Multi-ligamentous knee injuries** most commonly involve the ACL/MCL or PCL with posterolateral injuries. An operative treatment yields the best functional results in two complete ligament knee injuries.
E. **Knee dislocations**
  1. **Evaluation and treatment.** This relatively rare dislocation requires immediate reduction and evaluation for joint stability. Reduction under anesthesia is sometimes necessary (27,28). Immediate and continuous evaluation of vascular status of the leg reduction is important. If there is any question of the vascular supply, most specifically if pulses are diminished or absent in the affected limb, an arteriography must be performed immediately. Prophylactic fasciotomy should be considered to prevent a compartment syndrome following vascular repair, particularly if there is greater than 6 hours from injury to vascular repair. If a vascular repair is present combined with severe knee instability, an external fixator may be applied to protect the vascular construct until definitive surgical treatment of the torn ligaments ensues.
  2. **Early reconstruction** of torn ligaments offers the best outcomes (28). If the injury is associated with a vascular repair and/or significant disruption to the skin, a subacute reconstruction is indicated (0–3 weeks). Late surgical approach (more than 4 weeks) is more difficult secondary to soft tissue scarring, particularly if it involves a posterolateral corner, where individual structures can become more difficult to dissect. In dislocated knees that are approached late (more than 6 weeks), reconstructive efforts aimed at collateral ligament injuries are frequently necessary (in deference to a primary repair if done early). The cruciate ligament injuries are frequently reconstructed in acute and late surgeries in deference to a repair. Because of the typically severe nature of these injuries, allograft tissue in deference to autograft tissue from the same or contralateral knee is the norm.

     If the original injury has adequate joint surfaces and a competent vascular system, functional use of the leg will parallel the ability to get back satisfactory strength and motion. Acceptable function for day-to-day activities is common following these injuries. The ability to perform high-level activities following knee dislocations is rare.
F. **Extensor mechanism disruptions**
  1. **Anatomic considerations.** The extensor mechanism consists of the quadriceps muscle complex, quadriceps tendon, patella, patella tendon, and patella tendon insertion into the tibial tubercle. Disruption of the extensor mechanism along any one of its parts can result in failure of the patient to perform a straight leg raising effort. A partial tear frequently results in the patient's ability to lift his or her leg, but with a considerable lag (difference between passive and active extension of the leg).
  2. **Clinical considerations.** A quadricep tendon disruption is difficult to assess on physical examination unless one requests a straight leg raising effort by the patient. Quadricep tendon ruptures are a frequently missed cause of acute knee injuries.

     Patella tendon disruptions are often associated with an indirect trauma consisting of a forceful quadriceps contraction against a relatively fixed lower limb. These can be subtle injuries.

     If the rupture is below the inferior border of the patella (i.e., in the patella tendon or at the tibial tubercle), patella alta would be present, best seen on lateral knee x-rays.

     Extensor mechanism disruptions commonly occur in patients with systemic illness such as diabetes or renal failure, or with use of exogenous steroids (prednisone or anabolic steroids). Cortical steroid injections for treatment of patella tendinosis has been associated with an increased incidence of rupture.
  3. **Treatment.** The goal of treatment is to restore a functioning extensor mechanism to the knee. This is best accomplished surgically.

IV. SPECIAL CONCERNS IN THE GROWING ADOLESCENT

A. Physeal injuries. One cause of an acute knee injury in a growing adolescent is an injury to the physis.

1. A **distal femur physeal injury**, particularly if it is a non-displaced injury, can be confused with a collateral ligament injury. Pain is present, not only at the origin of the collateral ligaments, but across the anterior aspect of the femur or tibia, which is readily palpable in most children. X-rays can show some widening and, at times, displacement of the physis. Stress x-rays can confirm the diagnosis and assess the stability of the fracture construct. Surgical reduction and stabilization for any displaced physeal fracture is imperative. Stable injuries can be treated non-operatively (29).

2. The **tibial apophysis** can avulse in the adolescent with closing growth plates. The tibial growth plate fuses from posterior to anterior, and an avulsion of the tibial tubercle frequently involves an interarticular fracture into the joint. By history this injury is associated with a strong quadriceps contraction; radiographically this injury is associated with patella alta. Surgical reduction and fixation is advisable for the best outcome when the tubercle is displaced.

B. Ligament avulsion. Cruciate ligament avulsions, particularly the attachments of the ACL and PCL onto the tibia, occur in the growing adolescent. When these are associated with a large bony fragment, surgical reduction and fixation is advised. The rehab will follow the course of a bone healing rather than of a ligament reconstruction/revascularization.

C. Osteochondritis dissecans

1. **Definition.** Osteochondritis dissecans (OCD) is defined as an area of avascular bone commonly presenting in the medial femoral condyle of a skeletally immature child. The etiology of this area of avascularity is unknown. Most commonly accepted theories are trauma, abnormal ossification within the epiphysis, ischemia, or some combination of the above. Approximately 40% of patients with OCD have a history of prior knee trauma to a mild or moderate degree (21). The medial condyle is involved 85% of the time versus 15% of the lateral condyle. Fifty percent of loose bodies in the knee are associated with OCD.

2. **Natural history.** The majority of juvenile lesions (presenting before closure of growth plates) heal spontaneously. In the skeletally mature, there is a higher incidence of bone fragmentation (subchondral fracture). This bone collapse is in the area of the avascular bone and is felt to be because of faulty lead transmission of bone just below the cartilage. In its extreme form, the osteocartilaginous lesion can break away from the healthy bone forming a loose body. Once there is a fracture of bone in the area of avascularity, symptoms increase and the involved fragment may become disengaged.

3. **Treatment**

   a. **Juvenile osteochondral** lesions can generally be treated nonsurgically with rest or reduction from high impact activities and repetitive deep knee bending. The goal is to have the knee become pain free. The presence of an effusion is indicative of possible disruption of the articular surface, signifying the need for surgical evaluation. The patient and their family should be informed to return to the doctor if recurrent effusions are present. Following these patients in regular intervals (6–12 months) until resolution of the lesion on x-ray is advised.

   b. Surgical treatment for **adult OCD** (OCD after growth plate closure) is typically recommended. The type of surgical treatment depends on the size and location of the OCD site and the quality of the overlying cartilage. Options include drilling, debridement, fixation, replacement, or excision. The discussion of this is beyond the scope of this review (6).

V. OVERUSE SYNDROMES

A. Definition. Repetitive submaximal or subclinical trauma that results in macro- and/or microscopic damage to a tissue's structural unit can result in pain and/or dysfunction. Although clinicians refer to it as an "itis," an inflammatory response is not seen histologically. It is thought that damage to a tissue's structural unit and/or blood supply is a frequent cause of overuse injuries.

The most common form of overuse injury is from an endogenous source, that being mechanical circumstances in which the musculoskeletal tissue is subjected to greater tensile force or stress than the tissue can effectively absorb.

B. History. Overuse injuries are characterized by the absence of an acute injury, or at least no injury significant enough to explain the current clinical situation. The most important feature to look for in the patient's history is a "change" in functional demand. A transitional athlete/worker, defined as a person with a change in his or her internal or external environment, is at high risk for development of overuse injuries. These include:
  1. Change in intensity of repetitive activity (distance/time)
  2. Change in frequency or duration of repetitive activity
  3. Changes in equipment (footwear/surface changes including material composition and/or slope)
  4. Changes in competitive climate/work climate/activity level
  5. Changes in weather
  6. Changes in lifestyle (puberty, aging, significant weight gain, and, for women, pregnancy and menopause)

C. Physical examination
  1. Inspection
     a. **Alignment** of the limb is a must in evaluating any overuse injury of the lower extremity. This includes tilt of the pelvis, rotation of the femur, varus or valgus alignment of the knee, and pronation or supination at the foot. Any change in "normal alignment" can cause tissue overload anywhere along the kinetic chain. Some limb alignment features are constitutional and cannot be changed short of surgery; others can be modified. The two most common forms of modification are:
        i. An **orthotic** may change the position of a flexible foot and thus can affect the entire kinematic chain. Particularly, a flexible pronated foot can be restored to normal alignment with the use of an orthotic.
        ii. An anteriorly tilted pelvis is associated with **increased internal femoral rotation** and functional **knee valgus**. This can frequently be altered by appropriate hip abductor and extensor strengthening exercises (30).
     b. **Redness or warmth** is not common in overuse injuries but may indicate the presence of an injured bursa or tendon.
     c. **Joint effusion** is not common in overuse injuries. It indicates an intraarticular source of pathology.

D. Investigational tests
  1. **Strength tests.** These can include:
     a. **Weakness** compared to the contralateral limb
     b. **Concentric** (muscle shortens while contracting) muscle strength versus eccentric (muscle lengthens while contracting) muscle strength in same muscle group (see **H.1.b**).
     c. **Agonist** (joint motion in one plane due to muscle contraction) versus antagonist (the muscle group opposing or resisting joint motion caused by agonist muscle) strength in same limb (i.e., quad to hamstring strength)
     d. **Absolute strength** and **peak torque** to body weight ratio compared to population norms
     e. **Endurance strength** with a measure of muscle fatigability
  2. Evaluation of **flexibility**, especially in key muscle groups, including quadriceps, hamstring, hip flexors, and Achilles tendon

E. Radiographs
  1. **Plain radiographs** are infrequently necessary for evaluation of overuse injuries. Radiographic views of the patellofemoral joint, in particular axial views, may be helpful to assess patella position. Standing knee views show arthritic changes including bone spurs and joint space narrowing.

2. **MRI.** The main advantage of an MRI is its ability to view intra- versus extraarticular pathology. Routine use of an MRI to diagnose overuse injuries is not advantageous, although significant tendinosis and bursal edema can be visualized by MRI.
F. **Blood work**
   1. When there is a knee effusion that arises spontaneously or is associated with other complaints (e.g., rash or fatigue), then it is important to consider systemic diseases. Evaluate for **systemic disease**, including collagen vascular disease and Lyme's disease (see **II.D.1**).
G. **Treatment**
   1. **Reduce tissue irritation and pain with:**
      a. **Analgesic non-narcotic medications [nonsteroidal anti-inflammatory drugs (NSAIDs), acetaminophen]**
      b. **Physical therapy** modalities (ultrasound, e-stim, massage)
      c. **Rest or relative rest** of the injured part (reduce activities, substitute activities, and protect the injured part)
      d. **Ice**
      e. **Elevation** and **compression** if swelling is present
   2. **Correct anatomical problems** when possible (patella sleeves, orthotics, braces, rarely surgery).
   3. **Correct biomechanical errors** when possible (training sequence, sport style and form, strengthening and stretching of musculoskeletal units, evaluation of workplace station).
   4. **Correct environmental concerns** when possible (new shoes, change to a more absorbent surface, adequate clothing).
H. **Sports-specific rehabilitation**
   1. **Recovery** of strength
      a. **Closed chain exercises** of the lower extremity are those exercises where the foot is supported or planted during the exercise thus "closing the loop." Leg press or stand-up exercises such as partial squats are examples of closed chain lower leg exercises. For **lower extremity activities**, closed chained techniques are more functional and can obtain comparable gains in quadriceps strength with less overuse of the patellofemoral joint (30).
      b. **Concentric/eccentric** muscle strength. **Concentric** muscle contractions occur when a muscle shortens as it contracts. In an eccentric contraction, the muscle lengthens as contraction occurs.

         Eccentric strengthening has long been favored for recovery of strength in the treatment of tendinosis. For the patellofemoral joint, eccentric muscle activity is an important part of functional use of the joint. Eccentric strength is the main decelerator of the body, an important function of the quadriceps complex.
I. **The physician.** The physician's role in diagnosing overuse injuries is to render an injury with its appropriate treatment as well as educating the patient. Patient education is the best treatment for the prevention of overuse injuries in the future.
J. **The patient.** The patient's role is to understand the causative factors in the injury and to understand the progression from injury to wellness. This includes activity modifications and their role in modifying their activities. The patient needs to implement a paced return to full activities.

VI. **OVERUSE INJURIES ABOUT THE KNEE**
A. **Patella tendonosis**
   1. Patella tendonosis is a common overuse injury that more typically affects the proximal attachment of the patella ligament to the inferior pole of the patella, but can also affect the distal end of the tendon. It is also called a jumper's knee because it occurs most frequently in athletes who require repetitive eccentric quadricep contractions, as is common in jumping athletes, and athletes who frequent heavy weight training.
   2. The case of **patella tendonosis** is generally considered to be chronic stress overload resulting in microscopic tears of the tendon with incomplete healing.

3. **Treatment** is conservative and is the cornerstone of treatment for tendonosis. In addition to the general scheme of treatment of overuse syndromes outlined previously, the primary treatment emphasizes maximizing quad strength and knee joint flexibility, reducing repetitive eccentric quadriceps contraction exercises, and re-adding them in a paced fashion. Infrequently, surgery is necessary for the patient with recalcitrant disease. An MRI or ultrasound can be used to define the area of the tendon affected by chronic tearing and subsequent degeneration. Excising this area of the tendon can be useful (31). Alternative schools of thought feel that the distal pole of the patella impinges on the patella tendon, and excision of the distal pole can be useful in treating this form of tendonosis (32).

B. **Iliotibial band syndrome**
   1. **Iliotibial band (ITB) syndrome (also known as ITB tendonosis)** is caused by excessive friction between the iliotibial band and the distal lateral femoral condyle. The ITB functions as a weak extender of the knee in near full extension, and a more powerful knee flexor after 30 degrees of knee flexion. The ITB is most stretched over the lateral femoral condyle at 30 degrees of knee flexion. This condition is common in runners and cyclists.
   2. **Anatomic factors** have been implicated in ITB syndrome and include excessive foot pronation, genu varum at the knee, tight lateral patella retinacular structures, and an anterior tipped pelvis. Treatment is directed at modification of the initiating causative factors and reducing the excessive friction. Stretching of the ITB, treating foot pronation with an orthotic, treating a tight lateral patella retinaculum with manual therapy, and repositioning of an anterior tilted pelvis all can be useful interventions when the patient has these physical examination features.

C. **Tibial tubercle apophysis (Osgood-Schlatter disease)**
   1. **Clinical diagnosis.** This syndrome is usually seen in the rapidly growing athletic adolescent with open growth plates at the knee. It is characterized by point tenderness and enlargement of the tibial tubercle at the site of the patella tendon insertion. A constant traction to this location produces overgrowth of the tibial tubercle apophysis. X-ray evaluation can be negative, or at times a prominent or irregular apophysis is seen. Once the apophysis has closed, there frequently can be a free bony particle anterior and superior to the tibial tubercle.
   2. **Treatment.** The symptoms usually abate when the tibial tubercle fuses to the diaphysis, and, therefore, every effort should be made to quiet this injury down until full maturation is present in the developing adolescent. Treatment depends on the severity of the disease. Nearly all cases are managed by the proper balancing of activities against the patient's symptoms. This can follow the general treatment pattern of overuse injuries as previously outlined. Surgical treatment is not indicated. Aggressive treatment might occasionally involve limited use of a knee immobilizer in recalcitrant cases where the patient is dysfunctional in day-to-day activities, or non-compliant in activity reduction.

D. **Patellofemoral pain syndrome**
   1. **Definition.** Patellofemoral pain syndrome is used to describe a constellation of symptoms that are related to the patellofemoral joint. Typically, this type of pain is considered an overuse syndrome, although the exact etiology and nature of pain continues to be poorly understood. Patellofemoral pain syndrome is that pain which originates in the anterior knee structures, in the absence of an identifiable acute injury (blunt trauma, dislocating or subluxing patella).

   Chondromalacia patella (CMP) is a term often used to describe anterior knee pain, though use of this term to describe clinical symptoms is not appropriate. CMP should be used only to describe the pathological entity of cartilage softening on the underneath side of the kneecap. Typically this could only be diagnosed by surgical observation or MRI. The presence of cartilage softening does not always result in the clinical symptom of pain.
   2. **Pre-existing conditions.** Anatomic factors that can predispose a patient to patellofemoral pain can include flexibility deficits of the limb, malalignment

of the lower limbs including excessive femoral anteversion, high Q-angle, rotation variations of the tibia, genu velgum at the knee, hind foot valgus, and pes planus. **Kneecap malalignment**, both static and functional, has been implicated in the etiology of patellofemoral pain. However, there are a few population-based studies to support the "malalignment theory kneecap pain." Any one abnormality may be trivial as a single entity. However, in combination with other anatomic variables and associated with overtraining and overuse, they frequently can lead to overuse injury (14).

The role of **malalignment** and the etiology of patellofemoral pain continue to be debated. Radiographic imaging studies can reveal a patella that is malaligned within the trochlear groove, as evidenced by a patella tilt and/or subluxation. Some malalignment syndromes of the patella are residual from a previous subluxing or dislocating event. However, other malalignment syndromes can be present in the absence of an acute event, and frequently are similar in both knees of the same person. It is felt that patella malalignment, when constitutional in a person, can become an overuse syndrome more readily and become a painful problem.

3. **Clinical presentation.** The most common clinical presentation of a patellofemoral pain syndrome patient is pain on the anterior aspect of the knee that is aggravated by prolonged sitting and stair climbing. Because the retinacular structures of the patella extend both medially and laterally from the patella, pain can also be associated with either medial- or lateral-sided knee pain, therefore, it can create a very confusing clinical presentation. It is infrequently associated with swelling. Giving-way episodes can be reported; typically the giving-way episode is with straight-ahead activities or stair-climbing, when one tries to engage the quad and the quad "fatigues." This should not be confused with giving-way episodes associated with ligamentous instability, which typically occur with planting, pivoting, or jumping activities. Patients can also present with catching or clicking phenomena. This can occur because of irritation of the knee-cap as it tracks in the trochlear groove. Another common patient complaint is that the knee "locks." If the knee "locks" in full extension, this is a manifestation of patellofemoral pain. The patient does not want to engage the knee cap in the groove because of pain, and, therefore, keeps his or her leg straight. If the knee is locked secondary to a loose body or torn meniscus, it is always locked in some degree of flexion.

4. **Treatment.** Historically, non-surgical treatment has been the cornerstone for most patellofemoral pain disorders. The primary goal of patellofemoral rehabilitation is to reduce the symptoms of pain. This is done by a combination of physical therapy modalities, improving quadriceps strength, and endurance (see **V. H**). Other tools such as orthotics, knee sleeves, and McConnell taping can be used (33). Pelvic muscle strength, especially hip abductor and hip extensor strength, is essential for rotational control of the limb (23,30,34).

E. **Pes anserinus bursitis**
1. **Definition.** The "pes" tendons are terminal insertions of three long thigh muscles, one from each muscle group. These tendons come together to insert on the anteromedial aspect of the proximal tibia, between the tibial tubercle and the distal (tibial) attachment of the medial (tibial) collateral ligament. The three tendons are sartorius (femoral innervation), gracilius (obturator innervation), and semitendonosis (sciatic innervation). They are powerful internal rotators of the leg (tibia) and also aide in knee flexion.
2. **Clinical presentation.** The patient will present with soreness just below the medial knee, which can be reproduced by direct palpation or resisted internal rotation of the leg. In middle age, it can represent a referred pain pattern from the knee due to medial knee arthritis.
3. **Treatment.** In addition to the rest, ice, compression, and elevation (RICE) principle and physical therapy with modalities of stretching and strengthening, a steroid injection at the bursa site can be helpful.

References

1. Arendt EA. Assessment of the athlete with an acutely injured knee. In: Griffin LU, ed. *Rehabiliation of the injured knee.* St. Louis, MO: Mosby, 1990:20–33.
2. DeHaven K. Diagnosis of acute knee injuries with hemarthrosis. *Am J Sports Med* 1980;8:9.
3. Carson WG, James SL, Larson RL, et al. Patellofemoral disorders—physical and radiographic examination. Part II, radiographic examination. *Clin Orthop* 1984;185:178–186.
4. Polly DW, Callaghan JJ, Sikes RA, et al. The accuracy of selective magnetic resonance imaging compared with the findings of arthroscopy of the knee. *J Bone Joint Surg (Am)* 1988;70:192–198.
5. Muller ME, Allgöwer M, Schneider R, Willenegger H, et al. *Manual of internal fixation*, 3rd ed. Berlin: Springer-Verlag, 1991:23–52.
6. Mandelbaum BR, Seipel PR, Teurlings L. Articular cartilage lesions: current concepts and results. In: Arendt E, ed. *Orthopaedic knowledge update.* Rosemont, IL: American Academy of Orthopaedic Surgeons, 1999:19–28.
7. Minas T, Nehrer S. Current concepts in the treatment of articular cartilage defects. *Orthopaedics* 1997;20:525–538.
8. Hughston JC, Deese M. Medial subluxation of the patella as a complication of lateral retinacular release. *Am J Sports Med* 1988;16:383–388.
9. Laurin CA, Levesque HP, Dussault R, et al. The abnormal lateral patellofemoral angle. *J Bone Joint Surg (Am)* 1978;60:55–60.
10. Laurin CA, Dussault R, Levesque HP. The tangential x-ray investigation of the patellofemoral joint: x-ray technique, diagnostic criteria and their interpretation. *Clin Orthop* 1979;144:16–26.
11. Merchant AC, Mercer RL, Jacobsen RH, et al. Roentgenographic analysis of patellofemoral congruence. *J Bone Joint Surg (Am)* 1974;56:1391–1396.
12. Fithian DC, Meier SW. The case for advancement and repair of the medial patellofemoral ligament in patients with recurrent patellar instability. *Oper Tech Sports Med* 1999;7:81–89.
13. Arendt EA, Fithian DC, Cohen E. Current concepts of lateral patella dislocation. *Clin Sports Med* 2002;21:499–519.
14. Solomon DH, Simel DL, Bates DW, et al. The rational clinical examination. Does this patient have a torn meniscus or ligament of the knee? Value of the physical examination. *JAMA* 2001;286:1610–1620.
15. Cheung LP, Li KC, Hollett MD, et al. Meniscal tears of the knee: accuracy of detection with fast spin-echo MR imaging and arthroscopic correlation in 293 patients. *Radiology* 1997;203:508–512.
16. Rappeport ED, Wieslander SB, Stephensen S, et al. MRI preferable to diagnostic arthroscopy in knee joint injuries. A double-blind comparison of 47 patients. *Acta Orthop Scand* 1997;68:277–281.
17. Cannon WDJ, Vittori JM. The incidence of healing in arthroscopic meniscal repairs in anterior cruciate ligament-reconstructed knees versus stable knees. *Am J Sports Med* 1992;20:176–181.
18. Bhattacharyya T, Gale D, Dewire P, et al. The clinical importance of meniscal tears demonstrated in magnetic resonance imaging in osteoarthritis of the knee. *J Bone Joint Surg (Am)* 2003;85:4–9.
19. Indelicato PA. Non-operative treatment of complete tears of the medial collateral ligament of the knee. *J Bone Joint Surg (Am)* 1983;65:323–329.
20. Arendt EA, Dick R. Knee injury patterns among men and women in collegiate basketball and soccer: NCAA data and review of literature. *Am J Sports Med* 1995;23(6):694–701.
21. Griffin LY, Agel J, Albohm MJ, et al. Noncontact anterior cruciate ligament injuries: risk factors and prevention strategies. *J Am Acad Orthop Surg* 2000;8(3):141–150.
22. LaPrade RF. The medial collateral ligament complex and the posterolateral aspect of the knee. In: Arendt EA, ed. *Orthopaedic knowledge update.* Rosemont, IL: American Academy of Orthopaedic Surgeons, 1999:327–340.

23. Timm K. Randomized controlled trial of Protonics on patellar pain, position, and function. *Med Sci Sports Exerc* 1998;30:65–70.
24. Losee RR, Johnson TR, Southwick WO. Anterior subluxation of the lateral tibial plateau. *J Bone Joint Surg (Am)* 1978;60:1015–1030.
25. Miller MD, Harner CD, Koshiwaguchi S. Acute posterior cruciate ligament injuries. In: Fu FH, Harner CD, Vince KG, eds. *Knee surgery*. Philadelphia, PA: Williams & Wilkins, 1994:749–767.
26. LaPrade RF, Terry GC. Injuries to the posterolateral aspect of the knee: association of anatomic injury patterns with clinical instability. *Am J Sports Med* 1997;25:433–437.
27. Moore TM. Fracture-dislocaton of the knee. *Clin Orthop* 1981;156:128–140.
28. Sisto DJ, Warren RF. Complex knee dislocations. A follow-up study of operative treatment. *Clin Orthop* 1985;198:94–101.
29. Canale ST. Physeal injuries. In: Green NE, Swiontkowski MF, eds. *Skeletal trauma in children*. Philadelphia, PA: WB Saunders Co, 1998:17–58.
30. Powers C. Rehabilitation of patellofemoral joint disorders: a critical review. *Am J Sports Med* 1998;28:345–354.
31. Popp JE, Yu JS, Kaeding CC. Recalcitrant patellar tendinitis: magnetic resonance imaging, histologic evaluation, and surgical treatment. *Am J Sports Med* 1997;25:218–222.
32. Johnson DP, Wakele CJ, Watt I. Magnetic resonance imaging of patellar tendonitis. *J Bone Joint Surg (Br)* 1996;78:452–457.
33. McConnell J. The management of chrondromalacia patellae: a long-term solution. *Aust J Physiother* 1986;32:215–223.
34. McConnell E. The physical therapist's approach to patellofemoral disorders. *Clin Sports Med* 2002;21(3):363–388.
35. Association AM. *Standard nomenclature of athletic injuries*. Chicago, IL: American Medical Assocation, 1966.

Selected Historical Readings

Green NE, Allen BL. Vascular injuries associated with dislocation of the knee. *J Bone Joint Surg (Am)* 1977;59:236–239.

Torg JS, Conrad W, Kalen V. Clinical diagnosis of anterior cruciate ligament instability in the athlete. *Am J Sports Med* 1976;4:84–93.

Wilkinson J. Fracture of the patella treated by total excision. *J Bone Joint Surg (Br)* 1977;59:352–354.

FRACTURES OF THE TIBIA   25

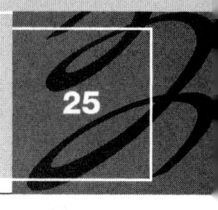

I. **FRACTURES OF THE TIBIAL PLATEAU** (1–4)
   A. For practical purposes, fractures of the tibial plateau are classified as follows:
      1. **Undisplaced** (a vertical fracture of the plateau)
      2. **Split** (a split fracture with displacement, with or without slight comminution)
      3. **Depressed** (centrally depressed fracture)
      4. **Split and depressed** with an intact tibial rim
      5. **Any of 1 through 4 with metaphyseal or even diaphyseal extension.** The elements of these descriptions are contained within **Schatzker's system** (**Fig. 25-1**).
   B. **Examination** is different from that for other knee injuries. It is wise to carry out a definitive examination only after roentgenographs have been obtained. Differential diagnosis includes a major ligamentous injury or knee dislocation (5–7). The examination should include inspection for wounds, evaluation of the distal circulation (pulses and capillary refill), and neurologic (motor or sensory) function. Motion and stability should not routinely be assessed in these injuries; however, this type of injury can be associated with ligamentous or meniscal damage (1).
   C. **Radiographs.** Oblique films in addition to the routine anteroposterior and lateral radiographs are often helpful in identifying fracture lines and articular displacement. Computed tomography demonstrates minor fractures and accurately depicts the degree of depression of the tibial plateau; axial cuts with sagittal reconstruction are the routine.
   D. Magnetic resonance imaging (MRI) can be helpful when there is clinical concern for associated ligamentous injury.
      1. **Undisplaced fractures.** In some settings, especially when multiple injuries are involved, fixation with two percutaneous cannulated cancellous lag screws is advisable to ensure maintenance of reduction. For isolated injuries, generally nonoperative management is selected. A splint is applied, and the leg is elevated for the first 24 to 48 hours. Knee aspiration is carried out if a significant hemarthrosis is present, and knee motion may be started with continuous passive motion (CPM) if available. As soon as the patient is comfortable and the range of motion is increasing, he or she can be followed up as an outpatient. Follow-up radiographs should be obtained shortly after motion is instituted to ensure that the fracture remains nondisplaced. Touch-down weight bearing should be maintained for 8 weeks to prevent displacement from shear forces.
      2. **Displaced fractures**
         a. **Split fracture.** Open reduction and fixation is generally done if there is a significant widening (lateral or medial displacement of more than 3–5 mm) of the plateau (8,9). The internal fixation must be rigid enough to allow movement of the joint as soon as there is soft-tissue healing. In this situation, the authors prefer to use the Association of the Study of Internal Fixation (ASIF) buttress plate (**Fig. 25-2**) or a dynamic compression or locking plate when the patient is osteoporotic (4). Recently, there has been a move toward use of smaller implants for all tibial plateau fixation. Specialized 3.5-mm T- and L-buttress plates allow the placement of more screws under the articular surface. If the patient is young and has dense bone, then multiple percutaneous cannulated lag screws can be inserted

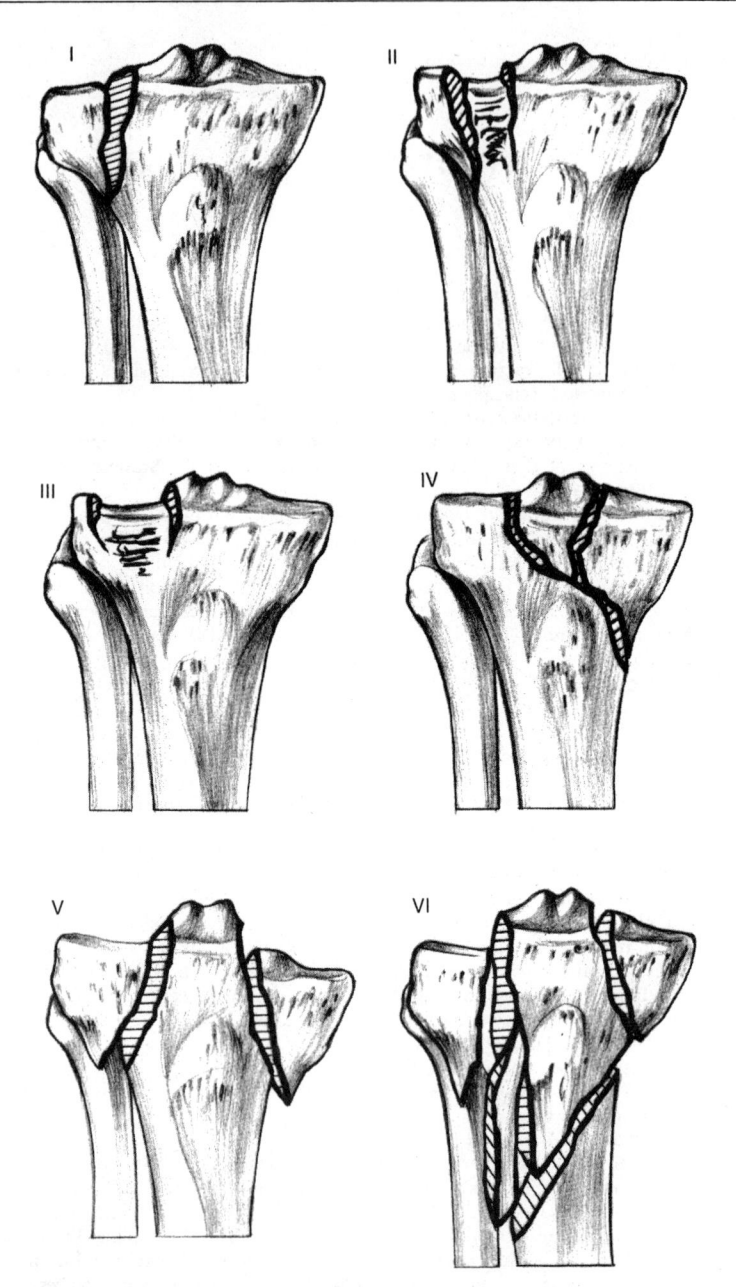

Figure 25-1. Schatzker's classification system. I, split; II, split with depression; III, depression; IV, medial condyle; V, bicondylar; VI, bicondylar with shaft extension. (From Hansen ST, Swiontkowski MF. *Orthopaedic trauma protocols.* New York: Raven, 1993:315.)

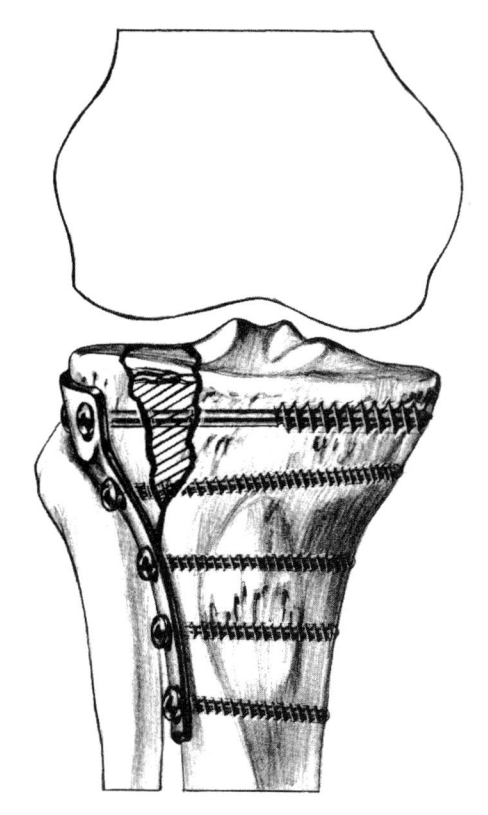

Figure 25-2. Internal fixation of a split depression fracture of the tibial plateau using L-buttress plate fixation with bone grafting of the elevated segment. (From Hansen ST, Swiontkowski MF. *Orthopaedic trauma protocols.* New York: Raven, 1993: 318.)

under fluoroscopic and/or arthroscopic control. Percutaneous placement of a large reduction clamp is often successful in providing reduction of the fracture. If open reduction and internal fixation are not feasible, then treatment should be as for comminuted fractures.

b. **Central depression of the plateau.** If depression is greater than 3 to 5 mm, especially with valgus stress instability of the knee greater than 10 degrees in full extension, then most authors currently recommend elevation with bone grafting and fixation (2,3,9,10). More recently, articular reductions have been done with arthroscopic visualization with percutaneous technique for elevation of the segment. Autogenous bone graft remains the treatment of choice, but allograft and cancellous substitutes such as corallin hydroxyapatite and calcium-phosphate cements have been successfully used (9). Generally, percutaneous lag screws are adequate for support of the elevated joint surface and bone graft or graft substitute material.

c. **Split-depressed fractures** with a displacement/depression of more than 3 to 4 mm are treated with reduction, fixation, and early motion in most young patients. Generally, this reduction is done with an open technique with an anterior or anterolateral approach, elevation, and bone grafting using buttress or locking buttress plates for older patients (**Fig. 25-2**) and lag screws or 3.5-mm small fragment T- or L-plates or one-third tubular plates (as washers) in younger patients. These fractures may be managed with arthroscopic reduction in skilled hands. Secure fixation is critical so that early motion with or without CPM can be initiated. Patients are generally limited to touch-down weight bearing for 12 weeks to prevent late fracture settling. If the patient's limb is stable to varus and valgus stress in an examination under anesthesia shortly after injury, then traction treatment with a tibial pin and early motion is an option (10,11). The patient is placed in a cast-brace (as described in **Chap. 7, III.H**) or a hinged knee brace after 3 to 4 weeks (1). This treatment is not currently recommended on a routine basis. If the instability exceeds 10 degrees, then reduction and fixation as described earlier is indicated (11).

d. **Fractures with metaphyseal/diaphyseal extension** are treated similarly to split-depressed fractures if the joint extension is significant. Generally, buttress plate fixation and bone grafting are required. When the injury is bicondylar, stripping the soft tissues off both condyles from an anterior approach should be avoided; this results in a high incidence of nonunion and deep infection. Instead, the most unstable condyle (usually lateral) is selected for the buttress fixation via an anterolateral approach and the other condyle is stabilized by percutaneous screw fixation, fixation with a posterior medial incision and small buttress plate, or neutralization with an external fixator for 4 to 6 weeks while motion is limited. With all tibial plateau fractures treated with operative stabilization, it is important to examine the knee for ligamentous stability after completing the fixation in the operating room to rule out ligamentous injury (see **II.B**) (1). The functional results of **treatment** are often better than the routine radiographs seem to predict. Early motion of the knee joint and delayed full weight bearing are the keys to maximum restoration of joint function (2–4).

   i. Apply a **cast-brace** (as described in **Chap. 7, III.H**) off the self-hinged knee braces, which are lightweight and limit varus and valgus stress and are more widely used. The same ambulation protocol, touch-down weight bearing, is followed.

   ii. In special situations, the patient is placed in a **long-leg cast** until the fracture is healed. Then the patient is placed in a rehabilitation program to regain full extension and flexion of the knee to beyond 90 degrees. The patient is kept on protected weight bearing for at least 3 or 4 months. This treatment is generally limited to patients with a severe neurologic condition or significant osteopenia.

E. **Complications**
  1. Significant **loss of range of motion** may occur, particularly if early movement is not instituted.
  2. **Early degenerative joint changes** with pain can occur regardless of the degree of joint reconstruction. In some instances, the pain may be severe enough to require arthroplasty or arthrodesis (8).
  2. The **infection rate** following operative treatment is reduced in experienced hands. Most infections occur because of excessive soft-tissue stripping.
  4. **Nerve and vascular injuries** that occur at the time of injury or subsequent to treatment are not uncommon (12). Nerve injuries are usually traction injuries, and recovery is unpredictable. Compartmental syndrome may be present and should be treated as described in **Chap. 2, III.**

II. **EXTRAARTICULAR PROXIMAL TIBIAL FRACTURES**
  A. **Classification.** Proximal tibial fractures are classified similar to diaphyseal fractures (see **III.C**).
  B. **Examination.** Initial examination should be comprehensive including inspection, palpation, and lower extremity neurovascular assessment. The integrity and condition of the soft tissues should be carefully inspected. The alignment of the lower extremity should also be noted. The compartments of the leg should be palpated and passive flexion and extension of the toes performed to assess for pain and possible compartment syndrome. Distal pulses may be palpable despite ischemia from increased compartment pressure. Definitive diagnosis may require measurement of intracompartmental pressures (see **Chap. 2, III**). The diagnosis of a compartment

syndrome is a surgical emergency and requires prompt release of pressure to preserve muscle and nerve viability. A careful examination of the extremity pulses is imperative to rule out potential vascular injury.

  C. Radiographs. Although a tibial diaphyseal fracture may be obvious from clinical examination, anteroposterior and lateral radiographs of the tibia (including the knee and ankle joints) are needed to plan management. Radiographs should be carefully reviewed to ensure fracture lines do not reveal intraarticular extension. Computed tomograms or plain tomograms can be helpful to identify intraarticular extension when plain x-rays are difficult to interpret.

  D. Treatment. Extraarticular proximal tibial fractures are often the result of high energy trauma with displacement and comminution. Most authors agree that operative management of such fractures is warranted to optimize patient outcomes. However, it remains unclear which surgical option (plate, nail, external fixator, or combination) is preferable. The rates of nonunion between implants did not appear to differ between treatment options (**Table 25-1**). Infection rates were significantly lower with intramedullary nails than with plates or external fixators ($p < 0.05$) (13). A trend towards increased rates of malunion with intramedullary nails was identified ($p = 0.06$). Pooled results across studies may be limited by heterogeneity between studies. Results should be interpreted with caution.

  E. Complications. Extraarticular fractures of the tibia are prone to infection, malunion (i.e., valgus and procurvatum deformities), nonunion, compartment syndrome, and implant failure (**Table 25-1**) (13).

    1. Infection: range 8% to 14% (deep infection rates 3%–5%)
    2. Malunion: range 2.4% to 20%
    3. Nonunion: range 2% to 8%
    4. Compartment syndrome: range 2% to 6%
    5. Implant failure: 8%

III. DIAPHYSEAL FRACTURES

  A. Epidemiology. Tibial fractures are the most common long bone fracture. They occur commonly in the third decade of life at a rate of 26 diaphyseal fractures per 100,000 population annually.

  B. Mechanism of injury. Five causes of injury include falls, sports related, direct blunt trauma, motor vehicle accidents, and penetrating injuries (e.g., gunshots).

  C. Classification. The most comprehensive classification for tibial fractures is the AO Association for the Study of Internal Fixation/Orthopaedic Trauma Association system that divides injury patterns into three broad categories: unifocal, wedge, and complex fractures.

    1. Unifocal fractures are further described as spiral, oblique, and transverse fractures (A).
    2. Wedge fractures are further described as intact spiral, intact bending, and comminuted wedge fractures (B).
    3. Complex fractures (i.e., multiple fragments) can be described as spiral wedge, segmental, and comminuted fractures (C).

  D. Examination. Initial examination should be comprehensive including inspection, palpation, and lower extremity neurovascular assessment. The integrity and condition of the soft tissues should be carefully inspected. The alignment of the lower extremity should also be noted. The compartments of the leg should be palpated and passive flexion and extension of the toes performed to assess for pain and possible compartment syndrome. The diagnosis of a compartment syndrome is a surgical emergency and requires prompt release of pressure to preserve muscle and nerve viability (see **Chap. 2, III**).

  E. Radiographs. Although a tibial diaphyseal fracture may be obvious from clinical examination, anteroposterior and lateral radiographs of the tibia (including the knee and ankle joints) are needed to plan management. Radiographs can provide information about fracture morphology, quality of the bone (i.e., osteopenia, osteoporosis), and gas in the tissues suggesting an open wound.

  F. Treatment. The selection of nonoperative or operative management must involve the consideration of many factors, including associated skeletal and ligamentous

TABLE 25-1 Proximal Extraarticular Tibial Fractures

	Point estimates and 95% confidence intervals				
	Infection	Nonunion	Malunion	CS	Implant failure
Plate	14% (8%–23%)	2% (0.3%–8%)	10% (5%–18%)	2% (0.3%–8%)	—
IM nail	2.5% (0.1%–3%)[a]	3.5% (1.7%–7%)	20% (1.5%–26%)[b]	5.5% (3.1%–9.6%)	7.5% (5%–12%)
Ex-fix	8% (4%–15%) DI: 3% (1%–8%)	8% (4%–15%)	4% (1.5%–10%)	—	—
Ex-fix Plate	+12% (5–26%) DI: 5% (1%–16%)	—	2.4% (0.4%–13%)	—	—

Ex-fix, external fixation; DI, deep infection; CS, compartment syndrome; IM, intramedullary.
[a]$p > 0.05$ when compared to plate.
[b]$p = 0.06$ when compared to plate.
Adapted from Busse J, Bhandari M, Kulkarni A, et al. The effect of low intensity, pulsed ultrasound on time to fracture healing: a meta-analysis. *CMAJ* 2002;166:437–441.

injuries, the degree of soft-tissue injury, injuries to other organ systems, the general condition of the patient, the skill and experience of the treating physician, and the resources of the facility. Options for treatment include: casting/functional bracing (nonoperative), external fixation, plate fixation, and intramedullary nailing.

1. **Nonoperative management** is commonly reserved for closed tibial diaphyseal fractures with less than 1.5 cm of shortening, axially stable transverse fractures, spiral oblique of comminuted fractures with less than 12 mm of initial shortening, angulations less than degrees initially, and less than 50% displacement (15). However, acceptable degrees of fracture shortening and translation are highly variable among surgeons (<5 mm to >15 mm). Surgeons' definitions of acceptable angular malunions (rotational, varus/valgus, and procurvatum/recurvatum) range from less than 5 degrees to 20 degrees (16). Sarmiento (17,18) developed a below-the-knee cast [patellar tendon bearing (PTB)] and prefabricated functional brace that allows knee motion while maintaining stability and length in the affected leg. This PTB cast is generally applied after 2 to 3 weeks in the long-leg bent knee cast that is applied following a closed reduction. Prefabricated braces are the most widely used. One of these two treatment methods should be chosen, and the particular technique should be strictly adhered to if the same excellent results reported in the literature are to be expected. These cast techniques are described in detail in **Chap. 4**. It must be re-emphasized that a below-the-knee total contact cast may not be applied immediately after the fracture; one must wait until the swelling has diminished. The authors suggest using a modified Robert Jones compression long-leg splint during the period of acute swelling. When the patient is ready for casting and following an appropriate spinal or general anesthetic, nearly all tibial fractures can be reduced by placing the leg over the end of the table. Adequate reduction and alignment are maintained in this position while the cast is applied. If shortening is minimal, then analgesia may suffice. The average healing time with closed treatment is approximately 18 weeks (range from 14.5–21.0 weeks). One of Sarmiento's principles is that, in general, the amount of final shortening is demonstrated on the initial radiograph, and the patient should be so informed. Good functional outcomes can be expected in 90% of cases (19–21). Closed treatment is recommended for children's fractures except when the physis or joint is involved (22).

2. **Operative management** is reserved for those fractures deemed unacceptable for nonoperative treatment. Most surgeons prefer intramedullary nails in the treatment of closed low energy fractures (95.5%), high energy fractures (96%), and those closed fractures with associated compartment syndrome (80.4%) (23). The majority of surgeons prefer intramedullary nails in the treatment of open tibial shaft fractures; however, there is a decline in the use of intramedullary nails as the severity of the soft tissue injury increases from Types I to IIIb (Type I, 95.5%; Type II, 88.1%; Type IIIa, 68.4%; Type IIIb, 48.4%) (23).

   a. **Closed fractures.** There have been three published meta-analyses evaluating treatment alternatives for closed tibial shaft fractures: two pooling data from primarily observational studies and one pooling data from on-use randomized trials (21,24,25). Littenburg and colleagues, in a comprehensive review of the available literature, identified 2005 patients treated with a cast or brace, 474 patients treated with a plate and screws, and 407 patients treated with intramedullary nails (21). Pooled infection rates were lower with casts (0%) and intramedullary nails (0%–1%) when compared to plates (0%–15%). While plate fixation achieved the fastest time to fracture union (median = 13 weeks) when compared to either casts (median = 13.7 weeks) or intramedullary nails (median = 20 weeks), there were no differences in the ultimate rates of nonunion between groups. Rates of deep infection were lower with casts and intramedullary nails than with plates (ranges: 0%–2%, 0%–1%, 0%–15%, respectively).

   In a review of prospective studies (eight observational and five randomized trials) evaluating treatment alternatives for tibial shaft fractures,

Coles and Gross found plate fixation to result in the lowest nonunion rates (2.6%) and highest infection rates (9%) compared to other treatment alternatives (24). Despite the apparent benefits of plate fixation in decreasing the time to fracture healing, only 2.1% to 7.4% of surgeon respondents to a survey preferred them in the treatment of closed tibial shaft fractures (low energy, high energy, and those with associated compartment syndrome). This likely reflects an assessment that the high risk of infection with plates outweighs their relative benefit in decreasing time to fracture union. It remains unclear whether surgeons from less industrialized countries, who prefer plate fixation in closed tibial shaft fractures, have similar access to intramedullary nails as those surgeons in developed nations.

A substantial proportion of respondents chose external fixation for high energy tibial shaft fractures and those associated with compartment syndrome. The role of external fixation in closed tibial shaft fractures has been evaluated in an observational study (26). Turen and colleagues, in a review of 68 closed fractures, identified a longer fracture healing time in fractures with compartment syndrome than those without (30.2 weeks versus 17.2 weeks, respectively)(26). Moreover, fracture healing times for closed fractures with compartment syndrome were similar to open fractures.

There remains considerable variability in their preference to ream the intramedullary canal or not. The evidence favoring reamed or nonreamed nail insertion is suggestive but not definitive. Bhandari and colleagues conducted a systematic review and found nine randomized trials ($n = 646$ patients) comparing reamed and nonreamed intramedullary nail insertion in tibial and femoral fractures (25). Reamed nailing resulted in a 56% reduction in the relative risk of nonunion compared to nonreamed nailing (95% confidence interval: 7%–79%).

b. **Open fractures.** An international survey suggests a progressive decline in the use of intramedullary nails as the severity of the soft tissue injury increases from Type I to IIIb. This is related to an increased use of external fixation with increasing soft tissue injury (3%–51%) (27). Surgeons rarely prefer plates in the treatment of open fractures (0.8%–1.1%). One study ($n = 56$) suggests external fixators that significantly decrease the risk of re-operation relative to plates (relative risk 0.13, 95% confidence interval 0.03–0.54, $p < 0.01$) (15). A meta-analysis found that nonreamed nails, in comparison to external fixators (five studies, $n = 396$ patients), reduced the risk of reoperation [relative risk (RR) 0.51, 95% confidence interval 0.31–0.69] (28). Nonreamed nails also offered advantages in decreasing the relative risk of malunion (RR 0.42, 95% confidence interval 0.25–0.71) and superficial infection (RR 0.24, 95% confidence interval, 0.08–0.73). While these studies shared methodologic limitations of lack of concealment, blinding, and loss to follow-up, the narrow confidence intervals make the results more definitive than those of the studies comparing reamed versus unreamed nailing. In the open tibial fracture trials, reamed nails, when compared to nonreamed nails, showed a trend toward decreasing the risk of reoperation (two studies, $n = 132$; RR 0.75, 95% confidence interval 0.43–1.32) (6). Because the confidence interval is very wide, the relative effect of reamed and unreamed nails in open tibial fractures remains unresolved.

G. **Complications.** Most patients experience some residual disability after a tibial fracture (21,24).
  1. **Compartment syndrome** has been discussed previously (see **Chap. 2, III**).
  2. **Joint stiffness** can be largely prevented by aggressive treatment to achieve early union. Flexion and extension exercises to the toes must not be neglected because these joints frequently stiffen and produce considerable postcasting dysfunction.
  3. **Complex regional pain syndrome** (reflex sympathetic dystrophy) can occur in 30% of patients with tibial diaphyseal fractures (29). Vigorous physical therapy and sympathetic may be required (see **Chap. 2**).

4. **Delayed union and nonunion** (30)
   a. The **following factors are related to delayed union or nonunion:**
      i. **Severe initial displacement** of the fracture fragments (probably indicating significant soft-tissue injury)
      ii. **Significant comminution**
      iii. **Associated soft-tissue injuries or open fractures**
      iv. **Infection**
      v. **Open management with inadequate stability**

      These complications can be minimized by adequate immobilization, early weight bearing (which is often delayed for 2 months if a dynamic compression plate is used), and early bone grafting where delayed union appears certain.
   b. Adjunctive therapies. **Low-intensity pulsed ultrasound** (30 mW/cm^2) given at 20 minutes per day has shown potential benefits in improving time to healing. A meta-analysis identified 138 potentially eligible studies, of which 6 randomized trials met inclusion criteria (31). Three trials, representing 158 fractures, were of sufficient homogeneity for pooling. The pooled results showed that time to fracture healing was significantly shorter in the groups receiving low-intensity ultrasound therapy than in the control groups. The weighted average effect size was 6.41 (95% confidence interval 1.01–11.81), which converts to a mean difference in healing time of 64 days between the treatment and control groups.

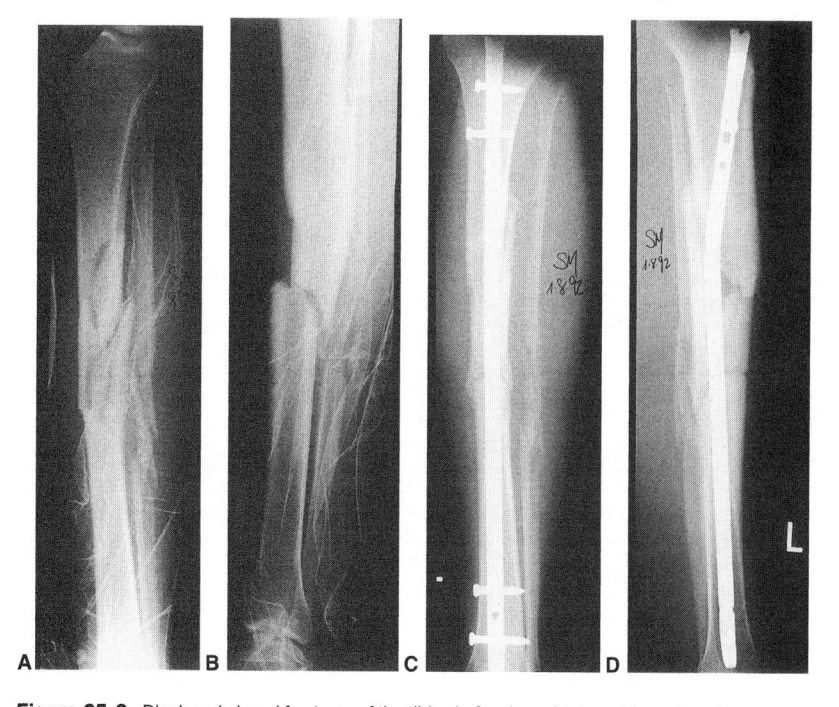

Figure 25-3. Displaced closed fractures of the tibia shaft, when shortened more than 1 cm or considered to be unstable, are best treated with interlocking nails. **A** and **B:** Preoperative radiographs of a shortened, unstable segmental fracture of the tibia shaft. **C** and **D:** The interlocking nail in place. The screws placed through the holes in the nail proximal and distal to the fracture provide length and rotational stability for the fracture. Nearly all fractures of the femoral shaft in skeletally mature individuals are treated with similar interlocking nails, allowing mobilization of the patient and early range of motion of adjacent joints.

5. **Infection** is a complication of open fractures or the opening of a closed fracture. The risk of infection is minimized by efficient surgical technique, by the proper use of antibiotics, and by a delayed primary closure for open fractures. For the most severe soft-tissue injuries, aggressive debridement and coverage with free or rotational muscle flaps minimizes this complication. Pin tract infection is common with the use of external fixators.
6. **Revision surgery.** An observational study of 192 patients with tibial shaft fractures identified three simple predictors of the need for reoperation within 1 year (32). Three variables predicted reoperation: the presence of an open fracture wound (RR 4.32, 95% confidence interval 1.76–11.26), lack of cortical continuity between the fracture ends following fixation (RR 8.33, 95% confidence interval 3.03–25.0), and the presence of a transverse fracture (RR 20.0, 95% confidence interval 4.34–142.86).

HCMC Treatment Recommendations
Tibial Plateau Fractures
   Diagnosis: Anteroposterior and lateral radiographs and physical examination. Computed tomography scans are helpful for assessment of displacement and for surgical planning.
   Treatment: Open reduction and internal fixation or percutaneous reduction with lag screw fixation aided by arthroscopy for fractures displaced more than 2 mm (depression or gapping). Knees that remain stable to varus/valgus stress in full extension may be treated nonoperatively.
   Indications for surgery: Knees with more than 10 degrees of instability in extension and/or joint displacement of greater than 2 mm
   Recommended technique: Joint visualization via open reduction or arthroscopy, reduction and fixation with lag screws and/or low profile plates and bone graft or bone graft substitute, early range-of-motion therapy and limited weight bearing for 8 to 12 weeks.

HCMC Treatment Recommendations
Tib-Fib Fractures
   Diagnosis: Anteroposterior and lateral radiographs of the leg and clinical examination. In 10% to 20% cases there is an open wound communicating with the fracture.
   Treatment: Nonoperative care for fractures that are isolated and not shortened more than 1 cm on initial radiographs, long leg splint for 2 to 3 weeks followed by fracture brace until fracture is united, operative stabilization for length unstable and/or open fractures. Interlocking nail, inserted with reaming is the procedure of choice.
   Indications for surgery: Fractures close to the joint or shortened on initial radiographs greater than 1 cm or failure to control angulation with nonoperative technique or open fracture
   Recommended technique: Interlocking nailing, statically locked. Insert with reaming: more reaming for larger diameter nails with closed fractures, less reaming for open fractures.

References
1. Delamarter RB, Hohl M, Hopp E. Ligament injuries associated with tibial plateau fractures. *Clin Orthop* 1990;250:226–233.
2. Honkonen SE. Degenerative arthritis after tibial plateau fractures. *J Orthop Trauma* 1995;9:273–277.
3. Honkonen SE. Indicators for surgical treatment of tibial condyle fractures. *Clin Orthop* 1994;302:199–205.
4. Keating JF. Tibial plateau fractures in the older patient. *Bull Hosp Joint Dis* 1999;58:19–23.

5. Frassica FJ, Sim FH, Staehl JW, et al. Dislocation of the knee. *Clin Orthop* 1991;263:200–205.
6. Rasul AT, Fischer DA. Primary repair of quadriceps tendon rupture: results of treatment. *Clin Orthop* 1993;289:205–207.
7. Rougraff BT, Reeck CC, Essenmacher J. Complete quadriceps tendon ruptures. *Orthopedics* 1996;19:509–514.
8. Volpin G, Dowd GSE, Stein H, et al. Degenerative arthritis after intraarticular fractures of the knee: long-term results. *J Bone Joint Surg (Br)* 1990;72:634–638.
9. Weale AE, Bannister GC. The management of depressed tibial plateau fractures. A comparison of non-operative treatment with operative treatment using allograft and autograft. *J Orthop Trauma* 1994;4:61–64.
10. Jensen DB, Rude C, Duus B, et al. Tibial plateau fractures: a comparison of conservative and surgical treatment. *J Bone Joint Surg (Br)* 1990;72:49–52.
11. Rasmussen PS. Tibial condyle fractures: impairment of knee joint stability as an indication for surgical treatment. *J Bone Joint Surg (Am)* 1973;55:1331.
12. Dennis JN, Jagger C, Butcher JL, et al. Reassessing the role of arteriograms in the management of posterior knee dislocations. *J Trauma* 1993;35:692–697.
13. Bhandari M, Audige L, Ellis T, et al. Evidence-Based Orthopaedic Trauma Working Group. Operative treatment of extraarticular proximal tibial fractures. *J Orthop Trauma* 2003;17:591–595.
14. Gustilo RB, Anderson JT. Prevention of infection in the treatment of one thousand and twenty-five open fractures of long bones: retrospective and prospective analyses. *J Bone Joint Surg [Am]* 1976;58:453–458.
15. Sarmiento A, Sharpe FE, Ebramzadeh E, et al. Factors influencing outcome of closed tibial fractures treated with functional bracing. *Clin Orthop* 1995;315:8–25.
16. Bhandari M, Guyatt GH, Swiontkowski MF, et al. A lack of consensus in the assessment of fracture healing among orthopaedic surgeons. *J Orthop Trauma* 2002;16:562–566.
17. Sarmiento A, Gersten LM, Sobol PA, et al. Tibial shaft fractures treated with functional braces. Experience with 780 fractures. *J Bone Joint Surg (Br)* 1989;71:602–609.
18. Sarmiento A, McKellop HA, Liinas A, et al. Effect of loading and fracture motion in diaphyseal tibial fractures. *J Orthop Res* 1996;14:80–84.
19. Faergemann C, Frandsen PA, Rock ND. Expected long-term outcome after a tibial shaft fracture. *J Trauma* 1999;46:683–686.
20. Gaston P, Will E, Elton RA, et al. Fractures of the tibia: can their outcome be predicted? *J Bone Joint Surg (Br)* 1999;81:71–76.
21. Littenberg B, Weinstein LP, McCarren M, et al. Closed fractures of the tibial shaft. A meta-analysis of three methods of treatment. *J Bone Joint Surg (Am)* 1998;80:174–183.
22. Spiegel PG, Cooperman DR, Laros GS. Epiphyseal fractures of the distal ends of the tibia and fibula. *J Bone Joint Surg (Am)* 1978;60:1046–1050.
23. Bhandari M, Guyatt GH, Swiontkowski MF, et al. Surgeons' preferences in the operative treatment of tibial shaft fractures: an international survey. *J Bone Joint Surg (Am)* 2001;83A:1746–1752.
24. Coles C, Gross M. Closed tibial shaft fractures: management and treatment complications. A review of the prospective literature. *Can J. Surg* 2000;43:256–262.
25. Bhandari M, Guyatt GH, Tong D, et al. Reamed versus non-reamed intramedullary nailing of lower extremity long bone fractures: a systematic overview and meta-analysis. *J Orthop Trauma* 2000;14:2–9.
26. Turen C, Burgess A, Vanco B. Skeletal stabilization for tibial fractures associated with acute compartment syndrome. *Clin Orthop* 1995;315:163–168.
27. Bach AW, Hansen ST Jr. Plate versus external fixation in severe open tibial shaft fractures. A randomized trial. *Clin Orthop* 1989;241:89–94.
28. Bhandari M, Guyatt GH, Swiontkowski MF, et al. Treatment of open fractures of the shaft of the tibia. *J Bone Joint Surg (Br)* 2001;83:62–68.
29. Sarangi PP, Ward J, Smth EJ. Algodystrophy and osteoporosis after tibial fractures. *J Bone Joint Surg (Br)* 1993;75:450–452.

30. Blick SS, Brumback RJ, Lakatos R, et al. Early prophylactic bone grafting of high-energy tibial fractures. *Clin Orthop* 1989;240:21–41.
31. Busse J, Bhandari M, Kulkarni A, et al. The effect of low intensity, pulsed ultrasound on time to fracture healing: a meta-analysis. *CMAJ* 2002;166:437–441.
32. Bhandari M, Guyatt G, Sprague S, et al. Predictors of re-operation following operative management of fractures of the tibial shaft. *J Orthop Trauma* 2003;17:353–361.

Selected Historical Readings

Burwell HN. Plate fixation of tibial shaft fractures. *J Bone Joint Surg (Br)* 1971;53:258–271.

Clancey GJ, Hansen ST Jr. Open fractures of the tibia. *J Bone Joint Surg (Am)* 1978;60:118–122.

Dehne E. Treatment of fractures of the tibial shaft fractures. *Clin Orthop* 1969;66:159–173.

Fernandez-Palazzi F. Fibular resection in delayed union of tibial fractures. *Acta Orthop Scand* 1969;40:105–118.

Karlstrom G, Olerud S. External fixation of severe open tibial fractures with the Hoffmann frame. *Clin Orthop* 1983;180:68–77.

Lottes JO. Medullary nailing of the tibial with the triflange nail. *Clin Orthop* 1974;105:253–266.

Nicoll EA. Fractures of the tibial shaft. *J Bone Joint Surg (Br)* 1964;46:373–387.

Olerud S, Karlstrom G. Secondary intramedullary nailing of tibial fractures. *J Bone Joint Surg (Am)* 1972;54:1419–1428.

Pare A. Compound fracture of leg. Pare's personal care (MII, 328). In: Hamby WB, ed. *The case reports and autopsy records of ambrose pare*. Springfield, IL: Charles C Thomas Publisher, 1960:82–87.

Sarmiento A. Functional bracing of tibial fractures. *Clin Orthop* 1974;105:202–219.

Schatzker J, McBroom R, Bruce D. The tibial plateau fractures. The toronto experience. *Clin Orthop* 1979;138:94–104.

Sorensen KH. Treatment of delayed union and nonunion of the tibia by fibular resection. *Acta Orthop Scand* 1969;40:92–104.

ANKLE INJURIES 26

I. **ANKLE SPRAINS.** The approach to ankle sprains should distinguish between the acute and chronic ankle sprain. The most common **ankle sprain** consists of an inversion injury of the foot with some degree of plantar flexion. Overall, the period of recovery is relatively short and uneventful. A more relevant injury with a completely different period of recovery is the injury while the foot is in eversion, the so-called **"high ankle sprain."** It accounts for 1% to 15% of the total ankle sprains (1). Therefore, the first issue when approaching a patient with an ankle sprain should be directed to identifying the mechanism of injury. Given the frequency of fractures, it is often recommended to obtain the history and do a brief exam using only palpation, and, if suspicion for a fracture is present, then obtain x-rays prior to extensive physical examination techniques.

   A. **Acute presentation**

   1. **Inversion injuries.** With inversion ligamentous injuries, there is tearing of the lateral ligaments in order from front to back. Thus, the anterior talofibular ligament (ATFL) is the most commonly injured ligament followed by the calcaneofibular ligament (CFL) and, in very rare instances, the posterior talofibular ligament (PTFL).

      Fig. 26-1 shows the anatomic location of the ligaments. Fractures can occur with simple inversion injuries. The most common sites are the distal fibula and the base of the fifth metatarsal.

      a. **Examination.** Palpation is the key to examining ankle injuries. Included in this is palpation of the bones around the ankle. Special attention should be drawn to the distal fibula, distal tibia, and the base of the fifth metatarsal as per the Ottawa criteria (**Table 26-1**). In more severe fractures, also palpate the proximal fibula as this can be broken (Maissoneuve fracture). All ankle ligaments should be palpated looking for tenderness. In the acute setting, pain is quite limiting; therefore, it is very difficult to stress the ankle joint or obtain ankle stress radiographs to confirm which ligaments are intact. In the absence of fracture, soft tissue swelling and pain will dictate the treatment.

      b. **Radiographic imaging.** The need for x-rays can be guided by consideration of the Ottawa ankle rules (**Table 26-1**). It is important to note that the rules do not apply to a pediatric population with open growth plates (to be safe, it is recommended to x-ray those under age 18). Although not specifically listed, we recommend strong consideration to obtain x-rays on people over the age of 50, especially women over the age of 50 due to lower bone mass and subsequent higher fracture rates. X-rays should include anteroposterior (AP), lateral, and mortise views.

      c. **Treatment.** If there is no medial tenderness, the ankle joint should be considered a **stable joint**. The traditional principles of rest, immobilization, compression, elevation, and icing should be applied followed by a functional return to activities while protected with any of the commercially available ankle braces until the pain allows proper muscle contraction of the dynamic stabilizers of the ankle (peroneal and deep compartment muscles of the lower leg). In rare occasions, due to pain with weight bearing, the patient will have to be protected for 6 to 8 weeks.

      If there is medial or anterior capsule tenderness, the possibility of developing **talar instability** is higher, and closer examination of the ankle

372 Chapter 26: Ankle Injuries

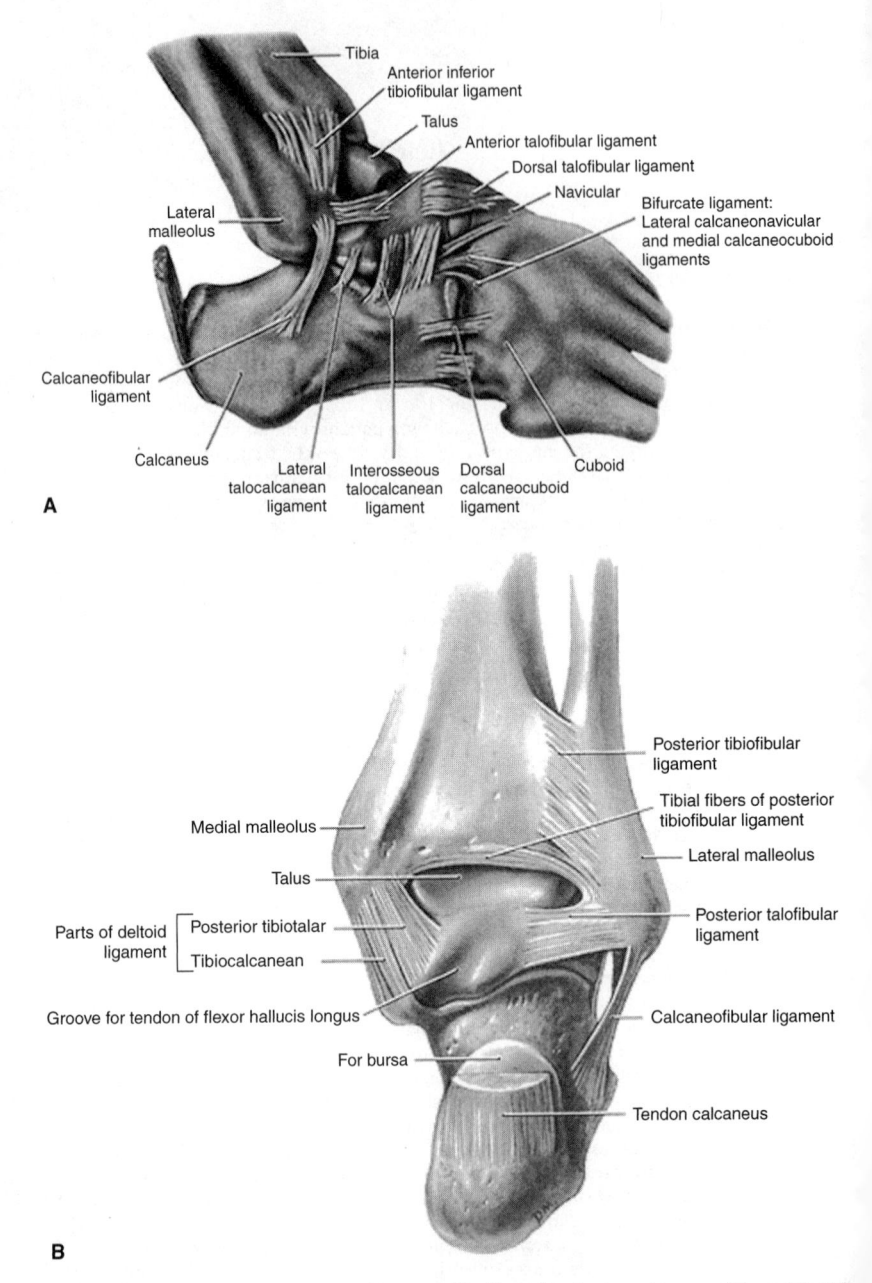

Figure 26-1. Anatomic description of the most significant ligaments and bones of the ankle and midfoot area.

TABLE 26-1 Ottawa Criteria to Perform Radiographic Examination

Ankle injuries
1. Pain along the posterior margin of the most distal 6 cm of the fibula
2. Pain along the posterior margin of the medial malleolus
3. Unable to bear weight immediately after the injury or to take four steps in the Emergency Department (even with a limp)
4. Age less than 18

Midfoot injuries
1. Pain along the base of the fifth metatarsal
2. Pain along the navicular
3. Unable to bear weight immediately after the injury or to take four steps in the Emergency Department (even with a limp)
4. Age less than 18

mortise for talar dome injuries and symmetry is warranted. If suspected, the period of immobilization in a walking cast or boot should be longer, for 6 to 8 weeks until the medial and anterior tenderness disappear. At that time it can be treated as a stable injury depending on the remaining discomfort within the ankle joint.

2. **Eversion injuries**
   a. **Examination.** The exam will show some tenderness along the most anterior and distal aspect of the syndesmosis of the ankle. Some tenderness along the lateral ligament complex may be present although to a much lesser degree than with true inversion ankle sprains. Any degree of external rotation, which stresses the ankle mortise, will increase or reproduce the pain. The external rotation can be applied directly by the examiner holding the lower leg with one hand and torquing on the foot with the opposite hand while keeping the ankle in a neutral position, so the talus is locked in the ankle mortise. If a fracture has been ruled out, a "squeeze test" (using both hands to push the mid-fibula and tibia together, noting pain distal to the area of compression) can be performed to assess syndesmotic injuries. If the patient can tolerate weight bearing, a more sensitive test for a syndesmosis injury consists of standing on the injured leg and applying an external rotation force to the ankle with an internal turn of the pelvis with the knee fully extended. If the patient can stand and perform some degree of external rotation, the suspicion for an unstable mortise should be low. If there is any tenderness in the proximal lower leg, full length tibia and fibula radiographs should be obtained to rule out a proximal fibula fracture (Maissonneuve fracture) or an unstable syndesmosis. This projection is taken as an AP view with 30° of internal rotation (when both malleolus are equidistant from the x-ray beam). A noncompetent syndesmosis is defined as the one that presents on an AP view of the ankle more than 6 mm of clear space between the tibia and the fibula measured at 10 mm proximal from the joint line (2) (**Fig. 26-2**). When it comes to x-ray measurements, the clear space in between the tibia and the fibula has been shown to be more reliable and less subjective to rotation than the overlap in between the tibia and fibula (<5 mm). If the syndesmosis appears intact on a static radiograph, but suspicion for syndesmotic injury remains high, consider stress views of the ankle (ideally under fluoroscopic dynamic examination) while applying external rotation to the foot. The best projection to assess the stability of the syndesmosis is the mortise view. The patient will have to be either sedated or injected with local anesthetic along the syndesmosis prior to its

374 Chapter 26: Ankle Injuries

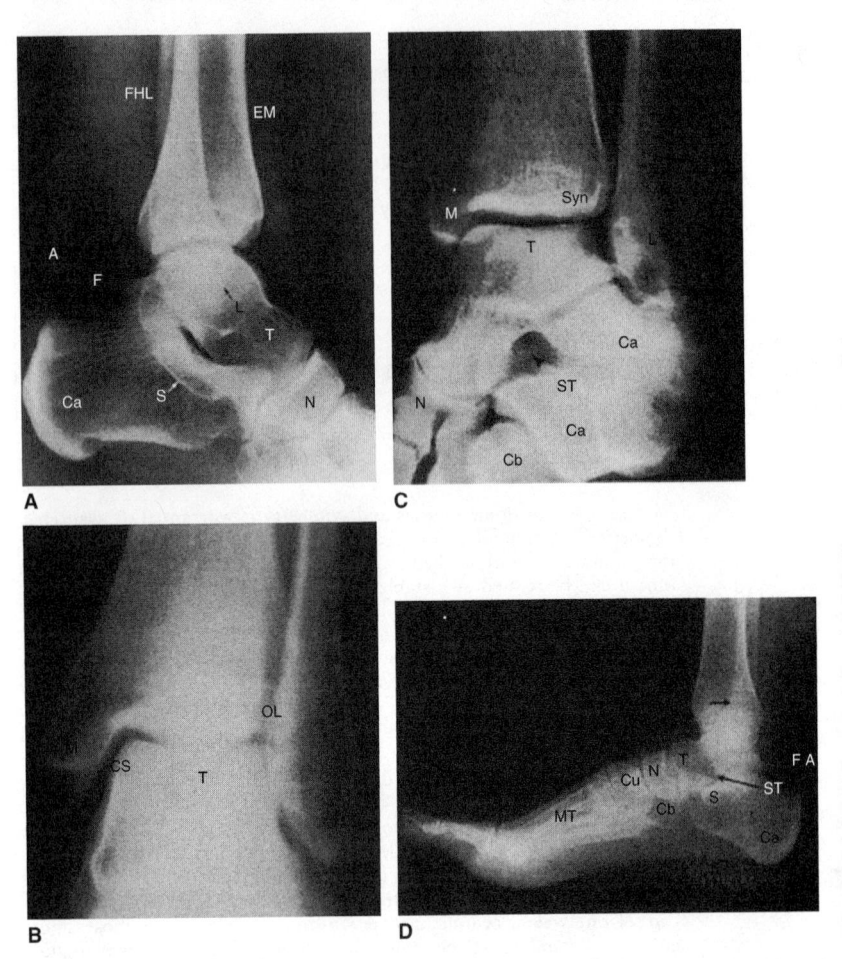

Figure 26-2. Radiographic appearance of the most common bony landmarks of the ankle and foot. **A:** Medial view of ankle region. **B:** Anterior view of ankle. **C:** Mortise view of ankle region. **D:** Lateral view of foot. M, medial malleolus; L, lateral malleolus; T, talus; Ca, calcaneus; S, sustentaculum tali; N, navicular; Cu, cuneiforms; Cb, cuboid; Mt, metatarsal; ST, sinus tarsi; A Achilles tendon; F, fat; arrowhead, superimposed tibia and fibula; Syn, Syndesmosis; FHL, flexor hallucis longus; EM, extensor muscles; CS, tibiofibular clear space; OL, tibiofibular overlap.

evaluation. A total of 5 to 15 cc of lidocaine 1% with epinephrine should suffice to anesthetize the syndesmosis. The injection is performed using a 25- or 22-gauge needle along the anterior aspect of the syndesmosis, starting immediately proximal to the joint line level and always "walking" along the lateral cortex of the tibia from distal to proximal. Special attention has to be paid to not angle the needle too posteriorly, never posterior to the plane of the fibula, to avoid damage into vital structures of the posterior compartment of the leg.

  b. **Treatment.** If the syndesmosis is **stable** or in the absence of fractures, the patient should be immobilized in a walking cast or boot for 6 to 8 weeks followed by a functional return to activities of daily living and sports. If the syndesmosis is **unstable** or in the presence of a proximal fibula fracture, the patient will require fixation of the syndesmosis with screws followed by immobilization for 6 to 8 weeks. Weight bearing should be started prior to removal of the screws and always after warning the patient about the possibility of screw breakage. A residual wide syndesmosis because of a misdiagnosis or improper treatment is a devastating sequelae that will lead to a very severe post-traumatic osteoarthritis of the ankle joint within 1 to 2 years.

B. **Subacute-chronic presentation**
1. **Inversion injuries.** The patient presents with some residual discomfort in areas where there may still be some healing taking place or where an injury has been missed. The physician has to rule out any residual instability, reported to be present in 20% to 40% of ankle sprains, or a chondral injury of the talus, present in 6.5% of ankle sprains (3). If the patient continues to report instability after a period of physical therapy, then one should consider stress views of the ankle. If the patient still presents enough pain that the ankle will be protected by contraction of the surrounding musculature, therefore making the exam for stability unreliable, the patient should have some intravenous sedation or local anesthetic injected into the ankle. A total of 5 cc of lidocaine 2% with epinephrine should be enough to anesthetize the ankle joint. The injection is performed with a 25- or 22-gauge needle along the most medial border of the ankle joint immediately distal to the medial shoulder of the tibial plafond and medial to the anterior tibialis tendon. The needle has to be angled at 45° from the coronal plane. The ankle can also be approached through the lateral aspect over the **"soft spot,"** which is defined as the junction of the tibia and fibula at the level of the joint line. However, the chances of damaging the dorsal cutaneous branch from the superficial peroneal nerve are relatively high. The best chance to identify the nerve branch is with gentle palpation of the skin, looking for a cord-like structure when the fourth toe is forced into plantar flexion.

    The stress views are obtained with a lateral radiograph while the foot is pulled forward (an anterior drawer test) in slight plantar flexion. The most commonly injured ligament, the ATFL, is stressed during this maneuver. A 10-mm difference of anterior displacement between the stress view and the resting view or a 3-mm difference of anterior displacement compared to the stressed opposite side is indicative of ankle instability. Treatment options for chronic instability include a formal physiotherapy program and, if that fails, the next reasonable step is a surgical repair/reconstruction of the lateral ligament complex of the ankle. In the absence of an obvious chondral injury of the talus on plain x-rays, a magnetic resonance imaging (MRI) scan is necessary to rule it out. A symptomatic chondral injury most likely will require some surgical treatment (i.e., arthroscopic debridement +/− subchondral drilling) to improve the symptoms.

2. **Eversion injuries.** The most common reason to present with residual pain after a syndesmosis sprain will be some degree of remaining instability. A careful and detailed evaluation of the patient has to be performed as surgical fixation of the syndesmosis will be the most likely treatment recommendation.

II. **ANKLE FRACTURES**

A. **Classification.** Ankle fractures are intraarticular injuries, and accurate reduction as well as maintenance of the reduction is required for a satisfactory long-term result. To achieve reduction by closed manipulation, it is necessary to know the direction of the forces producing the fractures. It must be emphasized that fractures about the ankle usually are not isolated injuries but have significant associated ligamentous ruptures. Ankle fractures may be classified by the Lauge-Hansen scheme (**Fig. 26-3**). This classification is useful because of the method used for its description. The first term makes reference to the position of the foot at the time of injury and the second term to the direction of the force applied to produce the fracture. That information is extremely valuable in planning closed reduction maneuvers.

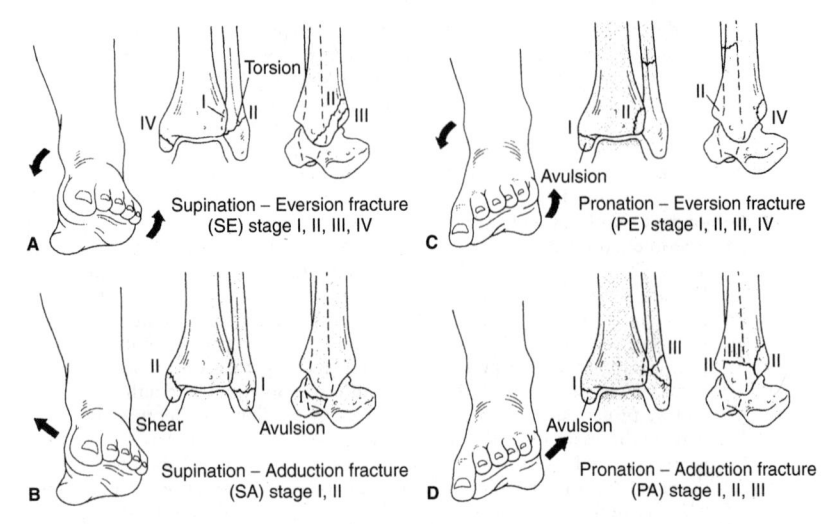

Figure 26-3. The Lauge-Hansen classification of ankle fractures. **A:** The supination-eversion fracture. Stage I: The avulsion of the anterior talofibular ligament from the tibia or simple rupture of the ligament. Stage II: The classic oblique fracture of the distal fibula, beginning anteriorly at the joint line and extending obliquely and posteriorly toward the shaft of the bone. Stage III: Avulsion or rupture of the posterior tibiofibular ligament. Stage IV: Avulsion fracture of the medial malleolus. **B:** The supination-adduction fracture. Stage I: Avulsion of the tip of the lateral malleolus or rupture of the associated ligaments. Stage II: Vertical fracture of the medial malleolus, usually beginning at the plafond. **C:** The pronation-eversion fracture. Stage I: Avulsion of the medial malleolus or ruptured deltoid ligament. Stage II: Rupture or avulsion of the anterior tibiofibular ligament. Stage III: A high short oblique fracture of the fibula. Stage IV: A posterior lip fracture of the tibia. **D:** The pronation-abduction fracture. Stage I: Avulsion of the medial malleolus or ruptured deltoid ligament. Stage II: Rupture or avulsion of the syndesmotic ligaments. Stage III: A short, oblique fracture of the distal fibula at about the level of the ankle joint. (From Weber MJ. Ankle fractures and dislocations. In: Chapman MW, Madison M, eds. *Operative orthopaedics*, 2nd ed. Philadelphia, PA: JB Lippincott, 1993:731–745, with permission).

The Danis-Weber or AO Association of Osteosynthesis classification system concentrates on the pattern of the fibular fracture (**Fig. 26-4**). The type A fracture is distal to the level of the syndesmosis and frequently transverse, the type B fracture is a spiral oblique fracture at the level of the syndesmosis, and the type C fracture is proximal to the syndesmosis level.

B. Examination. The ankle has to be palpated for tender areas. The Ottawa Criteria (**Table 26-1**) for evaluation and management of ankle injuries have been proven to be a practical way to approach these injuries. Recently, it has been shown to have a sensitivity of no less than 99.6% for detecting fractures (4). However, in spite of these reports, it does not seem to be used routinely for fear of missing ankle fractures and the potential legal consequences associated. The lack of soft tissue swelling in some situations may be misleading, especially in the elderly population.

C. Radiographs. AP, lateral, and oblique (the mortise view) films are essential for evaluating any ankle injury. A clearer delineation of the medial malleolar fracture may be achieved by an additional view obtained with the foot in 45 degrees of internal rotation. A lateral radiograph obtained at 50 degrees of external rotation is the best way to visualize the posterior malleolus (5).

D. Treatment. The main feature that determines the treatment plan is if the ankle fracture is a stable or unstable injury.

  1. Stable injuries. A stable ankle fracture is defined as the one that presents no widening of the medial or lateral mortise joint space. A fracture distal to the

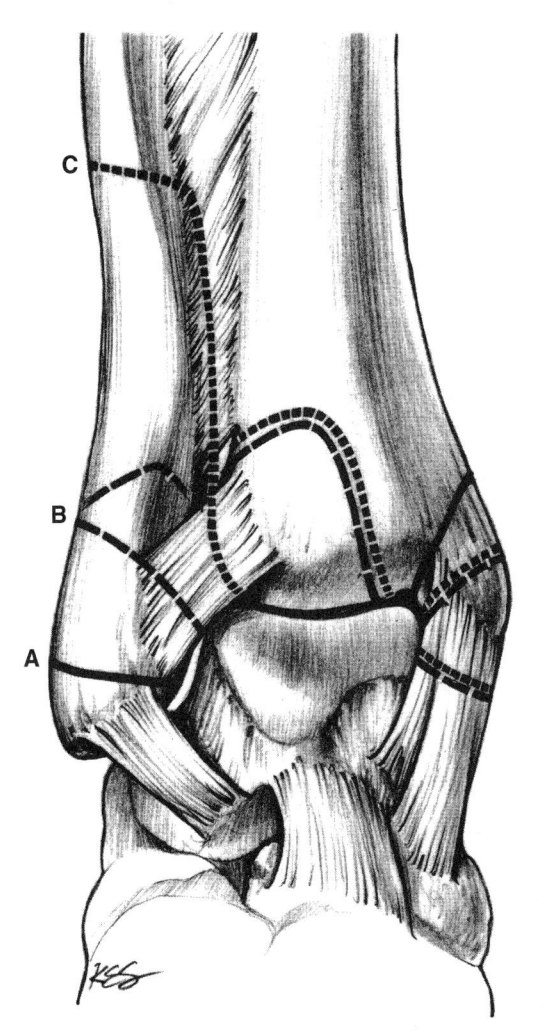

Figure 26-4. Diagrammatic representation of the Danis-Weber classification system. **A:** Transverse fracture of the distal malleolus. **B:** Spiral fracture at the level of the mortise. **C:** Fractures above the mortise with disruption of the syndesmosis. (From Hansen ST, Swiontkowski MF. *Orthopaedic trauma protocols.* New York: Raven, 1993: 340.)

syndesmosis with a ruptured deltoid ligament, which is suspected if there is significant medial tenderness, will represent an unstable ankle fracture with a stable syndesmosis. Therefore, the definition of stability should be an ankle joint where the fracture is distal to the syndesmosis with no injury to the medial stabilizers and consequently with no widening of the medial mortise. The immediate treatment consists of elevation, reduction of the fracture, and immobilization as soon as possible to reduce soft tissue swelling. If the fracture is merely a small avulsion off of the distal tip of the fibula without any involvement of the mortise, then treatment can be similar to that of the associated ligament sprain. For stable fractures that are larger and with some degree of displacement, a closed reduction maneuver can be attempted. For most oblique fractures of the fibula, the reduction is via plantar flexion and internal rotation. This can often be achieved by lifting the patient's limb (with the patient in the supine position) by the great toe. Immobilize the patient's leg in a short leg splint in this position. For long-term treatment (more than 4–6 weeks), the ankle must be maintained in a neutral position (90° from the long axis of the lower leg) to prevent any Achilles contracture and a longer than expected recovery time. The patient should be instructed in toe-touch weight bearing until there are radiographic signs of callus and lack of tenderness to pressure (3–4 weeks) over the lateral malleolus. Further protect the injury in a short leg cast with the foot in neutral position for another 3 to 4 weeks. Stable ankle fractures have equivalent results whether treated operatively or nonoperatively (6). Consequently, we recommend an attempt at nonoperative treatment whenever possible.

2. **Unstable injuries**
   a. These fractures should be reduced and internally fixed as an urgent procedure if the patient is seen **before significant swelling is apparent** (7,8). Preoperative planning is essential to minimize soft-tissue stripping and maximize fixation. Patients with open fractures should be managed with wound debridement and internal fixation; the results are generally equivalent to those for closed fractures (9). Significant improvement can be expected to continue 6 months after the fracture occurred (10,11).
      i. **Medial malleolar fragments** should be reattached with screws for larger fragments and with Kirschner wires with supplemental tension band wires for smaller fragments. With screw fixation, a length of 35 to 40 mm is appropriate so that the metaphyseal bone is engaged and the medullary canal is avoided with loss of screw purchase. The rate of nonunion with surgical treatment is reported to be as low as 1% compared with 15% with conservative treatment (12).
      ii. **Posterior malleolar fragments** are stabilized with screw fixation if they involve more than one fourth of the articular surface. Generally these fragments are reduced by reduction of the associated distal fibula fracture. The lag screw placement can be done from the anterior to posterior direction (frequently percutaneously). Formal open reduction, if required, must be done before definitive fixation of the lateral malleolus, which may limit the surgical exposure; the incision must be well posterior to the fibula.
      iii. **Lateral malleolar fractures** below the ankle joint (Danis-Weber A) may be reduced as medial malleolar fractures. If possible, an attempt should first be made to reduce and fix the fracture with a lag screw. Fractures with disruption of both anterior and posterior tibio-fibular ligaments can be held with a "position" (or syndesmosis) screw inserted parallel to the plafond into the tibia. This screw is generally placed after anatomic reduction of a type B or C fibula fracture, with the foot fully dorsiflexed (to prevent narrowing of the ankle mortise), through the plate, and after gaining purchase on one or both of the tibial cortices (see **iv** below). Spiral or oblique fractures with the tibiofibular ligament intact may be reapproximated by oblique lag screws and/or with a small, one-third tubular plate. Prophylactic antibiotics should be utilized (13). These plates could be placed on the posterior aspect of the fibula to prevent irritation from the plate when in the lateral aspect, a more subcutaneous position (14). More recently, success has been achieved with bioabsorbable implants (15,16). Repair to the deltoid ligament avulsion is generally not necessary (17). Postoperatively, the leg may be treated in a short-leg compression dressing with a plaster or fiberglass splint to control the position of the foot. As soon as the swelling is controlled, at 5 to 7 days, a removable splint can be used and early active motion started. The patient should remain partial weight bearing for 4 to 6 weeks. If the patient is unable to co-operate with the early, active range-of-motion protocol, then a short-leg cast is applied for 4 to 6 weeks (18,19). Weight bearing and strengthening exercises are initiated following this period.

      iv. If the tibio-fibular syndesmosis is widened, it is because the distal interosseous membrane is torn. This injury can be associated with a proximal fibula fracture (the Maissoneuve fracture). Authorities who report the best results treat this injury with a suture repair of a ligamentous rupture when feasible and with one or two position (or syndesmosis) screws placed parallel to the plafond. Some authors recommend the use of 4.5-mm cortical screws; we favor the use of one or two 3.5-mm screws with purchase through four cortices (exit the tibia slightly to allow removal if they break). Care must be taken to maintain the normal fibular length and, by keeping the foot in neutral position, the proper mortise width. Some authorities recommend delaying full weight bearing until the syndesmosis screws are removed. However, the authors have seen many more problems following early removal of the syndesmosis screws, and, currently, it is recommended to leave them in as weight bearing is progressed. The patient should be advised that the screws may break.

    b. When swelling is already significant, any gross malalignment should be corrected. Then the leg should be placed in a compression dressing with splints and elevated until the swelling has receded sufficiently for a safe open reduction. In order to avoid wound healing complications, patients should be seen and surgically treated as soon after the injury as possible (7). The operative complication rates are four times higher for diabetic (20,21) and obese patients managed operatively (22).

E. Complications
  1. Incomplete reduction is associated with a higher incidence of ankle joint symptoms than are seen when anatomic restitution is achieved. This situation can be improved by osteotomy and internal fixation even years after the fracture occurs (23). The results after restoring the original anatomy overall are worse than those with early anatomic reduction (12).
  2. Nonunion, although rare, can occur and is usually symptomatic. On the medial side, it may be associated with interposition of the posterior tibial tendon. Nonunion of either malleolus should be managed with internal fixation and bone grafting. Deep infection as the cause for the non-union has to always be ruled out with intraoperative cultures, especially after prior open reduction and internal fixation.

III. PILON FRACTURES. Fractures of the articular surface of the tibia are generally high-energy injuries from axial loads. They occur as a result of high speed motor vehicle accidents or falls from a height (24).
  A. Diagnosis is confirmed by radiographs, as for ankle fractures. The history of high-energy trauma or fall from a significant height should prompt a thorough examination of the heel, foot, and ankle paying special attention to swelling and tenderness. If the plain radiographs do not sufficiently document the fracture pattern, a computed tomographic (CT) scan is indicated to better delineate the size and location of the bony fragments.
  B. Treatment. Fractures of the joint surface with more than 2 to 3 mm of displacement, either gapping or impaction, are generally managed by reduction, fixation, and in some occasions with bone grafting. Significant swelling of the soft tissues occurs very rapidly with this type of injuries; therefore, operative management must be emergent or otherwise delayed for several days or weeks until the swelling subsides. Plating of an associated fibula fracture, application of an external fixator across the ankle joint, or a calcaneal pin traction on a Bohler frame are valid options in the interim to achieve indirect reduction of the joint fragments and expedite the resolution of the soft tissue swelling. All those options limit the amount of soft tissue stripping required in subsequent surgeries which will help to achieve bony consolidation and to decrease the potential complications. Acute compartment syndromes are not uncommon with this type of fracture. If open fasciotomy is performed, then the fibula should be plated to restore some stability to the fracture. Because of the high incidence of wound complications and deep infections,

there is a trend toward limited fracture exposure, indirect reduction and fixation of the joint surface with lag screws, and complete definitive treatment with an external fixator or percutaneous plates. Bone grafting may not be required if the fracture is not exposed, but it should be carried out if there is any doubt.

C. **Complications.** Deep infection may require multiple debridements, hardware removal, and muscle-flap (often free) coverage (24). If the problem is identified early, then the hardware can be generally left in place. Pilon fractures are associated with a very high rate of complications, and their management should be left to a specialist familiar with this type of injury. Frequently, the long-term result is a stiff, painful, and chronically swollen ankle that at some point may require an ankle arthrodesis to improve the function and symptoms of the patient.

IV. ACHILLES TENDON (TENDO CALCANEUS) RUPTURES

A. The **history** associated with an Achilles tendon rupture is often diagnostic. The patient profile is a middle-aged individual occasionally involved in recreational sports, also known as "the weekend warrior." Patients with a different profile are worth evaluating for risk factors (i.e., steroid use) because this pathology is fairly unusual in a young healthy individual. It cannot be emphasized enough that a healthy tendon will not rupture during exercise. However, unhealthy tendons do not necessarily cause symptoms. Usually, the patient was running or jumping when a sudden severe pain was felt behind the ankle, almost as if it had been struck by something. Patients will describe the episode as being "…kicked by somebody, I turned around, and there was nobody there…" or being hit by a rock or the opponent's racquet. Afterwards, the patient may be able to walk but usually with a significant difficulty.

B. **Examination** is most easily accomplished with the patient prone. By inspection and palpation, the defect in the Achilles tendon can be documented. Squeezing the calf in this position with an intact Achilles tendon causes passive plantar flexion to occur; this response is absent with tendon rupture (Thompson's test). Even if the plantar flexion is present but decreased, the diagnosis of Achilles tendon rupture can be made. Do not be misled by the patient's ability to plantar-flex the ankle actively because this can be done with the muscles from the deep posterior compartment of the lower leg. Neurovascular exam is normally intact. In case of doubt, depending on the expertise of the radiology department, an ultrasound will be definitive to demonstrate a gap within the tendon fibers. If ultrasound is not available, an MRI will be diagnostic. The treatment guidelines are the same for either a partial or a complete rupture and are more dependent on the patient's profile.

C. **Treatment**

1. Patients with low functional demands may undergo **nonoperative treatment**. The foot is held in equinus for 8 weeks in a short-leg cast. It is extremely important not to force the plantar flexion excessively as the posterior aspect of the most distal part of the lower leg may develop skin necrosis from lack of blood supply. This can be easily demonstrated by the blanching of the skin that takes place with forced plantar flexion. The acute swelling also decreases the tolerance of the skin to plantar flexion. The position chosen for immobilization cannot compromise the posterior skin, and normal color has to be seen along the posterior aspect of the leg. Ambulation with crutches using an elevated heel on the shoe for 8 to 12 weeks then follows. Finally, rehabilitation exercises are begun to increase strength and range of motion.

2. **Operative treatment** is often recommended, especially for the young, competitive athlete. The advantages of open treatment are that the proper strength-length relationship of the musculotendinous unit is re-established, the internal repair probably adds extra strength to the ruptured tendon, and immobilization can be limited. The risk of re-rupture of the tendon is lower with operative management (25). The incision should be made to one side of the tendon (not directly posteriorly) and should not extend distally into the flexor creases posterior to the ankle; this helps minimize adhesions of the tendon to the skin. A careful repair of the tendon sheath also limits these adhesions. The actual type of tendon repair is left to the discretion of the surgeon; numerous

materials and patterns of suture repair have been discussed. The plantaris tendon or the flexor hallucis longus tendon transfer may be used to augment the repair. Postoperatively, the ankle is kept in a slight equinus position with a short-leg cast or boot for 8 weeks. Ambulation and physical therapy are then allowed as tolerated to increase strength and range of motion.

D. Complications. The rate of complications with either treatment, conservative or surgical, is similar. The difference is the type of complications which occur. With conservative treatment, the most common complications include re-rupture and weakness of the Achilles complex with plantar flexion. The weakness is more noticeable during the practice of sports and very rarely during activities of daily living (ADLs). With surgical treatment, the complications are related to skin dehiscence/necrosis, neurologic damage, and infection. There is no good data to recommend either treatment based on the type of complications. The final decision must be left to the patient once all the information is presented to him or her in an objective manner.

References

1. Lewis JE, Marymont JV. Ankle arthroscopy and sports-related injuries. In: Mizel MS, Miller RA, Scioli MW, eds. *Orthopaedic knowledge update, foot and ankle 2.* Rosemont, IL: American Orthopaedic Foot and Ankle Society, 1998:39–54.
2. Pneumaticos SG, Noble PC, Chatziioannou SN, et al. The effects of rotation on radiographic evaluation of the tibiofibular syndesmosis. *Foot Ankle Int* 2002;23:107–111.
3. Dalton GP. Fractures of the talus. In: Mizel MS, Miller RA, Scioli MW, eds. *Orthopaedic knowledge update, foot and ankle 2.* Rosemont, IL: American Orthopaedic Foot and Ankle Society, 1998:39–54.
4. Bachmann LM, Kolb E, Koller MT, et al. Accuracy of Ottawa ankle rules to exclude fractures of the ankle and mid-foot: systematic review. *BMJ* 2003;326(7386):417.
5. Nabil A, Ebraheim NA, Mekhail AO, et al. External rotation—lateral view of the ankle in the assessment of the posterior malleolus. *Foot Ankle Int* 1999;20:379–383.
6. Bauer M, Bergstrom B, Hemborg A, et al. Malleolar fractures: non-operative versus operative treatment: a controlled study. *Ankle Fractures* 1985;199:17–27.
7. Carragee EJ, Csongradi TZ, Bleck EE. Early complications in the operative treatment of ankle fractures: influence of delay before operation. *J Bone Joint Surg (Br)* 1991;73:79–82.
8. Phillips WA, Schwartz HS, Keller CS, et al. A prospective, randomized study of the management of severe ankle fractures. *J Bone Joint Surg (Am)* 1985;67:67–78.
9. Franklin JL, Johnson KD, Hansen ST. Immediate internal fixation of open ankle fractures. *J Bone Joint Surg (Am)* 1984;66:1349–1356.
10. Belcher GL, Radomisli TE, Abate JA, et al. Functional outcome analysis of operatively treated malleolar fractures. *J Orthop Trauma* 1997;11:106–109.
11. Ponzer S, Nasell H, Bergman B, et al. Functional outcome and quality of life in patients with type B ankle fractures: a two year follow-up study. *J Orthop Trauma* 1999;13:363–368.
12. Donatto KC. Fractures of the ankle. In: Mizel MS, Miller RA, Scioli MW, eds. *Orthopaedic knowledge update, foot and ankle 2.* Rosemont, IL: American Orthopaedic Foot and Ankle Society, 1998:39–54.
13. Paiement GD, Renaud E, Dagenais G, et al. Double-blind randomized prospective study of efficacy of antibiotic prophylaxis for open reduction and internal fixation of closed ankle fractures. *J Orthop Trauma* 1994;8:64–66.
14. Winkler B, Weber BG, Simpson LA. The dorsal antiglide plate in the treatment of Danis-Weber type-B fractures of the distal fibula. *Clin Orthop Rel Res* 1990;259:204–209.
15. Bostman OM. Osteoarthritis of the ankle after foreign-body reaction to absorbable pins and screws: a three to nine year follow-up study. *J Bone Joint Surg (Br)* 1998;80:333–338.

16. Dijkema ARA, van der Elst M, Breederveld RS, et al. Surgical treatment of fracture-dislocations of the ankle joint with biodegradable implants: a prospective randomized study. *J Trauma* 1993;34:82–84.
17. Stromsoe K, Hoqevold HE, Skjeldal S, et al. The repair of a ruptured deltoid ligament is not necessary in ankle fractures. *J Bone Joint Surg (Br)* 1995;77:920–921.
18. Hedstrom M, Ahl T, Dalen N. Early postoperative ankle exercise. *Clin Orthop Rel Res* 1994;300:193–196.
19. Sondenaa K, Hoigaard U, Smith D, et al. Immobilization of operated ankle fractures. *Acta Orthop Scand* 1986;57:59–61.
20. Flynn JM, Rodriguez-del Rio F, Pizá PA. Closed ankle fractures in the diabetic patient. *Foot Ankle Int* 2000;21:311–319.
21. McCormack RG, Leith JM. Ankle fractures in diabetics: complications of surgical management. *J Bone Joint Surg (Br)* 1998;80:689–692.
22. Bostman OM. Body-weight related to loss of reduction of fractures of the distal tibia and ankle. *J Bone Joint Surg (Br)* 1995;77:101–103.
23. Marti RK, Raaymakers EL, Nolte PA. Malunited ankle fractures. The late results of reconstruction. *J Bone Joint Surg (Br)* 1990;72:709–713.
24. Ovadia DN, Beals RK. Fractures of the tibial plafond. *J Bone Joint Surg (Am)* 1986;68:543–551.
25. Bomler J, Sturup J. Achilles tendon rupture. An 8-year follow-up. *Acta Orthop Belg* 1989;55:307–310.

Selected Historical Readings

Black HM, Brand RL, Eichelberger MR. An improved technique for the evaluation of ligamentous injury in severe ankle sprains. *Am J Sports Med* 1978;6:276–282.

Brantigan JW, Pedegana LR, Lippert FG. Instability of the subtalar joints. *J Bone Joint Surg (Am)* 1977;59:321–324.

Goergen TG, Danzig LA, Resnick D, et al. Roentgenographic evaluation of the tibiotalar joint. *J Bone Joint Surg (Am)* 1977;59:874–877.

Jacobs D, Martens M, van Audekercke R, et al. Comparison of conservative and operative treatment of Achilles tendon rupture. *Am J Sports Med* 1978;6:107–111.

Mast JW, Spiegel PG, Pappas JN. Fractures of the tibial pilon. *Clin Orthop* 1988;230:68–82.

Nistor L. Surgical and non-surgical repair of Achilles tendon rupture. *J Bone Joint Surg (Am)* 1981;63:394–399.

Ramsey P, Hamilton W. Changes in tibiotalar area of contact caused by lateral talar shift. *J Bone Joint Surg (Am)* 1976;58:356–357.

Yablon IG, Keller FG, Shouse L. The key role of the lateral malleolus in displaced fractures of the ankle. *J Bone Joint Surg (Am)* 1977;59:169–173.

FRACTURES AND DISLOCATIONS OF THE FOOT

27

I. **FRACTURES OF THE CALCANEUS**
   A. **Mechanism of injury.** Calcaneal fractures are more frequent than any other fracture of the tarsal bones and comprise 1% to 2% of all fractures. These fractures, which are often bilateral, are likely to occur when a person falls from a height and lands on the heels. Associated injuries include compression fractures of the lumbar spine and occasionally fractures about the knee or pelvis.
   B. **Classification.** Although there are many classification systems (Sander's classification is the most widely utilized) (1), a description of the fracture location provides the most information.
      1. **Avulsion fractures** occur in the posterior process of the tubercle as a result of increased tension in the Achilles tendon. This tension causes a fracture of the calcaneus rather than a ruptured tendon. If the avulsion fracture is large and runs into the body of the calcaneus (into or beyond the posterior facet), it is termed a **tongue-type fracture** (**Fig. 27-1**).
      2. **Fractures into the body of the calcaneus**
         a. **Fractures not involving the subtalar joint**, with or without disruption of the plantar surface of the calcaneus, can result in heel shortening and varus.
         b. **Fractures involving the subtalar joint** typically involve a triangular-shaped subarticular fragment that remains in place medially, the fractured and impacted posterior facet (generally the anterior portion is driven down into the body of the calcaneus to a greater degree than the posterior portion), and displacement of the lateral wall or the calcaneus under the fibula. This is termed a **joint depression fracture** (**Fig. 27-1**).
   C. **Examination.** Pain and tenderness in the heel are present, with associated broadening of the heel and ecchymosis. Ecchymosis on the posterior sole of the foot with calcaneal tenderness is nearly diagnostic of a calcaneal fracture. When open fractures are occurring, the wound is most often medial near the sustentaculum talus. A foot compartmental syndrome can occur in 2% to 5% of patients and must be treated with urgent decompression (see **Chap. 2**). Because of the risk of associated injuries, the spine and pelvis must be thoroughly evaluated.
   D. **Radiographs.** Fractures are identified on roentgenograms by a fracture line of increased (impaction) or decreased bone density. Consideration must be given to any distortion of the normal shape of the calcaneus. In addition to the lateral radiographs, calcaneal (axial) views and computed tomography (CT) are valuable to clarify the fracture pattern and to assess any increased width of the calcaneus. As with any severe fracture, analgesics often are required for the patient's comfort during the radiographs examination.
   E. **Treatment.** All fractures should initially be treated in a well-padded splint for the first 7 to 10 days until the swelling begins to resolve.
      1. **Isolated avulsion fractures** do not usually involve the subtalar joint.
         a. Those with **minimal displacement** may be treated by a short-leg, non–weight-bearing cast with the ankle in a neutral position for 4 to 6 weeks (1). The lack of displacement should be confirmed by a roentgenogram after the cast is applied.
         b. Avulsion fractures (tongue type) with **major displacement** require reduction and internal fixation of the displaced bone to reattach the Achilles tendon.

383

Tongue type

Joint depression type

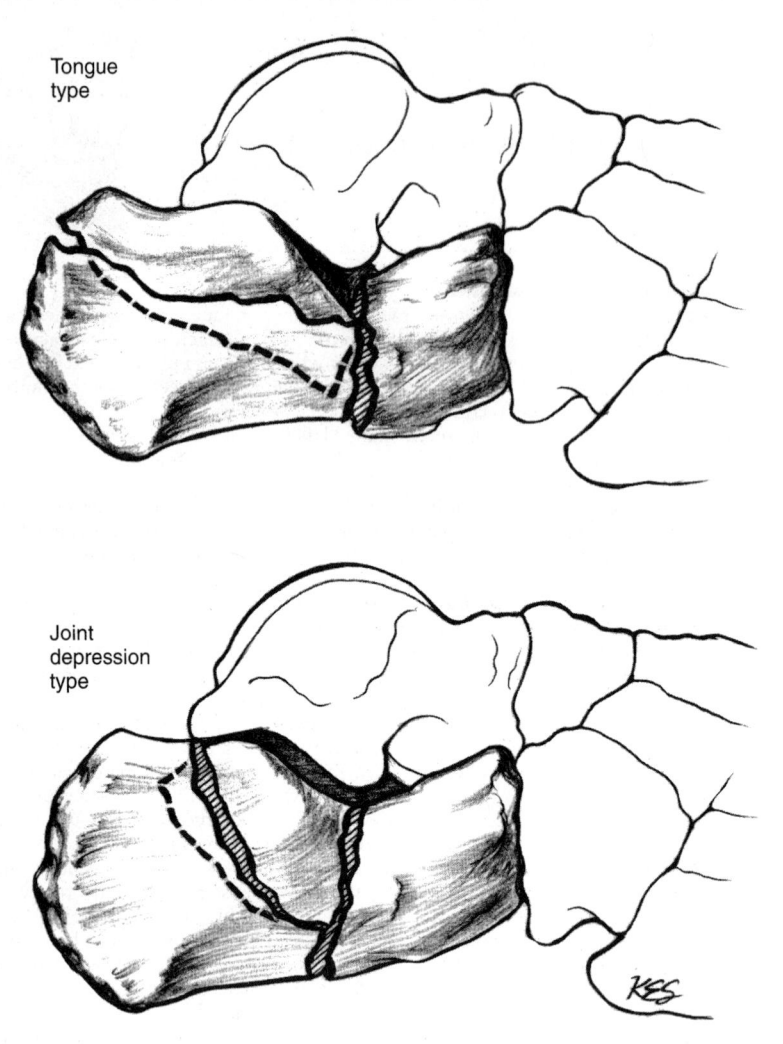

Figure 27-1. Diagrammatic representation of tongue type and joint depression type calcaneal fractures. (From Hansen ST, Swiontkowski MF. *Orthopaedic trauma protocols.* New York: Raven, 1993:355, with permission.)

This procedure, generally accomplished with two lag screws, is followed by non–weight-bearing immobilization in a short-leg cast. The foot is held in slight plantar flexion for the first 3 to 4 weeks and then in a neutral position for an additional 3 to 4 weeks. Alternatively, a percutaneous reduction maneuver as described by Essex-Lopresti provides excellent reduction (2).

2. **Fractures into the body of the calcaneus**
   a. **Treatment**
      i. The **tuber (Böhler) angle should be restored** with treatment whenever possible. The tuber angle, which is established by the lateral roentgenogram, is formed by the intersection of one line along the superior aspect of the tuber of the calcaneus with a second line

along the superior aspect of the middle and anterior portions of the calcaneus. The angle is normally 30 degrees, but it could also be compared to the uninjured side.

    ii. **With conservative treatment, restoration** of this angle is thought to be **unnecessary**, and **treatment consists of compression** to prevent edema and decrease hemorrhage, **followed by early subtalar motion** and 6 to 12 weeks of no weight bearing.

    iii. **Open reduction** for anatomic restoration is desirable to realign articular fragments and prevent peroneal impingement while allowing for normal shoe wear (**Fig. 27-2**). There is no solid evidence to suggest that patients who have open reduction and internal fixation (ORIF) have better functional results (3–5). Most experienced surgeons believe that the risk of infection that accompanies ORIF is outweighed by better foot shape and heel position.

    iv. **Early subtalar arthrodesis** may be appropriate in very severely comminuted articular fractures, but such treatment is rarely advocated.

b. The **authors advocate** a surgical reduction for intraarticular fractures only when the fracture can be anatomically reduced and held in that reduced position (4). The calcaneus is cancellous bone, and fractures of the calcaneus usually are comminuted. Attempts at reconstruction require a great deal of operative skill and knowledge of internal fixation with specialized implants. Referral to an experienced surgeon is recommended. When the surgeon is inexperienced and referral is not possible, these fractures should be treated by compression and early motion under proper supervision (1,3,6). Early motion should be started within the first 72 hours. Short-term hospital treatment appears to be worth the cost in improving the end result and shortening the period of disability following this serious and frequently disabling injury (7). The **authors recommend the following treatment program:**

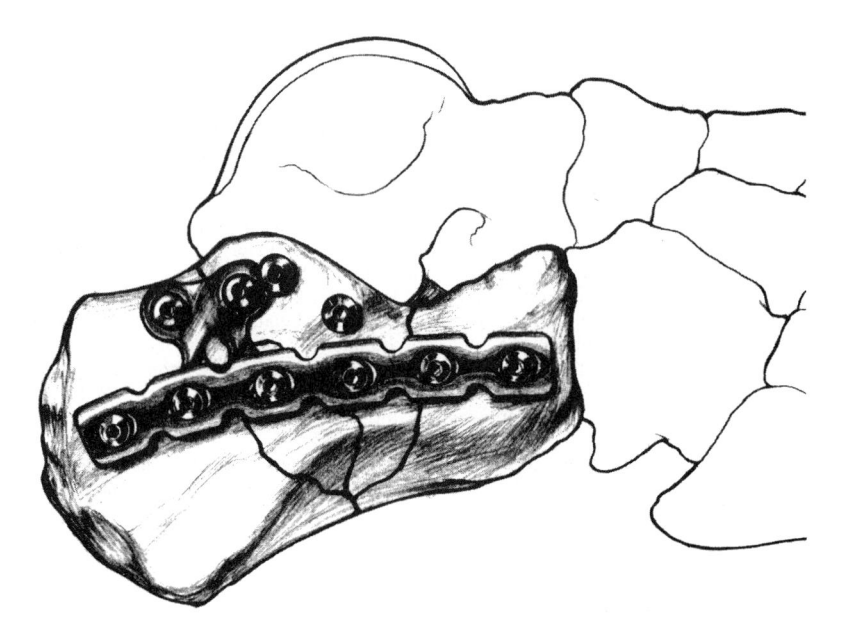

Figure 27-2. Postoperative view of standard internal fixation for a joint depression fracture. (From Hansen ST, Swiontkowski MF. *Orthopaedic trauma protocols.* New York: Raven, 1993:359, with permission.)

i. The **patient is admitted to the hospital** when necessary for adequate pain medication, elevation of the foot, and a proper compression dressing.
ii. After control of pain and **within 2 to 3 days, motion** is begun, with emphasis on inversion and eversion. Once the patient is comfortable with the therapy and after outside follow-up therapy is arranged, the patient is discharged.
iii. **Weight bearing** may be started as soon as the fracture is consolidated (usually 8–10 weeks). When partial weight bearing is begun, a sponge placed in the heel is helpful. A wheelchair is generally required for 8 to 12 weeks for patients with bilateral fractures.

F. **Complications**
  1. **Fracture blisters** and skin loss can occur.
  2. Persistent pain can arise from swelling (the **sequela of a compartmental syndrome**), deformity, and stiffness.
  3. **Problems with shoe fitting** occur because of heel widening and varus. A pedorthotist should be consulted for specialized shoes and inserts.
  4. **Persistent pain,** usually associated with loss of subtalar motion, can be severe enough to require a triple arthrodesis. This procedure does not always produce a pain-free foot and should be undertaken with caution (8). Pain frequently occurs beneath the lateral malleolus because of widening of the calcaneus with impingement of the peroneal tendons and loss of heel height. Surgical relief involving the decompression of the peroneal tendons can improve symptoms and should be considered.

G. **Calcaneal fractures in children** (9)
  1. Calcaneal fractures in children follow the same pattern and are caused by the **same mechanisms as in adults.**
  2. The **treatment** program follows the same general plan as for the adult.
  3. Unreduced intraarticular fractures persist in limiting subtalar joint motion but have **minimal symptoms** in short-term follow-up.

II. **SUBTALAR AND TALAR DISLOCATIONS**
A. **Definition**
  1. A **subtalar dislocation** occurs through the subtalar joint with the ankle and foot displaced medially or laterally. The talus can snap back by itself inside the mortise, leaving the foot displaced medially or laterally relative to the toes (10–12).
  2. In a **talar dislocation**, the talus is completely dislocated from its position within the mortise and tarsus. This is a rare injury.

B. **Mechanism of injury.** Progressive degrees of inversion forces applied to the foot cause rupture of progressively more ligaments around the talus, resulting in a subtalar-talonavicular or a complete talar dislocation. Inversion, internal rotation, and equinus forces cause rupture of the talonavicular ligament. More displacement ruptures the medial, interosseous, and lateral talocalcaneal ligaments; finally, the lateral ligaments (anterior talofibular, calcaneal-fibular, and posterior talofibular ligaments) can rupture. The talus can ultimately be forced from its major attachments and dislocate. The skin often breaks; in this event, the talus may extrude from the foot. This injury can also be associated with a fracture of the neck of the talus, which is also commonly an open injury (8,13).

C. **Examination**
  1. A **subtalar dislocation** shows a classic positioning of the foot medially or laterally on the ankle. There is always marked tenting of the skin on the side opposite the foot.
  2. With a closed **talar dislocation**, the talus comes to rest under the skin on the dorsolateral aspect of the ankle.
  3. With both injuries, swelling is always severe. These are **true emergencies.**

D. **Radiographs.** The diagnosis may be made on physical examination, but the extent of injury and the exact position of the involved bones should be confirmed by multiple roentgenographic views. Do not delay. Arrange for anesthesia even before obtaining roentgenograms.

E. **Treatment**
   1. It may be advisable to carry out a **manual reduction** by slow but firm traction in the line of the deformity with analgesia, but only if there are delays with gaining access to the operating room for anesthesia services. Reduction is easy unless there is trapping of the posterior tibial tendon around the neck of the talus in a lateral subtalar dislocation where open reduction is necessary.
   2. **After reduction**, a short-leg Jones compression splint is applied until swelling is controlled; then active range-of-motion exercises are begun.
   3. An **associated fracture must be reduced anatomically** and the reduction rigidly maintained, preferably with small fragment lag screws. Where fixation is stable, early active motion may be started using a removable posterior splint.

F. **Complications**
   1. **Ischemic skin loss** can be seen.
   2. **Avascular necrosis of the body of the talus** can occur with a talar dislocation (3,11).
   3. **Pain and stiffness** can ensue.
   4. **Subtalar arthritis** can develop.

III. **FRACTURE OF THE TALUS**
   A. **Neck of the talus** (13). Talus neck fractures are generally classified by the Hawkins' system (**Fig. 27-3**). Type I is nondisplaced and type II is displaced with associated subtalar joint subluxation. In type III, the talar body is dislocated from the ankle mortise, and in type IV the talonavicular joint is also subluxated.

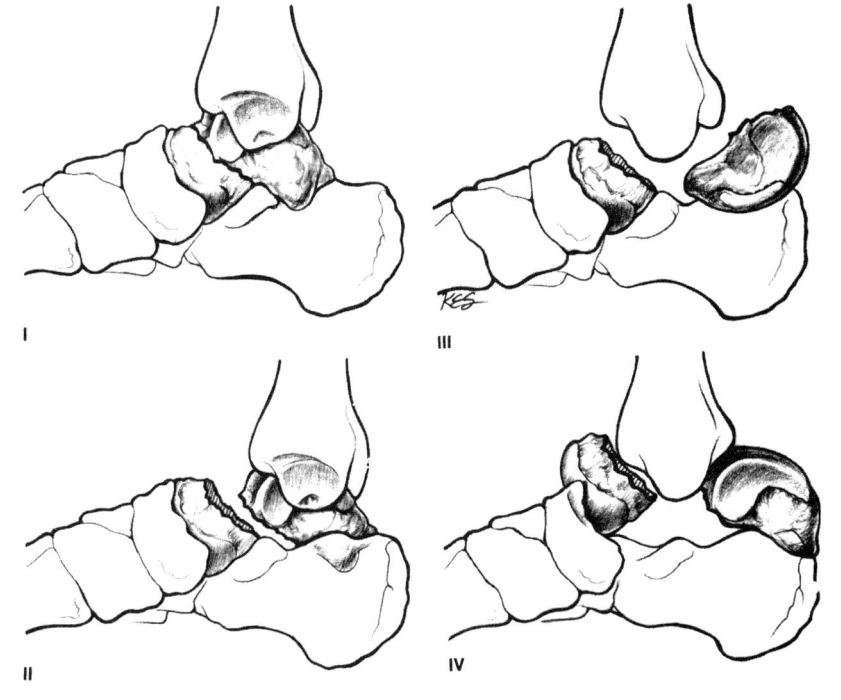

Figure 27-3. Diagrammatic representation of Hawkins' classification of talar neck fractures. **I**, nondisplaced; **II**, displaced with associated subtalar joint subluxation; **III**, talar body dislocated from the ankle mortise; **IV**, talonavicular joint subluxated also. (From Hansen ST, Swiontkowski MF. *Orthopaedic trauma protocols*. New York: Raven, 1993:340, with permission.)

1. **Mechanism of injury.** This injury is most commonly the result of forceful ankle dorsiflexion. Historically, it occurred with biplanes impacting the ground (the "aviator's astralagus"). The talus impinges on the anterior portion of the tibia, causing a fracture through the talar neck. The fracture, which may not be displaced, is easily overlooked without adequate radiographs.
2. **Treatment.** Accurate reduction and rigid immobilization are important. To preserve the function of the hind foot joints, open anatomic reduction and internal fixation are recommended. Placement of small fragment lag screws across the fracture site is advisable. Because post-traumatic avascular necrosis of the body of the talus occurs commonly, most surgeons recommend waiting for subchondral resorption of the body of the talus to be apparent in the mortise radiographs before allowing full weight bearing (Hawkins' sign). This complication is less frequent with emergent reduction and fixation of widely displaced fractures.
3. **Complications**
   a. **Dislocation of the peroneal tendons** occurs as an associated injury that should be ruled out and treated if present.
   b. **Avascular necrosis** is the most serious complication. Ankle arthrodesis can be difficult in this setting, and specialized techniques must be used (2).
B. **Other talar fractures.** Fractures may involve the body of the talus as well as the neck. Anatomic reduction is necessary for fractures involving the articular surfaces (14). Whenever the fragments are large enough and it is technically possible, ORIF usually is required. (See the foregoing discussion of Hawkins' sign.)

IV. **Fractures of the navicular, cuneiform, and cuboid bones** occur rarely as isolated injuries; the navicular is the most common. Whenever there is displacement of greater than 2 mm, the authors recommend open anatomic reduction and screw fixation (15). When associated with midfoot fractures or subluxations, reduction and fixation can be difficult. Referral to a surgeon experienced in the management of the fractures should be considered. Swelling can be severe, as with calcaneus fractures, so the procedure may be delayed 7 to 10 days while swelling subsides. Postoperative treatment involves 6 weeks in a non–weight-bearing cast or brace followed by 6 weeks in a short-leg weight-bearing boot or cast.

V. **SUBLUXATION, DISLOCATION, AND FRACTURE-DISLOCATION OF THE MIDTARSAL, TARSAL-METATARSAL, OR PHALANGEAL JOINTS** (16)
A. **Radiographs.** The usual deformities can be masked in massive swelling. Anteroposterior, lateral, and oblique radiographs of the foot are essential. It is frequently helpful to compare these with films of the normal foot. Midfoot subluxations can be subtle, and a high index of suspicion is necessary when there is a history of axial loading of the foot and midfoot tenderness. Standing films, when possible, may expose Lisfranc joint subluxation as the bones separate when force (weight bearing) is applied. Stress radiographs of the midfoot are indicated when the diagnosis is not clear.
B. **Treatment.** Manipulative reduction is done; **anesthesia** is usually used for **forefoot** dislocations. If reduction is possible and if stability is sufficient, plaster immobilization for 4 weeks is adequate. If reduction is incomplete or if there is instability, then displacement may occur, leading to malunion, persistent subluxation, and a painful planovalgus forefoot. If the reduction is unstable, then open reduction may be required and internal fixation is generally necessary.
   1. For **midtarsal dislocations and subluxations (The Lisfranc joint injury)**, accurate anatomic reduction is required to prevent the sequelae of forefoot abduction and collapse of the medial arch. Open reduction and fixation with screws is recommended (16). This allows arthrofibrosis of the injured joints, which preserves the normal slope of the foot. Although screw breakage can occur, it is generally advisable to leave the screws in place because removal can lead to planovalgus deformity. Although nearly all patients experience long-term discomfort and swelling, the normal shape of the foot makes the management of these complaints easier.

2. **Phalangeal dislocations** require only reduction and symptomatic treatment. Stiff-soled shoes are often helpful for 4 to 6 weeks postinjury. Taping of injured toes to the adjacent uninjured toe can be helpful.

VI. **FRACTURES OF THE FOREFOOT**
  A. The **diagnosis** of a forefoot fracture is usually suspected when localized bony tenderness or deformity is found.
  B. Anteroposterior, oblique, and lateral **roentgenograms** of the foot generally confirm the diagnosis.
  C. **Treatment**
   1. **Metatarsals**
      a. **Avulsion fractures of the base of the fifth metatarsal** (the insertion of the peroneus brevis) should be treated symptomatically unless there is gross (>3 mm) displacement, in which case the treatment of choice is ORIF. Symptomatic treatment usually consists of a compression dressing and elevation until the swelling is controlled, followed by a short-leg weight-bearing cast with a well-molded arch. Anything more distal than avulsion fractures have the risk of nonunion and must be managed much more carefully. This fifth metatarsal proximal neck shaft **junction** fracture (Jones fracture) is prone to delayed union and nonunion (17,18). Therefore, no weight bearing for 10 to 12 weeks is indicated. Open reduction and bone grafting is required for nonunions (17) and may be considered as a primary option in others. For example, athletic individuals may choose this option, as well as certain elderly patents who may not tolerate 10 to 12 weeks of non–weight bearing. For surgical fixation, intramedullary screw fixation is preferred.
      b. **Fractures of the metatarsal shaft** are caused by a crushing injury. As a rule, the soft-tissue injury is more severe than the fracture. Initial treatment should include a compression dressing and elevation to control swelling, which is followed by reduction if the fracture is displaced. If the great toe remains cocked up or the first web space remains widened with **fractures to the first metatarsal**, then the reduction is incomplete or unstable. Open reduction with small fragment plates for this type of unstable first metatarsal fracture is recommended. If the second through fifth metatarsal fractures are seen to have the metatarsal heads at the same level without excessive (>5 mm) shortening, then the reduction is satisfactory. If displacement is more severe, then closed reduction with axial Kirschner wire fixation may be necessary to prevent long-term transfer metatarsalgia. After proper reduction, the foot is placed in a short-leg plaster cast with well-contoured longitudinal and metatarsal arches. No weight bearing is allowed on the affected foot for 4 to 6 weeks. An additional 6 weeks is spent in a walking cast or fracture boot. Open reduction rarely is indicated for lesser metatarsal fractures unless there is marked shortening or plantar angulation.
      c. **Fractures of the metatarsal necks** can be associated with displacement of the metatarsal head toward the weight-bearing surface of the foot, which disrupts the normal mechanics of proper weight bearing.
         i. **Fractures of the first metatarsal neck or of multiple metatarsal necks** must be reduced and are usually held with some type of percutaneous wire fixation because they are often unstable. Pins can be placed through the plantar surface of the foot, through the metatarsal heads, and into the shaft of the metatarsals. Roentgenographic image intensification aids in the placement of these pins, but with proper palpation and anesthesia, it can ordinarily be accomplished percutaneously.
         ii. **An isolated metatarsal neck fracture** should be grossly aligned to avoid abnormal pressure of the metatarsal head on the sole of the foot (transfer metatarsalgia) and to avoid forcing the toe against the top of the shoe. Immobilize in a short-leg walking cast for 6 to 10 weeks.

2. **Toes**
   a. **Fractures of the toes** are treated by taping them to the adjacent toe, which acts as an adequate splint. Avoid maceration by using dry cotton or Webril between the toes.
   b. A **fracture of the great toe** often requires a short-leg cast with a platform under the toes for comfort as well as immobilization.
   c. **Fractures of the sesamoids of the great toe**
      i. **Mechanism of injury.** These fractures are usually the result of a direct force applied to this area of the foot either from a fall with landing on the metatarsal heads or from a weight being dropped on the foot. Occasionally, these injuries occur as avulsion fractures from forceful hyperextension of the great toe or from traction injuries to the flexor hallucis brevis. The fractures are usually transverse.
      ii. **Examination.** The patient experiences localized pain over the area. Differential diagnosis takes into account a congenital bipartite sesamoid. Local pain and irregular surfaces on the roentgenogram are the distinguishing features for a fracture. It is sometimes difficult to visualize on plain x-ray and a CT may be needed.
      iii. **Treatment.** No weight bearing is allowed as long as the area is painful. After initial treatment, a metatarsal pad can help relieve pressure. Occasionally, pain persists; sesamoid resection and reconstitution of the tendon are then indicated.

HCMC Treatment Recommendations
Calcaneus Fractures
   Diagnosis: Lateral and axial views of the heel, CT scan, clinical examination
   Treatment: Non–weight bearing for 12 weeks with early subtalar motion where nonoperative treatment is selected, ORIF with non–weight-bearing and passive subtalar motion for 12 weeks where ORIF indicated
   Indications for surgery: Significant widening of the heel with lateral wall "blow out," depression or gapping of the subtalar joint more than 2 to 3 mm
   Recommended technique: ORIF via lateral incision

HCMC Treatment Recommendations
Talus Fractures
   Diagnosis: Lateral and mortise radiographs, clinical examination
   Treatment: ORIF for any displaced fracture
   Indications for surgery: Fractures with more than 2-mm gapping, loose osteochondral fragment
   Recommended technique: ORIF with small fragment lag screws via medial and lateral approaches; subtalar joint must be debrided of bone/cartilage fragments; non–weight bearing for 8 to 12 weeks

---

HCMC Treatment Recommendations
Subtalar Dislocations
   Diagnosis: Lateral and axial views of the hindfoot, clinical examination
   Treatment: Closed reduction with follow-up radiographs with or without CT scan
   Indications for surgery: Irreducible dislocation, significant debris in subtalar joint
   Recommended technique: Incision on the side of the deformity, exploration of the subtalar joint after removing tissue blocking reduction—ORIF with small or minifragment screws of larger fragments

HCMC Treatment Recommendations
Tarsometatarsal (Lisfranc) Fracture/Dislocations
  Diagnosis: Lateral, oblique anteroposterior radiographs of the foot; clinical examination
  Treatment: ORIF of displaced fractures
  Indications for surgery: Displacement of first, second, third metatarsal bases with ligament disruption or major displacement of base of the first, second, third metatarsals
  Recommended technique: ORIF with small fragment screws, K wire fixation for displaced base of fifth metatarsal ligament disruptions

HCMC Treatment Recommendations
Metatarsal Fractures
  Diagnosis: Anteroposterior, lateral, oblique foot radiographs; clinical examination
  Treatment: 4 to 6 weeks of limited weight bearing
  Indications for surgery: Open fractures, shortening/comminution of first metatarsal or fifth metatarsal, multiple metatarsal fractures
  Recommended technique: ORIF with small or minifragment plates, K wires for metatarsal neck fractures

HCMC Treatment Recommendations
Toe Fractures
  Diagnosis: Anteroposterior, lateral, oblique foot radiographs; clinical examination
  Treatment: Protective orthosis or shoe wear for 6 to 8 weeks, progressive weight bearing as tolerated, buddy taping of lesser toe fractures
  Indications for surgery: Open fractures, displaced intraarticular fracture of the great toe
  Recommended technique: ORIF with K wires or minifragment screws

References

1. Sanders R. Current concepts review—displaced intra-articular fractures of the calcaneus. *J Bone Joint Surg (Am)* 2000;82:225–249.
2. Tornetta P. The Essex-Lopresti reduction for calcaneal fractures revisited. *J Orthop Trauma* 1998;12:469–473.
3. Csizy M, Buckley R, Tough S, et al. Displaced intra-articular calcaneal fractures: variables predicting late subtalar fusion. *J Orthop Trauma* 2003;17:106–112.
4. Parmar HV, Triffitt PD, Gregg PJ. Intra-articular fractures of the calcaneum treated operatively or conservatively—a prospective study. *J Bone Joint Surg (Br)* 1993;75:932–937.
5. Thordarson DB, Krieger LE. Operative vs. non-operative treatment of intra-articular fractures of the calcaneus: a prospective randomized trial. *Foot Ankle Int* 1996;17:2–9.
6. Stephenson JR. Treatment of displaced intraarticular fractures of the calcaneus using medial and lateral approaches, internal fixation and early motion. *J Bone Joint Surg (Am)* 1987;69:115–130.
7. Pozo JL, Kirwan EOG, Jackson AM. The long-term results of conservative management of severely displaced fractures of the calcaneus. *J Bone Joint Surg (Br)* 1984;66:386–390.
8. Sanders R, Pappas J, Mast J, et al. The salvage of open grade IIIB ankle and talus fractures. *J Orthop Trauma* 1992;6:201–208.

9. Wiley JJ, Profitt A. Fractures of the os calcis in children. *Clin Orthop* 1984;188:131–138.
10. DeLee JC, Curtis R. Subtalar dislocation of the foot. *J Bone Joint Surg (Am)* 1982;64:433–437.
11. Goldner JL, Polett SC, Gates HS III, et al. Severe open subtalar dislocations—long-term results. *J Bone Joint Surg (Am)* 1995;77:1075–1079.
12. Monson ST, Ryan JR. Subtalar dislocations. *J Bone Joint Surg (Am)* 1981;63:1156–1158.
13. Canale ST, Kelly FB. Fractures of the neck of the talus: long-term evaluation of seventy-one cases. *J Bone Joint Surg (Am)* 1978;60:143–156.
14. Pettine KA, Morrey BF. Osteochondral fractures of the talus. *J Bone Joint Surg (Br)* 1987;69:89–92.
15. Sangeorzan BJ, Benirschke SK, Mosca V, et al. Displaced intraarticular fractures of the tarsal navicular. *J Bone Joint Surg (Am)* 1989;71:1504–1510.
16. Arntz CT, Veith RG, Hansen ST Jr. Fractures and fracture-dislocations of the tarsometatarsal joint. *J Bone Joint Surg (Am)* 1988;70:173–181.
17. Kavanaugh JH, Brower TD, Mann RV. The Jones fracture revisited. *J Bone Joint Surg (Am)* 1978;60:776–782.
18. Torg JS, Balduini FC, Zelko RR, et al. Fractures of the base of the fifth metatarsal distal to the tuberosity. *J Bone Joint Surg (Am)* 1984;66:209–214.

Selected Historical Readings

Barnard L, Odegard JK. Conservative approach in the treatment of fractures of the calcaneus. *J Bone Joint Surg (Am)* 1970;52:1689.

Canale ST, Belding RH. Osteochondral lesions of the talus. *J Bone Joint Surg (Am)* 1980;62:97–102.

Essex-Lopresti P. The mechanism, reduction technique and results in fractures of the os calcis. *Br J Surg* 1952;39:395–419.

Hawkins LG. Fractures of the talus. *J Bone Joint Surg (Am)* 1970;52:991–1002.

Mindell ER, Cisek EE, Kartalian G, et al. Late results of injuries to the talus. *J Bone Joint Surg (Am)* 1963;45:221–245.

Noble J, McQuillan WM. Early posterior subtalar fusion in the treatment of fractures of the os calcis. *J Bone Joint Surg (Br)* 1979;61:90–93.

OVERUSE AND MISCELLANEOUS CONDITIONS OF THE FOOT AND ANKLE

28

I. **ACHILLES TENDINOPATHY** encompasses both inflammation and degeneration if present in the peritenon.
   A. **Insertional** type may be associated with a Haglund deformity or retrocalcaneal bursitis. This is a typical overuse injury caused by accumulated impact load (1), which occurs most often in runners and repetitive jumpers. Insertional type occurs more in an older age group than does noninsertional tendinopathy.
      1. **Treatment** should be **conservative** in 95% of cases. Rest, analgesics, cross training, physiotherapy, orthotics with a heel lift, and, occasionally, casting should be used. Steroid injections are very seldom indicated. (2,3).
      2. **Surgery** is indicated after 6 to 12 months of failed conservative treatment. Surgery consists of the following: excise retrocalcaneal bursa, resect superior prominence, and debride diseased or calcified portion of the tendon. Reattach if necessary. The patient should be non–weight bearing for 6 to 8 weeks. Rehabilitation is resumed but recovery might take up to 1 year. Success rate is 70% to 86%. (4)
   B. **Noninsertional** type is associated with typical hypovascular zone 2 to 6 cm proximal to insertion. The etiologic profile includes repetitive microtrauma, more common in males, older athletes, tight gastrosoleus and hamstrings, functional overpronation. Extrinsic factors include improper training, improper shoe wear, systemic or injected steroids, and fluoroquinolone antibiotics (5). There are various classification systems that could be simplified into peritendinitis (sheath only), tendinosis (tendon only), or pantendinitis (sheath and tendon) (6). Diagnosis is primarily by history and clinical evaluation and is confirmed with ultrasound (operator dependent) or magnetic resonance imaging (MRI). Typical signs and symptoms are morning stiffness or pain, start-up pain, postexercise pain, and tendon fullness or nodule.
      1. **Treatment** in **acute** situations includes pain relief, analgesics, ice, and restriction of activities. A heel lift or boot brace can be used until symptoms subside (2), followed by a rehabilitation program (7). Other measures include stretching and strengthening of the Achilles and gastrosoleus, eccentric muscle-tendon strengthening review, and modification of training regimens (reduce frequency, duration, and intensity and focus on low-impact activities), correction of structural abnormalities (overpronation), and modifications in foot wear. Treatment is 90% to 95% successful, but it usually takes 2 to 6 months to recover from an Achilles tendinopathy.
      2. **Treatment** of **chronic** cases (>3 months) depends on severity. Peritendinitis is treated with mechanical "brisement" or surgical debridement followed by an early rehabilitation program (7). Chronic pantendinitis is treated with debridement, longitudinal tenotomy (8), or tendon transfer depending on the clinical situation. It appears from the literature that surgical treatment of chronic tendinitis might do better than nonoperative treatment.

II. **PLANTAR HEEL PAIN** is a common foot problem in the athlete. Running and jumping place repetitive stress on the heel and create an overuse syndrome with chronic inflammation.
   A. **Differential diagnosis.** To differentiate, a thorough history and examination is required. This should include exact location and duration of pain and the relationship

to athletic activity. Chronic pain at rest is unusual and might be due to a tumor. The differential diagnosis includes the following:
1. Plantar fasciitis—by far the most common reason for plantar heel pain
2. Nerve entrapment
3. Fat pad atrophy
4. Heel bruise
5. Tendinopathy of flexor hallucis longus or flexor digitorum brevis
6. Stress fracture
7. Tumor

B. **Plantar fasciitis** could be at insertion into medial calcaneal tuberosity or midfoot and may be due to repetitive traction and microtears. Usually, plantar fasciitis has an insidious onset as an overuse condition in long distance runners. Midfoot plantar fasciitis is more common in sprinters who run on their toes.
   1. **Symptoms and signs** include pain during the first minutes of walking, especially when first getting out of bed. Pain may subside with low-intensity walking but then recur with prolonged or more vigorous activities.
   2. Always evaluate for **leg length discrepancy**. Heel pain is more common in the shorter leg and may be treated with an appropriate lift. Also inquire about a functional short leg syndrome from running on the same tilt of the road. Plantar fasciitis is frequently caused by a shortened Achilles tendon because limited ankle dorsiflexion increases the stress on the plantar fascia. Fasciitis at the insertion has localized deep tenderness. It is usually not associated with increased pain or with passive dorsiflexion of the toes (windlass mechanism). Midfoot fasciitis has tenderness in midfoot and increased pain with passive dorsiflexion of the toes. Passive dorsiflexion of the big toe aggravates both plantar fasciitis and flexor hallucis longus tendinopathy. Resisted flexion of the big toe is painful only with involvement of the tendon.

C. **Treatment**
   1. **Conservative.** The cornerstone of treatment is modification in training, for example, reducing mileage, shortening workouts, and alternating activities such as low resistance cycling and swimming pool running (9). There is not a single entity that works for everyone, but conservative measures usually include the following:
      a. A shock-absorbing heel cup for heel pain or a full length orthotic or UCBL (University of California Berkeley Laboratory) orthotic for midsubstance pain.
      b. Though not proven uniquely effective, analgesics, as they do decrease pain.
      c. Physical therapy to include Achilles and plantar fascia stretching, hindfoot taping, contrast baths, and ultrasound treatment.
      d. A night dorsiflexion splint might help to keep the fascia under tension to reduce early morning weight-bearing pain.
      e. Injections may be used in refractory cases. This has historically been done with steroids, although steroids pose a risk of plantar fascia rupture. Consistent with the fact that this has been noted to be a degenerative rather than an inflammatory process, there is no data demonstrating that the anti-inflammatory component of the steroid is necessary. For these reasons, many physicians are moving away from injections, or injecting but without the steroid component.
      f. Shockwave therapy, which tries to spur on inflammatory response, might prove to be helpful in the future.

      The heel spur seen on roentgenograms is seldom, if ever, the cause of heel pain.
   2. **Surgical.** Plantar fascia release should be avoided in competitive athletes because it may increase the compressive forces to the dorsal aspect of the midfoot and decrease flexion forces on the metatarsophalangeal joint complex (10). When indicated, the plantar fascia is released from the calcaneus through a medial incision. The patient is allowed to bear weight as tolerated with crutches, and rehabilitation is started after 2 weeks.

D. **Calcaneal fat pad trauma.** The patient complains of diffuse plantar heel pain that is exacerbated with weight bearing and with activities on hard surfaces.
  1. **Examination** reveals diffuse tenderness localized to the fat pad. There is no radiation of the pain. The heel pad feels soft and thin, and the underlying calcaneus is palpable.
  2. **Treatment** is nonsurgical. A cushioned heel cup and shock-absorbing shoes might help. The patient should reduce activities and avoid hard running surfaces.
E. **Nerve entrapment syndromes**
  1. Entrapment of the **first branch of the lateral plantar nerve** is a common cause of chronic heel pain in athletes (11). The site of compression is between the deep fascia of the abductor hallucis muscle and the medial margin of the quadratus plantae muscle. This injury is more common in athletes who spend a significant amount of time on their toes such as ballet dancers, figure skaters, and sprinters.
     a. **Diagnosis** is made on clinical grounds. Exclude the more common reasons for heel pain. Early morning pain is less problematic; the pain increases as the day goes on. Tenderness is specific over the area of compression and may radiate down toward the toes (the Tinel sign).
     b. **Treatment** is similar to that for other causes of heel pain. If conservative treatment fails, a release of the nerve may be done through a medial incision.
  2. **Tarsal tunnel syndrome** could also be a source of heel pain. Compression of the posterior tibial nerve within the tarsal tunnel results in tenderness over the area that may shoot down toward the toes on the plantar aspect of the foot. Excessive pronation in long-distance runners may place repeated stress on the medial structures of the hindfoot.
     a. On **examination**, there might be burning, pain, or tingling on the plantar aspect of the foot. Pain is more diffuse than with the other causes of heel pain. Electromyography and nerve conduction studies can be helpful but are not always sensitive enough.
     b. **Treatment.** A medial heel wedge or an arch support may decrease the tension on the medial side of the ankle and therefore the nerve. Physical therapy can also improve the biomechanics. Steroid injection into the tarsal tunnel might give short-term pain relief. Tarsal tunnel release is helpful in recalcitrant cases.
  3. **Metatarsalgia**
     a. Metatarsalgia or pain over the metatarsal heads is the most common forefoot problem. It typically occurs on the second metatarsal head and can have numerous etiologies.
        i. A **tight or shortened Achilles tendon** limits ankle dorsiflexion, which, in turn, increases the forces on the forefoot. A person compensates by using the long toe extensors to augment dorsiflexion power, but this pulls the plantar fat pad away from the weight-bearing surface under the metatarsal heads, further aggravating forefoot pain.
        ii. Similarly, **idiopathic claw toe deformities** could displace the fat pad and cause metatarsalgia.
        iii. **Metatarsophalangeal joint capsulitis** might cause pain over the plantar aspect of the joint. This is more common at the second metatarsophalangeal joint and is associated with a long second metatarsal or instability of the first ray.
        iv. A **Morton (or common digital nerve) neuroma** causes pain in the web space and is most common in the third web space (between the third and fourth metatarsals).
     b. The differential diagnosis of midfoot to forefoot pain always includes **stress fractures** (see **IV** below).
     c. **Treatment.** The goal is to unload the metatarsal area. Orthotics, metatarsal bars, cushioned shoes, analgesics, and Achilles stretching are the cornerstones of initial management. If conservative management does not help, surgical correction of claw toes or excision of neuroma might be indicated.

III. **TIBIALIS POSTERIOR DYSFUNCTION SYNDROME.** Rupture of the tibialis posterior (TP) tendon is a cause of a painful, acquired flatfoot deformity in adults. It is more common in women 40 years of age and older (12–14). Numerous reports describing the condition have been published over the past 20 years, but it still remains a condition that is not commonly recognized. This could be due to the insidious nature of the condition, usually without a history of acute trauma (12).

A. **Anatomy.** By virtue of its lever arm length and muscle strength, the TP tendon is the main dynamic stabilizer of the hindfoot against valgus deformity. It also plays a major role in maintaining the medial longitudinal arch. Insufficiency of the TP results in excessive strain on the static ligament–bone hind- and midfoot constraints. The soft tissue gradually elongates, the arch flattens, and the peroneus longus and brevis tendons have an unopposed abduction force on the forefoot.

B. **Etiology of TP tendon rupture.** To understand the etiology of TP tendon tears, it is important to remember its function. It resists considerable forces in maintaining the medial longitudinal arch. It also helps lock the mid- and hindfoot to allow a solid lever arm during the push-off part of the gait cycle. Approximately 20% of TP ruptures are associated with rheumatic conditions (12). An estimated 80% of TP tendon ruptures develop spontaneously. There are several theories to explain this phenomenon.

1. **Mechanical.** The acute angle around the medial malleolus could lead to excessive friction that leads to slow deterioration over many years. This also explains the age predilection of this condition.
2. **Vascular.** Laboratory studies have identified an area of poor blood supply to the tendon behind the medial malleolus. This could lead to a decrease in healing potential after minor trauma.
3. **Achilles tendon contracture.** Either due to gastrocnemius alone or in combination with soleus, a contracture or shortness of the Achilles tendon increases the workload and force on the TP during the gait cycle.

C. **Clinical presentation.** Contrary to popular belief, TP tendon rupture or insufficiency is common in American society. A proper history and thorough physical examination is usually all that is needed to make this a straightforward diagnosis.

1. **History.** Onset is insidious, with discomfort reported on the medial side of the foot without any preceding acute trauma. Women are affected more often then men, and persons in their 40s are most often affected. There is not necessarily a relation to activity level.
2. **Symptoms.** Initially, patients complain of only mild to moderate pain and of swelling and discomfort on the medial side of the foot and ankle. It is usually not incapacitating; rather, there is a chronic medial weight-bearing ache that limits physical activities. Without treatment, the symptoms might increase over a variable length of time. In a late stage, the patient might complain of additional weight-bearing pain on the lateral aspect of the ankle, a progressive deformity, and an abnormal gait.
3. **Signs**
   a. In an early stage, one can see and palpate the swelling behind the medial malleolus and over the course of the TP tendon to its insertion in the navicular. The tenderness is usually over the same area.
   b. In a more advanced stage, the hallmark deformity becomes apparent. This is a combination of hindfoot valgus, forefoot abduction, and flattening of the medial longitudinal arch.
   c. Much information can be gathered by observing the patient. When viewed from posterior, the amount of heel valgus above the normal neutral to 5 degrees in the weight-bearing position can be noted. The "too many toes" sign is indicative of forefoot abduction. The patient is also asked to raise on the toes. A normal TP locks the hindfoot in varus to give a solid lever for push-off. With an insufficient TP, the heel does not move into varus, and it is impossible to raise oneself on the toes.
   d. Frontal and side views confirm the forefoot abduction and loss of medial arch. An apropulsive, antalgic gait is usually noticed if the patient is asked to walk at a rapid pace.

e. Physical examination further confirms the clinical suspicion. Tendon and muscle power around the ankle is tested. The TP is evaluated with the foot in plantar flexion, and the patient is asked to invert the foot against resistance. Look for recruitment of the tibialis anterior to augment this action.
f. The flexibility of the Achilles tendon is tested with the knee first extended to determine the role of the gastrocnemius in possible tightness, and then with the knee flexed to isolate the soleus by eliminating the influence of the gastrocs.
g. Range of movement of the ankle, especially the subtalar joint, is evaluated, and any pain is noted. In advanced cases, there might be tenderness on the lateral aspect of the ankle as a result of impingement of the fibula on the calcaneus.

4. **Diagnostic workup.** Thorough history and clinical examination is usually all that is needed to make the diagnosis.
    a. **Plain roentgenographs.** In most cases beyond stage 1, weight-bearing radiographs show specific changes. The most obvious is the change in the talo-first metatarsal alignment on the anteroposterior and lateral views. In a normal foot, the talo-first metatarsal alignment is in a straight line. In TP tendon ruptures, the alignment is altered to varying degrees because of the peritalar subluxation.
    b. **MRI** confirms a tear or degeneration in the TP tendon and shows the abnormal alignment of the bony elements, but it is costly and usually unnecessary. It is helpful in early, subtle injuries of the tendon and to rule out other causes of medial midfoot pain such as navicular stress fractures.
    c. **Computed tomography** (CT) is not necessary as a primary diagnostic tool, but it can be helpful to determine the integrity of the peritalar joints and, therefore, in **planning** the surgical procedure. It is of great value in the continuing study of the changes in the foot secondary to TP tendon ruptures.

5. **Classification**
    a. **Stage 1a: mild, occult (13%).** Symptoms last less than 1 year, there is mild swelling and tenderness over the TP tendon and slight weakness in inversion power, and there is minimal hindfoot valgus on weight bearing.
    b. **Stage 1b: moderate (44%).** Symptoms last up to 18 months, and there is definite tenderness, swelling, and weakness of the TP tendon. Moderate pes planus and heel valgus occur as a result of dorsolateral peritalar subluxation.
    c. **Stage 2: advanced (17%).** Symptoms last for 1.5 to 2.5 years. There is more pronounced flatfoot deformity caused by peritalar subluxation, and there is considerable heel valgus and moderate prominence of the talar head medially. The subtalar joint is usually still mobile and the deformities passively correctable.
    d. **Stage 3a: complete (15%).**
    e. **Stage 3b: peritalar dislocation (11%).** Progressive dorsolateral peritalar subluxation reaches the point of dislocation in the neglected case. Symptoms last between 4 and 20 years. Pain occurs also on the lateral side as a result of impingement of the calcaneus on the distal fibula. The fibula takes an increasing amount of load on weight bearing. It becomes hypertrophic, and stress fractures are not uncommon. The talocalcaneal relation is completely distorted, with minimal actual articular contact. The majority of these deformities are fixed and not passively correctable.

6. **Treatment**
    a. Nonsurgical. Other than certain grade 1a tears, nonsurgical management of TP tendon tears is essentially palliative. In most cases, it will neither result in healing of the tendon nor correction of the deformity. Noninvasive means are therefore only useful if there are factors present that contraindicate surgical intervention. This includes advanced age, significant medical problems, low activity level, and minimal discomfort. It is still advisable to start most patients on conservative treatment before electing to do surgery.

Treatment should be directed to control pain, inflammation, and development of deformity. Options include the use of crutches, minimal weight bearing, or casting in a recent onset case. Nonsteroidal anti-inflammatory drugs (NSAIDs) might help relieve pain and swelling. In more advanced cases, orthotics come into play. These include heel or sole lifts, inserts, UCBL type heel cups, and modified, accommodative shoes. In severe deformities, shoe modifications that incorporate calipers could be used.

    b. **Surgical.** Surgical treatment options include tendon repair, tendon augmentation, and bony stabilization of both nonessential and essential joints.

        i. Stage 1. A tendon repair is still feasible. The TP tendon is usually augmented with a second tendon. A multitude of augmenting techniques have been described (12,14). This includes the use of the flexor digitorum longus, flexor hallucis longus, or peroneus longus that serve as dynamic stabilizers. Free tendon grafts are also used to repair the TP tendon, although the results are variable. It is of utmost importance to evaluate for tightness of the Achilles tendon and to lengthen it if necessary.

        ii. Stage 2. In more advanced cases, tendon repair and augmentation is usually not sufficient to relieve pain and prevent deformity. The surgical option is dependent upon the degree and mobility of the deformity. If the peritalar subluxation is still correctable, the bony stabilization is done in nonessential joints. This includes the lateral column distraction fusion that reduces the peritalar subluxation and heel valgus without compromising the important subtalar and talonavicular movement. Other options include a medial column or a subtalar fusion, with or without an Achilles lengthening.

        iii. Stage 3. The surgical treatment of subtotal peritalar dislocation with a fixed hindfoot deformity (grade 3b) usually requires a triple arthrodesis.

IV. STRESS FRACTURES

A. Description. The foot and ankle are the most common areas for stress fractures. A stress fracture is defined as a partial or complete fracture resulting from its inability to withstand repetitive stress applied in a repeated, subthreshold manner. It is, therefore, a series of events causing stress fractures. Ninety-five percent of stress fractures are in the lower extremities, +/− 50% are of the foot and ankle. All the bones of the foot and ankle can sustain stress fractures. The metatarsals, though, are involved in 55% of cases, whereas the sesamoids and talus are involved in less than 1%. Stress fractures occur in all sports but especially in running and running-based sports (15). Sedentary people starting a fitness program are more prone to stress fractures. This is a well-demonstrated phenomenon in new military recruits. Stress fractures are more likely to develop in women. Leg length discrepancy, malalignment, prior injury, cavus feet that lack normal pronation, as well as poor physical condition, predispose to stress fracture.

B. Diagnosis

1. The history is fairly typical, with pain being intensified by ongoing training. There might be an association with a recent increase in duration and intensity of training. It is usually insidious with an increase of pain over a period of time.
2. There should always be a high index of suspicion for stress fractures with insidious onset of pain. Physical examination should localize the involved area.
3. **Standard radiographs** should be the first-line imaging test for evaluation of possible stress fractures. However, one must be aware of their lack of sensitivity. Callous formation is the abnormality seen on plain films and represents the active bone healing the injury. Plain films will thus be normal for the first few weeks. Furthermore, a large percentage will always appear normal on x-rays. Thus, if one's clinical evaluation is suspicious for stress fracture, further imaging is often necessary (16).
4. **Bone scans.** The gold standard for recognizing a stress reaction in bone used to be a technetium bone scan. The bone scan becomes positive after a week of ongoing stress reaction in the bone. A negative bone scan effectively rules out a stress fracture (16).

5. **MRI.** It is useful to list the indication, as special short time inversion recovery (STIR) images may be helpful. It is the most sensitive and specific method of diagnosing and grading stress fractures and is especially helpful in the feet (17).
6. The combination of a negative roentgenogram and positive bone scan represents an early fracture, and treatment at this stage may prevent longstanding problems. CT scan has a place in diagnosing talus and midfoot fractures because these bones are cancellous in structure and stress fractures are difficult to identify on plain radiographs.
7. The most critical or at-risk stress fractures of the foot are of the navicular, proximal second metatarsal (18) and intraarticular fractures, and the great toe sesamoids. The navicular is particularly difficult to diagnose (19). Workup should include plain films, MRI bone scan, and CT scan. Significant disability can result from delayed diagnosis.

C. Treatment
1. Treatment greatly depends on the location of the stress fracture. Treatment should include 6 weeks of casting followed by verification of union by CT. Resumption of leg-based athletics is at 12 to 18 weeks after initiation of treatment. Custom orthotics should be used when the patient returns to athletics (16).
2. Noncritical fractures include distal metatarsals 2, 3, and 4, the lateral malleolus, and the calcaneus (20). Treatment should be aimed at keeping the level of activity below that which causes pain. This implies decreasing the level of activity or substituting swimming, biking, circuit training, or other low impact activities. Orthotics within shoes can limit stress in the involved area (19). Activities can progress as long as they are not painful. There are reasons to try to limit NSAIDs as their anti-inflammatory properties can inhibit bone healing and their pain relief properties may give the patients a false level of reassurance (21).

V. GREAT TOE METATARSOPHALANGEAL JOINT PROBLEMS

A. Turf toe is defined by some as a sprain of the plantar capsuloligamentous complex. Others use the term to be more encompassing for a variety of injuries around the first metatarsophalangeal joint. Differential diagnosis includes injury to the medial or lateral ligamentous structures, the phalangeal sesamoid ligament, a fractured sesamoid, osteochondral or chondral injury, chondral contusion caused by direct linear impact, and dislocations and injury to the interphalangeal joint (22). This injury is common in football players but is also seen in basketball and track athletes. Careful history and clinical evaluation is necessary to localize injury. Anteroposterior, lateral, oblique, and sesamoid views should be obtained.
1. Initial **conservative treatment** consists of the general approach: rest, ice, compression, and elevation. A postoperative shoe with firm sole to limit movement helps in ligamentous injuries. The patient's foot is immobilized for 3 weeks and rehabilitation is started as tolerated. Sesamoid fractures are treated with a cast shoe with the great toe in 10 degrees of flexion for 8 to 10 weeks.
2. **Surgical treatment** consists of debridement and drilling of articular surface if pain persists in a case of chondral fracture. Partial excision or internal fixation of sesamoid fracture is undertaken when the fracture does not heal.

B. Hallux rigidus is degenerative arthritis of the first metatarsophalangeal joint. In most cases, there is no specific predisposing factor.
1. Possible etiologies include congenital flattening of the metatarsal head, metatarsus primus elevatus, osteochondritis of the head, a long hallux, pes planus, and osteochondral injuries (turf toe).
2. Hallux rigidus presents a significant problem for an athlete. Dorsiflexion of the big toe plays an important role in activities such as accelerating and jumping. Compensation by rolling onto the lateral aspect of the foot might cause stress and strain on the ankle, knee, and hip.
3. **Diagnosis.** Enlargement around the metatarsophalangeal joint is usually obvious. This is due to a combination of bony prominences and synovitis. Dorsiflexion is limited and reproduces the patient's pain. Radiographic findings might be minimal in early stages. With time, obvious degenerative changes and osteophytes within the joint become apparent. Sesamoids are generally not involved.

4. Differential diagnosis includes gout or other inflammatory arthritis.
5. **Treatment**
   a. **Conservative.** Pressure against the toe is alleviated by modifying foot wear, incorporating a higher and wider toe box, a stiffer shoe, a rigid insert, or a rocker bottom sole. NSAIDs or injected steroids might give symptomatic relief.
   b. **Surgical.** Fusion is a good option in older people but would significantly impair athletic performance. In athletes, a cheilectomy with or without a dorsiflexion osteotomy of the proximal phalanges (Moberg procedure) is preferred (23,24). The patient is permitted to ambulate weight bearing as tolerated in a postoperative shoe. Rehabilitation starts 7 to 10 days after surgery with active and passive range-of-motion exercises. The patient should wear a soft shoe to allow motion at the metatarsophalangeal joint with walking. Athletes could resume cycling, swimming, and any activity that avoids significant impact against the metatarsophalangeal joint, but should avoid running, jumping, and similar activities for 10 to 12 weeks. Metatarsophalangeal joint arthroplasties (excision or prosthetic replacement) have very limited application in the young, active population.

VI. **HALLUX VALGUS (BUNIONS).** The etiology of hallux valgus is still debated, but there appears to be a significant hereditary component. Shoe wear has been suggested as an etiological factor, as a tight toe box and a high heel will place an increased laterally and distally directed force on the great toe. Joint laxity is associated with an increased rate of hallux valgus. Not all hallux valgus deformities are symptomatic. Typically, patients will describe pain over the medial bunion that corresponds to bursal inflammation. In more severe deformities the main complaint is that of second and third ray metatarsalgia.
   A. **Evaluation**
      1. History
         a. What causes pain?
         b. Shoe wear: type and any recent changes?
         c. What activities does it affect?
      2. Physical exam
         a. Compare shoe size to foot size. Any change in shoes due to bunions?
         b. Evaluate callus pattern: lesser metatarsal overload, great toe pronation
         c. Evaluate gait: excessive pronating, → more force on the medial rays, → increased valgus angulation of first Metatarsophalangeal (MTP) joint. Evaluate kinetic chain of gait from the pelvis down.
      3. X-rays
         a. Angle of long axis of first and second metatarsals
   B. **Treatment**
      1. **Conservative**
         a. Shoe modification is the most important. The shoes should be big enough, have a low heel, and a wide and high toe box.
         b. Orthotics to support the medial arch and unload the lesser metatarsal heads might be of benefit.
         c. Bunion pads might help for medial eminence pain.
         d. Silastic spacers could be used between the toes.
         e. Physical therapy if biomechanical factors seem to be resulting in excessive foot pronation
      2. **Surgical**
         a. Should never be for cosmetic reasons
         b. Refer to an orthopaedic surgeon or podiatrist if there is not adequate pain relief after 6 months of appropriate conservative care.

VII. **CLAW AND HAMMER TOES.** The claw toe represents a hyperextension deformity of the MTP joint and a flexion deformity of the proximal interphalangeal (PIP) joint. This frequently involves multiple toes and is usually an indication of a muscle imbalance between the intrinsic or extrinsic muscles of the toes. The most common complaint is pain and friction over the dorsum of the PIP joint. With time, the plantar fat pad dislocates distally and exposes the metatarsal heads. This results in significant metatarsalgia.

A hammer toe deformity consists of a flexion deformity of the PIP joint; often with this the MTP joint and the distal interphalangeal (DIP) joint are spared. The most common cause of a hammer toe deformity is a result of the toe hitting against the tip of the shoe resulting in a flexion deformity. These patients typically will have symptoms as a result of a painful corn at the tip of the toe or a callus along the dorsum of the toe as indicated in this patient.

A. Evaluation
1. General
   a. Neurologic abnormalities
   b. Muscle imbalance, specifically gastrosoleus contracture
   c. Intrinsic muscle imbalance
   d. Diabetes
   e. Vascular compromise
2. Local
   a. Flexible (correctible) deformity: usually does well with conservative treatment
   b. Rigid (impossible to passively correct the PIP or DIP deformity)

B. Conservative treatment
1. Shoe modifications: should be big enough, low heel, wide and high toe box. This is especially important for the rigid deformities.
2. Orthotics with a metatarsal bar might help to reduce the plantar fat pad and reduce the metatarsal pain.
3. Silatic spaces and claw toe splints might be helpful.

C. Surgical treatment. Only indicated if conservative measures fail

References

1. Clain MR, Baxter DE. Achilles tendinitis. *Foot Ankle Int* 1992;13:482–487.
2. Mohr RN. Achilles tendonitis—rationale for use and application or orthotics. *Foot Ankle Clin* 1997;2:439–456.
3. Shrier I, Matheson GO, Kohl HW III. Achilles tendonitis: are corticosteroid injections useful or harmful?. *Clin J Sport Med* 1996;6:245–250.
4. McGarvey WC, Palumbo RC, Baxter DE, Leibman BD. Insertional Achilles tendinosis: surgical treatment through a central tendon splitting approach. *Foot Ankle Int* 2002;23:19–25.
5. McCarvey WC, Singh D, Trevino SG. Partial Achilles tendon rupture associated with fluoroquinolone antibiotics: a case report and literature review. *Foot Ankle Int* 1996;17:496–498.
6. Clement DB, Taunton JE, Smart GW. Achilles tendinitis and peritendinitis: etiology and treatment. *Am J Sports Med* 1984;12:179–184.
7. Johnston E, Scranton P, Pfeffer GB. Chronic disorders of the Achilles tendon: results of conservative and surgical treatments. *Foot Ankle Int* 1997;18:570–574.
8. Maffulli N, Testa V, Capasso G, et al. Results of percutaneous longitudinal tenotomy for Achilles tendinopathy in middle-and long-distance runners. *Am J Sports Med* 1997;25:835–840.
9. Pfeffer G, Bacchetti P, Deland J, et al. Comparison of custom and prefabricated orthotics in the initial treatment of proximal plantar fasciitis. *Foot Ankle Int* 1999;20(4):214–221.
10. Daly PJ, Kitaoka HB, Chao EYS. Plantar fasciotomy for intractable plantar fasciitis: clinical results and biomechanical evaluation. *Foot Ankle* 1992;13:188–195.
11. Baxter DE, Pfeffer GB. Treatment of chronic heel pain by surgical release of the first branch of the lateral plantar nerve. *Clin Orthop* 1992;279:229–236.
12. Johnson KA. Tibialis posterior tendon rupture. *Clin Orthop* 1983;177:140–147.
13. Sangeorzan BJ, Smith D, Veith R, et al. Triple arthrodesis using internal fixation in treatment of adult foot disorders. *Clin Orthop* 1993;294:299–307.
14. Thordarson DB, Schmotzer H, Chon J. Reconstruction with tenodesis in an adult flatfoot model. A biomechanical evaluation of four methods. *J Bone Joint Surg (Am)* 1995;77:1557–1567.

15. Ting A, King W, Yocum L, et al. Stress fractures of the tarsal navicular in long-distance runners. *Clin Sports Med* 1988;7:89–101.
16. Santi M, Sartoris DJ. Diagnostic imaging approach to stress fractures of the foot. *J Foot Surg* 1991;30:85–97.
17. Arendt EA, Griffiths HJ. Use of MR imaging in the assessment and clinical management of stress reactions of bone in high-performance athletes. *Clin Sports Med* 1997;16:291–306.
18. Micheli LJ, Sohn RS, Solomon R. Stress fractures of the second metatarsal involving lisfranc's joint in ballet dancers. *J Bone Joint Surg (Am)* 1985;67:1372–1375.
19. Schwellnus MP, Jordaan G, Noakes TD. Prevention of common overuse injuries by the use of shock absorbing insoles. *Am J Sports Med* 1990;18:636–641.
20. DeLee JC, Evans JP, Julian J. Stress fracture of the fifth metatarsal. *Am J Sports Med* 1983;11:349–353.
21. Dahners LE, Mullis BH. Effects of nonsteroidal anti-inflammatory drugs on bone formation and soft-tissue healing. *J Am Acad Orthop Surg* 2004;12(3):139–143.
22. Rodeo SA, O'Brien S, Warren RF, et al. Turf-toe: an analysis of metatarsophalangeal joint sprains in professional football players. *Am J Sports Med* 1990;18:280–285.
23. Mann RA, Clanton TO. Hallux rigidus: treatment by cheilectomy. *J Bone Joint Surg (Am)* 1988;70:400–406.
24. Mulier T, Steenwerckx A, Thienpont E, et al. Result after cheilectomy in athletes with hallux rigidus. *Foot Ankle Int* 1999;20(4):232–237.

Selected Historical Readings

Anzel SH, Covey KW, Weiner AD, et al. Disruption of muscle and tendons. An analysis of 1,014 cases. *Surgery* 1959;45:406–414.

Astrom M, Gentz CF, Nilsson P. Imaging in chronic Achilles tendinopathy: a comparison of ultrasonograpy, magnetic resonance imaging and surgical findings in 27 histologically verified cases. *Skeletal Radiol* 1996;25:615–620.

Bennett GL, Graham CE, Mauldin DM. Triple arthrodesis in adults. *Foot Ankle* 1991;12(3):138–143.

Bonney G, McNab I. Hallux valgus and hallux rigidus. *J Bone Joint Surg (Br)* 1952;34:366–385.

Dameron TB Jr. Fractures and anatomical variations of the proximal portion of the fifth metatarsal. *J Bone Joint Surg (Am)* 1975;57:788–792.

Key JA. Partial rupture of the tendon of the posterior tibial muscle. *J Bone Joint Surg (Am)* 1953;35:1006–1008.

Leach RE, Seavey NS, Salter DK. Results of surgery in athletes with plantar fasciitis. *Foot Ankle* 1986;7:155–161.

Lehman RC, Torg JS, Pavlov H, et al. Fractures of the base of the fifth metatarsal distal to the tuberosity: a review. *Foot Ankle* 1987;7:245–252.

Lutter LD. Surgical decisions in athletes' subcalcaneal pain. *Am J Sports Med* 1986;14:481–485.

Puddu G, Ippolito E, Postacchini F. A classification of Achilles tendon disease. *Am J Sports Med* 1976;4:145–150.

ASPIRATION AND INJECTION OF UPPER AND LOWER EXTREMITIES

29

I. **GENERAL GUIDELINES**
   A. For any injection, consider infiltrating the subcutaneous skin of the entry site. It will improve the patient's comfort, and it will allow one to make several attempts without extra discomfort for the patient.
   B. When using corticosteroids, be aware of the possibility of subcutaneous atrophy or skin color changes if the medication is left subcutaneously.
   C. In an obese patient, be prepared to use spinal needles.
   D. Use larger gauge needles with large syringes (20 cc and above) if an aspiration of a joint is going to be performed as blood or pus presents a thicker texture than synovial fluid.
      When trying to rule out a septic joint, avoid having the entry site over the area of cellulitis as this will contaminate the joint and eventually the sample sent to the lab.
II. **THE SHOULDER JOINT** (i.e., the glenohumeral joint) may be entered either anteriorly or posteriorly as depicted in **Fig. 29-1**. When using the anterior approach,

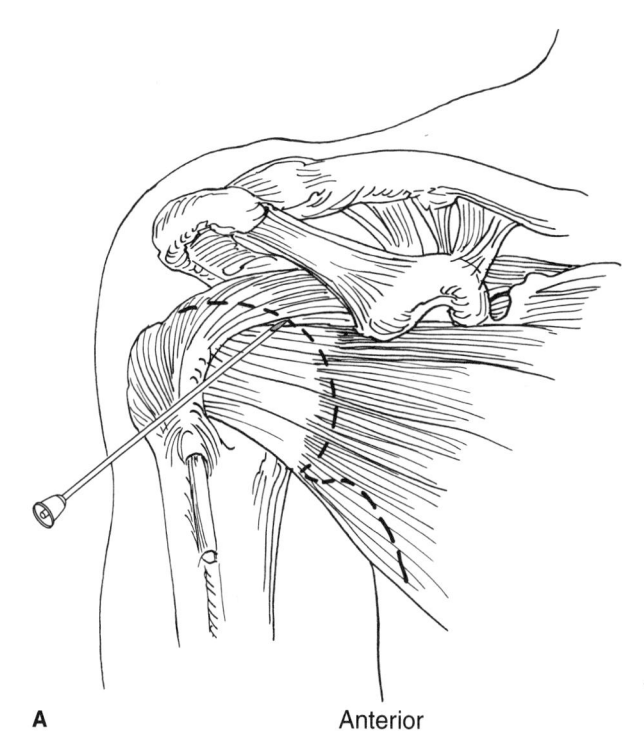

A   Anterior

Figure 29-1. Shoulder joint and subacromial space.

403

404 Chapter 29: Aspiration and Injection of Upper and Lower Extremities

— 2 cm
— 1 cm

B

Posterior

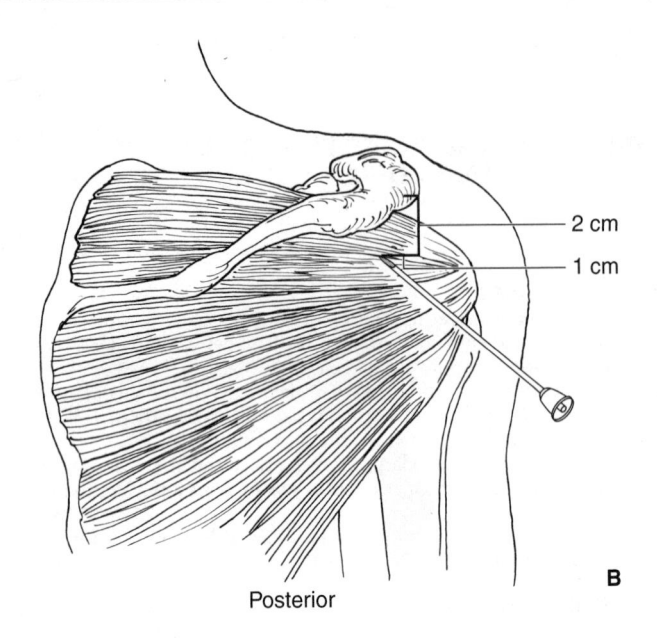

Figure 29-1. *(continued)*

palpate the medial aspect of the humeral head and enter just medial to this. In our experience, more physicians now prefer a posterior approach. A posterior aspiration or infiltration of the shoulder is performed with an entry site located approximately 2 cm distal and 1 cm medial to the posterior corner of the acromion (**Fig 29-1B**). At this level the "soft spot" of the shoulder can be felt. The needle will be placed perpendicular to the posterior chest wall and aiming for the coracoid process, which is felt over the anterior aspect of the shoulder with the opposite hand. A "pop" will be felt when the capsule is penetrated with a medium-sized needle. Slight rotation of the arm may be used to confirm if the needle tip is over the glenoid rim versus the humeral head and the need for any relocation of the needle.

Using the same entry site and with an angle of approximately 30 degrees cephalad, the subacromial space can be reached. Sometimes if the needle is angled too superiorly, or in an obese patient, the needle will hit the posterior margin of the acromion and it will have to be "walked" into the subacromial space.

III. **THE ELBOW JOINT (Fig. 29-2).** The elbow will present a semi-flexed position secondary to the pain and increased intraarticular fluid. The entry site will be located at the center of the triangle formed by the lateral epicondyle, the radial head, and the most lateral corner of the olecranon. At this level the "soft spot" of the elbow joint is felt and the elbow joint can be easily reached. A second approach can be done immediately proximal to the superior margin of the olecranon and centered over the middle third of the olecranon through a transtendinous approach for the triceps tendon. This would provide full access to the olecranon fossa.

An injection of the extensor carpi radials brevis (ECRB) for "tennis elbow" will be performed after identifying the most tender spot. For the most part it will be located just a few centimeters proximal to the lateral epicondyle. With an angle of 30 degrees, the painful spot is reached with the tip of the needle, and after backing out a few millimeters the medication is injected. Multiple "hits" with the tip of the needle

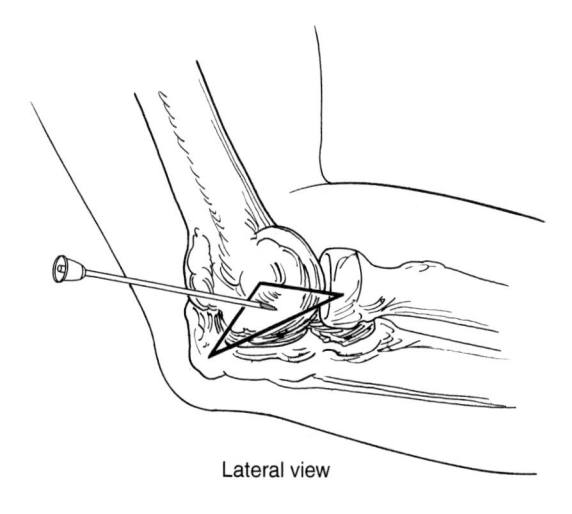

Chapter 29: Aspiration and Injection of Upper and Lower Extremities 405

Figure 29-2. Elbow joint.

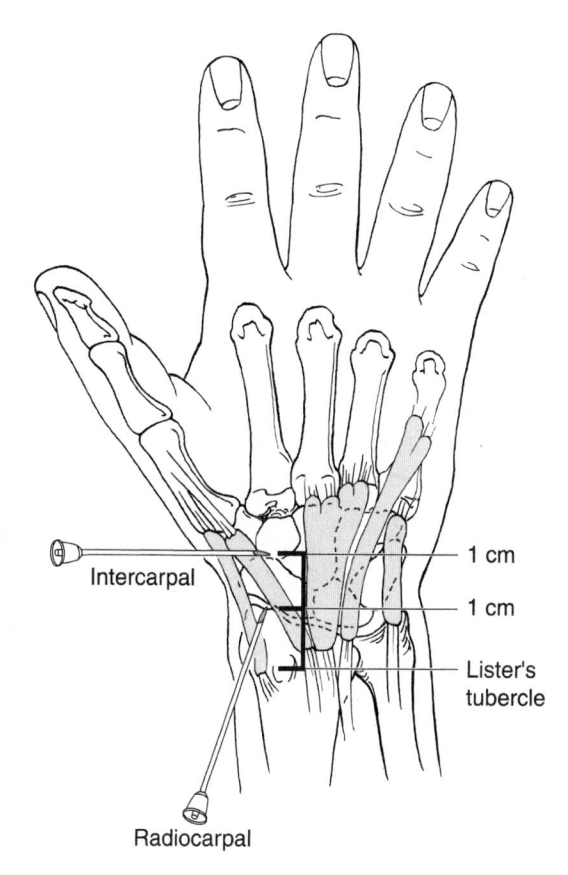

Figure 29-3. Wrist joint.

against the lateral cortex of the humerus will be made to "agitate" the attachment site of the ECRB.

IV. **THE WRIST JOINT (Fig. 29-3).** The wrist would be approached from the dorsal aspect. Most commonly, we can access the proximal radiocarpal joint in between the third and fourth extensor tendon compartments. This is located approximately 1 cm distal to Lister's tubercle which is easily palpable. On the same direction and moving 2 cm distal from the tubercle, we will have access to the intercarpal joint. The joint space in between the carpal bones is quite limited, and most of the time the medication will be placed in between the capsule and bony structures and not in between the carpal bones. The distal radioulnar joint can be approached in between the fourth and fifth extensor tendon compartments. The entry site for the needle is located over a divot which may be felt radial to the most prominent portion of the ulna.

V. **THE HIP JOINT (Fig. 29-4).** Intraarticular hip injections are safest when done with fluoroscopic guidance. A lateral or anterolateral approach can be recommended to access the hip joint. With any hip aspiration/injection, the femoral pulse must be palpated and marked to get a good sense of the location of the femoral neurovascular bundle and the chances for injury after different maneuvers. Spinal needles must be used to reach a joint as deep as the hip joint. The anterolateral approach will have an

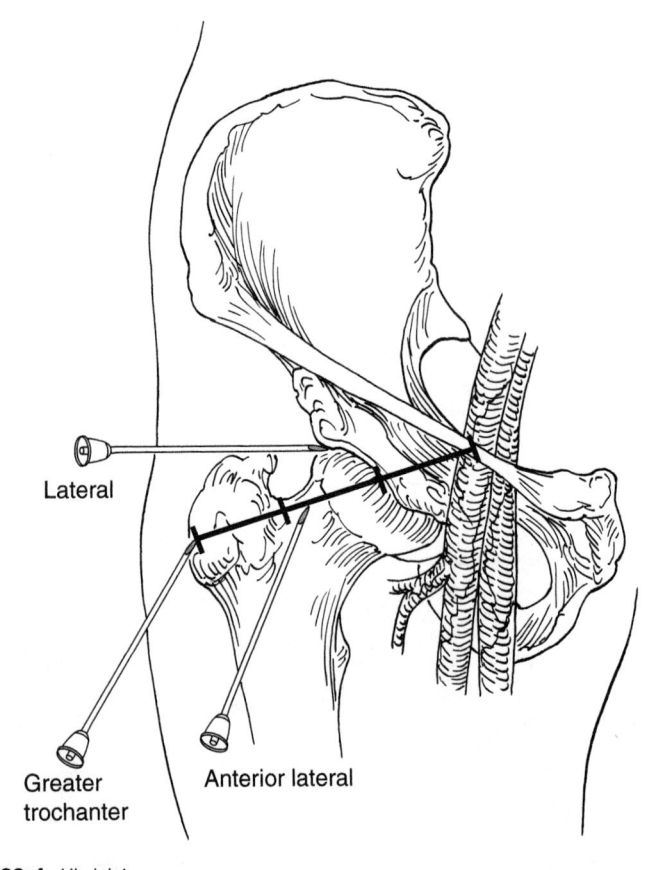

Figure 29-4. Hip joint.

entry site located approximately over the junction of the lateral with the middle third of the total distance between the greater trochanter and the inguinal ligament. With this entry site, the needle will be angled approximately 45 degrees cephalad and 45 degrees medially. It is recommended to proceed with imaging intensification in order to guarantee full access to the hip joint. The lateral approach consists of performing an injection right above the tip of the greater trochanter and aiming straight medial to reach the junction of the femoral head with the femoral neck. The needle will be angled slightly anteriorly in order to correct for the femoral anteversion. An alternative to this is to place the extremity in internal rotation by 15 degrees to 20 degrees and the needle parallel to the coronal plane.

The greater trochanter bursa can be injected easily within the office, without any fluoroscopic assistance. The needle is placed slightly distal to the most prominent or painful area, and angled 30 degrees to 40 degrees from inferior to superior until the lateral cortex of the femur is touched with the tip of the needle. At this level, pull back a few millimeters and proceed with the injection of the area. The medication should go without much resistance as a confirmation of being in a virtual space (i.e., greater trochanter bursa).

VI. **THE KNEE JOINT (Fig. 29-5).** A knee with a moderate to large effusion will present an increased space between the patella and the femur as the patella is translated anteriorly by the increased intraarticular pressure. Therefore, under those circumstances, the easiest approach is to proceed laterally. The needle will be placed at a 90 degrees angle with the long axis to the limb. The entry site will be located at the level of the proximal pole of the patella. Laterally, a void between the patella and the femur may be felt and the needle will be easily introduced at that level. Aspiration of the joint can be performed with subsequent "milking" of the intraarticular effusion.

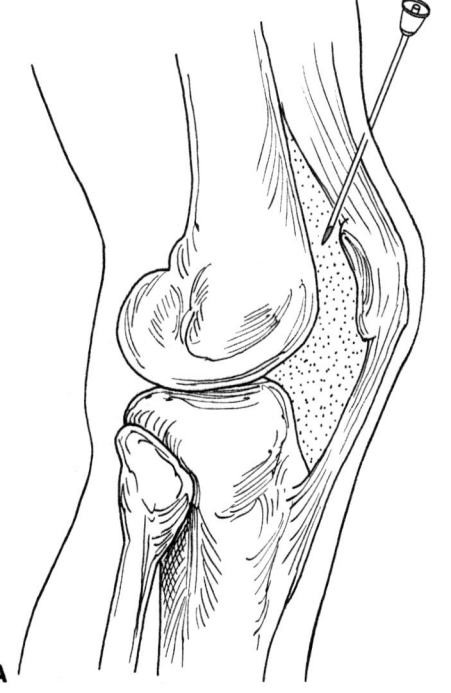

Figure 29-5. Knee joint.

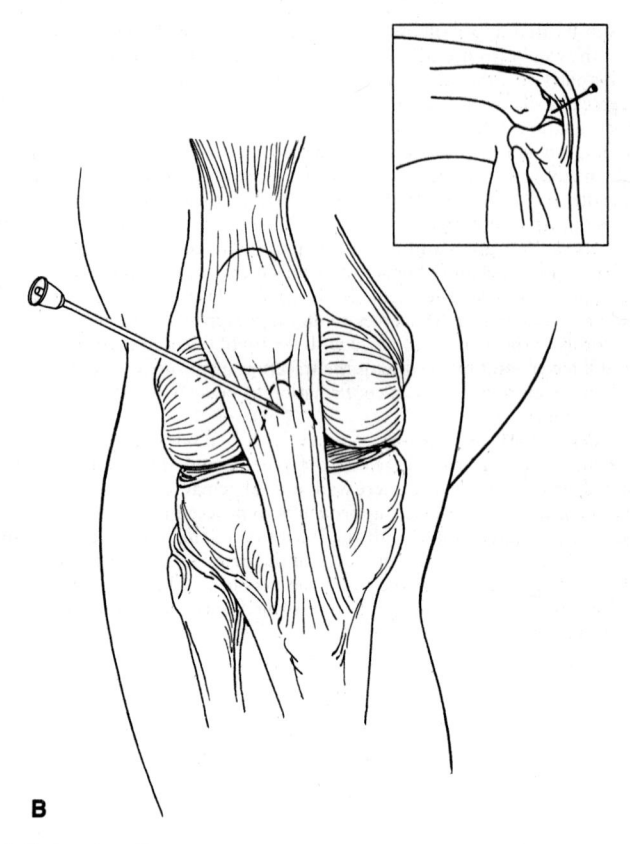

Figure 29-5. *(continued)*

An injection of a knee joint without an effusion through this approach is slightly more difficult as there is no virtual space created between the patella and the femoral trochlea. In an attempt to inject the knee joint through the already described lateral approach, the non-trained physician most likely will hit and damage the articular surface of the patella and/or femur. Therefore, the authors prefer to proceed with a lateral approach, similar to the one performed during knee arthroscopy (**Fig 29-5B**). This is located at the level of the inferior pole of the patella and a few millimeters lateral to the border of the patellar tendon. The needle is aimed at 30 degrees caudad and 30 degrees medially, toward the trochanteric notch. The knee will be flexed at 90 degrees when this is performed. During the injection of the medication, some resistance may be felt, which is related to the presence of the retropatellar fat pad. This will be avoided by moving the needle either forward or backward until the injection becomes easier to perform.

VII. **THE ANKLE JOINT (Fig. 29-6).** The safest approach to the ankle joint is through the medial aspect. The needle will be placed at approximately 60 degrees from the sagittal plane with an entry site immediately medial to the anterior tibial tendon. A "soft spot" can be felt which corresponds to the tibiotalar joint. The "shoulder" of the tibial plafond will be easily identified at that level. Special attention is required to direct the needle to be oblique enough to avoid any scuffing of the cartilage as the ankle joint is a very superficial joint. An alternative approach is to proceed with a lateral aspiration or

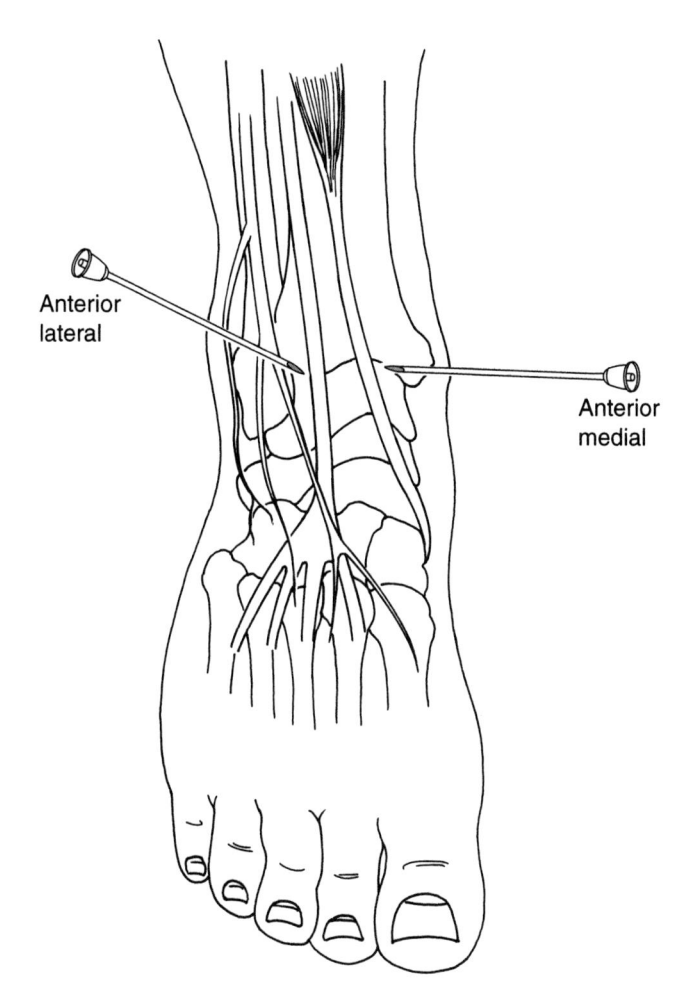

Figure 29-6. Ankle joint.

injection which will be done lateral to the extensor digitorum longus tendon. Also, 60 degrees of obliquity is recommended. The level for the entry site is similar to the one described for the medial approach. The dorsal cutaneous branch of the superficial peroneal nerve is at risk for an injury with the use of the lateral approach. In most occasions it can be seen or felt with forced plantar flexion of the foot and the fourth toe, which places the superficial nerve under tension.

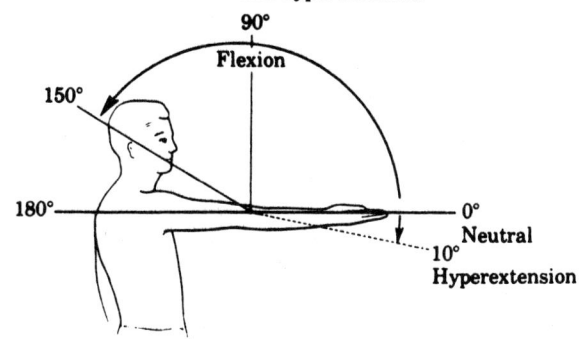

JOINT MOTION MEASUREMENT   A

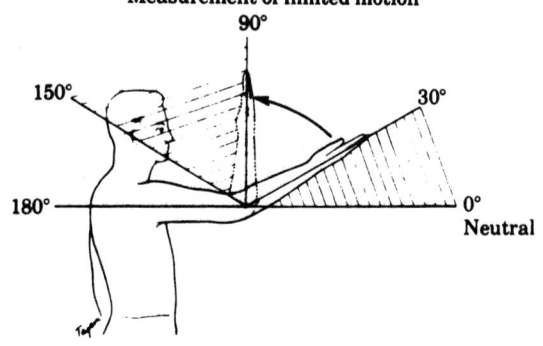

Figure A-1. Elbow.

412 A: Joint Motion Measurement

Pronation and supination

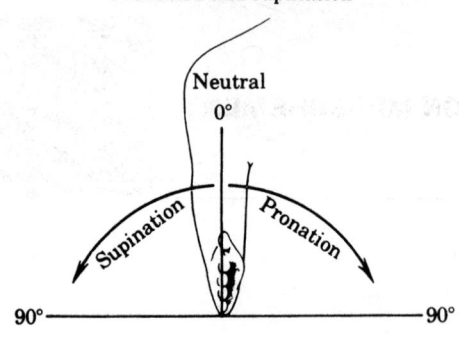

90° — Supination — Neutral 0° — Pronation — 90°

Figure A-2. Forearm.

Flexion and extension

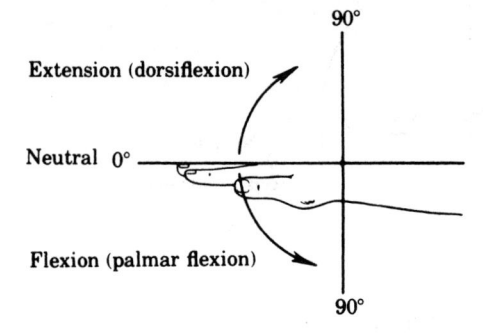

90°

Extension (dorsiflexion)

Neutral 0°

Flexion (palmar flexion)

90°

Radial and ulnar deviation

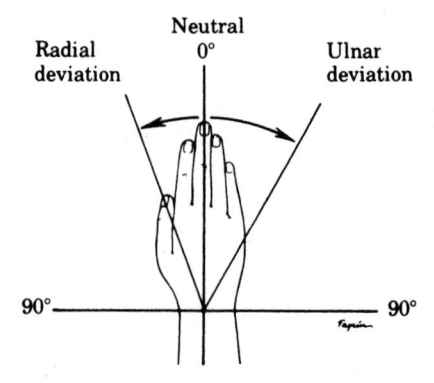

Radial deviation — Neutral 0° — Ulnar deviation

90° — 90°

Figure A-3. Wrist.

A: Joint Motion Measurement 413

Zero starting position

Interphalangeal joint

Metacarpophalangeal joint

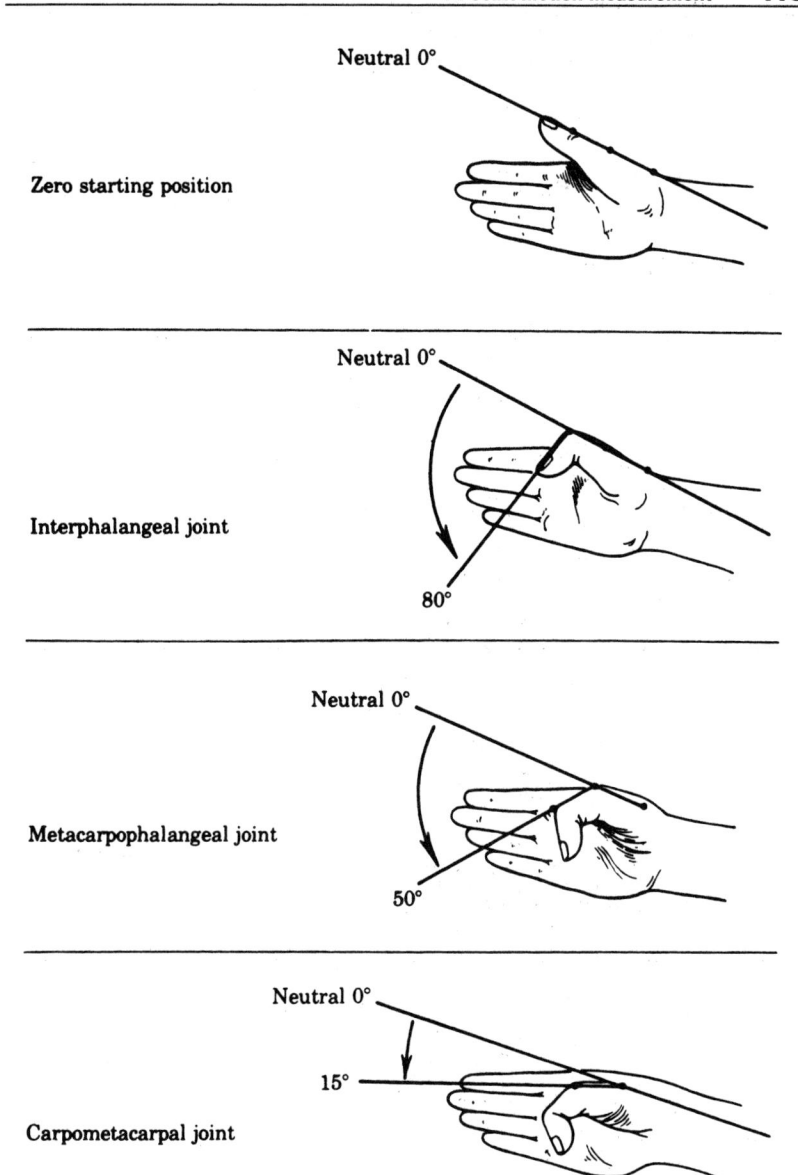

Carpometacarpal joint

Figure A-4. Thumb (flexion).

A: Joint Motion Measurement

Measurement of limitation of opposition

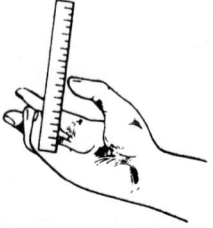

By distance between thumbnail and top of little finger

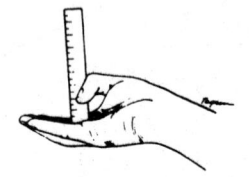

By distance between thumb and base of little finger

(Advice: Use fifth finger when present.)

Figure A-5. Thumb (opposition).

A: Joint Motion Measurement 415

Distal interphalangeal joint

90°

0°
Neutral

0°
Neutral
Proximal interphalangeal joint

100°

0°
Neutral
Metacarpophalangeal joint

90°

Composite motion of flexion

Fingertip to distal palmar crease

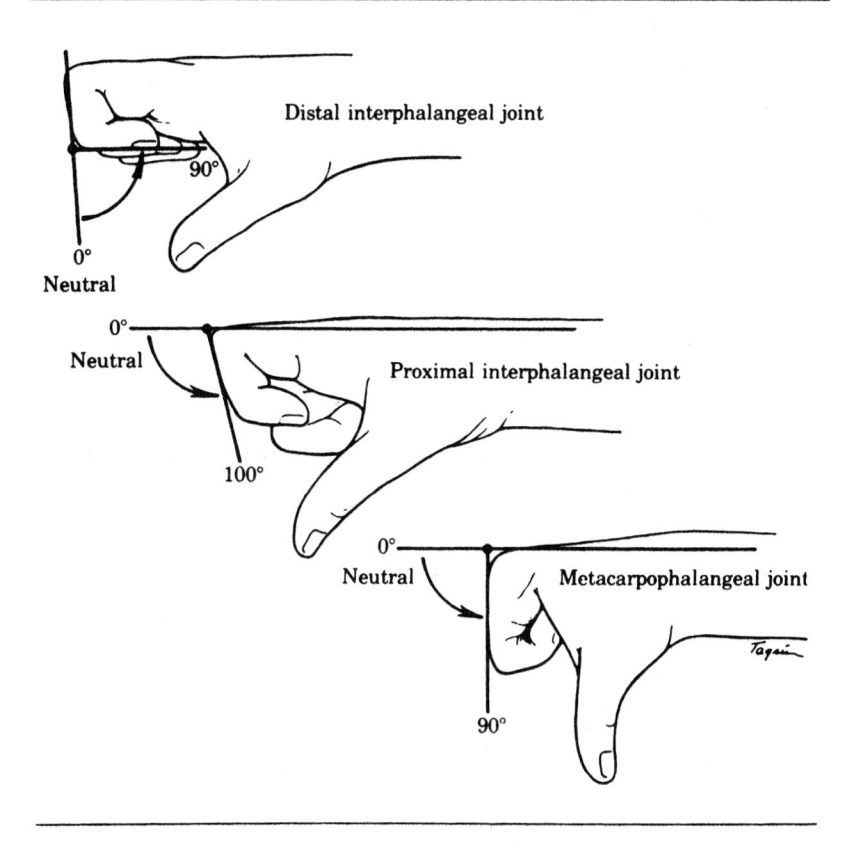

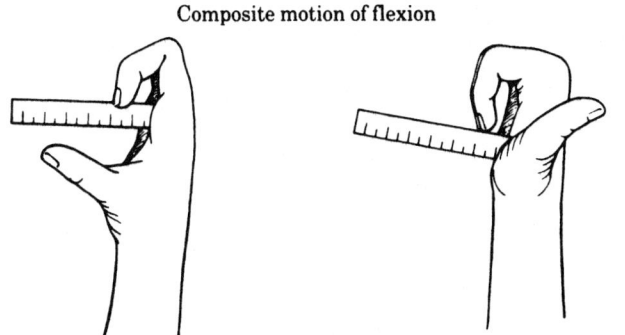

Fingertip to proximal palmar crease

Figure A-6. Fingers (flexion).

416 A: Joint Motion Measurement

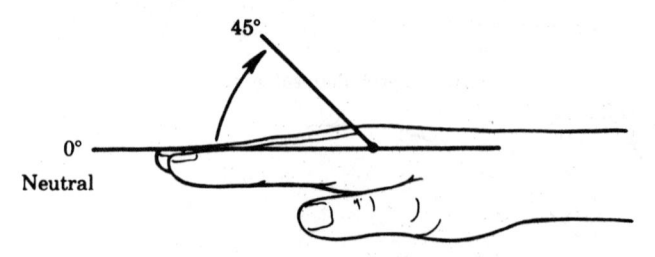

Extension—metacarpophalangeal joint

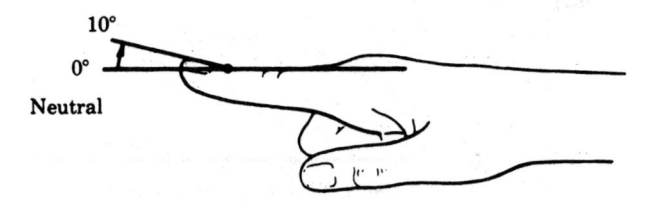

Hyperextension—distal interphalangeal joint

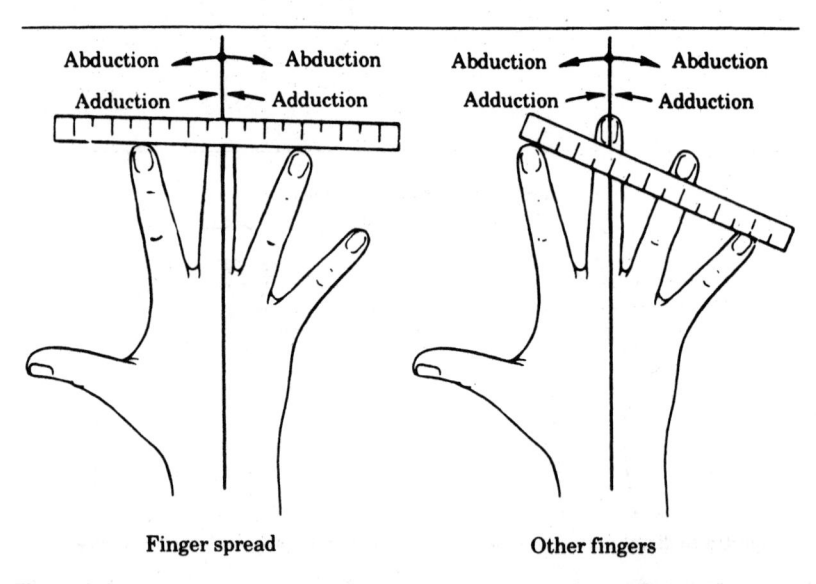

Finger spread

Other fingers

Figure A-7. Fingers (extension, abduction, and adduction).

A: Joint Motion Measurement 417

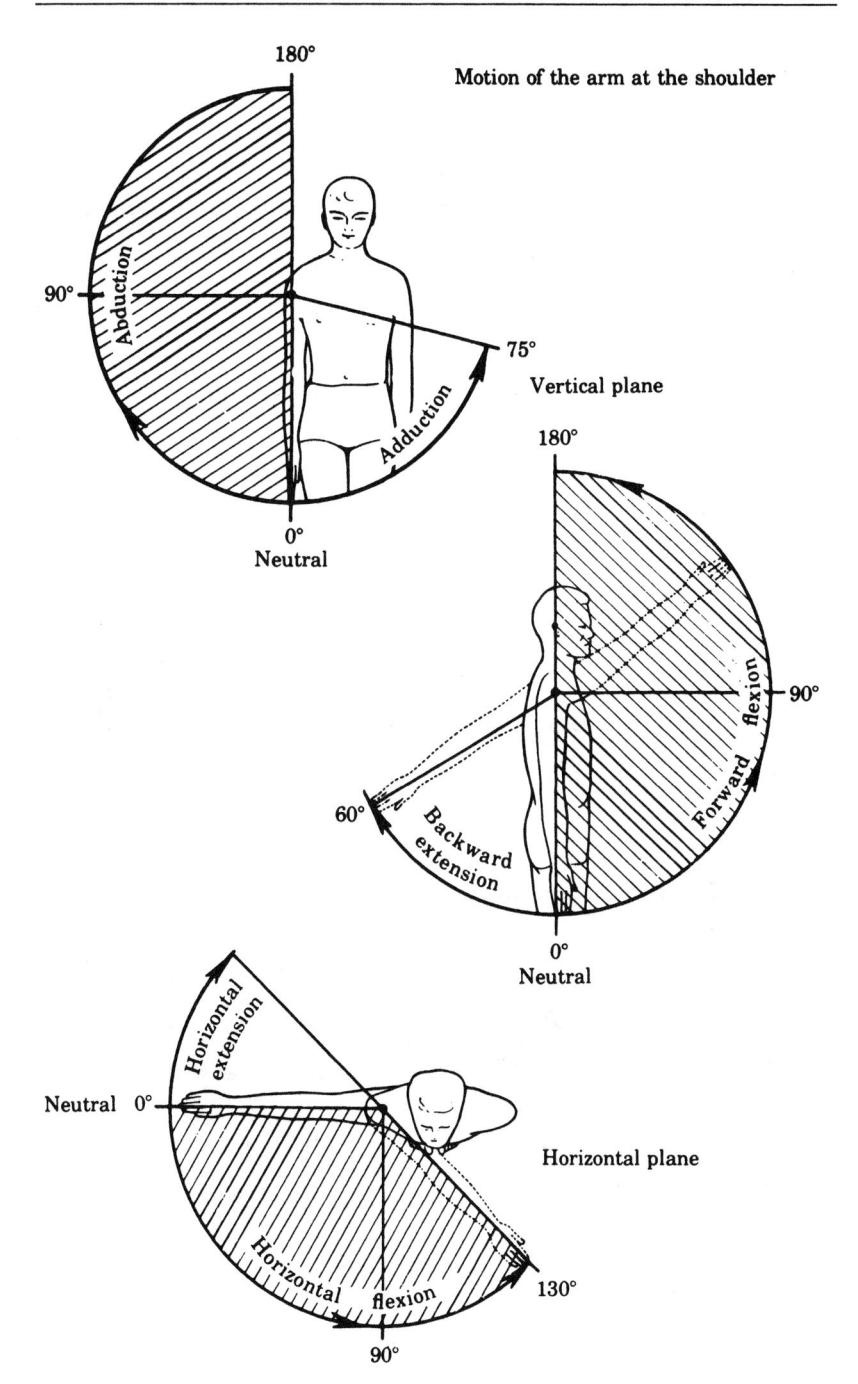

Figure A-8. Shoulder (abduction, adduction, flexion, and extension).

418 A: Joint Motion Measurement

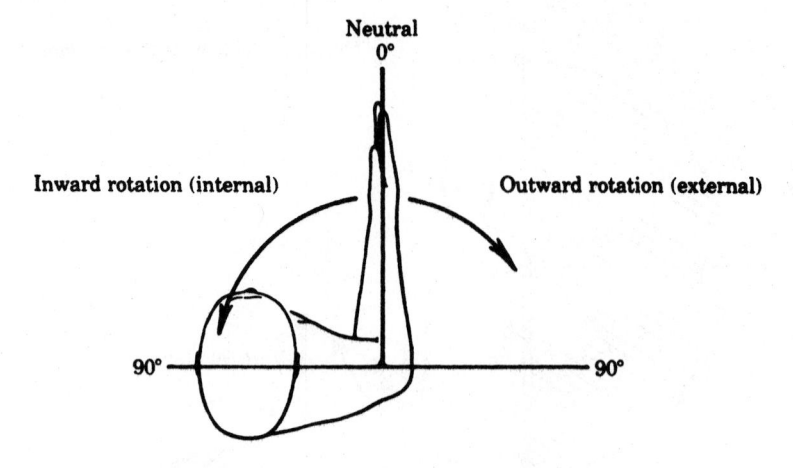

Neutral 0°

Inward rotation (internal)   Outward rotation (external)

90° — 90°

Rotation with arm at side

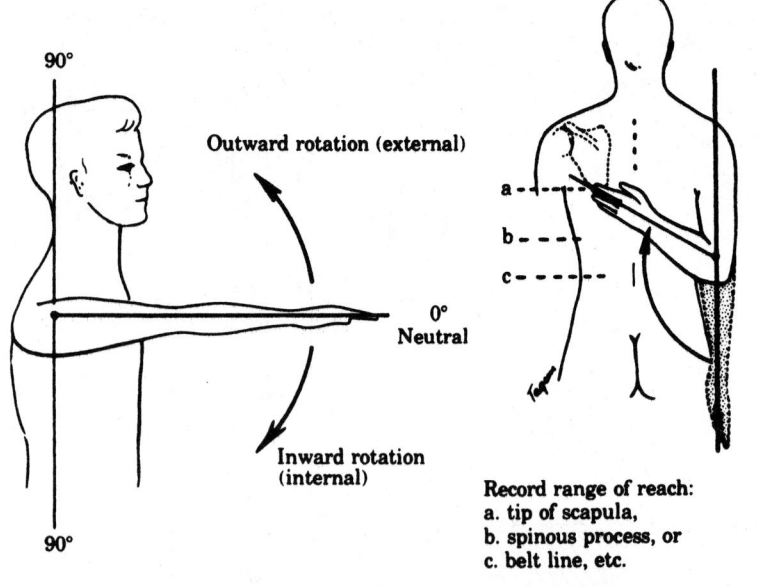

90°

Outward rotation (external)

0° Neutral

Inward rotation (internal)

90°

Rotation in abduction

Record range of reach:
a. tip of scapula,
b. spinous process, or
c. belt line, etc.

Internal rotation posteriorly

Figure A-9. Shoulder (rotation).

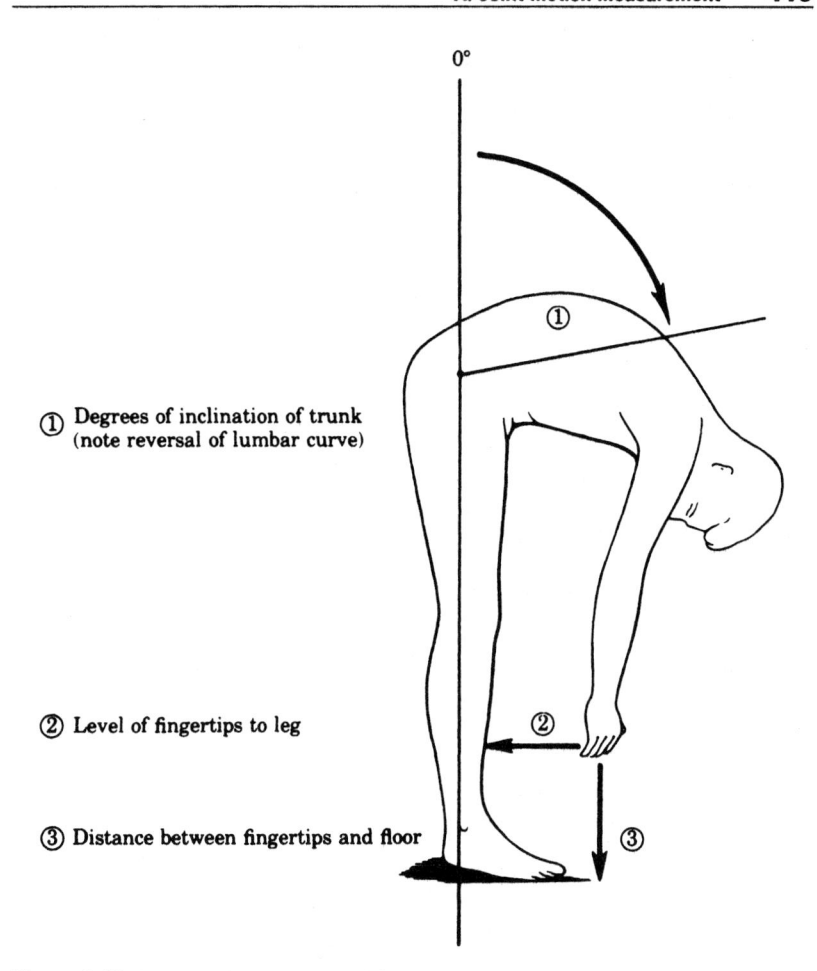

① Degrees of inclination of trunk (note reversal of lumbar curve)

② Level of fingertips to leg

③ Distance between fingertips and floor

Figure A-10. Methods of measuring spinal flexion.

420 A: Joint Motion Measurement

④ The steel tape measuring method

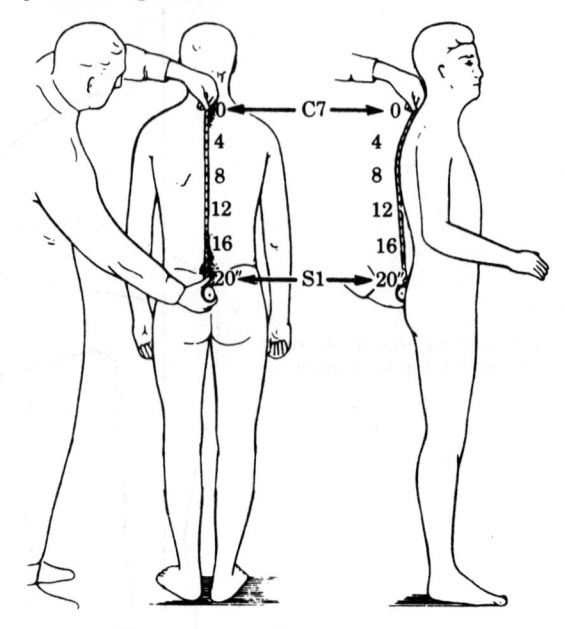

The patient standing erect

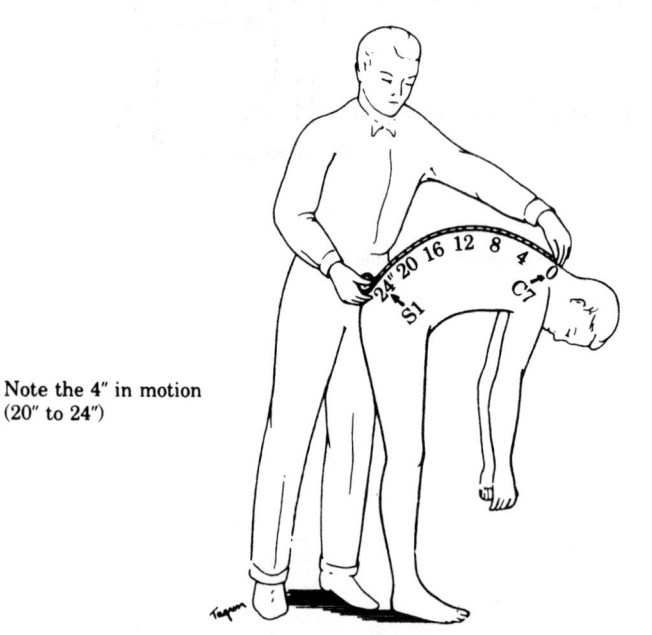

Note the 4" in motion
(20" to 24")

The patient bending forward

Figure A-10. *(continued)*

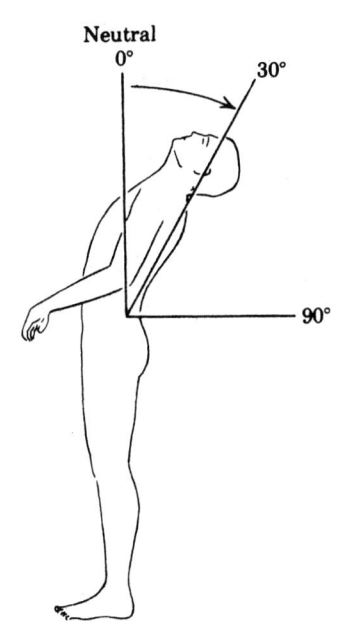

Figure A-11. Thoracic and lumbar spine (extension).

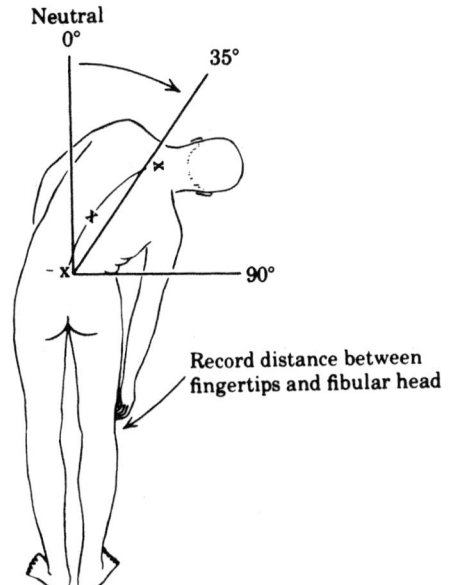

Figure A-12. Thoracic and lumbar spine (lateral bending).

422 A: Joint Motion Measurement

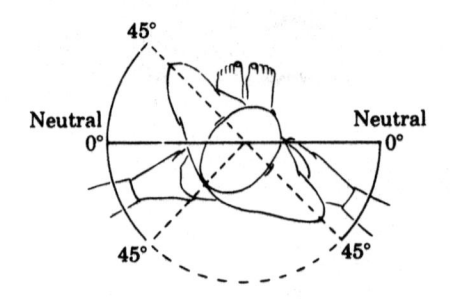

Figure A-13. Spine (rotation).

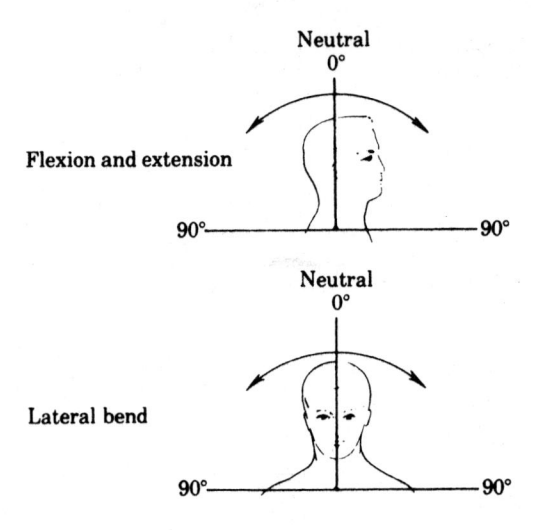

Flexion and extension

Lateral bend

Rotation

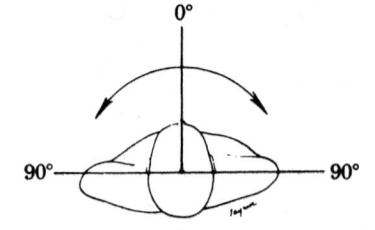

Figure A-14. Cervical spine.

A: Joint Motion Measurement 423

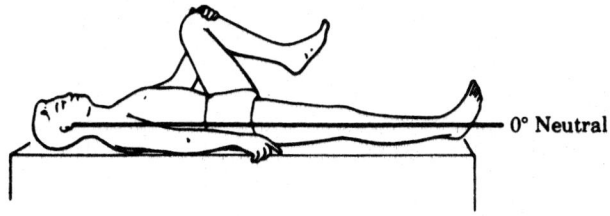

Zero starting position

0° Neutral

Flexion

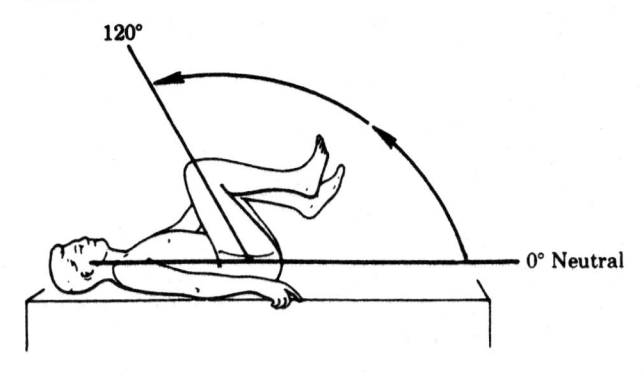

120°

0° Neutral

Limited motion in flexion

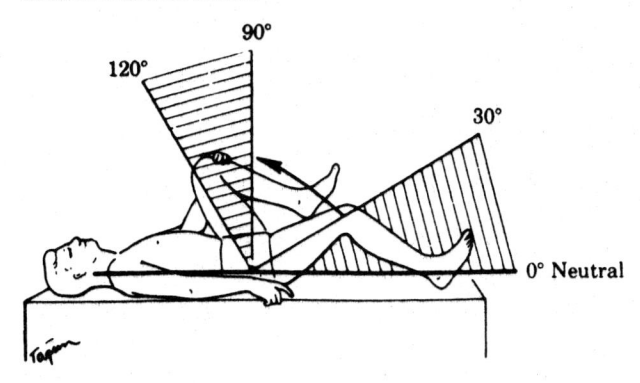

90°
120°
30°

0° Neutral

Figure A-15. Hip (flexion). Always keep opposite hip flexed to flatten lumbar spine.

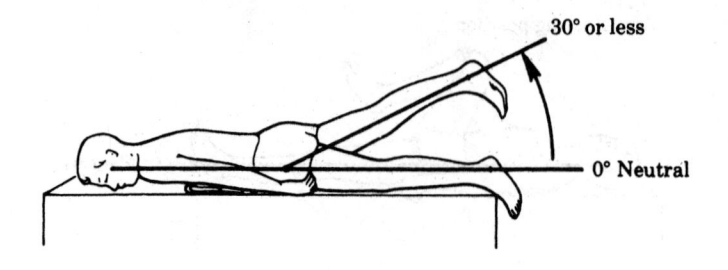

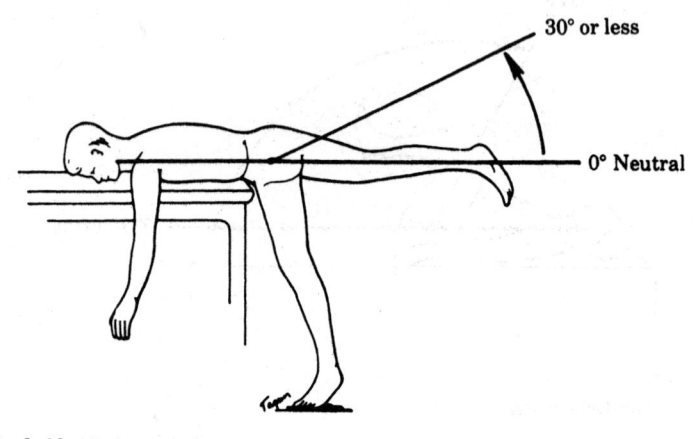

Figure A-16. Hip (extension).

A: Joint Motion Measurement   **425**

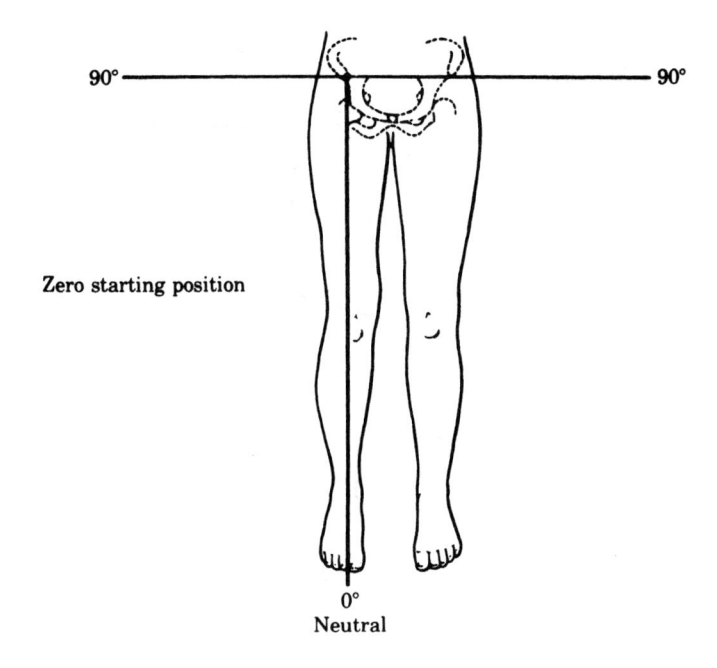

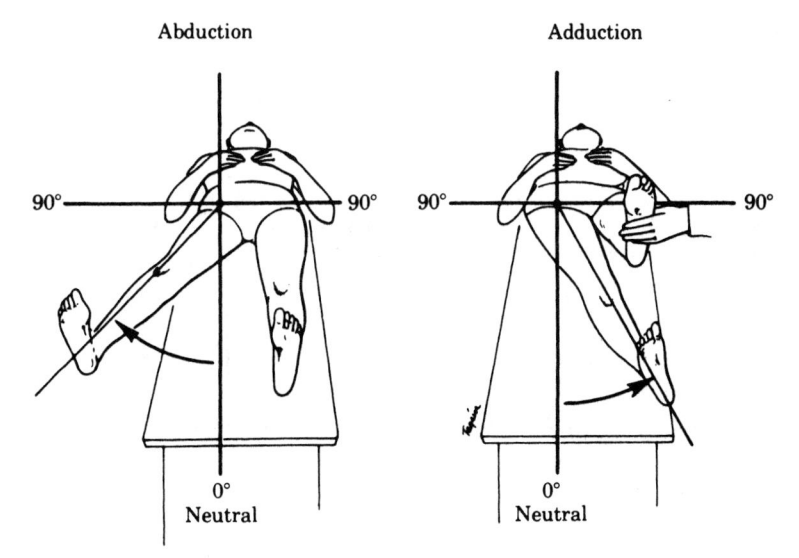

Figure A-17. Hip (abduction and adduction).

426 A: Joint Motion Measurement

Rotation in flexion

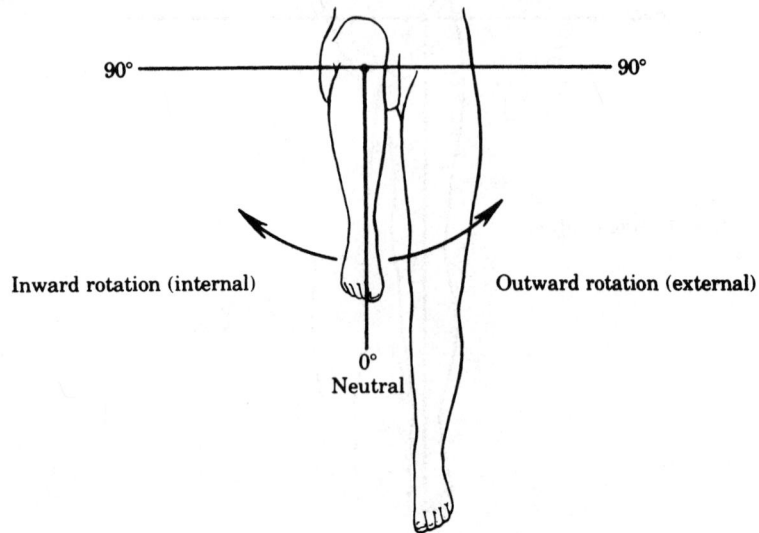

90° — 90°

Inward rotation (internal) — Outward rotation (external)

0° Neutral

Rotation in extension

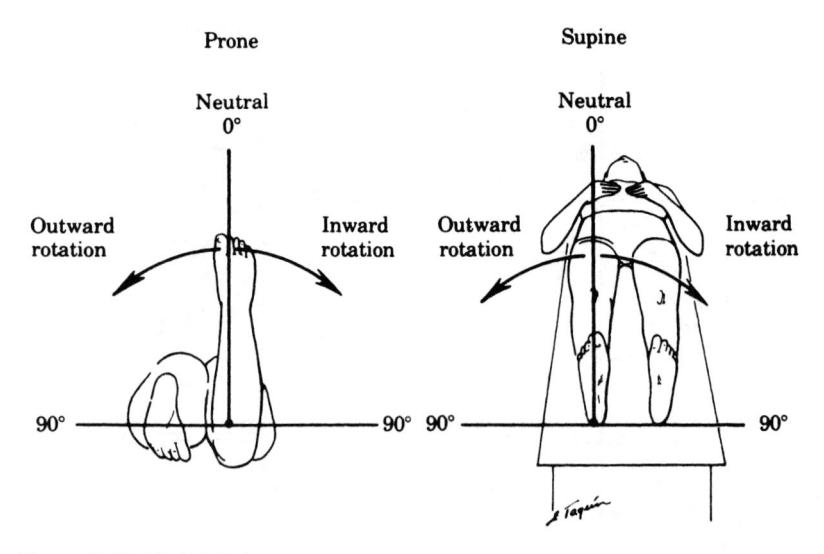

Prone

Neutral 0°

Outward rotation — Inward rotation

90° — 90°

Supine

Neutral 0°

Outward rotation — Inward rotation

90° — 90°

Figure A-18. Hip (rotation).

A: Joint Motion Measurement   **427**

Flexion and hyperextension

Hyperextension

0°
Neutral

Flexion

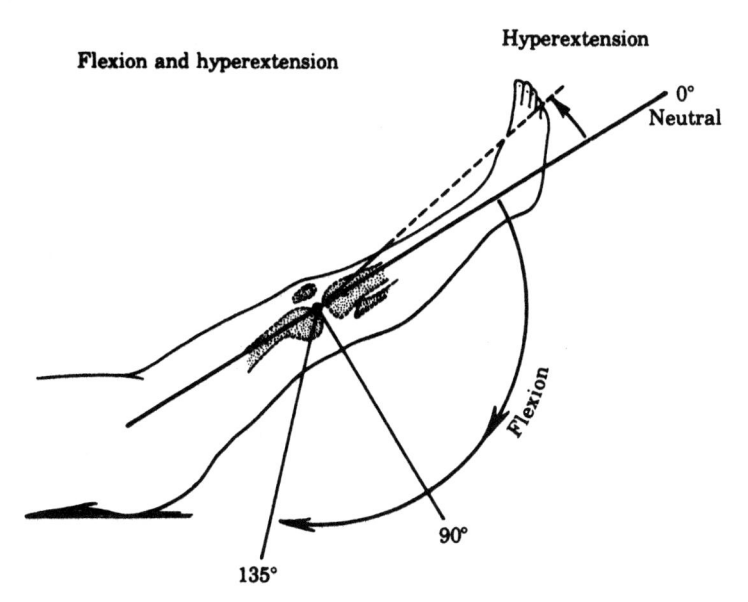

90°

135°

Figure A-19. Knee.

Flexion and extension

90°

20°
Extension
(dorsiflexion)

Neutral
0°

Flexion
(plantar flexion)

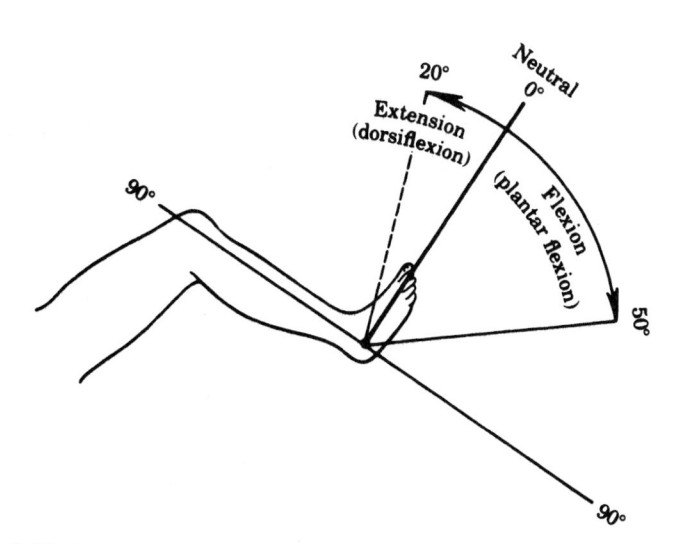

50°

90°

Figure A-20. Ankle. Always note position of knee when recording ankle extension and flexion.

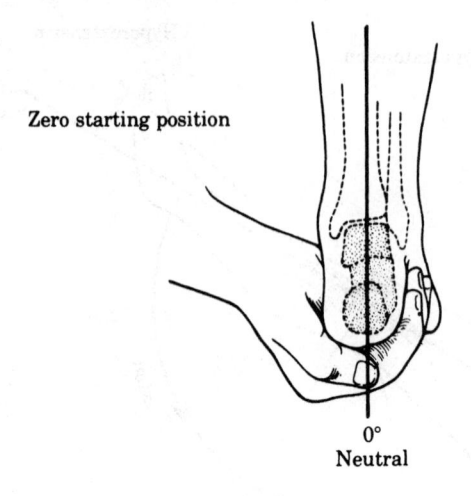

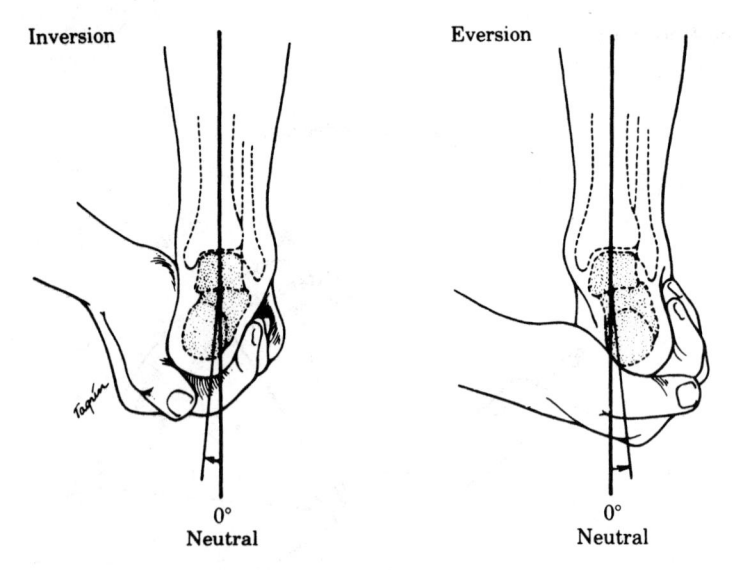

Figure A-21. Hind part of the foot (passive motion).

A: Joint Motion Measurement   **429**

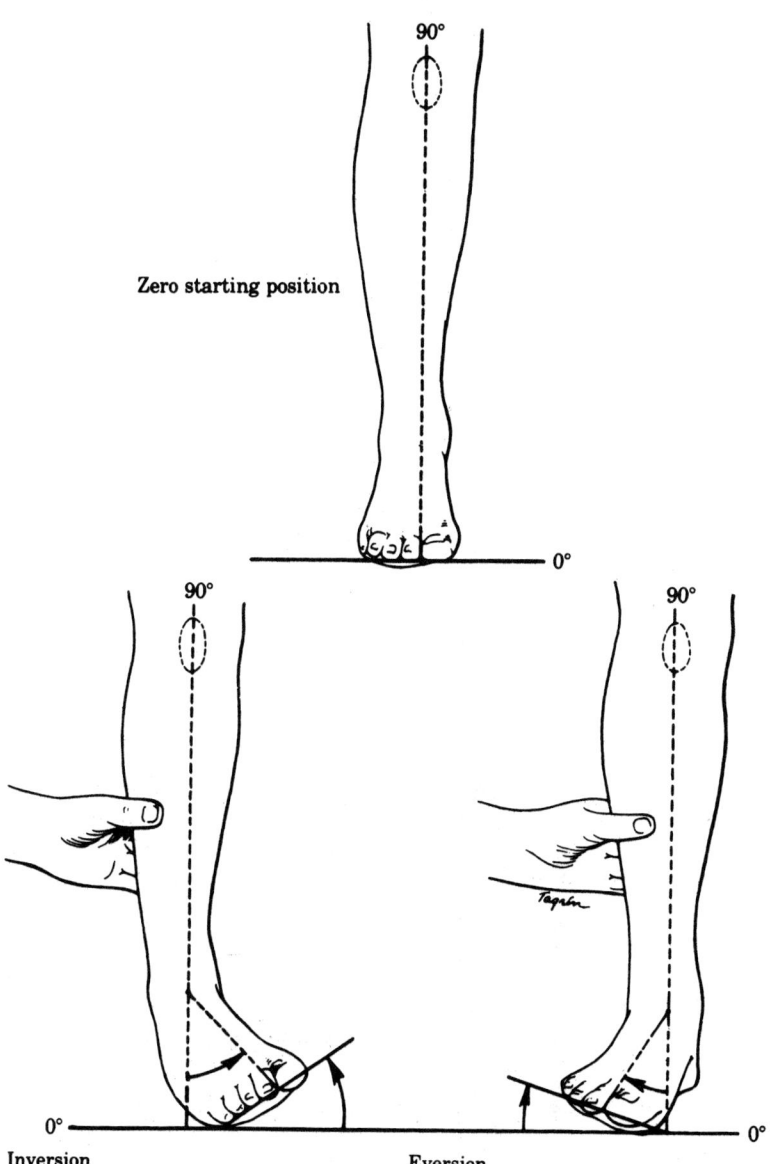

Zero starting position

Inversion
(supination, adduction, and plantar flexion)

Eversion
(pronation, abduction, and dorsiflexion)

Figure A-22. Forepart of the foot.

TABLE A-1 Normal Range of Joint Motion in Male Subjects: Comparison of Estimated Ranges of Motion (Degrees)

Joint	Average ranges of joint motion[a]	This study[b,c] (N = 109)	This study <19 years[b,c] (N = 53)	This study >19 years[b,c] (N = 56)
SHOULDER				
Horizontal flexion	135	140.7 ± 5.9	140.8 ± 6.8	140.7 ± 4.9
Horizontal extension		45.4 ± 6.2	47.3 ± 6.1[d]	43.7 ± 5.8[d]
Neutral abduction	170	184.0 ± 7.0	185.4 ± 3.6	182.7 ± 9.0
Forward flexion	158	166.7 ± 4.7	168.4 ± 3.7[d]	165.0 ± 5.0[d]
Backward extension	53	62.3 ± 9.5	67.5 ± 8.0[d]	57.3 ± 8.1[d]
Inward rotation	70	68.8 ± 4.6	70.5 ± 4.5[d]	67.1 ± 4.1[d]
Outward rotation	90	103.7 ± 8.5	108.0 ± 7.2[d]	99.6 ± 7.6[d]
ELBOW				
Flexion	146	142.9 ± 5.6	145.4 ± 5.3[d]	140.5 ± 4.9[d]
Extension	0	0.6 ± 3.1	0.8 ± 3.5	0.3 ± 2.7
FOREARM				
Pronation	71	75.8 ± 5.1	76.7 ± 4.8	75.0 ± 5.3
Supination	84	82.1 ± 3.8	83.1 ± 3.4[d]	81.1 ± 4.0[d]
WRIST				
Flexion	73	76.4 ± 6.3	78.2 ± 5.5[d]	74.8 ± 6.6[d]
Extension	71	74.9 ± 6.4	75.8 ± 6.1[d]	74.0 ± 6.6[d]
Radial deviation	19	21.5 ± 4.0	21.8 ± 4.0	21.1 ± 4.0
Ulnar deviation	33	36.0 ± 3.8	36.7 ± 3.7	35.3 ± 3.8

TABLE A-1 (Continued)

HIP			
Beginning position flexion	113	2.1 ± 3.6	0.7 ± 2.1[d]
Flexion	28	122.3 ± 6.1	3.5 ± 4.3[d]
		123.4 ± 5.6	121.3 ± 6.4
Extension	48	9.8 ± 6.8	7.4 ± 7.3[d]	12.1 ± 5.4[d]
Abduction	31	45.9 ± 9.3	51.7 ± 8.8[d]	40.5 ± 6.0[d]
Adduction	45	26.9 ± 4.1	28.3 ± 4.1[d]	25.6 ± 3.6[d]
Inward rotation	45	47.3 ± 6.0	50.3 ± 6.1[d]	44.4 ± 4.3[d]
Outward rotation		47.2 ± 6.3	50.5 ± 6.1[d]	44.2 ± 4.8[d]
KNEE			
Beginning position flexion	134	1.6 ± 2.7	2.1 ± 3.2[d]	1.1 ± 2.0[d]
Flexion		142.5 ± 5.4	143.8 ± 5.1[d]	141.2 ± 5.3[d]
ANKLE			
Flexion (plantar)	48	56.2 ± 6.1	58.2 ± 6.1[d]	54.3 ± 5.9[d]
Extension (dorsiflexion)	18	12.6 ± 4.4	13.0 ± 4.7	12.2 ± 4.1
FOREPART OF THE FOOT			
Inversion	33	36.8 ± 4.5	37.5 ± 4.7[d]	36.2 ± 4.2[d]
Eversion	18	20.7 ± 5.0	22.3 ± 4.6[d]	19.2 ± 4.9[d]

[a] Averages of estimates from four sources used by The American Academy of Orthopaedic Surgeons.
[b] Mean ± one standard deviation (SD).
[c] Average age (± SD) = 22.4 ± 2.7, 9.2 ± 1.7,   and 34.9 ± 3.4 years, respectively; average leg length (± S.D.) = 81.2 ± 5.6, 68.7 ± 7.1, and 93.1 ± 3.6 cm, respectively.
[d] Significant differences, $p < 0.01$.
From Boone DC, Azen SP. Normal range of motion of joints in male subjects. *J Bone Joint Surg* 1979;61A:756.

MUSCLE STRENGTH GRADING   B

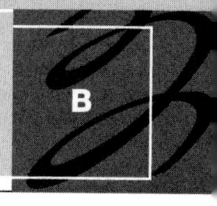

Grade 5: **Normal.** Normal power is present. The muscle can move the joint through a full range of motion against full resistance applied by the examiner or by any other test methods.
Grade 4: **Good.** The muscle can move the joint through a full range of motion against gravity and against some resistance but cannot overcome normal resistance.
Grade 3: **Fair.** The muscle can move the joint through a full range of motion only against gravity.
Grade 2: **Poor.** The muscle can move the joint through a complete range only when gravity is eliminated.
Grade 1: **Trace.** Contraction of the muscle is felt but no motion of the joint is produced.
Grade 0: **Zero.** Complete paralysis is present with no visible or palpable contractions.

DERMATOMES AND CUTANEOUS DISTRIBUTION OF PERIPHERAL NERVES

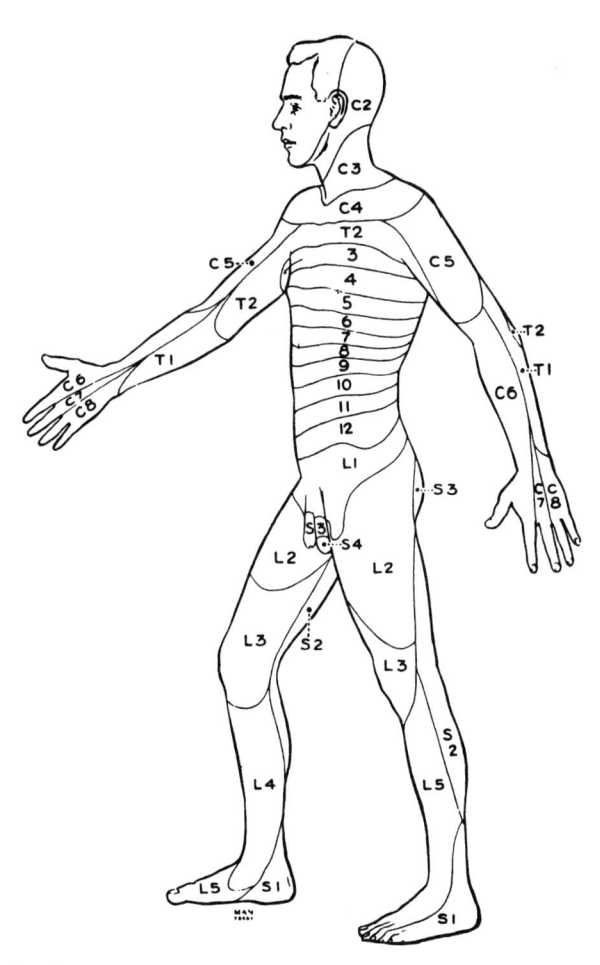

Figure C-1. Anterior view of the dermatomal innervation of spinal segments. (From Haymaker W, Woodhall B. *Peripheral nerve injuries,* 2nd ed. Philadelphia, PA: WB Saunders, 1953:26, with permission.)

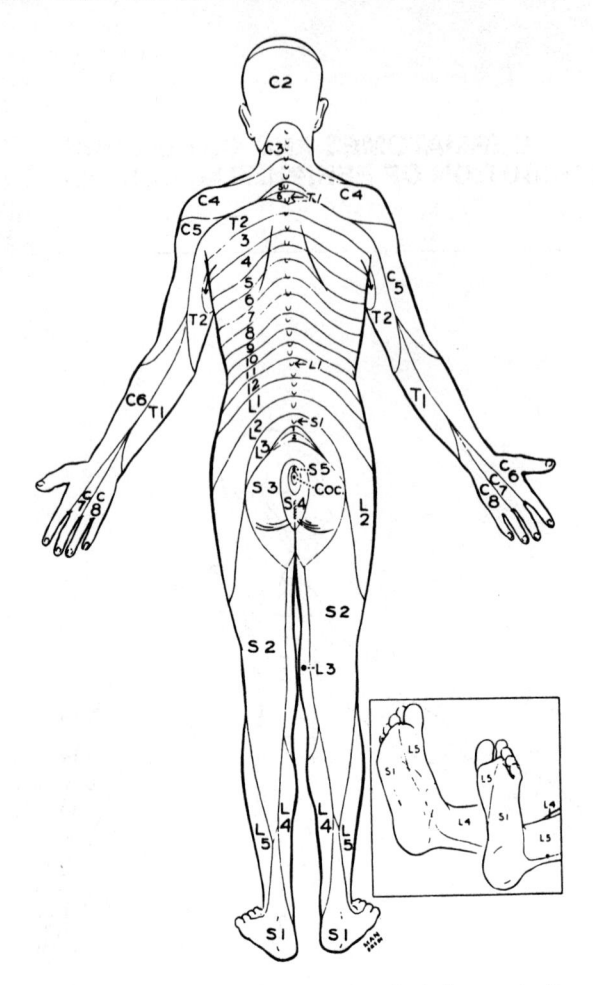

Figure C-2. Posterior view of the dermatomal innervation of spinal segments. (From Haymaker W, Woodhall B. *Peripheral nerve injuries,* 2nd ed. Philadelphia, PA: WB Saunders, 1953:27, with permission).

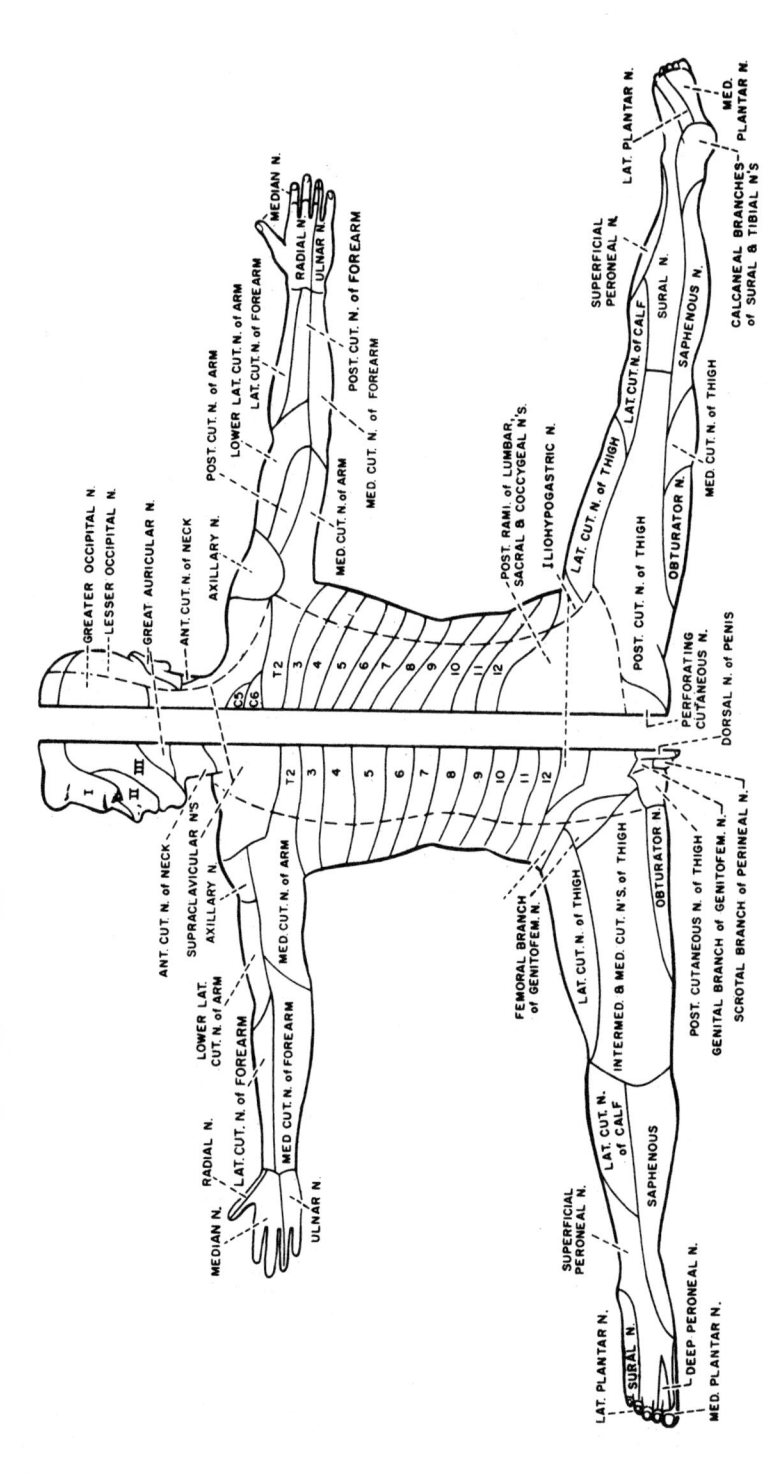

Figure C-3. The cutaneous distribution of peripheral nerves. (From Wright PE, Simmons JCH. Peripheral nerve injuries. In: Edmonson AS, Crenshaw AH, eds. *Campbell's operative orthopaedics*, 6th ed. St. Louis, MO: Mosby, 1980:1644, with permission).

DESIRABLE WEIGHTS OF ADULTS

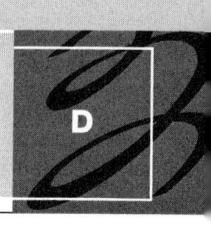

TABLE D-1 Height (ft) and Weight (lb) Tables[a]

Men

Height Feet	Height Inches	Small frame[b]	Medium frame	Large frame
5	2	128–134	131–141	138–150
5	3	130–136	133–143	140–153
5	4	132–138	135–145	142–156
5	5	134–140	137–148	144–160
5	6	136–142	139–151	146–164
5	7	138–145	142–154	149–168
5	8	140–148	145–157	152–172
5	9	142–151	148–160	155–176
5	10	144–154	151–163	158–180
5	11	146–157	154–166	161–184
6	0	149–160	157–170	164–188
6	1	152–164	160–174	168–192
6	2	155–168	164–178	172–197
6	3	158–172	167–182	176–202
6	4	162–176	171–187	181–207

Women

Height Feet	Height Inches	Small frame	Medium frame	Large frame
4	10	102–111	109–121	118–131
4	11	103–113	111–123	120–134
5	0	104–115	113–126	122–137
5	1	106–118	115–129	125–140
5	2	108–121	118–132	128–143
5	3	111–124	121–135	131–147
5	4	114–127	124–138	134–151
5	5	117–130	127–141	137–155
5	6	120–133	130–144	140–159
5	7	123–136	133–147	143–163
5	8	126–139	136–150	146–167
5	9	129–142	139–153	149–170
5	10	132–145	142–156	152–173
5	11	135–148	145–159	155–176
6	0	138–151	148–162	158–179

440

TABLE D-1 (Continued)

Men		Women	
Height in 1" heels	Elbow breadth	Height in 1" heels	Elbow breadth
5'2"–5'3"	$2_{1/2}"–2_{7/8}"$	4'10"–4'11"	$2_{1/4}"–2_{1/2}"$
5'4"–5'7"	$2_{5/8}"–2_{7/8}"$	5'0"–5'3"	$2_{1/4}"–2_{1/2}"$
5'8"–5'11"	$2_{3/4}"–3"$	5'4"–5'7"	$2_{3/8}"–2_{5/8}"$
6'0"–6'3"	$2_{3/4}"–3_{1/8}"$	5'8"–5'11"	$2_{3/8}"–2_{5/8}"$
6'4"	$2_{7/8}"–3_{1/4}"$	6'0"	$2_{1/2}"–2_{3/4}"$

[a]Weights at ages 25–29 years based on lowest mortality rate. Weight in lb according to frame (in indoor clothing weighing 5 lb for men and 3 lb for women; shoes with 1 inch heels).

[b]To approximate frame size: Bend forearm upward at a 90-degree angle. Keep fingers straight and turn the inside of the wrist toward body. Place thumb and index finger of other hand on the two prominent bones on either side of the elbow. Measure space between fingers on a ruler. (A physician uses a caliper.) Compare with elbow measurements for *medium-framed* men and women. Measurements lower than those listed indicate small frame. Higher measurements indicate large frame.

From Metlife Height and Weight Tables. Courtesy of Metropolitan Life Insurance.

SURGICAL DRAPING TECHNIQUES

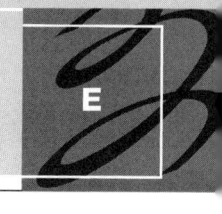

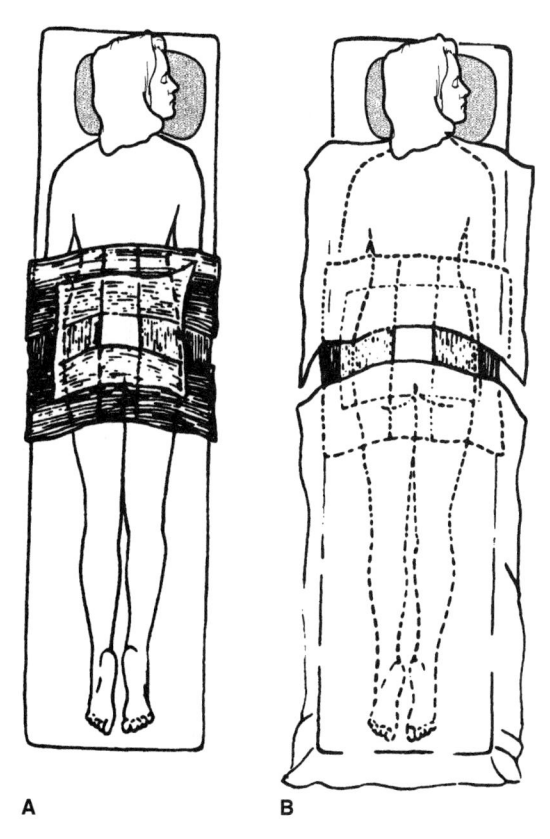

Figure E-1. A back drape. **A:** Four towels are used to square off the operative site. A plastic adherent sheet is then applied to the skin and towels. **B:** One sheet is placed over the superior portion of the body. A lap or split sheet is used last. An easier alternative is to use a commercially available impervious sheet after toweling off the operative area.

444 E: Surgical Draping Techniques

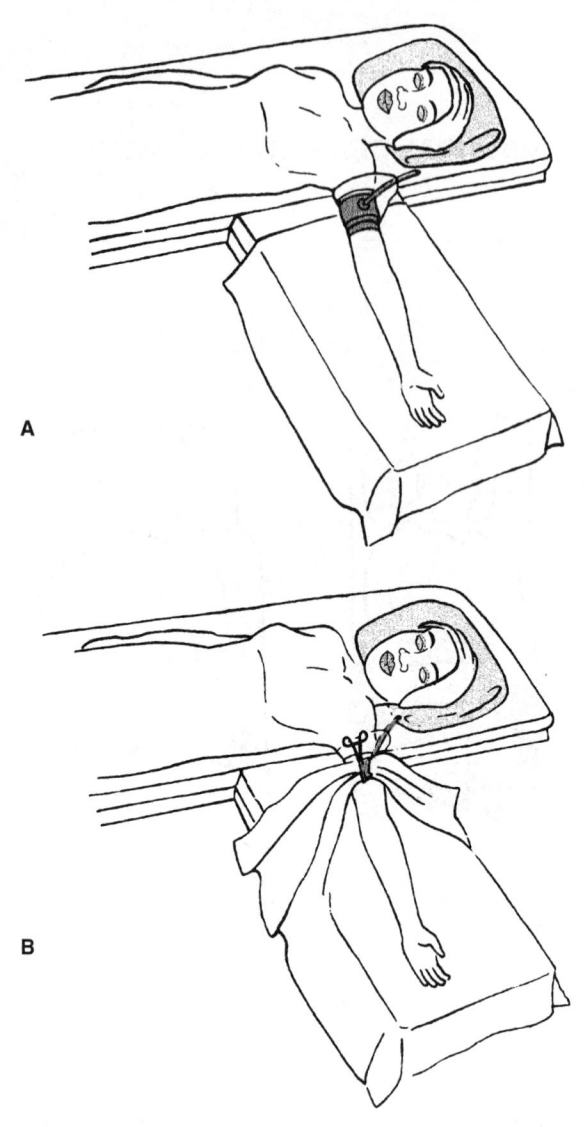

Figure E-2. An extremity drape. **A:** Place a small waterproof sheet under the extremity. If a cloth or nonwaterproof sheet is used, place a plastic or waterproof sheet over the first sheet. **B:** A second small sheet is placed under the extremity with the proximal edge brought around the extremity and clipped just distal to the tourniquet. **C:** If the skin has been prepared with a germicidal antiseptic, two layers of tubular stockinet are rolled over the extremity up to the tourniquet, but any unprepared skin must also be wrapped with sterile bias-cut stockinet. The third small sheet is placed proximal to the extremity and is clipped beneath the extremity just distal to the tourniquet. **D:** A lap or split sheet is applied last. Commercial extremity sheets with a tight waterproof rubberized cuff to seal off the extremity are now available.

E: Surgical Draping Techniques   **445**

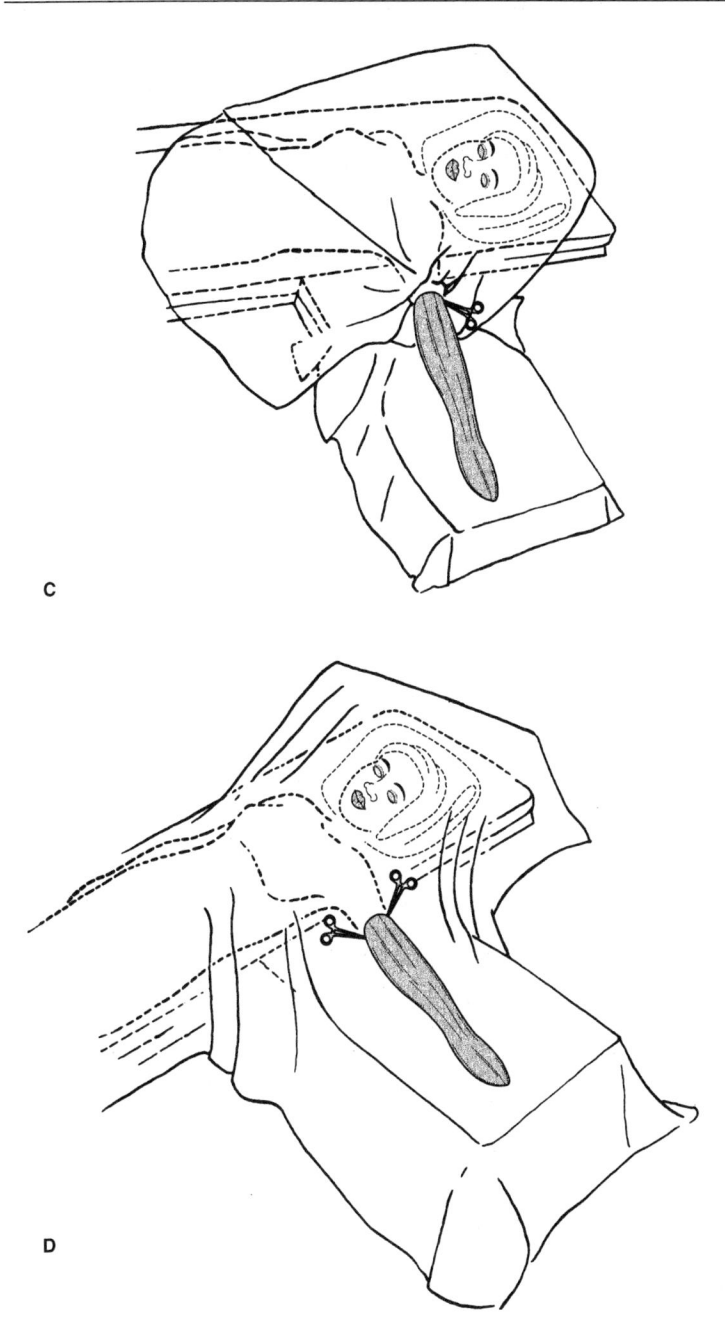

Figure E-2. *(continued)*

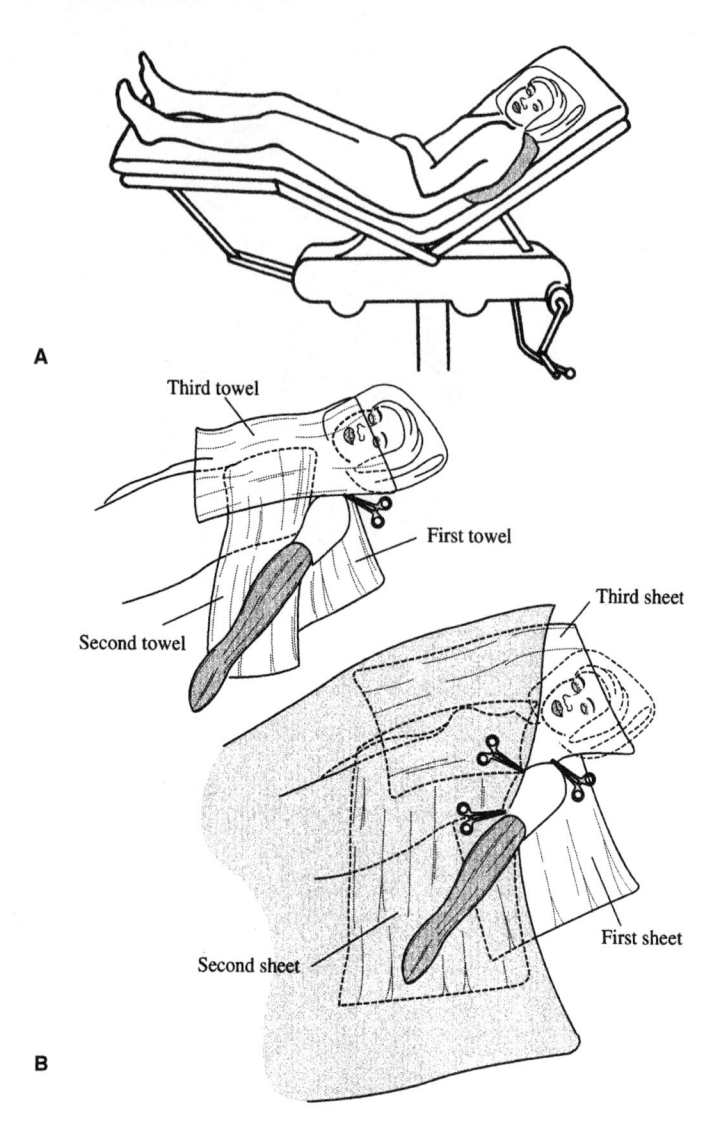

Figure E-3. A shoulder drape. **A:** This is the basic position. A plastic sheet with an adherent edge may be placed just inferior to the hairline. A sandbag is placed under the appropriate shoulder. A neurologic headrest may be used. If necessary, the surgical table can be adjusted to make the upper body more upright. **B:** The arm is squared off with towels that are clipped to each other. A plastic split sheet with an adherent edge may be placed over the towels. Two layers of tubular stockinet are rolled up the arm. Three or four small sheets are placed over the towel edges and are clipped, or a split sheet may be used. The head and neck need to be properly sealed off. One large sheet is placed over the inferior portion of the body. The stockinet can be kept secure by overwrapping with a sterile 4-in. elastic compression (Ace) wrap.

E: Surgical Draping Techniques 447

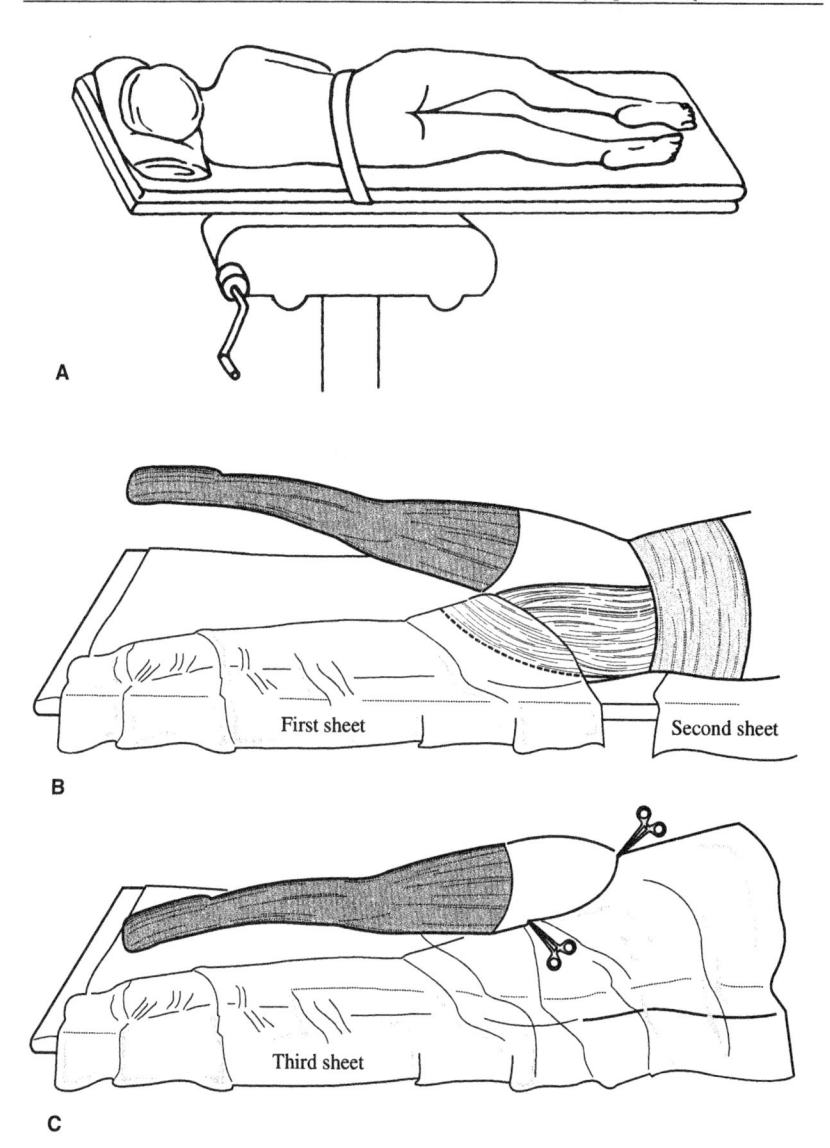

Figure E-4. A lateral hip drape. **A:** The patient is carefully positioned lateral on the table (perpendicular to the table). **B:** Three towels are used to drape the hip and are clipped together. The anterior and posterior towels must cover the pubic area. The first sheet is placed between the legs, and two layers of stockinet are rolled up the leg, which has been prepared first with a germicidal antiseptic, and overwrapped with a 6-in. elastic compression (Ace) wrap. A split sheet with an adhesive edge is applied next, sealing off the perineum snugly, but allowing for proper posterior exposure. **C:** An adhesive plastic sheet is placed over the exposed skin. The completed draping system must have two layers of sterile sheets superior, inferior, and around the hip.

ELECTROMYOGRAPHY AND NERVE CONDUCTION STUDIES

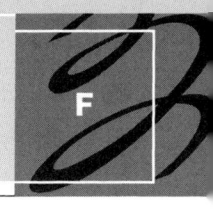

I. **ELECTROMYOGRAPHY**
   A. **Usage.** An electromyelogram (EMG) assists in the differential diagnosis of diseases affecting the lower motor neuron and its motor unit. The muscle action potentials are picked up by three electrodes: a recording or positive electrode; an indifferent electrode, which subtracts out extraneous electrical disturbances; and a ground. The electrical activity is displayed on an oscilloscope, as shown in **Fig. F-1**, and is played through a loudspeaker. It takes 7 to 21 days for denervation to occur, and studies performed during the first week following injury or onset of symptoms are usually unrevealing.
   B. **Findings**
      1. **When denervated, a muscle at rest has fibrillation potentials and positive "sharp waves."** Both potentials are shown in **Fig. F-2**. The fibrillation potentials have a voltage of 10 to 300 μV, a duration of 1 to 5 msec, and a frequency of 1 to 30/second. They sound like raindrops falling on a tin roof. The positive sharp waves have a great variability of voltage, a duration exceeding 10 msec, and a frequency of 2 to 100/second. The sound is that of a dull, loud thumping.
      2. **In partially denervated muscles under voluntary contraction, a polyphasic unit** (highly complex motor unit voltages) often develops. It has a voltage of 50 to 500 μV, a duration of 5 to 25 msec, and usually six or more spikes (**Fig. F-3**).
      3. The **nascent** (just born) **motor unit activity (Fig. F-4) is the early evidence of nerve regeneration.**
      4. **Myotonia dystrophica and myotonia congenita produce high-frequency discharges** that sound like a dive bomber in the loudspeaker. They are precipitated by needle insertion, percussion, or voluntary contraction (**Fig. F-5**). **Pseudomyotonic potentials** have no waxing or waning of the sound and are found in **polymyositis, alcoholic neuropathy,** and so on.
      5. **In primary muscle disease,** voluntary contraction produces small polyphasic units of short duration (**Fig. F-6**).
      6. A **complete nerve lesion** has **no action potentials;** a **partial lesion** has at least **a few action potentials with voluntary contraction.**
      7. The localization of a nerve lesion is made by the application of a thorough knowledge of neuromuscular anatomy. A **summary of EMG findings and their interpretation is found in Table F-1.**
II. **NERVE CONDUCTION STUDIES** are done by stimulating a nerve trunk at two points with an electrical pulse strong enough to activate all of the motor axons. The pulse required is 0.1 to 0.5 msec in duration with 60 to 300 V. The sweep of the oscilloscope is calibrated so the time between each shock and the beginning of each evoked muscle action potential (picked up by another set of electrodes) can be measured. By dividing the distance between the two stimulating points by the difference in time to activate the muscle, the motor conduction velocity is obtained:

Conduction velocity = distance/latency$_2$ − latency$_1$

   A. **Motor**
      1. In general, **motor conduction velocities in excess of 45 m/second in the arms and in excess of 40 m/second in the legs are considered normal.** Conduction velocity of a nerve increases 2.4 m/second/1°C elevation in temperature. This increase must be considered when studying a limb with impaired

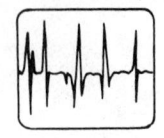

Figure F-1. Normal innervated muscle contracted. Action potential 5 to 10 msec, 500 to 2,000 μV.

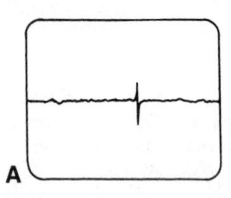

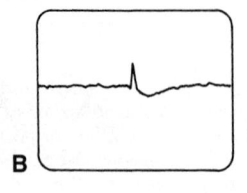

Figure F-2. Denervation.
A: Fibrillation potential.
B: Positive sharp wave.

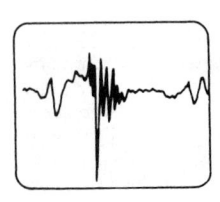

Figure F-3. Complex polyphasic motor unit.

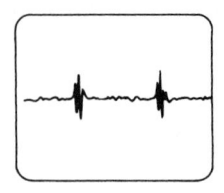

Figure F-4. Nascent motor unit activity.

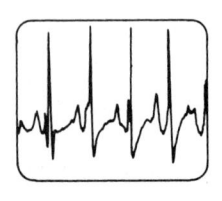

Figure F-5. Myotonia.

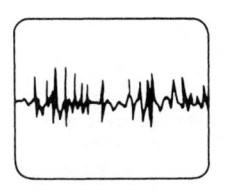

Figure F-6. Myopathic activity.

TABLE F-1 Presumptive Diagnoses from EMG Findings

EMG findings	Presumptive diagnoses
Fibrillation potentials with the muscle at rest	Muscle at least partially denervated
Positive sharp waves	Muscle at least partially denervated
Polyphasic motor unit voltages	Chronic denervation
Nascent motor units	Nerve regeneration
Myotonic voltage discharges	Myotonia dystrophica or myotonia congenita
Pseudomyotonic discharges	Polymyositis, alcoholic neuropathy, etc.
Small polyphasic units	Primary muscle disease
No action potential	A complete nerve lesion

vascularity. Also, conduction velocities are faster in the proximal segments of a nerve than in the distal segments. This difference is a function of temperature and of the diameter of the nerve. The newborn has conduction velocities of one half the adult value, with the adult range reached by age 3 years. Conduction velocity gradually decreases with aging, slowing by 6% between the third and seventh decades.

2. **Distal motor latencies are normally lower than 5 msec except in the posterior tibial and peroneal nerves where latency should be less than 7 msec.**

B. **Sensory nerve conduction studies are often the most sensitive to detect nerve abnormalities.** They are done by stimulating the sensory fibers of a digit and recording the sensory nerve's electrical activity with electrodes placed more proximally on the extremity so as to measure both the conduction velocity and latency. An absent response is a positive finding and indicates significant abnormality. The sensory nerve conduction studies require more expertise by the examiner.

1. **Sensory nerve conduction velocities in the upper extremities are normally greater than 35 m/second in the wrist to elbow segment.**
2. **The upper limit for normal distal sensory latencies is 4 msec.**

INDEX

ABCs (airway, breathing, circulation), 3
Abdominal injury, 6
Abduction
  fingers, 416f
  forepart of foot, 429f
  hip, 425f
  shoulders, 417f
Acetabular fracture, 312–313, 314
Achilles tendinopathy, 393
Achilles tendon rupture, 380–381
Anterior cruciate ligament (ACL) injuries, 348–351
Acromioclavicular (AC)
  dislocation, 218
  injuries, 218–221
  joint, 218, 219f
  joint disorders, 234–235
Acromion, 229
Adduction
  fingers, 416f
  forepart of foot, 429f
  hip, 425f
  shoulder, 417f
Adherent materials, 102
Adhesive capsulitis, 234
Adhesive strapping, 115–116
Adolescent idiopathic scoliosis, 209
Adolescent kyphosis, 211
Adolescent round back, 210
Adult respiratory distress syndrome (ARDS), 27
Advanced trauma life support (ATLS), 2
Air splints, 95, 98
Allopurinol, 63
American Spinal Injury Association (ASIA) classification, 185
Aminoglycoside, 16
Ampicillin, 44t
Amputation
  hand injury, 279
  wrist injury, 276
Amyloidosis, 65
Analgesics, 122–123
Ancef, 155t
Anectine, 160
Ankle arm index (AAI), 9
Ankle brachial index (ABI), 9

Ankle fracture, 379–380
Ankle injuries, 371–382, 393–402. *See also* Foot injuries
  Achilles tendinopathy, 393
  Achilles tendon rupture, 380–381
  ankle fracture, 379–380
  ankle sprain, 371–375
  injection site, 408–409
  joint motion measurement, 427f
  Ottawa ankle rules, 371, 373t
  pilon fracture, 379–380
Ankle sprain, 371–375
Ankylosing spondylitis, 58, 58t, 64
Anterior compartmental syndrome of leg, 30f
Anterior cord syndrome, 186
Anterior knee pain syndrome, 76
Anterior talofibular ligament (ATFL), 371
Anterior tibial syndrome, 29
Antibiotics, 42–46t, 122, 153–154, 155t
Antimalarial drugs, 65
Anvils, 171
Apert syndrome, 285
Apprehension sign, 341
Aravan, 60
ARDS (adult respiratory distress syndrome), 27
Arterial pressure index (API), 9
Arthritis. *See also* Joint conditions, acute nontraumatic
  glenohumeral joint, 233–234
  gonorrheal, 53t
  infections, 56t
  JRA. *See* Juvenile rheumatoid arthritis (JRA)
  Lyme, 42
  psoriatic, 53t, 57
  rheumatoid. *See* Rheumatoid arthritis
  septic. *See* Septic arthritis
  wrist/hand, 292
Arthrodesis, 62
Aspiration and injection techniques, 403–409
  ankle joint, 408–409
  elbow joint, 404–406
  general guidelines, 403
  hip joint, 406–407

453

Aspiration and injection techniques (*Continued*)
  knee joint, 407–408
  shoulder joint, 403–404
  wrist joint, 405*f*, 406
Aspirin
  rheumatic fever, 64
  rheumatoid arthritis, 59
  thromboembolism, 124
Assessment. *See* Evaluating the trauma patient
Association of Osteosynthesis (AO) classification system, 376, 377*f*
Atabrine, 64
Auranofin, 60
Autologous chondrocyte transplantation, 63
Autosomal dominant metabolic disease, 159
Avascular necrosis (AVN), 12–13, 81, 292, 310, 321
Aviator's astralagus, 388
Avulsion fracture of vertebral ring apophysis, 87
Axonotmesis, 22
Azathioprine, 60

Back drape, 443*f*
Back pain, 85–89, 203–209
Backboard, 93, 94*f*
Bamboo spine, 58
Bandaging, 116–117. *See also* Cast and bandaging techniques
Bankart repair, 225
Barlow test, 78
Barton fracture, 257*f*, 260
Baseline blood replacement requirements, 3
Baumann angle, 243
Bending irons, 171, 172*f*
Bending press, 170–171, 172*f*
Bent drill bit, 164
Betamethasone, 64
Bias-cut, 102
Bicortical grafts, 176
Bigliani classification of acromial morphology, 230*f*
Bilateral short-leg spica, 109
Bimalleolar axis, 70
Bimanual pelvic examination, 6
Bivalving casts, 115
Bladder catheterization, 124
Bloodborne pathogens, 157
Blount disease, 72
Board splints, 98*f*
Body casts, 106–108
Body jacket, 106*f*
Böhler bow, 139*f*
Bone and joint infections. *See* Musculoskeletal infections, acute
Bone cutting instruments, 162–164

Bone file, 164
Bone graft material, 176
Bone-muscle origin interface failure, 289
Bone saws/files, 164
Bone scan, 207, 398
Bone screw
  biomechanics, 164–166
  cancellous, 165
  cannulated cancellous, 165
  cortical, 165, 166*f*
Bone tumors involving spine, 87
Bony mallet fracture, 278, 278*f*
Boutonierre deformity, 271
Bowed legs, 71–72
Bowel problems, 124–125
Bowen wire tightener, 173, 174*f*
Box suture, 177*f*
Boxer's fracture, 278, 280*f*
Brachial plexus, 22, 285
Brachial plexus injuries, 285–286
Brief review. *See* HCMC recommendations and protocols
Brown-Séquard syndrome, 186
Bunions, 74–75, 400
Bursitis, 56*t*
Burst fracture, 193–194
  stable, 193, 194*f*
  unstable, 193–194, 195*f*
Buttonhole effect, 308

C-reactive protein (CRP), 40, 42, 43
Cal hypertension, 29
Calcaneal fat pad trauma, 395
Calcaneal fractures, 383–386, 390
Calcaneonavicular coalition, 74
Calcific bursitis, 233
Calcific tendonitis, 56*t*
Captain of the ship, 3
Carpal tunnel syndrome (CTS), 28, 259, 287–288
Carpometacarpal (CMC), 292
Cast
  benders, 103
  brace, 114
  cutters, 102
  dryers, 103
  knives, 103
  padding, 102
  spreaders, 102
Cast-cutting electric saw, 102
Cast and bandaging techniques, 101–118
  adhesive strapping, 115–116
  bandaging, 116–117
  basic principles, 103–105
  below-the-knee total contact, 113–114, 113*f*
  bivalving casts, 115
  body casts, 106–108
  cutting casts, 114

Dehne/Sarmiento casting techniques, 112–114
equipment, 102–103
joint immobilization, 117–118
knee cast-brace, 114
knee cylinder casts, 110, 112
long-leg cast, 112
lower extremity, 106
materials, 101–102
short-leg cast, 112
spica, 108–110
splitting casts, 115
upper extremity, 105–106
Catterall classification system, 79
Cefazolin, 44t, 155t
Ceftazidime, 45t, 46t
Ceftriaxone, 45t
Cefuroxime, 45t
Central cord syndrome, 186
Cephalosporin, 46t
Cephalosporins, 16, 44t
Cephazolin, 122
Cerclage, 171–174
Cerebral palsy, 89–90, 286
Cervical spine traction, 141–144
Cervicotrochanteric fractures, 322
Chance fracture, 194, 196f
Charnley traction unit, 148, 149f
Chilblain, 23
Childhood foot conditions, 73–75
Childhood hip disorders, 78–82
Childhood knee disorders, 75–78
Children. *See* Pediatric orthopedic conditions
Chip fractures, 345
Chisels, 163
Chlorhexidine gluconate, 158
Chloroquine, 60, 64
Chondrocalcinosis, 56
Chondrolysis, 81
Chondromalacia patella (CMP), 76, 355
Chondrosarcoma, 297
Chronic osteomyelitis, 47
Chronic patella instability, 76
Chronic regional pain syndrome (CRPS), 34
Circular cast, 104
Clavicle fractures, 213–215
Claw toe, 395, 400
Clindamycin, 44t, 47, 122
Clinical viscosity test, 57n
Closed antegrade interlocking nailing, 330, 367f
Closed chain exercises, 354
Closed tibial shaft fractures, 365–366
Cloth masks, 158
Club foot, 73
Club hand, 284
COBB method, 210, 211

Colace, 124
Colchicine, 63, 64
Collarbone, 213–215
Colles, Abraham, 257
Colles' fracture, 257–259
Collins hitch, 97f
Common digital nerve neuroma, 395
Compartment syndrome, 10–11, 29–34
clinical approach, 31–34
defined, 29
diagnostic factors, 32t
etiologies, 29–30
increased tissue pressure, 31, 32–34
locations, 29
other terms for, 29
tibial shaft fracture, 366
wrist and hand, 281
Complete spinal cord injuries, 185
Complex regional pain syndrome, 366
Complications, 27–37
ankle fractures, 379
calcaneal fracture, 386
Colles' fracture, 259
compartment syndrome, 29–34. *See* Compartment syndrome
CRPS, 34
elbow dislocation, 253
extraarticular proximal tibial fracture, 363
femoral diaphyseal fracture, 331
fracture of odontoid process, 189
fractures of tibial plateau, 362
hangman fracture, 190
humeral shaft fractures, 243
intertrochanteric fracture, 324–326
lateral condyle fractures, 247
malignant hyperthermia, 160
medial epicondyle fractures, 247
myositis ossificans, 35–36
nerve compression syndromes, 28–29
patella dislocations, 347
pelvic fracture, 304
pilon fractures, 380
proximal humerus fractures, 241
RSD, 34
shoulder dislocation, 225
SIRS, 27–28
sternoclavicular injuries, 221
subtalar/talar dislocation, 387
subtrochanteric fracture, 330
supracondylar humeral fractures, 246
talar neck fractures, 388
tibial shaft fracture, 366–368
tourniquet, 157
traction, 150–151
venous thromboembolism, 34–35
Compression fracture, 193
Computed axial tomography, 19

Concentric/eccentric muscle strength, 354
Congenital spondylolisthesis, 207
Contouring internal fixation plates, 170–171, 172f
Corticosteroids, 61, 65
Coxa vara, 72, 322
Cranial trauma, 5–6
Cruciate ligament avulsions, 352
Crutchfield's rule of 5lb/level, 142
Crystal-induced arthritis, 55–56, 56t, 63
CT scan, 19. *See also* Roentgenograms
   knee injury, 344
   low back pain, 207
   pelvic fracture, 302
   spinal injury, 185
   TP tendon rupture, 397
Cubital tunnel, 288
Cubital tunnel syndrome, 288
Cutaneous distribution of peripheral nerves, 437f
Cutting casts, 114

D-Penicillamine, 60, 65
Danis-Weber classification system, 376, 377f
Dantrium, 160
Dantrolene, 160
de Quervain's tenosynovitis, 291
Debridement, 62
Decompression, 233
Deep vein thrombosis (DVT), 34–35
Deformities of the spine, 209–211
Degenerative joint disease, 52t, 59t
Degenerative spondylolisthesis, 207
Dehne/Sarmiento casting techniques, 112–114
Demerol, 122
Dermatomes, 435f, 436f
Dermatomyositis, 53t
Developmental dysplasia of the hip (DDH), 78–79
Deyerle technique, 319
Diagnostic imaging. *See* CT scan; Magnetic resonance imaging (MRI); Roentgenograms
Diamond-shaped point, 138
Diaphyseal fracture of radius and ulna, 256
Digitalis, 64
Dilaudid, 122
Disability exam, 5
Disc degeneration, 204
Disc herniation, 205
Discharge summary, 121
Discitis, 86–87
   acute, 41
Discoid meniscus, 77
Displaced femoral neck fractures, 318
Displaced tuberosity fracture, greater/lesser, 240–241
Displaced intraarticular/supracondylar fractures, 333
Displaced surgical neck fractures, 239–240
Displaced unicondylar fractures, 332
Distal radioulnar joint (DRUJ), 268–269
Distal radius fractures, 276
Distraction, 151
Diuretics, 64
Docusate sodium, 124
Donati skin suture, 179
Dorsal splint, 105
Dorsal triquetral avulsion fractures, 273
Dorsiflexion
   ankle, 427f
   forepart of foot, 429f
   wrist, 412f
Dow Corning medical adhesive, 102
Draping techniques. *See* Surgical draping techniques
Drill bits, 164–165
Drill guide, 164
Dumbbells, 125
Dunlop traction, 144
Durkin's compression test, 287
Dynamic compression plate (DCP), 167
Dynamic compression plate with lag screw, 169f
Dynamic fluoroscopy, 185

Eccentric/concentric muscle strengthening, 354
Elbow, 283
Elbow and forearm injuries, 251–263
   Barton fracture, 257f, 260
   Colles' fracture, 257–259
   diaphyseal fracture of radius and ulna, 256
   distal epiphyseal separation, 260
   distal radial/ulnar fractures, 259–260, 262
   elbow dislocation, 251–253, 261
   epiphyseal fracture of proximal radius, 254–255
   fracture of olecranon, 253–254
   Galeazzi fracture, 257
   HCMC treatment recommendations, 261–262
   injection site, 404–406
   isolated ulna fracture, 257
   joint motion measurement, 411f, 412f
   Monteggia fracture-dislocation, 255–256
   proximal ulna fractures, 261
   radial head fracture, 255, 261
   rupture of distal biceps, 251
   Smith fracture, 257f, 260
Elbow dislocation, 251–253, 261
Elevators, 161

Emergencies, 7–13
Emergency splints, 93–99
  backboard, 93, 94f
  lower extremity splinting, 95–98
  make-do splints, 99
  precautions, 99
  upper extremity splinting, 93–95
Enbrel, 60
Enchondromas, 295
Epicondylitis, 289
Epiphyseal fracture of proximal radius, 254–255
Epiphyseal plate fracture, 18
Epiphyseal separation, distal, 260
Erb's disease, 285
Erythrocyte sedimentation rate (ESR), 40, 42, 43
Esmarch bandage, 156
Etanercept, 60
Evaluating the trauma patient, 2–7
  history, 4
  physical examination, 5–7
  primary survey, 3
  secondary survey, 5–7
  trauma x-ray series, 3–4
Eversion, foot, 428f, 429f
Everting suture, 177, 178f
Ewing's sarcoma, 295
Exercise ischemia, 29
Exercise myopathy, 29
Extension
  ankle, 427f
  cervical spine, 422f
  fingers, 416f
  hip, 424f
  shoulder, 417f
  thoracic and lumbar spine, 421f
  wrist, 412f
Extensor mechanism, 351
  disruptions, 351
  instability, 341–342
Extensor tendon lacerations, 277
External skeletal fixation, 175–176
Extraarticular distal femur fractures, 333
Extraarticular proximal tibial fractures, 362–363, 364t
Extremity arterial injury, 8
Extremity drape, 158, 444–445f

Familial hypophosphatemic rickets, 72
FANA, 58
Fasciotomy, 34
Fat embolism syndrome (FES), 27
Felon, 276, 277f
Felt, 102
Femoral anteversion, 70
Femoral diaphyseal fracture, 330–332
Femoral fractures, 317–338

  displaced femoral neck fractures, 318
  distal femur fractures, 334
  femoral diaphyseal fracture, 330–332
  femoral head fracture, 311–312, 313
  femoral neck fracture, 12, 317–322, 333
  femoral shaft fractures, 334
  greater trochanteric fractures, 326–327
  HCMC treatment recommendations, 333–334
  impacted femoral neck fractures, 318
  intertrochanteric fracture, 322–326, 330, 334
  intracondylar fracture, 332–333
  isolated avulsion fractures of lesser trochanter, 327–328
  stress fractures, 318
  subtrochanteric fractures, 328–330, 334
  supracondylar fracture, 332–333
  unicondylar fracture, 332–333
Fiberglass cast, 101
Fiberglass-free masks, 158
Fight bites, 280
Finger spread, 416f
Fingers, 271–273. See also Wrist and hand
First-degree strain, 20, 21
Fixed-angle devices, 323
Fixed skeletal traction, 150, 151f
Flat feet, 73–74
Flexible flat feet, 74
Flexion
  ankle, 427f
  cervical spine, 422f
  elbow, 411f
  fingers, 415f
  hip, 423f
  knee, 427f
  palmar, 412f
  shoulder, 417f
  thumb, 413f
  wrist, 412f
Flexion-distraction injury, 194, 195f
Flexor tendon lacerations, 276
Flexor tendon sheath, 273
Floating shoulder, 214
Flow sheets, 121
Fluothane, 160
Foot disorders, 73–75
Foot injuries, 383–402. See also Ankle injuries
  bunions, 400
  calcaneal fat pad trauma, 395
  calcaneal fractures, 383–386, 390
  claw toe, 395, 400
  fractures of forefoot, 389–390
  fractures of navicular, cuneiform, cuboid bones, 388
  hallux rigidus, 399–400

Foot injuries (*Continued*)
  hammer toe, 401
  HCMC recommendations, 390–391
  joint motion measurement, 428*f*, 429*f*
  Lisfranc joint injury, 388, 391
  metatarsal fractures, 389, 391
  metatarsalgia, 395
  midfoot subluxations, 388
  nerve entrapment syndromes, 395
  phalangeal dislocations, 389
  plantar fasciitis, 394
  plantar heel pain, 393–395
  stress fracture, 398–399
  subtalar dislocation, 386–387, 390
  talar dislocation, 386–387
  talar neck fractures, 387–388
  talus fractures, 387–388, 390
  tarsal tunnel syndrome, 395
  tarsometatarsal (Lisfranc) fracture, 388, 391
  toe fracture, 390, 391
  TP tendon rupture, 396–398
  turf toe, 399
Foot progression angle, 71*f*
Forearm, 284
Forearm casts, 105
Forearm injuries. See Elbow and forearm injuries
Forefoot adductus, 70, 71*f*
Forefoot surgery, 62
Fracture of clavicle, 213–215
Fracture
  femur, 317–318. See also Femoral fractures
  humerus, 239–249. See also Humeral fractures
  lower cervical spine, 190–192
  odontoid process, 188–189
  olecranon, 253–254
  pelvis, 299–305. See also Pelvic fractures
  stress fractures, 19–20, 318, 398–399
  thoracic/thoracolumbar/lumbar spine, 193–198
  tibia, 359–370. See also Tibial fractures
Frostbite, 22–23
Frostnip, 22–23
Frozen shoulder, 234
Functional short leg syndrome, 394

Galeazzi fracture, 78, 257
Gamekeeper's thumb, 272, 275*f*
Gamma nail, 324
Gangrene, 47
Gardner-Wells skull traction tongs, 142
Gas gangrene, 47
Gentamicin, 45*t*, 46*t*
Genu valgum, 71
Genu varum, 71

Gigli saw, 164
Glasgow coma score, 5
Glenohumeral disorders, 233–234
Glenohumeral joint, 223
Gold, 60, 65
Goldwaithe iron, 106, 107*f*
Gonorrheal arthritis, 53*t*
Gouges, 163
Gouty arthritis, 55–56, 56*t*, 63
Grading muscle strength, 433
Greater trochanteric fractures, 326–327
Grip strength, 266
Group A streptococcal myonecrosis, 47
Growth plate injuries, 18
Gunshot wounds, 16
Gustilo and Anderson classification of open fractures, 14
Guyon's canal, 287*f*

Haglund deformity, 393
Hallux rigidus, 399–400
Hallux valgus, 74–75, 400
Halo ring, 142, 143*f*
Halo traction, 108
Halothane, 160
Hamilton-Russell traction, 145, 147*f*
Hand. See Wrist and hand
Hand cutters, 102
Hand dressing, 281*f*
Hand press, 170–171, 172*f*
Hangman fracture, 189–190
Hard signs of arterial injury, 8
Hare splints, 96
Hawkins' classification of talar neck fractures, 387*f*
Hawkins' sign, 388
HBV immunization, 157
HCMC (Hennepin County Medical Center) recommendations and protocols
  AC injuries, 221
  acetabular fractures, 314
  calcaneus fractures, 390
  clavicle fractures, 215
  distal femur fractures, 334
  distal humerus fractures, 248
  distal radius fractures, 262
  elbow and forearm injuries, 261–262
  elbow dislocations, 261
  femoral fractures, 333–334
  femoral head fractures, 313
  femoral neck fractures, 333
  femoral shaft fractures, 334
  foot injuries, 390–391
  forearm shaft fractures, 261
  hip dislocations, 313
  humeral fractures, 247–248
  humeral shaft fractures, 248
  intertrochanteric hip fractures, 334

Lisfranc fracture, 391
metatarsal fractures, 391
pelvic ring fractures, 304
proximal humerus fractures, 247
proximal ulna fractures, 261
radial head fractures, 261
shoulder injuries, 227
subtalar dislocations, 390
subtrochanteric femur fractures, 334
talus fractures, 390
tarsometatarsal fracture/dislocations, 391
tib-fib fractures, 368
tibial plateau fractures, 368
toe fractures, 391
Head-to-torso ratio, 198–199
Heel pain, 393–395
Height and weight tables, 440–441t
Hematogenous osteomyelitis, 40, 41
Hematoma, 22
Hemiarthroplasty of the hip, 320
Hemolytic disorders, 42
Hemothorax, 6
Heparin, 124
Hepatitis B virus (HBV) immunization, 157
Herniated intervertebral disc, 87
Herring classification system, 79
Hibiclens, 158
High ankle sprain, 371
High-velocity weapons, 16
Hill-Sachs lesion, 226
Hip
  aspiration/injection, 406–407
  dislocation, 307–311, 313
  disorders, 78–82
  external (lateral) rotation, 70, 71f
  hemiarthroplasty of, 320
  internal (medial) rotation, 70, 71f
  replacement, 320
  total hip arthroplasty, 312, 320
History, 4
Hole drilling, 164
Hooded surgical exhaust systems, 159
Hooked acromion, 229
Hospital care. See Orthopedic unit care
Humeral epiphyseal slips, distal, 246
Humeral fractures, 239–249
  diaphyseal fractures, 241–243
  distal humerus fractures, 248
  HCMC treatment recommendations, 247–248
  humeral shaft fractures, 241–243, 248
  intercondylar fractures, 246
  lateral condyle fractures, 246–247
  medial epicondyle fractures, 247
  proximal humeral epiphyseal separation, 241
  proximal humerus fractures, 239–241, 247
  supracondylar fractures, 243–246

Hydraulic principle, 112
Hydrocortisone, 63
Hydroxychloroquine, 60, 64, 65
Hydroxyzine, 123
Hyperextension
  elbow, 411f
  fingers, 416f
  knee, 427f
  whiplash injury, 192
Hyperthermia, 159–160
Hypnotics, 123
Hypothermia, 23
Hydromorphone, 122

Idiopathic adolescent scoliosis, 87–88
Idiopathic claw toe deformities, 395
Iliotibial band (ITB)
  syndrome, 355
  tendinosis, 355
Imaging techniques. See also CT scan; Magnetic resonance imaging (MRI); Roentgenograms
Impending ischemic contracture, 29
Impingement syndrome, 229
Increased femoral anteversion, 70
Indocin, 63
Indomethacin, 63
Infection of bone, acute (hematogenous osteomyelitis), 40
Infections. See Musculoskeletal infections, acute
Infectious arthritis, 56t
Inferior dislocation, 226
Inflammatory bowel disease, 58t
Inflammatory polyarthritis, 53–54t, 57–58, 64
Inflammatory spondyloarthropathy, 58, 58t, 64
Infusion technique (tissue pressure measurement), 32f
Injection technique (tissue pressure measurement), 33f
Injections, 403–409. See also Aspiration and injection techniques
Inpatients. See Orthopedic unit care
Intercondylar distance, 72
Intercondylar fractures, 246
Interlocking nail, 175
Intermalleolar distance, 72
Internal fixation plates, 170–171, 172f
Internal tibial torsion, 70
Interns. See Students/interns
Intertrochanteric hip fractures, 322–326, 330, 334
Intoeing, 70
Intraarticular distal clavicle fractures, 214
Intracondylar femur fracture, 332–333
Intradermal (subcuticular) suture, 177, 178f

Intramedullary nailing, 174–175
Inversion, foot, 428f, 429f
Isolated avulsion fractures of lesser trochanter, 327–328
Isolated meniscus tear, 347
Isolated ulna fracture, 257
Isthmic spondylolisthesis, 207

Jefferson fracture, 187–188
Jersey finger, 276
Jewett brace, 197
Joint arthrodesis, 62
Joint aspiration, 84
Joint conditions, acute nontraumatic
  differential diagnosis, 53–54t, 55–58
  examination, 51, 51t
  history, 51, 51t
  JRA. *See* Juvenile rheumatoid arthritis (JRA)
  laboratory data, 52, 52t, 55
  roentgenographic findings, 51–52, 52t
  synovial fluid analysis, 52t
  treatment, 59–65
Joint-depression calcaneal fracture, 383, 384f
Joint immobilization, 117–118
Joint infections. *See* Musculoskeletal infections, acute
Joint motion measurement, 411–431
  ankle, 427f
  cervical spine, 422f
  elbow, 411f
  fingers, 415f, 416f
  foot, 428f, 429f
  forearm, 412f
  hip, 423f, 424f, 425f, 426f
  normal range of motion, 430–431t
  shoulder, 417f, 418f
  spinal flexion, 419–420f
  spine, 421f, 422f
  steel tape measuring method, 420f
  thoracic and lumbar spine, 421f
  thumb, 413f, 414f
  wrist, 412f
Joint replacement, 62
Joint resurfacing or replacement, 62
Jones compression splint, 96
Juvenile rheumatoid arthritis (JRA), 56t
  examination, 58
  history, 57–58
  laboratory tests, 58
  treatment, 65

Kefzol, 155t
Kienböck disease, 292
Kinking, 171
Kirschner bow, 138
Kirschner wire, 138, 169

Kirschner wire traction bows, 173–174
Kite angle, 73
Klumpke's paralysis, 285
Knee cast-brace, 114
Knee cylinder casts, 110, 112
Knee dislocation, 351
Knee disorders, 75–78
Knee immobilizer, 344
Knee injuries, 339–358
  ACL injuries, 348–351
  adolescents, 352
  chondromalacia patella, 355
  diagnostic tests, 342–344
  differential diagnosis, 340
  extensor mechanism disruptions, 351
  history, 339–340
  immobilization/crutches, 344
  injection site, 407–408
  ITB syndrome, 355
  knee dislocation, 351
  ligament avulsion, 352
  ligamentous injury, 348–351
  locked knee, 341
  MCL injuries, 348–351
  meniscus injury, 340, 347–348
  osteochondritis dissecans, 352
  Osgood-Schlatter disease, 355
  overuse injury, 339, 352–356
  patella dislocation, 345–347
  patella fractures, 344–345
  patella tendinosis, 354–355
  patellofemoral pain syndrome, 355–356
  PCL tear, 348–351
  pes anserinus bursitis, 356
  physeal injuries, 352
  physical exam, 340–342
  range of motion, 340–341
  rehabilitation, 354
  stability testing, 341–342
  treatment, 344
Knee joint swelling, 340
Kneecap malalignment, 356
Knock knees, 71–72
Knot strength, 174
Kocher-Langenbach posterolateral approach, 312
Kyphosis, 88–89, 210–211

Lace-up canvas ankle supports, 98
Lachman's exam, 349, 350f
Lag screw fixation, 165
Lag screws, 169
Lag sign, 341
Laminar air flow systems, 159
Lateral bend
  cervical spine, 422f
  thoracic and lumbar spine, 421f
Lateral condyle fractures, 246–247

Lateral epicondylitis, 289
Lateral hip drape, 447f
Lateral skeletal traction, 144–145, 146f
Lauge-Hansen classification of ankle fractures, 376f
Leflunomide, 60
Leg and ankle braces, 98
Leg casts, 105
Leg length discrepancy, 394
Legg-Calvé-Perthes disease, 79–81
Level of consciousness, 5
Ligamentous injury, 21–22
Light bulb sign, 225
Limping child, 67–68
Lipoma, 295
Lippert, FG, III, 160
Lisfranc joint injury, 388, 391
Local ischemia, 29
Locked knee, 341
Long bone, 19
Long head of biceps tendinitis, 233
Long-leg casts, 112
Long-leg hip spica, 109–110, 111f
Long-leg total contact cast, 112–113
Long-leg walking cast, 112
Long-leg weight-bearing cast, 114
Lordosis, 89
Low back pain, 203–209
Low-contact dynamic compression plate (LCDCP), 167
Low-molecular-weight dextran, 124
Low-molecular-weight heparin, 124
Low velocity gunshot, 16
Lower extremity alignment conditions, 70–72
Lower extremity splinting, 95–98
Lower extremity traction, 145–150
Lumbar-Scheuermann disease, 87, 211
Lumbar spinal stenosis, 208
Lyme arthritis, 42

Madelung's deformity, 285
Magnetic resonance imaging (MRI)
  bone tumors, 295
  knee injuries, 343–344
  limping child, 68
  low back pain, 207
  osteomyelitis, 83
  rotator cuff disorders, 229–230, 230t
  spinal injury, 185
  stress fracture, 20, 399
  TP tendon rupture, 397
  wrist, 249
Make-do splints, 99
Malignant hyperthermia, 159–160
Mallet, 163
Mallet finger, 291
Mangled extremity, 11

Mangled Extremity Severity Score (MESS), 11, 12t
Masks, 158
MAST trousers, 299
Master sling, 150
McElvenny's technique, 319
Medial collateral ligament (MCL) injuries, 348–351
McMurray test, 347
Measuring joint motion, 411–431. *See also* Joint motion measurement
Mechanical low-back pain, 86
Medial epicondyle fractures, 247
Medial patellofemoral ligament (MPFL), 340
Medial tibial syndrome, 29
Medical students. *See* Students/interns
Medicated bandage, 117
Meniscus injury, 340, 347–348
Mental status, 5
Mepacrine, 64
Meperidine, 122
MESS (Mangled Extremity Severity Score), 11, 12t
Metacarpalphalangeal joint (MCPJ), 271
Metatarsal fractures, 389, 391
Metatarsalgia, 395
Metatarsophalangeal joint capsulitis, 395
Metatarsus adductus, 70, 71f
Metatarsus primus varus, 74
Methicillin, 44t
Methotrexate, 60, 64, 65
Methylprednisolone, 64, 186
Metronidazole, 47
Metzenbaum dissecting scissors, 161
Meyerding grading system, 207
Midfoot fasciitis, 394
Midfoot subluxations, 388
Milwaukee brace, 211
Minerva body jacket, 107, 108f
Missed injury rate, 2
Mixed connective tissue disease, 53t
Moberg procedure, 400
Modified Dunlop traction, 144, 145f
Modified Jones compression splint, 96–98
Moleskin adhesive, 102
Monteggia fracture-dislocation, 255–256
Morphine, 122
Morton neuroma, 395
MRI. *See* Magnetic resonance imaging (MRI)
Mucin clot, 57n
Multi-ligamentous knee injuries, 351
Multidirectional instability (MDI), 226
Multiple screw fixation, 320
Munster cast, 257
Muscle strength grading, 433

Musculoskeletal infections, acute, 39–49
  adjunctive treatment, 43
  antibiotic treatment, 42–46t
  bacterial considerations, 41
  chronic osteomyelitis, 47
  diagnosis, 40–41
  differential diagnosis, 41
  gas gangrene, 47
  hemolytic disorders, 42
  Lyme arthritis, 42
  prevention, 39–40
  puncture wound, 42
  special considerations, 41–42
  summary, 48
  surgical intervention, 43, 47
Musculoskeletal trauma
  assessment, 5–7
  defined, 1
  emergencies, 7–13
  epidemiology, 1
  urgencies, 13–17
Myelogram, 207
Myochrysine, 60
Myositis ossificans, 35–36, 253
  circumscripta, 35
  paralytica, 35
  progressiva, 35
  traumatica, 35

Nafcillin, 44t, 46t
Nail plate and pulp, 276
Narrative notes, 121
Near-far/far-near suture, 178–179, 179f
Neck halter traction, 141
Necrotizing fasciitis, 47
Needle holder, 161
Neer's anatomic concept, 240f
Nerve compression syndromes, 28–29
Nerve injuries, 22
Neurapraxia, 22
Neurogenic back pain, 203
Neurologic mental status, 5
Neurology of lower extremities, 206, 206t
Neuromuscular disorders, 89–90
Neurotmesis, 22
Neurovascular bundle, 223
Neurovascular exam, 11
Neutralization plates, 166
Nightstick fracture, 257
95-degree fixed-angle device, 329
Nonsteroidal antiinflammatory drugs. See NSAIDs
Nontraumatic joint conditions. See Joint conditions, acute nontraumatic
Nonunion, 321, 331, 379
Normal range of motion, 430–431t. See also Joint motion measurement

NSAIDs
  aspirin. See Aspirin
  cubital tunnel syndrome, 288
  hallux rigidus, 400
  inflammatory spondyloarthropathy, 64
  Legg-Calvé-Perthes disease, 81
  low back pain, 208
  orthopedic unit care, 122
  PIN syndrome, 289
  rheumatoid arthritis, 59–60

Occult infection, 64
Olecranon, 283
Olecranon pin traction, 146f
One doctor, one manipulation, 17, 245
Open fractures, 13–16
Open joint injuries, 16
Open reduction and internal fixation (ORIF), 385
Open tibial shaft fractures, 366
Operating room, 153–181. See also Orthopedic unit care
  antibiotics, 122, 153–154, 155t
  bloodborne pathogens, 157
  bone cutting instruments, 162–164
  bone graft material, 176
  bone saws/files, 164
  bone screw biomechanics, 164–166
  cerclage, 171–174
  day of surgery, 154
  external skeletal fixation, 175–176
  hyperthermia, 159–160
  infection control, 157–159
  intramedullary nailing, 174–175
  plating, 166–171
  scheduling surgery, 153
  skin suture, 176–179
  surgical exposure instruments, 160–161
  surgical prep, 121, 153–160
  tourniquet, 156–157
Opposition (thumb), 414f
Orthopaedic emergencies, 7–13
Orthopedic trauma. See Musculoskeletal trauma
Orthopedic unit care, 119–135. See also Operating room
  activities/physical therapy, 125
  analgesics, 122–123
  antibiotics, 122, 153–154, 155t
  bowel problems, 124–125
  hypnotics, 123
  postoperative orders, 126
  preoperative orders, 125–126
  rounds, 119–120, 131–133
  sedatives, 123
  skin, 125
  students/interns. See Students/interns
  surgical prep, 121, 153–160

thromboembolism, 123–124
urinary retention, 124
workup routines, 120–121
Orthopedic urgencies, 13–17
Ortolani maneuver, 78
Osgood-Schlatter disease, 76, 355
Osteoarthritis, 55, 62
Osteochondral fracture, 343f, 345
Osteochondritis dissecans (OCD), 77, 352
Osteogenesis imperfects, 207
Osteolysis, 235
Osteomyelitis, 41, 46t, 47, 69, 83–84
Osteosarcoma, 297
Osteotome, 162, 163
Osteotomy, 62
Ottawa ankle rules, 371, 373t
Overbody traction, 144–145, 146f
Overview of treatment recommendations. *See* HCMC recommendations and protocols

Palindromic rheumatism, 56t
Palmar flexion (wrist), 412f
Panner's disease, 292
Partial cord syndromes, 186
Passive muscle stretch, 31
Patella, 344
  dislocation, 345–347
  dislocation, acute, 76
  fractures, 344–345
  subluxation/dislocation, 340
  tendon disruptions, 351
  tendinosis, 354–355
  tendon-bearing cast, 113
Patellofemoral pain syndrome, 76, 355–356
Pavlik harness, 78
Pearson attachment, 149
Pediatric orthopedic conditions, 67–91
  back pain, 85–89
  bowed legs, 71–72
  bunions, 74–75
  calcaneal fracture, 386
  child who refuses to walk/bear weight, 68–69
  club foot, 73
  diaphyseal femur fractures, 331–332
  distal radial/ulnar fractures, 259–260
  femoral neck fracture, 322
  flat feet, 73–74
  foot disorders, 73–75
  general principles, 17–18
  growth plate injuries, 18
  head-to-torso ratio, 198–199
  hip disorders, 78–82
  infections and inflammatory conditions, 83–85
  intertrochanteric fractures, 322
  intoeing, 70
  knee disorders, 75–78
  knock knees, 71–72
  limping child, 67–68
  lower extremity alignment conditions, 70–72
  neuromuscular disorders, 89–90
  pitfalls, 18
  spinal injuries, 198–199
  spine-related disorders, 85–89
  subtrochanteric fractures, 322
Pelvic fractures, 299–305
  classification, 299
  complications, 304
  examination, 299
  HCMC treatment recommendations, 304
  incidence/mechanism of injury, 299
  pelvic hemorrhage, 299–302
  roentgenograms, 302
  treatment, 302, 304
Penicillin, 47, 64
Penicillin G, 44t
Percutaneous pinning *in situ*, 81
Perineal inspection, 6
Periosteal elevators, 161, 162f
Peripheral nerves, cutaneous distribution, 437f
Periscapular muscles, 223
Peroneal nerve palsy, 28
Pes anserinus bursitis, 356
Pes planus, 73–74
Phalangeal dislocations, 389
Phalangeal fractures, 279
Phalen's test, 287
Physeal injuries, 352
Physical examination, 5–7
Pillow splint, 98f
Pilon fracture, 379–380
Pin breakage, 151
Pinch strength, 266
Planovalgus deformity, 388
Plantar fascitis, 394
Plantar flexion
  ankle, 427f
  forepart of foot, 429f
Plantar heel pain, 393–395
Plaquenil, 60
Plaster splints, 101, 105
Plate benders, 170–171, 172f
Plate contouring, 173f
Plating, 166–171
Pneumatic tourniquets, 156–157
Pneumothorax, 6
Point contact plate (PCP), 167
Polyarteritis nodosa, 53t
Polydactyly, 285
Polyethylene jacket, 109f
Polymyalgia rheumatica, 54t

Polymyositis, 53t
Popeye sign, 227
Postaxial duplication, 285
Posterior compartmental syndrome of leg, 30f
Posterior cord syndrome, 186
Posterior cruciate ligament (PCL) tear, 348–351
Posterior drawer test, 349
Posterior interosseous (PIN) syndrome, 288–289
Posterior talofibular ligament (PTFL), 371
Postoperative orders, 126
Postural kyphosis, 210
Preaxial duplication, 285
Prednisone, 63, 64
Preiser's disease, 292
Preoperative orders, 125–126
Presenting at rounds, 131–133
Pressure sores, 125
Primary curve, 209
Primary survey, 3
Primum non nocere, 133
Probenecid, 63
Problem-oriented style of progress notes, 120
Progress notes, 120–121
Pronation
 forearm, 412f
 forepart of foot, 429f
Prone reduction, 224
Protocols. See HCMC recommendations and protocols
Proximal hand, 271
Proximal humeral epiphyseal separation, 241
Proximal humerus fractures, 239–241, 247
Proximal interphalangeal joint (PIPJ), 271
Proximal tibial fractures, 362–363, 364t
Proximal ulna fractures, 261
Pseudo locked knee, 341
Pseudo-winging of the scapula, 235
Pseudogout, 54t, 56, 63–64
Pseudosubluxation, 18, 198
Psoriatic arthritis, 53t, 57, 64
Psoriatic spondylitis, 58t
Psychogenic back pain, 203
Puncture wound, 42

Quads active test, 349

Radial agenesis, 284
Radial club hand, 284
Radial deviation, wrist, 412f
Radial head fracture, 255, 261
Radial nerve injury, 243
Radial/ulnar fractures, distal, 259–260, 262
Radiographic diagnosis, 19

Radiography. See CT scan; Magnetic resonance imaging (MRI); Roentgenograms
Radioisotopic bone scanning, 40
Range of motion (ROM), 430–431t. See also Joint motion measurement
 ankle, 431t
 elbow, 430t
 forearm, 430t
 forepart of foot, 431t
 hip, 431t
 knee, 431t
 shoulder, 430t
 wrist, 430t
Ratchet teeth, 161
Recommendations. See HCMC recommendations and protocols
Rectal examination, 6
Referred pain, 77
Reflex sympathetic dystrophy (RSD), 34
Reiter syndrome, 53t, 57, 58t
Respiratory problem, 39
Reston, 102
Retrocalcaneal bursitis, 393
Reverse Bankart lesion, 225
Reverse Colles' fracture, 257f, 260
Reverse Hill-Sachs lesion, 225, 226
Reverse obliquity fracture, 324, 326–328f
Review of treatment recommendations. See HCMC recommendations and protocols
Revision surgery, 368
Rhabdomyolysis, 29
rhBMP-2, 209
Rheumatic fever, 53t, 57, 64
Rheumatoid arthritis, 53t
 diagnostic criteria, 54t, 55
 JRA. See Juvenile rheumatoid arthritis (JRA)
 roentgenographic findings, 52t
 synovial fluid analysis, 52t
 treatment, 59–62, 59t
Rib hump, 210
Rickets, 72
Rigid flat feet, 74
Risser cast, 107, 197
Risser classification, 210
Rocker walker, 112
Roentgenograms
 AC joint disorders, 235
 Colles' fracture, 257–258
 distal radial/ulnar fractures, 260
 elbow dislocation, 251
 fracture of odontoid process, 188–189
 glenohumeral disorders, 234
 hangman fracture, 190
 intercondylar fractures, 246
 Jefferson fracture, 187–188

joint conditions, 51–52, 52t
lateral condyle fractures, 246
MDI, 226
medial epicondyle fractures, 247
pelvic fracture, 302
radial head/neck fractures, 255
rotator cuff disorders, 229–230
rotator cuff tear, 226
shoulder dislocation, 225
spinal injury, 83, 184f, 196
TP tendon rupture, 397
Roller splints, 96
ROM. *See* Range of motion (ROM)
Rotation
   cervical spine, 422f
   hip, 71f, 426f
   shoulder, 418f
   spine, 422f
Rotator cuff disorders, 229–233
Rotator cuff muscles, 223
Rotator cuff tears, 226, 233, 266
Rounds, 119–120, 131–133
Roundsmanship, 133
Rubber rocker walker, 112
Rupture of distal biceps, 251
Rupture of long head of biceps brachii, 226–227
Rupture of pectoralis major, 227

Salicylates, 65
Salter classification of epiphyseal separations, 18
Saw-cutting technique, 115f
Scaphoid fractures, 273, 281
Scaphoid lunate ligament tears, 281
Scapular dyskinesia, 235
Scapular fractures, 227
Scapular winging, 235–236
Scapulothoracic bursitis, 235
Scapulothoracic disorders, 235–236
SCFE (slipped capital femoral epiphysis), 69, 81, 82f
Schatzker's classification system, 360f
Scheduling surgery, 153
Scheuermann disease, 88
Scheuermann disease (adolescent kyphosis), 211
Schmorl nodes, 87, 88
Sciatic nerve injury, 311
Sciatic nerve neurapraxia, 29
Sciatica, 203–209
Scleroderma, 53t
Scoliosis, 87–88, 209–210
"Scottie dog" sign, 208
Screws, 165–166
Second-degree strain, 20, 21
Secondary survey, 5–7
Sedatives, 123

Selective dorsal rhizotomy, 90
Self-compression plate, 168f
Self-tapping screw, 166
Selter-Thompson classification system, 79
Sentinel compartment, 34
Septic arthritis, 46t, 69
   bacterial considerations, 41
   children, 84–85
   differential diagnosis, 55
   roentgenographic findings, 52t
   synovial fluid analysis, 52t
   treatment, 59t, 62
Serrated biopsy needle, 40
Shoe covers, 102
Short-leg cast, 112
Short-leg spica, 109
Short-leg splint, 96–98
Short-leg walkers, 98
Shortened Achilles tendon, 395
Shoulder dislocation, 223–226
Shoulder drape, 446f
Shoulder girdle, 223
Shoulder immobilizers, 95
Shoulder injuries, 223–237
   AC joint disorders, 234–235
   acute injuries, 223–238
   anatomy, 223
   arthritis, 233–234
   differential diagnosis, 223
   dislocation, 223–226
   frozen shoulder, 234
   glenohumeral disorders, 233–234
   HCMC treatment recommendations, 227
   injection site, 403–404
   joint motion measurement, 417f, 418f
   MDI, 226
   nonacute disorders, 229–237
   pain, anterior, 232t
   rotator cuff disorders, 229–233
   rupture of long head of biceps brachii, 226–227
   rupture of pectoralis major, 227
   scapular fractures, 227
   scapulothoracic disorders, 235–236
   shoulder dislocation, 223–226
   torn rotator cuff, 226, 233
Shoulder separation, 218
Shoulder spica, 110
Sinding-Larsen-Johansson syndrome, 76
SIRS (systemic inflammatory response syndrome), 27–28
Skeletal dysplasia, 72
Skeletal traction, 138–141
Skin
   contamination, 158
   suture, 176–179
   tenting, 99
   traction, 137

Skull tong traction, 141–142
SLE (systemic lupus erythematosus), 53t, 57, 64
Sliding hip screw, 324
Sliding hip screw fixation, 320
Sliding screw plate, 325f
Sling-and-swathe bandages, 93–95, 96f
Slipped capital femoral epiphysis (SCFE), 69, 81, 82f
Small finger base fracture, 279
Smith fracture, 257f, 260
Smith-Petersen anterior approach, 319
Snapping scapula, 235
Sof-Roll, 102
Soft signs of arterial injury, 8
Soft tissue injuries, 20–22
Solganal, 60
Spanish windlass, 96
Specialist, 102
Spica, 108–110
Spina bifida, 90
Spinal cord injury without radiographic abnormality (SCIWORA), 199
Spinal deformity, 209–211
Spinal imbalance, 209
Spinal injury/disease, 183–212
  acute spinal injury, 183–201
  ASIA classification, 185
  children, 198–199
  clearance of spine in trauma patients, 183
  complete/incomplete spinal cord injuries, 185
  deformities of the spine, 209–211
  diagnostic studies, 183–185
  fracture/dislocation of lower cervical spine, 190–192
  fracture of odontoid process, 188–189
  fractures of thoracic/thoracolumbar/lumbar spine, 193–198
  hangman fracture, 189–190
  hypertension whiplash injury, 192
  initial evaluation/management, 183
  joint motion measurement, 419–420f, 421f, 422f
  Jefferson fracture, 187–188
  kyphosis, 210–211
  low back pain, 203–209
  partial cord syndromes, 186
  pharmacologic management, 186
  sciatica, 203–209
  scoliosis, 209–210
  spondylolisthesis, 207–208
Spinal stenosis, 205
Spine-related disorders, 85–89. See also Spinal injury/disease
Splints. See Cast and bandaging techniques; Emergency splints
Split-depressed fractures, 361
Split fracture, 359
Split Russell traction, 148, 148f
Splitting casts, 115
Spondyloarthropathy, 58
Spondylogenic back pain, 203, 204t
Spondylolisthesis, 86, 207–208
Spondylolysis, 86, 207
Steel rule of thirds, 187
Steel tape measuring method, 420f
Steinmann pins, 138
Steri-Strips, 177
Sternoclavicular injuries, 217–218
Stirrup walker, 112
Stockinet, 102
Straight leg raise, 203
Stress fractures, 19–20, 318, 398–399
Stress radiographs, 344
Structural curve, 209
Structural kyphosis, 210
Stryker Quickstick, 11
Students/interns, 126–134
  dealing with patients, 128
  final thoughts, 133–134
  general principles, 128–131
  involvement, 126
  maturation, 127–128
  patient care/ward decisions, 126–127
  presenting at rounds, 131–133
  usefulness, 127
  working with others, 131, 133
Subacromial space, 403f
Subcuticular suture, 177, 178f
Subtalar dislocation, 386–387, 390
Subtrochanteric femur fractures, 328–330, 334
Succinylcholine, 160
Sudeck atrophy, 34
Sugar-tong splint, 276
Sulfasalazine, 60, 64
Sulfinpyrazone, 63
Summary treatment recommendations. See HCMC recommendations and protocols
Supination
  forearm, 412f
  forepart of foot, 429f
Supracondylar femur fracture, 332–333
Supracondylar humeral fractures, 243–246
Surgery. See Operating room
Surgical draping techniques, 443–447
  back drape, 443f
  extremity drape, 444–445f
  lateral hip drape, 447f
  shoulder drape, 446f
Surgical exposure instruments, 160–161
Surgical scissors, 161
Swayback, 89

Index

Sympathetically maintained pain syndrome, 34
Syndactyly, 285
Systemic inflammatory response syndrome (SIRS), 27–28
Systemic lupus erythematosus (SLE), 53t, 57, 64

T plate, 169
Talar dislocation, 386–387
Talar neck fractures, 387–388
Talipes equinovarus, 73
Talocalcaneal coalition, 74
Talus fractures, 17, 387–388, 390
Tardy ulnar nerve palsy, 28
Tarsal tunnel syndrome, 395
Tarsometatarsal (Lisfranc) fracture, 388, 391
TcMDP bone scans, 344
Tendon, 20–21
Tendon-bone insertion failure, 291
Tendon sheath, 21
Tendonitis, 56t
Tennis elbow, 404
Tension band
   fixation, 169
   plating, 169
   wire internal fixation, 169
   wiring technique, 253–254, 254f
Tension fractures, 317
Tetanic muscle contractions, 159
Tetanus immunization, 265
Thigh-foot angle, 71f
Thigh-foot axis, 70
Third-degree strain, 20, 21
Thomas splint, 95–96, 97f, 150
Thompson's test, 380
Three-phase bone scan, 68
Three-point plaster fixation, 103f
Thromboembolism, 123–124
Thumb base fracture, 279
Thumb carpometacarpal (CMC), 292
Tib-fib fractures, 368
Tibial apophysis, 352
Tibial diaphyseal fracture, 363–368
Tibial fractures, 359–370
   diaphyseal fractures, 363–368
   extraarticular proximal, 362–363, 364t
   HCMC treatment recommendations, 368
   tib-fib fractures, 368
   tibial plateau fractures, 359–362, 368
   tibial shaft fractures, 363–368
Tibial plateau fractures, 359–362, 368
Tibial shaft fractures, 363–368
Tibial tubercle apophysis, 355
Tibialis posterior (TP) dysfunction syndrome, 396–398

Tibialis posterior (TP) tendon rupture, 396–398
Tight Achilles tendon, 395
Tinel's test, 287
Tissue pressure, 32–34
   measurement, Wick technique, 33f
Tobacco use disorder, 265
Tobramycin, 45t, 46t
Toe fracture, 390, 391
Toes. *See* Foot injuries
Tong traction, 141–142
Tongue-type calcaneal fracture, 383, 384f
Torn rotator cuff, 226, 233
Total hip arthroplasty, 312, 320
Tourniquet, 156–157
Toxic shock syndrome, 47
Traction, 137–152
   acetabular fracture, 312, 313
   balanced suspension skeletal, 148–149
   buck extension skin traction, 145, 147f
   cervical spine, 141–144
   complications, 150–151
   fixed halo skull traction, 142–144
   fracture of lower cervical spine, 191
   lower extremity, 145–150
   materials, 137
   objectives, 137
   shoulder dislocation, 224–225
   skeletal, 138–141
   skin, 137
   tongs, 141–142
   upper extremity, 144–145
Traction bows, 139f
Transepiphyseal fractures, 322
Transient synovitis, 85
Transient/toxic synovitis, 69
Translational injuries, 194, 197f
Transverse fractures, 344–345
Trauma x-ray series, 3–4
Traumatic amputation, 11–12
Traumatic tension in muscles, 29
Treatment recommendations. *See* HCMC (Hennepin County Medical Center) recommendations and protocols
Trenchfoot, 23
Triamcinolone, 63
Triangular fibrocartilage complex (TFCC), 268–269
Trigger digits, 291
Trocar, 138
Tuber angle, 384
Tubular stockinet, 102
Tumors, hand, 294–297
Turf toe, 399
Type III acromion, 229

Ulnar deviation, wrist, 412f
Ulnar fractures, distal, 259–260, 262

Ulnar nerve compression at elbow, 28
Ulnar palsy, acute, 28
Ultrasound, 68
Undisplaced supracondylar fractures, 332
Unicondylar femur fracture, 332–333
Unna boot, 117
Unreamed nail, 175
Upper extremity splinting, 93–95
Upper extremity traction, 144–145
Uricosuric agents, 63
Urinary retention, 124

Valgus reduction, 319
Vancomycin, 16, 122, 155*t*
Varus/valgus stress testing, 349
Vascular back pain, 203
Velpeau bandage, 93, 95*f*
Vena cava filter, 35
Venous thromboembolism, 34–35
Vertical fractures of patella, 345
Viscerogenic back pain, 203
Vistaril, 123
Volar compartmental syndrome of forearm, 29*f*
Volkmann ischemia, 29

Walking cast, 112
Wandering off center, 164
Warfarin, 124
Watson-Jones anterolateral approach, 319–320
Webril, 102
Wedge compression fracture, 193
Weekend warrior, 380
Weight and height tables, 440–441*t*
Whiplash injury, 192
Wick technique (tissue pressure measurement), 33*f*
Winging of the scapula, 235–236
Wire cerclage, 171
Wire tighteners, 173–174
Workman's compensation, 297
Workup routines, 120–121
Wrist and hand, 265–298
  acute injuries, 265–282
  amputation, 276, 279
  arthritic conditions, 292
  bone damage, 292
  carpal tunnel syndrome, 287–288
  cubital tunnel syndrome, 288
  developmental birth conditions, 284–286
  hand injuries, 276–280
  history, 266, 283
  injection site, 405*f*, 406
  injury site characteristics, 265
  joint motion measurement, 412*f*, 413*f*, 414*f*, 415*f*, 416*f*
  muscle/tendon damage, 289–291
  nerve damage, 286–289
  nonacute conditions, 283–298
  normal range of motion, 267*f*, 268*t*
  patient's habits/addictions, 265–266
  pearls/pitfalls, 280–281
  physical exam, 268–273, 283–284
  PIN syndrome, 288–289
  tetanus immunization, 265
  tumors, 294–297
  workman's compensation, 297
  wrist injuries, 273–276

X-ray series, 3–4

Zosyn, 16
Zyloprim, 63